Textbook of International Health

THIRD EDITION

Textbook of International Health: Global Health in a Dynamic World

THIRD EDITION

ANNE-EMANUELLE BIRN, ScD

Canada Research Chair in International Health,
University of Toronto, Canada

YOGAN PILLAY, PhD

Deputy Director-General, Strategic Health Programmes,
National Department of Health, Pretoria, South Africa

TIMOTHY H. HOLTZ, MD, MPH, FACP

Assistant Professor of Global Health and
Assistant Clinical Professor of Family and Preventive Medicine,
Emory University, Atlanta, USA

New York Oxford
OXFORD UNIVERSITY PRESS
2009

Oxford University Press, Inc., publishes works that further
Oxford University's objective of excellence
in research, scholarship, and education.

Oxford New York
Auckland Cape Town Dar es Salaam Hong Kong Karachi
Kuala Lumpur Madrid Melbourne Mexico City Nairobi
New Delhi Shanghai Taipei Toronto

With offices in
Argentina Austria Brazil Chile Czech Republic France Greece
Guatemala Hungary Italy Japan Poland Portugal Singapore
South Korea Switzerland Thailand Turkey Ukraine Vietnam

Copyright (c) 2009 by Oxford University Press, Inc.

Published by Oxford University Press, Inc.
198 Madison Avenue, New York, New York 10016
www.oup.com

Oxford is a registered trademark of Oxford University Press

Library of Congress Cataloging-in-Publication Data
Birn, Anne-Emanuelle, 1964-
Textbook of international health : global health in a dynamic
   world / / Anne-Emanuelle Birn, Yogan Pillay, Timothy H. Holtz. — 3rd ed.
   p. ; cm.
Rev. ed. of: Textbook of international health / Paul F. Basch. 2nd ed. 1999.
Includes bibliographical references and index.
ISBN 978-0-19-530027-7 (cloth : alk. paper)
1. World health.   I. Pillay, Yogan.   II. Holtz, Timothy H.
III. Basch, Paul F., 1933- Textbook of international health.   IV. Title. [DNLM:
1. World Health.   2. International Cooperation.   3. Quality of Health Care.
WA 530.1 B619t 2009] RA441.
B38 2009 362.1—dc22   2008022619

9 8 7 6 5 4 3 2 1
Printed in the United States of America
on acid-free paper

To our children, and to children everywhere

Foreword by Archbishop Emeritus, Desmond Mpilo Tutu

Protecting and nurturing the health of all peoples is fundamentally important. This fully revised edition of Oxford University Press's *Textbook of International Health* could not be published at a more critical moment. On one hand, medico-scientific, administrative, and political changes have enabled great improvements in life expectancy over the past century. On the other hand, health conditions have stagnated or even deteriorated in many developing and transitional countries, as well as among marginalized populations in developed countries. Each year millions of people experience premature death and disability that could and should be prevented through concerted human action. Even the well-off are touched by the global spread of health problems. New and re-emerging diseases—tuberculosis, diabetes, Ebola—are as much a reflection of global economic processes and living patterns as they are of biological phenomena. They require the collective attention of the world community.

This textbook, appropriately, takes a critical approach to the determinants of health and disease and the role of local and national authorities and international donors and agencies in addressing health problems. Key to a full understanding of international health is knowledge of how economies are structured and function in local and global contexts, and how economic factors and political forces are intertwined to produce the conditions of health within and across societies. In other words, political, social, and economic power are vital underlying factors in determining who lives shorter or longer lives and how national and international entities respond to the challenges of global health. As such, this book does not merely describe international health activities or prescribe technical solutions to particular diseases, but it compels us to better understand the contexts in which health problems emerge and the forces that underlie and propel them. It also discusses the various ways in which governments, organizations, and peoples can work together more effectively to improve health and enable us all to live more fulfilling, productive and, dare I say, happier lives. Herein lies the value of this book for international health students and professionals.

I fully sympathize with and subscribe to this type of analysis as it has also guided my own work and life. We live in an increasingly unequal world—with burgeoning inequities within developing countries, as well as between industrialized and underdeveloped settings. Inequity in resource allocation, inequity in gender relations, inequity in services and living conditions all fuel disharmony at interpersonal, community, and larger levels. There is an urgent need for international commitment to combat these inequities through social justice efforts that replace the slavish focus on consumption, profit-making, and individualism propagated by neoliberal ideology, especially since the 1980s. The principles of social justice have been and continue to be the cornerstone of my life and work, both in the Church and in civic life.

A fundamental ingredient of equitable development, peace, social justice, and human well-being is the empowerment of the most vulnerable and the marginalized. Unless we build societies that take social justice seriously, we will continue to suffer the effects of poverty, inequities, racism and sexism, interpersonal and civil conflict, and general social disintegration and their social, economic, and health consequences—all issues discussed in this book.

In my 1984 Nobel Peace Prize acceptance speech, I pleaded with the international community to divert resources used to purchase armaments and instead put these resources to ending misery to ensure global security. I also called on the international community to ensure that human beings everywhere can enjoy basic human rights, the right to a fulfilled life, the right of movement, the right to work, and the freedom to be fully human.

I was honored to be invited to deliver a keynote lecture during the 2008 World Health Assembly in Geneva, Switzerland—honored because here I was a layperson speaking to leaders of public health from over 180 countries that belong to the UN family. However, given that I am a survivor of tuberculosis and cancer, as well as the ravages of poverty and the tyrannical system of apartheid, I considered myself somewhat qualified to speak to this gathering. In my lecture I noted the toll that disease takes on families, communities, and nations:

> And you would be particularly aware of the devastation caused by disease—TB, malaria, HIV/AIDS, river blindness, polio, cholera, infant mortality, maternal illnesses, many fuelled by poverty—children dying of easily preventable diseases if they could but get the inexpensive vaccination/inoculation; many illnesses resulting from a lack of clean water, proper sanitation, and decent housing. There is also evil when we refuse or become immobilized by bureaucracies or corruption to provide the needed remedy to heal the nations. We must never forget that as government leaders, we have a calling

to dispel ignorance, restore justice, and defend liberty. We have this calling to ensure peace and build good health. Much disease and heartbreak is preventable if governments had the political will—the 15% Now Campaign seeks to urge African Heads of State to honour their pledges and so prevent unnecessary deaths of 8 million of their citizens.

Then there are those leaders playing havoc with the well-being, the health of their people. In these places, even the children are enlisted into the ranks of soldiers. Likewise, parents watch helplessly as their children succumb, either because medication is rendered useless because of lack of electricity and so of refrigeration, or they are held up at check points and may fail to reach the hospital in time, if at all. Health cannot be de-linked or separated from the killing effects of living under the bonds of terror, oppression, and tyranny.

In parallel fashion, this volume focuses on international health, but at bottom it is about understanding and transforming societies and their political, social, and public health conditions to enable the improvement of human well-being.

The textbook covers a range of complex public health, medical, and sociopolitical issues and is written in a clear and highly organized fashion, making it accessible to students and professionals who have not had previous exposure to these fields. The authors' arguments and conclusions—while passionately presented—are carefully and thoroughly researched and well balanced. Case studies that show how progressive social policies adopted by particular societies affect all aspects of people's lives, including their health, offer powerful testimony to the possibility of mutual learning and the enormous contributions of various developing countries. For example, the democratic involvement of communities in policy making is a powerful mechanism to improving people's lives.

The book is also important for development "partners," including the aid agencies of former colonial governments and imperial powers, philanthropic foundations financed by corporate profits, and international organizations. Assistance by developed countries to developing countries has long been seen as a moral issue for which the poorer partners were expected to be grateful. However, as this book illustrates, the traditional purveyors of aid have amassed their wealth largely through the exploitation of workers and resources—in both underdeveloped and industrialized countries. The authors capture the challenges and dilemmas of development aid and cogently outline proposals on how international health (aid) should be conducted in the short term and how the historic legacies and ongoing inequities of the aid system might be redressed in the long term.

Development aid must reach its intended beneficiaries and not just benefit highly paid international consultants and technical advisors. We must ask the people—the intended beneficiaries—what assistance they require and how this assistance should be provided. All too often, others make decisions for the intended beneficiaries with the result that that aid often does not reach them and even when it does, sustainable solutions do not result from such interventions.

In sum, I highly recommend this textbook to students and professionals of international health, as well as to anyone who is interested in the ingredients of human health and well-being in an international context.

Cape Town, South Africa

Preface

The 20th century, as historian Eric Hobsbawm has characterized it, was an "age of extremes." The world underwent extraordinary social and scientific developments: huge increases in population, productivity, and economic growth; the decolonization of subjugated peoples across Africa, Asia, and the Caribbean; a remarkable rise in life expectancy; and vast improvements in living conditions for much of the global population. But the 20th century also witnessed two World Wars—the deadliest in human history—the rise and fall of the Cold War, and hundreds of regional conflicts, and was punctuated by two pandemics—influenza in 1918–1919 and HIV/AIDS starting in the 1980s—that each killed tens of millions of people. Moreover, despite decreases in economic and social inequality in the mid-20th century and notable improvements in child health and well-being, the last decades of the century saw growing inequities between developed and underdeveloped countries, as well as within most countries, together with soaring rates of food, housing, economic, health, and social insecurity.

The new millennium brought shared hope that a better and longer life could be attained by the majority of the world's population, especially the most vulnerable and marginalized—the more than 2 billion people who live on less than US$2/ day. Despite this hope, the first decade of the 21st century has already witnessed two major wars (in Afghanistan and Iraq), a U.S.-led war on terror, riots in many countries due to food shortages and the rising cost of basic foodstuffs, and growing income inequality and poverty in high, medium, and low income societies. Furthermore, a range of infectious diseases has emerged and re-emerged in recent decades, threatening populations across the world, and there are millions of premature deaths each year due to entirely preventable causes. Added to these problems is a global financial crisis and recession, which is generating widespread unemployment and impoverishment.

These forces and issues are part of the broader context of international health, which practitioners, decision makers, activists, and researchers need to understand and contemplate in their work and advocacy. Of course, those involved in international health must also learn about the policies, practices, institutions, and interventions that are central to addressing global health. This *Textbook of International Health* aims to describe, explain, and analyze these dimensions of international health from a political economy perspective; that is, how health, locally and globally, relates to the organization of economic activity and the distribution of power and wealth.

This book would not exist were it not for the first two editions written by the late Paul F. Basch. Described by his colleagues as a "man of singular purpose," Basch made his *Textbook of International Health* into *the* basic textbook of the field, even in its first edition. In revising and, ultimately, rewriting Paul Basch's marvelous second edition, we have sought to follow his lead in "fram[ing] some of the larger issues in international health in ways that serve the needs of students, scholars, and workers in this and related fields and to provide a base from which to expand knowledge wherever interest and opportunity may lead." As Basch noted in the second edition's preface (p. vi),

> Each major topic contains enough complexity to consume a lifelong career... [and requires a] balance between principles and specifics to satisfy both planners and technicians; between the past and the present to build an appreciation of why we are where we are; and between advocates and critics of various approaches to highlight the challenges of fulfilling the best of intentions...[all the while] maintain[ing] the attitude of an observer who is both passionately interested and earnestly disinterested.

We hope to have honored Paul Basch's legacy in building on his *chef d'oeuvre* and in pursuing our own approach to the writing of the textbook. While the second edition of the textbook was a basic primer, a sort of "traveler's guide to international health," this third edition is part primer and part analytic tool for the international health practitioner to use to better understand the social, political, and economic systems that contribute to the state of health of a nation, a city, a village, and the world as a whole. It will not be surprising to dedicated readers of this book that after almost a decade since the second edition was published, both the format of the text and much of its content have changed. For example, we have elaborated significantly on the impact of global climate change and environmental conditions on health, on the underlying determinants of health within and across countries, on the political economy of health and development aid, and on health under crisis conditions. Most notably, we have made significant changes to the book's critical perspective on global political and social forces, and expanded on what can be done at local, national, and international levels to improve health and foster lasting positive change. While each chapter of the book stands alone, many threads run through

the text, including the role of the societal determinants of health, of social and economic policies, and of the redistribution of resources within and across societies.
This perspective helps us to better understand why the populations living in some
societies have better health than others.

This book has benefited from the wisdom and experiences of countless international health practitioners, scholars, and activists. While we have tried to be as comprehensive as possible, the field of international health is vast and one book cannot
pretend to be encyclopedic, as Basch noted in the preface of the second edition.
However, we believe that any international health practitioner (novice or not) will
find something useful in this textbook.

Acknowledgments

All books are ultimately collective endeavors, but this one is especially so. We have drawn from the research, knowledge, and camaraderie of literally thousands of community health workers, scholars, activists, administrators, friends, students, and colleagues. Many are cited directly in the references. Here we gratefully acknowledge the people who enabled this project to come to fruition, with our apologies to those whose names were inadvertently left out.

Several cohorts of University of Toronto students, both graduate students in the Dalla Lana School of Public Health and undergraduates from the Department of Social Sciences, provided outstanding research and editing assistance, withstanding tight deadlines and complex requests with composure and humor. Thanks especially to Melisa Dickie, Bronwyn Underhill, Danielle Schirmer, Sarah Jacobs, Franziska Satzinger, Sarah Stranks, Giulia El-Dardiry, René Guerra Salazar, Klaudia Dmitrienko, Ilan Alleson, Katharine Hagerman, Angela Daust, Angela Loder, Zahra Khoja, and Krista Lauer. Whitney Pyles in Atlanta purveyed similar excellent research assistance.

We were fortunate to enlist an esteemed set of colleagues to review individual, and in some cases multiple, chapters of the textbook. We are grateful to Robert Chernomas, Meredith Fort, Albert Berry, Ardeshir Sepehri, Lucy Gilson, Rick Brennan, Daniel Bausch, Catherine Cubbin, Alison Katz, Kent Buse, Donald Cole, Nikolai Krementsov, Barbara Starfield, Theodore Brown, Brandon Kohrt, and Joanne Corrigall for their generosity of time and expertise. All errors of commission or omission remain, of course, our own.

Many, many others helped us secure information or images and researched or reviewed chapter sections. Our appreciation goes to Juliana Martínez Franzoni, Abhijit Das, Joan Hsiao Bromley, Joan Benach, Jillian Clare Cohen Kohler, Maria Hamlin Zúniga, Vera Marques, Mary O'Hara, Henry Kahn, Simon Szreter, Lisa Forman, Colin Leys, Camara Jones, Judith Richter, Nancy Krieger, Anthony

Robbins, Phyllis Freeman, Wanda Cabella, Andrea Vigorito, Suzanne Marks, Steve Gloyd, Steve Morse, Victoria Gammino, David Parker, Ann Langford, Alex Scott-Samuel, Myer Glickman, Shankar LeVine, Reed Brody, Leslie London, Carles Muntaner, Theresa Betancourt, Claudia Chaufan, Robert Gould, Tanya Keeble, Daniel Tarantola, Nadia Nijim, Dick Clapp, Alan Berkman, Basia Tomczyk, Leisel Talley, Tom Handzel, Wendy Johnson, Jennifer Kasper, Christina Chan, Vera Ngowi, Holly Solberg, Brad Woodruff, Dabney Evans, Lorna Thorpe, Patrick Kachur, Aun Lor, and others we may have unintentionally omitted.

At Oxford University Press, executive editor William Lamsback and his staff expertly shepherded us and the textbook through all phases of preparation. Anupama Gopinath and her colleagues from Newgen Imaging Systems led us through the editing and production process with grace and patience. We also thank retired Oxford editor Jeffrey House, who had the vision to bring out a third edition of Paul Basch's *Textbook of International Health* and the confidence in the three of us to fully revise and rewrite, update, and reshape the text.

During the preparation of this book, the Canada Research Chairs Program provided support to Anne-Emanuelle Birn and to many of the above-named research assistants. Doctors for Global Health supported Timothy Holtz in his work on this project.

Finally, we are indebted to Esperanza, Irina, Jackie, Nadia, Nikita, Nikolai, and Vishay, who provided us the time, space, and inspiration to complete the book.

Contents

Some Abbreviations and Acronyms Used in International Health   *xix*
List of Illustrations   *xxv*
    Figures   *xxv*
    Tables   *xxix*
    Boxes   *xxxiii*

1   Introduction   3

2   The Historical Origins of Modern International Health   17

3   International Health Agencies, Activities, and Other Actors   61

4   The Political Economy of Health and Development   132

5   What Do We Know, What Do We Need to Know,
    and Why it Matters—Data on Health   192

6   Epidemiologic Profiles of Global Health and Disease   242

7   Societal Determinants of Health and Social Inequalities in Health   309

8   Health under Crisis   365

9   Globalization, Trade, Work, and Health   417

10 Health and the Environment   470

11 Health Economics and the Economics of Health   537

12 Understanding and Organizing Health Care Systems   583

13 Toward Healthy Societies: From Ideas to Action   656

14 Doing International Health   694

    Appendix   741

    Index   761

Some Abbreviations and Acronyms Used in International Health

AIDS	Acquired Immunodeficiency Syndrome
AKF	Aga Khan Foundation
ARI	Acute Respiratory (Tract) Infection
ARVs	Antiretroviral Drugs
BCG	Bacille Calmette-Guèrin (TB vaccine)
BW	Biological Weapons
BWC	Biological Weapons Convention
CBA	Cost–Benefit Analysis
CBW	Chemical and Biological Weapons
CDC	Centers for Disease Control and Prevention
CEA	Cost-Effectiveness Analysis
CFCs	Chlorofluorocarbons
CHD	Coronary Heart Disease
CHE	Complex Humanitarian Emergency
CHW	Community Health Worker
CIDA	Canadian International Development Agency
CIS	Commonwealth of Independent States
CMH	Commission on Macroeconomics and Health
COPD	Chronic Obstructive Pulmonary Disease
CRC	Convention on the Rights of the Child

CSDH	Commission on Social Determinants of Health
CTBT	Comprehensive Test Ban Treaty
CVD	Cardiovascular Disease
CW	Chemical Weapons
CWC	Chemical Weapons Convention
DAC	Development Assistance Committee (OECD)
DALY	Disability Adjusted Life Year
DDT	Dichlorodiphenyltrichloroethane
DFID	Department for International Development (UK)
DHS	Demographic and Health Survey
DOTS	Direct Observed Therapy, Short-course
DPT	Diphtheria, Pertussis, Tetanus (immunization)
DRC	Democratic Republic of the Congo (formerly Zaire)
EIA	Environmental Impact Assessment
EID	Emerging Infectious Diseases
EPI	Expanded Program on Immunization (WHO)
EPZ	Export Processing Zones
EU	European Union
FAO	Food and Agriculture Organization (UN)
FDA	Food and Drug Administration (US)
FDI	Foreign Direct Investment
FEMA	Federal Emergency Management Agency (US)
GBD	Global Burden of Disease
GBV	Gender-Based Violence
GDP	Gross Domestic Product
GIS	Geographic Information System
GMO	Genetically Modified Organism
GNH	Gross National Happiness
GNI	Gross National Income
GNP	Gross National Product
GOBI	Growth Monitoring, Oral Rehydration, Breast feeding, Immunization (UNICEF)
GOBI/FFF	GOBI plus Family Planning, Food Production, Female Education
GP	General Practitioner

HAART	Highly Active Antiretroviral Treatment
HCP	Healthy Cities Program
HDI	Human Development Index
HFA	Health for All (WHO)
HFA2000	Health for All by the Year 2000
HIA	Health Impact Assessment
HIV	Human Immunodeficiency Virus
HMO	Health Maintenance Organization
HNP	Health, Nutrition, and Population division (World Bank)
HPV	Human Papilloma Virus
IBRD	International Bank for Reconstruction and Development (World Bank)
ICCPR	International Covenant on Civil and Political Rights
ICD	International Classification of Diseases
ICDDR,B	International Centre for Diarrhoeal Disease Research, Bangladesh
ICESCR	International Covenant on Economic, Social, and Cultural Rights
ICHI	International Classification of Health Interventions
IDA	International Development Association (World Bank)
IDB	Inter-American Development Bank
IDRC	International Development Research Centre (Canada)
IFI	International Financial Institution
IFPMA	International Federation of Pharmaceutical Manufacturers & Associations
IHR	International Health Regulations
ILO	International Labour Organization
IMCI	Integrated Management of Childhood Illness
IMF	International Monetary Fund
IMR	Infant Mortality Rate
INCLEN	International Clinical Epidemiology Network
INGO	International Nongovernmental Organization
IRB	Institutional Review Board
ISI	Import Substitution Industrialization
LASM	Latin American Social Medicine

LGBT	Lesbian, Gay, Bisexual, and Transgendered
LNHO	League of Nations Health Organization
MCH	Maternal and Child Health
MCO	Managed Care Organization
MDG	Millennium Development Goals
MMR	Maternal Mortality Ratio
MMRate	Maternal Mortality Rate
MOH	Ministry of Health
MSF	Médecins Sans Frontières
MTCT	Mother-to-Child Transmission
NGO	Nongovernmental Organization
NHA	National Health Accounts
NHS	National Health Service (UK)
NIEO	New International Economic Order
NIH	National Institutes of Health (US)
NTD	Neglected Tropical Diseases
ODA	Official Development Assistance
OECD	Organization for Economic Cooperation and Development
OIHP	Office Internationale d'Hygiène Publique
OPEC	Organization of Petroleum Exporting Countries
ORT	Oral Rehydration Therapy
PAHO	Pan American Health Organization
PASB	Pan American Sanitary Bureau
PEPFAR	President's Emergency Plan for AIDS Relief (US)
PHC	Primary Health Care
PHM	People's Health Movement
PHS	U.S. Public Health Service
PIH	Partners In Health
PPPs	Public-Private Partnerships
PQLI	Physical Quality of Life Index
QALY	Quality Adjusted Life Years
RF	Rockefeller Foundation
SADC	Southern African Development Cooperation

SAL	Structural Adjustment Loan
SAP	Structural Adjustment Policy (or Program)
SARS	Severe Acute Respiratory Syndrome
SES	Socioeconomic Status
SPHC	Selective Primary Health Care
STD	Sexually Transmitted Disease
STI	Sexually Transmitted Infection
SWAP	Sector-Wide Approach
TB	Tuberculosis
TBA	Traditional Birth Attendant
TNC	Transnational Corporation
TRIPS	Trade-Related Intellectual Property Rights (Agreement)
UDHR	Universal Declaration of Human Rights
UN	United Nations
UNCTAD	United Nations Conference on Trade and Development
UNDP	United Nations Development Programme
UNEP	United Nations Environment Program
UNFCCC	United Nations Framework Convention on Climate Change
UNFPA	United Nations Population Fund
UNHCR	United Nations High Commissioner for Refugees
UNICEF	United Nations Children's Fund
UNRRA	United Nations Relief and Rehabilitation Agency
USAID	United States Agency for International Development
VA	Verbal Autopsy
WDR	World Development Report (World Bank)
WHA	World Health Assembly (WHO)
WHO	World Health Organization
WHOSIS	WHO Statistical Information System
WSF	World Social Forum
YPLL	Years of Potential Life Lost

List of Illustrations

Figures

2–1   The Demographic Transition   31
2–2   Tuberculosis Mortality and Medical Interventions   37
2–3   Epidemiologic Transition   40
2–4   Yellow Fever Patient Segregated in a Screened Cubicle in the
        Gorgas Hospital, Ancon, Canal Zone   44
2–5   Caribbean Laborers Felling Trees for Swamp Drainage and
        Canal Construction at New Market Creek Swamp, Panama,
        Circa 1910   45
2–6   House-to-House Administration of Antihelminthics,
        Rockefeller Foundation International Health Board's
        Cooperative Hookworm Campaign in Rural Mexico, 1920s   51
3–1   DAC Members Net ODA 1990–2004 and DAC Secretariat
        Simulation of Net ODA to 2006 and 2010   94
3–2   Net ODA in 2006: Amounts   95
3–3   Net ODA in 2006 as a Percentage of GNI   95
3–4   Development Assistance for Health by Source, 1997–2003   122
4–1   Understanding Health and Illness: The Interplay of Host, Agent,
        and Environment   136
4–2   Political Economy of International Health Framework   138
4–3   Trends in Life Expectancy by Region   145
4–4   Changes in Life Expectancy, 1962–2002   145
4–5   Annual Life Expectancy in EU Member States and the
        Commonwealth of Independent States   146
4–6   Political Economy-Based Classification of Countries   154

4–7   Long-Term Trends of ODA as a Percentage of GNP by DAC
           Countries   159
4–8   Long-Term Trends of Net ODA Disbursements by DAC
           Countries   160
4–9   Net Resource Flows on Debt from Developing
           Countries   166
4–10   Net Resource Flows on Debt from Developing Countries by
           Region, 2002   167
4–11   World Poverty Rates, 1990–2003   175
5–1   Age Pyramids for Populations of Five Countries   206
5–2   Population Size Estimates with and without the Effect of AIDS,
           South Africa, 2000 and 2025   207
5–3   International Form of Medical Certificate of Cause
           of Death   215
5–4   Coverage of Vital Registration of Deaths, World,
           1995–2003   221
5–5   Distribution of Disease Burden (in DALYs) by Age Group
           and Region, 2002   230
6–1   Leading Causes of Death in the World, 2002   245
6–2   Leading Causes of Death in Denmark, 2002   246
6–3   Leading Causes of Death in Egypt, 2002   247
6–4   Leading Causes of Death in Nigeria, 2002   248
6–5   Age-Standardized Mortality Rate between Selected
           Countries, 2002   249
6–6   Rates of Change in Under-5 Mortality Rate by Income   252
6–7   Major Causes of Childhood Deaths in Developing Countries,
           2002   253
6–8   Global Population Pyramid in 2002 and 2025   256
6–9   Estimates of Maternal Mortality Ratios   260
6–10   Coverage of Maternal Health Services   260
6–11   Reported Number of Cholera Cases and Case Fatality Rates,
           1950–1998   267
6–12   Number of Estimated Cases of Malaria in Proportion to
           Population of Each Country   274
6–13   Estimated Deaths Caused by Acute Respiratory Infection
           Worldwide   276
6–14   Estimated TB Incidence Rates, by Country, 2005   284
6–15   Estimated Number of People Living with HIV and Adult
           HIV Prevalence (Globally and in Sub-Saharan Africa,
           1990–2007)   288
6–16   Number of People Receiving ARV Therapy in Low- and
           Middle-Income Countries by Region, 2002–2007   293

6–17   Unmet Need for ARV Therapy among Adults in Developing
            and Transitional Countries in Sub-Saharan Africa,
            2002–2005   294
7–1   Water Connection Rates and Infant Mortality Rates, 2006   314
7–2   All-Cause Mortality among Men 40–59 in St. Petersburg,
            Russia, by Education Level   323
7–3   Cardiovascular Mortality among Men 40–59 in St. Petersburg,
            Russia, by Education Level   324
7–4   Infant Mortality by Wealth Quintile, Selected Countries   329
7–5   Maternal and Child Health Indicators in Developing Countries,
            by Wealth Quintile   329
7–6   Social Class and Infant Mortality in the United Kingdom: The
            Black Report and Beyond   343
7–7   Life Expectancy by Social Class for Men (England and Wales)
            since the Black Report   344
7–8   Whitehall All-Cause Mortality over 25 Years According to
            Level in Occupational Hierarchy   345
7–9   Schematic Representation of Psychosocial Pathways   348
8–1   New Orleans, Post Katrina, 2005   368
8–2   Damage from the Earthquake in Balakot, Pakistan, 2005   372
8–3   Map of Complex Humanitarian Emergencies Causing
            Displacement   376
8–4   UNICEF Framework for Malnutrition   380
8–5   The Impact of Conflict and Emergencies on Health and Health
            Services   383
8–6   Child Landmine Survivor, Sierra Leone, 1990s   385
8–7   Military Expenditures 1996–2005   387
8–8   Number of IDPs and Refugees, 1990–2004   400
9–1   Child Laborers at Indiana Glass Works, at Midnight, 1908   419
9–2   Child Stone Quarry Worker, India   420
9–3   Pathways of Neoliberal Globalization and Effects
            on Health   427
9–4   Applying Pesticides without Protective Equipment,
            Tanzania   446
10–1   Political Economy of Environmental Health Determinants,
            Effects, and Responses   475
10–2   Ecological Footprints: A Global Snapshot   481
10–3   Environmental Disease Burden by WHO Subregion, 2002   483
10–4   Number of Passenger Vehicles by Region   492
10–5   Passenger Vehicles as a Proportion of Population by
            Region   493
10–6   Aral Sea Shrinkage   496

10–7   Percentage of Population with Access to "Improved Sanitation,"
            1990 and 2006   497
10–8   Drinking Water Coverage by Region, 2006   497
10–9   Curitiba Transit Stop, Estação Central   522
11–1   The Preston Curve Applied to Health Spending: Life
            Expectancy at Birth (2006) and Annual Per Capita
            Expenditure on Health (2005) (for 193 Countries)   571
11–2   Real GDP and Genuine Progress Indicator (GPI) Per Capita,
            1950–2004 for the United States in US$ 2000   572
12–1   Total Expenditure on Health Per Capita, 2004 (in US$)   590
12–2   Global Health Worker Density   633
14–1   Schoolchildren in Santa Marta, El Salvador, Awaiting their
            Annual Check-Up (Doctors for Global Health)   721
14–2   Well-Baby Clinic Outside a Public Health Center
            in Nhamatanda, Sofala Province, Mozambique
            (Health Alliance International)   721
14–3   The Bangladeshi Delegation at the Ceremony of the Native
            Peoples of the World, Savar, First People's Health Assembly,
            Held Near Dhaka, 2000   732

Tables

3–1   Typology of International Health Actors, Agencies, and Programs 68

3–2   Selected UN Organizations 70

3–3   Selected Autonomous UN Specialized Agencies 70

3–4   Major UN Conferences and Summits Relating to Health 72

3–5   WHO Regional Offices 74

3–6   Major WHO Activities 76

3–7   Voting Power as a Function of Shareholding 82

3–8   Recent IFI Development Strategies 87

3–9   Selected Bilateral Agency Budgets and Priorities 91

3–10   Endowments and Priorities of Selected Foundations 100

3–11   Private Health Insurance Penetration in 2006 104

3–12   Leading Pharmaceutical Companies by Revenues and Profits 105

3–13   Selected Religious Agencies—Spending and Activities 108

3–14   Largest Current International Health Funders 121

4–1   Key Analytic Questions from the Writings of Vicente Navarro 143

4–2   Causes and Treatment of Diarrhea According to Contrasting Approaches to Health 147

4–3   Causes and Treatment of Obesity According to Contrasting Approaches to Health 148

4–4   Human Rights Instruments as a Baseline for the "Right to Health" 178

4–5   Pathways to Health and Human Rights 179

5–1   Some Uses and Limitations of Statistical Health Data 195

5–2   Some Questions about Health Data 200

5–3   Commonly Used Health Indicators   201
5–4   Some Topics Recommended by the UN World Population
             and Housing Census Programme and Various National Census
             Agencies for Inclusion in a National Population Census   202
5–5   Some Personal and Administrative Uses of Vital Records   210
5–6   Major Subdivisions of the International Classification of
             Diseases, Tenth Revision   214
5–7   Countries with Highest and Lowest Infant Mortality Rates
             (IMR), 2006   217
5–8   Infant Mortality in India by State, 2001   218
5–9   Infant Mortality Rate by Region, Brazil, 2004   219
5–10   The 12 Leading Causes of Death in the World, 2002   227
5–11   The 10 Leading Causes of Death by Country Income Level,
             2002   229
5–12   Leading Causes of Disease Burden (in DALYs) for Males and
             Females Aged 15 Years and Older, Worldwide, 2002   231
6–1   Public Health Epidemiologic Terms   243
6–2   Global Distribution of Cause-Specific Mortality Among
             Children Under the Age of 5 (2006)   251
6–3   Some Functional Consequences of Deficiency of Selected
             Micronutrients   253
6–4   Selected Indigenous Populations and Related Health
             Indicators   263
6–5   Some Enteric Agents that Can Cause Acute or Chronic
             Diarrhea   268
6–6   Descriptions of "Neglected Tropical Diseases"   270
6–7   Some Emerging Infections and Probable Factors in Their
             Emergence   295
6–8   Some Factors in the Emergence of Infectious Diseases   297
8–1   Famine Scale Based on Joint Criteria of Mortality,
             Malnutrition, and Food Security   375
8–2   Main Sources of the World's Refugees, January 2005   378
8–3   Prevalence of Mental Health Disorders in Adult Populations
             Affected by Complex Emergencies   381
8–4   Selected Antipersonnel Toxic and Infective Agents and Their
             Health Effects, Whose Hostile Use has Been Verified   391
8–5   Comparison of Mortality in Violent and Nonviolent Zones
             in the Democratic Republic of Congo   398
8–6   Total Population of Concern to UNHCR, January 2005   400
9–1   Key Definitions Relating to Globalization, Trade, and
             Work   424
9–2   Trade Treaties and Their Influence on Health   430

9–3   Examples of Human Rights Violations Linked to Transnational
            Corporate Activity   435

9–4   Challenges for Occupational Health in Some Developing
            Countries   444

9–5   Estimated Number of Children Exploited through Prostitution
            (Worldwide)   452

10–1   World CO_2 Emissions (Billion Metric Tons) by Region   477

10–2   The Impact of Environmental Problems and Conditions
            on Health   482

10–3   Agents of Environmental Health Problems   484

10–4   Selected Pollution Hotspots   488

10–5   Actions to Confront Environmental Hazards   509

10–6   Technologies and Practices to Improve Environmental
            Conditions   520

11–1   Spending on Health: Some Examples of the Extent of Inequities
            (in US$)   538

11–2   How the Health Care Sector Differs from Markets   544

11–3   Organization and Effects of Single-Payer and Multiple-Payer
            Systems Compared   548

11–4   Economic Evaluation Techniques for Health   555

11–5   Using CEA to Determine Health Priorities   556

11–6   GNI, Debt, Health Expenditures, and Donor Funding in
            Selected Countries (2006–2007)   563

11–7   Neoliberal and Social Justice Approaches to Health
            Compared   569

11–8   International Comparisons of Health Measures, Health
            Expenditures, and Inequalities   573

12–1   Public versus Private Financing and Delivery of Health Care
            Services   587

12–2   Roemer's Health System Typology   588

12–3   Comparison of Health Indicators: Cuba, the United States, and
            Sweden, 2006   591

12–4   Private Expenditures as % of Total Health Spending in Selected
            Countries, 2006   592

12–5   Evolution of Health Systems   594

12–6   Characteristics of Health Sector Reform   609

12–7   Health System Principles and Building Blocks   617

12–8   Drug Pipeline for TB as Compared to Cancer and
            Cardiovascular Diseases   629

12–9   Provider Remuneration Mechanisms   637

13–1   Cost of the Smallpox Eradication Program   659

13–2   Mortality Rates for Selected Welfare States   667

13–3   Data on Selected Determinants of Health and Mortality Rates
                for Three Developing Countries and the United States   668
13–4   Selected Health Outcomes, Kerala and India   673
Appendix   Some World Wide Web Sites of Interest for
                International Health   741

Boxes

1–1   Ways of Conceptualizing International Health   11
2–1   Motives for Imperial Health   30
2–2   The Demographic Transition   31
2–3   The McKeown Thesis   37
2–4   The Epidemiologic Transition   40
2–5   International Health Imperatives   50
2–6   Early International Health Organizations, Location, and Year of Founding   52
3–1   Eras of International Health Activity   64
3–2   Functions of the WHO   73
3–3   Primary Health Care and its Fates   79
3–4   International Health Aid in Nicaragua   85
3–5   PEPFAR   92
3–6   Role of "Big Pharma" in International Health   103
3–7   Rockefeller Foundation Principles of International Health Cooperation   123
4–1   Categorizing Countries: Income and Redistribution   153
4–2   Water Privatization   168
4–3   MDGs and Selected Targets   173
4–4   Governmental Obligations for Health Under International Human Rights Law   180
5–1   Additional Information to be Included in Routine Data Collection to Enable Measurement of Social Inequalities in Health and Societal Determinants of Health   203
5–2   Age-Adjustment   220
5–3   Some Vital Events as Defined by the UN   222

5–4   Registrar General of India (RGI) Million Death Study in
        India   223
6–1   The Health of Children over Five and Young Adults:
        Unique Realities and Issues   254
6–2   Disability   255
6–3   Injecting Drug Use   258
6–4   Dental Health   258
6–5   Mental Health of Adults   261
6–6   Cholera   267
6–7   Measles   275
6–8   Social Cost of HIV/AIDS in Sub-Saharan Africa   290
6–9   Brazilian National AIDS Program   291
7–1   Definitions   310
7–2   Interactions of the Determinants of Health: Living
        Conditions   313
7–3   Food Quality and the Societal Determinants of Health   316
7–4   Immigrant, Migrant, and Refugee Status   334
7–5   Differences between Inequalities and Inequities in Health   341
7–6   The Commission on Social Determinants of Health's
        Overarching Recommendations and Principles of Action   353
7–7   Ten Tips for American Public Health Researchers and
        Workers   354
8–1   Definitions and Classifications   366
8–2   Root Causes of Food Insecurity   373
8–3   Landmine Effects on Health   388
8–4   War and the Environment   392
8–5   A Code of Conduct for Humanitarian Relief   405
9–1   The Precautionary Principle and the WTO   430
9–2   Water Privatization   431
9–3   Transnationals, the WTO, and Infant Formula: A Case Study
        of Unethical Practices   433
9–4   The Tragedy of Union Carbide in Bhopal   441
9–5   The Organization of Work, Increased Risk of HIV,
        and Opportunities for Prevention   445
9–6   Export of Hazards: The Case of Canadian Asbestos
        Production   447
10–1   Definitions   470
10–2   Climate Change and Human Development   478
10–3   Four Environmental Worldviews, as Identified by Jennifer
        Clapp and Peter Dauvergne   479
10–4   Child Health and the Environment   483
10–5   Environmental Racism   489

10–6   Lead Contamination   491
10–7   Asthma and Air Pollution   494
10–8   The Aral Sea Crisis   495
10–9   Food Safety   498
10–10   Biodiversity and Human Health   501
10–11   Deforestation of the Amazon   502
10–12   Exxon Valdez Oil Spill   507
10–13   Key International Environmental Conferences and
            Agreements   511
10–14   Environmental Health Cooperation and CFCs   513
10–15   Environmental Protection and Health Promotion: EIA, HIA,
            and the Precautionary Principle   516
10–16   Alternative Energy Sources   518
10–17   Curitiba, Brazil—"The Green City"   521
10–18   Principles of Sustainable Cities   523
11–1   Georgia's Experiences with Changes in Health Financing   539
11–2   Covered Health Care Services and the Limits to Access
            in South Africa   546
11–3   The Bamako Initiative   549
11–4   Lack of Harmonization of Development Assistance,
            Vietnam   564
11–5   Corruption in the Health Sector   565
11–6   Kerala   575
12–1   Basic Features of Germany's Social Insurance System   596
12–2   Basic Features of the NHS   599
12–3   Basic Features of the Former Soviet Model   602
12–4   Basic Features of Health Care under China's "Market
            Socialism"   604
12–5   Basic Features of Health Care Delivery in the United
            States   608
12–6   Maternal and Child Health Example: Bureaucratic
            and Resource Barriers   618
12–7   Maternal and Child Health Example: Poor Quality Care   620
12–8   Maternal and Child Health Example: Infrastructural
            and Economic Barriers   621
12–9   Long-Term Care Facilities and Hospices   622
12–10   Maternal and Child Health Example: Inequalities
            in Health Care Facilities   623
12–11   Maternal and Child Health Example: Health Human Resources
            Shortages   625
12–12   The Political Economy of Big Pharma   628

12–13   Maternal and Child Health Example: Lack of Insurance
           Coverage   632
12–14   The "Brain Drain," the Shortage of Health Workers,
           and Cuba's Solution   634
12–15   Medical Tourism   636
12–16   Maternal and Child Health Example: Provider Reimbursement
           Incentives   638
12–17   Encouraging Publication of Health Research by Developing
           Country Researchers   638
12–18   Maternal and Child Health Example: Health Planning within
           Larger Societal Reforms   641
12–19   Decentralization and District Health Systems   643
12–20   Selections from the *Declaration of Alma-Ata*   644
12–21   Maternal and Child Health Example: Primary Health Care   646
13–1   Scaling Up Versus Building Stairs, Bridges, and
           Foundations   662
13–2   Why Vertical Programs Do Not Work: The Case of TB in
           Assam   664
13–3   Limits to Technical Approaches to International Health   665
13–4   Factors Contributing to the Success of Cuba's Social
           Services   670
13–5   Creating Healthy Societies through Cooperation: Health
           Alliance International   674
13–6   ALAMES's Guiding Principles and Key Aspects
           of its Political Agenda   676
13–7   Components of Mexico City's Integrated Territorial Social
           Program   677
13–8   A Critique of "Pro-Poor" Approaches to Policy Making:
           Why Not Antipoverty Instead?   680
13–9   Wherefore International Efforts? Promise and Limitations of the
           Framework Convention on Tobacco Control   683
13–10   Challenges of National and International Approaches
           to Combating Female Genital Cutting   685
14–1   Trypanosomiasis in East Africa   698
14–2   Personal Motivations for Working in International Health   700
14–3   Voices from the Ground   701
14–4   Key Questions to Consider in Carrying Out International
           Health Work   723

Textbook of International Health

THIRD EDITION

Introduction

In recent years, the challenges of international health have captured the attention of politicians, business executives, the United Nations, celebrities, magnates, and the media. Suddenly, it seems, international health has surfaced as a pressing global priority. Yet many of the problems of international health—such as high rates of infant and maternal mortality, tuberculosis, heart disease, and other causes of premature mortality—are not new. Health workers, activists, and community members have long struggled to improve health conditions within and across societies. Moreover, the spread of disease from one place to another has been a recurring economic and political concern.

So what is new, what is old, what is ongoing, and, most importantly, what is vital to improving international health? This third edition of Oxford University Press's *Textbook of International Health* examines international health's historical origins, the patterns and underlying causes of leading health problems, approaches to resolving these issues, the political context of international health, as well as the development of international health as a field of study, research, and practice. This introductory chapter begins by defining public health, international health, global health, and what distinguishes them. We then discuss why international health matters and some of the persistent dilemmas of the field. Next, we explore the ideologies, elements of, and approaches to international health policy making and practice. We end with a guide to the textbook as a whole.

KEY DEFINITIONS

According to the World Health Organization (WHO), "Health is a state of complete physical, mental, and social well-being and not merely the absence of disease or infirmity" (Preamble to the Constitution of the World Health Organization as adopted by the International Health Conference 1946). This idealistic and comprehensive definition—which nonetheless leaves out the important dimension of spiritual well-being—is much cited but little followed by major international health actors. As we will see in Chapter 3, these organizations typically frame international health in terms of disease control. Numerous international agencies sponsor programs and campaigns against particular diseases; indeed, a range of agencies and organizations are named after the diseases they pursue, most prominently the Global Fund to Fight AIDS, Tuberculosis and Malaria. Even those that support health systems often view the elimination of disease as the ultimate purpose, with particular disease-control activities prioritized.

We experience good and poor health at a personal level, but illness and death are also social phenomena shared by households, friends and kin, classmates and work colleagues, caregivers and healers, and the larger society. At the same time, the social context—how people live, work, and recreate, and the differences between rich and poor—greatly affects who becomes ill (and of what diseases), disabled, or dies prematurely.

As we will discuss in subsequent chapters, there is an emerging consensus that addressing the social determinants of health (which are closely linked to human rights, as laid out in the 1948 *Universal Declaration of Human Rights*) is essential to ensuring the highest attainable state of health and well-being (WHO Commission on Social Determinants of Health 2008). These determinants include adequate housing, access to clean water, sanitation, nutrition, education, broad social policies and protections, safe working conditions, and living wages. Underlying these factors are the political and economic forces that shape the distribution of power and resources and influence the extent of inequality and the existence and/or nature of social security systems in particular societies and globally.

International health is closely connected to the field of "public health," a concept coined in the early 19th century to distinguish government efforts for the preservation and protection of health from private actions. A century later, U.S. public health leader C.-E.A. Winslow famously defined public health as:

> the science and art of preventing disease, prolonging life, and promoting physical health and efficiency through organized community efforts for the sanitation of the environment, the control of community infections, the education of the individual in principles of personal hygiene, the organization of medical and nursing service for the early diagnosis and preventive treatment of disease, and the development of the social machinery which will ensure to every individual in the community a standard of living adequate for the maintenance of health (Winslow 1920, p. 23).

This ample definition might be taken as a basis for international actions and cooperation for health, yet what constitutes public health remains contested. This is especially true in recent years, as the preeminence of public health as a social good is being increasingly displaced by profit-driven agendas (Lexchin 2007; Puliyel and Madhavi 2008).

Because public health has at times been interpreted in narrow, medicalized terms (Lantz, Lichtenstein, and Pollack 2007) and because the field of public health has (had) both repressive and progressive strands (Krieger and Birn 1998), several other conceptions have come to the fore. As we will see in Chapter 4, "social medicine" developed in the 19th century as a form of integrating political action and health efforts; this approach still resonates today among doctor-activists, a range of local health departments, and certain national programs (Holtz et al. 2006).

In 1989, the Canadian Institute for Advanced Research introduced the concept of "population health" (later officially endorsed by Canada's federal and regional health ministers), "proposing that individual determinants of health do not act in isolation" (Public Health Agency of Canada 2004) but rather interact in a complex fashion. For example, unemployment can lead to social isolation, poverty, and homelessness, with profound effects on health.

In Brazil and elsewhere in Latin America, the concept of "collective health" was developed in the 1970s, and accelerated in the 1990s, to emphasize the role and agency of ordinary people and social movements in shaping health outcomes (Nunes 1996; Almeida Filho and Paim 1999). While the field and actors of collective health emphasize the political dimensions and determinants of health, they challenge the exclusive role of, and reliance on, the public sector, especially in contexts where governments are repressive, unrepresentative, or unresponsive to the collective needs of the population.

These various movements and spheres of action—public health, social medicine, population health, collective health—have all influenced ideas, institutions, and practices internationally, yet international health is also a separate field, with its own traditions, organizations, and trajectory.

International Health

As we will cover in greater detail in Chapter 2, the term "international health" first came into use in the early 20th century after sovereign countries began to recognize the value of intergovernmental cooperation and established permanent bodies to address health issues that crossed national borders. Although somewhat distinct from the concerns of tropical medicine (which addressed the health problems in Europe's colonies in Asia, Africa, the Caribbean, and other "tropical" settings), this new arena of international health nonetheless reflected the interests of imperial powers to protect international commerce and fend off epidemics of diseases, such as cholera and plague, that might cause social unrest or reduce worker productivity (Bashford 2006). As such, an early priority of international health organizations was disease surveillance, standardization, and sanitary treaties calling for mandatory reciprocal notification of, and measures to combat, particular diseases, including ship and passenger inspection and quarantine. Colonial authorities and some nongovernmental entities, most notably the Rockefeller

Foundation, also undertook international public health campaigns against yellow fever, hookworm, and other ailments in the Americas, Asia, Africa, and the Pacific, as well as Europe.

When the WHO was founded after World War II, this flagship multilateral, intergovernmental health organization crafted the optimistic and unifying term "world health" to reflect its singularity of purpose rather than retain the more politically wrought "international" nomenclature. As we will discuss in Chapter 3, the idealism undergirding the founding of the WHO was quickly enveloped in Cold War rivalries between the Soviet Union and the United States and their respective allies. International cooperation became characterized by continued economic and political domination of industrialized powers over developing countries, many of which had newly acquired independence. In concrete terms, then, the notion of world health never gained firm grounding; instead, international health principally covered the problems of health in underdeveloped countries and the efforts by industrialized countries and international agencies to address these problems. As such, the term international health retained its primacy.

Global Health

More recently, international health has been reconceptualized as "global health," a term that may seem more familiar to some readers than international health. The U.S. Institute of Medicine has defined global health as "health problems, issues, and concerns that transcend national boundaries, may be influenced by circumstances or experiences in other countries, and are best addressed by cooperative actions and solutions" (Institute of Medicine 1997, p. 2). Global health is portrayed as going beyond prior understandings of communication and accords regarding health issues between governments to refer to the health needs of people across the world, irrespective of borders, thus depoliticizing the field.

The term *global health*—adopted broadly over the past decade[1]—is meant to rise above past ideological uses of the term international health (as a "handmaiden" of colonialism or a pawn of Cold War political rivalries) to imply a shared global susceptibility to, experience of, and responsibility for health (Birn 2006). As such, global health aims to address the health problems of both rich countries and poor countries. The concept of global health allows international health practitioners to apply a critical analysis of public health problems wherever they occur. In its more collective guise, then, global health refers to health and disease patterns in terms of the interaction of global, national, and local forces, processes, and conditions in political, economic, social, and epidemiologic domains.

However, the term global health has also been used to assert U.S. "global unilateralism," that is, a tailoring of the world's health agenda to meet hegemonic U.S. national interests and undercut bona fide internationalist efforts (Kickbusch 2002). While the national self-interest of leading countries has long shaped the international health field, the post–Cold War geopolitical realignment in the 1990s paved the way for a single "superpower"—the United States (together with key allies)—to dominate the international health agenda.

The idea of global health is inevitably tied to arguments around globalization—the growing political, social, and cultural relations among individuals, communities, and countries that occur as business interests, people, goods, ideas, and values travel around the globe—and economic (or neoliberal) globalization, the increasing connectedness of the world economy via the removal of barriers to trade and capital flows. Not only are money and goods globalized, but so are people—as migrants, immigrants, or transnationals moving back and forth between countries—and health problems (and their underlying determinants) (Sreenivasan and Benatar 2006). The health dimensions of globalization are also typically linked to the opening of new disease reservoirs; global travel, migration, and ineffective border control; the problems of wars, refugees, and social disruption; and the dangers of bioterrorism and biological warfare. In terms of global health governance, the following issues and players are deemed central: international agreements and protocols; international agencies and nongovernmental organizations (NGOs); human rights issues (e.g., privacy, the right to health, discrimination); and international trade and development of pharmaceuticals (including matters of patents).

While worldwide exchange and interdependence have always accompanied trade, today's globalization is exceptional due to the unprecedented integration of markets, unfettered financial transactions, the concomitant spread of neoliberal ideology (favoring privatization, free trade, deregulation, and a shrinking of the public sector), the increased role of transnational corporations in global commerce, and the role of international financial institutions in social policy making.

According to some analysts, the globalization of public health is a promising development, allowing for diffusion of technologies, ideas, and values, with enlightened self-interest and altruism converging as all nations cooperate in areas of public health surveillance, research, and intersectoral action (Yach and Bettcher 1998b). Others, however, believe that the World Bank, International Monetary Fund (IMF), and World Trade Organization—together with corporate interests writ large—exert enormous and excessive influence over global and domestic social and economic policy making, with international health policy, in turn, dominated by a market-led paradigm that fosters privatization and overlooks the underlying determinants of disease (Navarro 1998; Pappas, Hyder, and Akhter 2003; Koivusalo 2006). Even its proponents recognize that a more globalized public health is unable to fend off all of the deleterious effects of diminished social safety nets, unequal economic prosperity, and the environmental, work-related, and social problems of unfettered economic growth (see Chapter 9 for details) (Yach and Bettcher 1998a).

Notwithstanding the invoked distinctions, there is considerable conflation between international health and global health, and the "new" definition of global health bears many similarities to early 20th century understandings of international health. This textbook will use the nomenclature international health and global health according to general usage in the sources cited, but we favor the term international health because we believe that the notion of global health is not substantively different from the predecessor term international health as it has been used for more than a century. Moreover, we hold that public health practitioners, scholars, and activists may take on a critical perspective while maintaining affiliation with more traditional public health fields and institutions.

We also refrain from employing the term "international public health," defined as "the application of the principles of public health to health problems and challenges that affect low- and middle-income countries and to the complex array of global and local forces that affect them" (Merson, Black, and Mills 2006, p. xix), because of its inaccurate generalizations concerning nonindustrialized countries and their "inadequate health systems" (ibid). Indeed, we argue that international health by definition encompasses all countries and the intertwined political and economic forces that create poor or favorable health conditions wherever they occur. We recognize as well that all countries, institutions, researchers, and practitioners can learn from others as well as share their own experiences and knowledge, regardless of levels of development or political, social, and economic trajectory.

What, Then, Is International Health?

On one level, the international health field is built upon the health-related agreements to which most countries are signatories, whether they call for international notification of disease outbreaks and routine vital statistics, the protection of the rights of children, or access to needed medicines. The ethical, human rights, and legal dimensions of these agreements provide a framework of state obligations, cooperation, and shared global governance in the name of improving international health (Buchanan and DeCamp 2006; Nixon and Forman 2008).

On another level, international health is characterized by the activities that are carried out by international, bilateral, multilateral, regional, and transnational health organizations. Many of these agencies have been active in promoting health as a development issue since World War II and earlier. These efforts and agencies often regard international health as a global public good upon which all people depend. As we shall see in Chapter 3, there are many other entities—small and large, well financed and those supported only through volunteer labor, supranational institutions and social movements—whose work affects health at local and global levels. Certainly, the present proliferation of transnational health actors, such as NGOs, has drawn renewed attention to international health.

Simultaneously, there are countless people—mothers; activists struggling for access to water, food, and housing; local primary health care workers; conscientious leaders; and so on—who contribute every day to addressing international health problems. Yet these key players remain little recognized as they are typically not considered part of the international health response; international health "experts" have a lot to learn from people whose advice they rarely seek.

On yet another level, international health deals with the worldwide dimensions of the new appearance, ongoing spread, and recrudescence of diseases, together with their causes and consequences. These include sensationalized potential or actual "pandemics," such as avian influenza; burgeoning rates of diabetes related to food production and marketing; stress-related mortality in factories where exploitation and the absence of worker protections feed on one another; and a range of preventable ailments that are nonetheless decimating populations, including HIV/AIDS, many cancers, and malaria.

International health is also a topic of importance to various other fields including international development, political science, international relations, economics, and social work, in part because health serves as an indicator of how well societies are faring.

A further, central facet of international health deals with organizing a humanitarian response to disasters and emergencies, especially those involving large numbers of people whose lives are disrupted by ecological, economic, or military calamity.

Security concerns around potential bioterrorist threats as well as the social and political threats posed by health crises—often accompanied by lurid media coverage—have helped drive international health upwards on the foreign policy agenda of various countries. The other face of this geopolitical interest in international health has to do with protection of the contemporary world economic order: market capitalism. In this sense, international health efforts are concerned with disease outbreaks that could interrupt commerce, manufacturing, tourism, and other sectors—representing the interests of powerful economic actors. They may also be focused on maintaining the health of military personnel, the productivity of workers in multinational enterprises, and protecting the health of expatriate populations and travelers.

At the same time, as we shall see, international health has also become big business, whether in terms of private markets for health insurance and pharmaceutical sales or subcontractors for health and development initiatives. The emergence of public–private partnerships in health is thus a double-edged sword—on one hand furnishing needed funding to the field, on the other hand subjecting public matters and resources to private interests or even profiteering.

Another strain of international health views health systems financing and organization and health economics as central priorities of the field. Spearheaded by the World Bank, this perspective regards health needs primarily as deriving from health systems (with health-financing policies the main motor of activities), and health's importance stemming from its effects on poverty and the economy as a whole (see Chapters 4 and 11). A variant on this approach has to do with the indirect role of international agencies, treaties, loans, and experts in international health. For example, IMF loan conditionalities have pervasively required cuts in social sector spending: austerity measures on most African countries restrict the number of health care workers who can be hired and limit the amount of public funds that can be spent on schools, all with enormous implications for health. Some health donors, such as the United States, proscribe payment to local health workers (Pillay and Mahlati 2008). Here we note that although the World Bank and other leading financiers of international health activities operate under the assumption that health is a function of health care (systems), this textbook argues, based on a vast body of evidence, that health is shaped by a range of political, economic, and other societal factors, of which the provision of health care is but one element.

International health is also often understood in terms of the diffusion of ideas, practices, and technologies, principally from developed to developing countries. This understanding includes missionary, charitable, philanthropic, or development work that ranges from infrastructure-building to disease campaigns, programs focused on household and health behavior, nanotechnology, and the distribution of bed nets to prevent malaria, among a myriad of other approaches. Some of these activities follow a welfare assistance or donation model; numerous others employ incentives, providing only partial funding and thus requiring local governments to contribute considerable financial, human, and physical resources to international health endeavors. Most projects make use of transnational personnel, that is, country nationals who have been trained overseas or foreigners, typically from donor countries, working in "recipient country" settings. Many of these efforts presuppose that the health problems of developing countries stem from lack of resources, knowledge, and particular tools (as well as unhealthy behaviors) and that it is the role of international health agencies to decide which of these to purvey and how.

The social justice perspective on international health, by contrast, sees cooperation around health issues as a collective concern of people "on the ground" and their *representative* organizations, movements, and elected officials. What makes health *international* resides in the shared problems and aspirations of ordinary peoples and efforts, supported by like-minded movements in other settings and those transnational NGOs that respond to priorities and modalities defined locally. From a theoretical perspective, the social justice approach to international health draws from the field of political economy (see ahead) whereby the distribution of power and resources—social, economic, political, scientific—are key to understanding and addressing the challenges of international health. Human well-being, health, and dignity derive, accordingly, from just and equitable societies; the political struggle for universal social rights and protections is thus central to human progress. The social justice model counters neoliberal ideology, which holds that the competitive pursuit of profits under free-market capitalism, locally and globally, is the motor of human advancement. These ideas, movements, and efforts will be discussed throughout the book.

Box 1–1 Ways of Conceptualizing International Health

- Humanitarian/human rights/ethical imperative
- Global public good
- Security
  ◦ Fear of pandemics and "exotic/deadly" diseases
  ◦ Social unrest
  ◦ Bioterrorism
- Protect and preserve markets/capitalism
- International agreements
- Disease control and research
- Business interests: pharmaceutical companies/insurance markets
- Economic development/technology diffusion
- Foreign policy issue
- Social justice

Readers may be wondering about the significance of the graphics on the front cover of the textbook. The frames of slums, microbes, and people holding hands in solidarity may be interpreted quite literally in terms of their relevance to international health. But the main image of a small Brazilian fishing craft bobbing on choppy waters beneath an overcast sky requires further elaboration. Some may see it as portending the uncertain future of international health, with its bareness suggesting the bankruptcy of the field. Others may see this picture of a boat named *Saúde Global* ("global health" in Portuguese) more optimistically, with bright colors enveloping an empty vessel open to a world of possibilities. Regardless of one's a priori perspective, we are about to embark on an international health voyage, one that may take us to unexpected places and that will undoubtedly, like all journeys, leave us challenged and changed.

ONGOING CHALLENGES AND DILEMMAS IN INTERNATIONAL HEALTH

There will be a series of questions interspersed throughout the textbook. Readers will be able to respond to some of these based on the material presented; others are meant to stimulate additional contemplation and study. Those posed here are meant in this latter spirit: there are no right answers, but the questions should leave you hungry for further reading.

Who bears responsibility for preserving and protecting health within and across countries? How should these entities be held accountable?

Who should set health priorities?

What should be the role of international entities in shaping domestic and local policies concerning health and well-being?

How are dominant economic policies (today or in the past) related to the international health agenda?

Should international health efforts be universal or targeted?

Do economic stability and/or growth need to precede public health development?

What is the relationship between the distribution of power and resources—within and between countries—and patterns of morbidity and mortality?

Why are health indicators deteriorating in some regions/countries of the world whereas others have made great strides in reducing mortality and disease in recent years?

How important is population control as compared to other health needs?

What is the contribution of trained clinicians to improving health? What other skills are needed in addressing international health problems?

Can a balanced mixture of modern biomedical science and traditional medicine be achieved?

What constitutes success in international health?

OVERVIEW OF THE TEXTBOOK

This textbook is designed for a semester-long advanced undergraduate or first-year graduate course. The chapters are meant to flow logically from week to week, but ample cross-referencing allows for material to be presented in a different order or for students to read ahead. This third edition of the *Textbook of International Health*, unlike its predecessors, is written by a trio of authors. As a South–North/East–West/underdeveloped–developed/local–transnational/female–male/academic–practitioner/government–NGO affiliated crew, we have been fortunate to draw from the erudition and vast knowledge base of the late Paul Basch and his first two editions of the text. At the same time, we have reshaped much of the text based on our own research, practical experience, and theoretical understanding in the arenas of policy making, epidemiology, politics, international cooperation, and historical analysis at local, national, and international levels.

Political Economy Framework

Because dominant approaches to addressing public health problems based on disease-control campaigns and the diffusion of medicalized technologies have failed in much of the world—with public health problems and indicators having worsened in many regions in spite of concerted international health efforts—we have written this book from a contrasting perspective. The international public health community has laid out lofty goals: we need to critically and collectively (i.e., among professionals, agencies, *and* local health workers and community members) analyze what we are doing well and what we are doing poorly and recognize the urgency in tackling the underlying determinants of premature death and ill health.

For this reason we have chosen to write the *Textbook of International Health* from a political economy approach (see Chapter 4 for further explanation) which analyzes health in the context of the political, economic, and social structures of societies, that is, who owns what, who controls whom, and how these factors are shaped by and reflect the social and institutional fabric (i.e., class, racial/ethnic/gender structure, existence of a welfare state, etc.). A political economy perspective views health not solely in terms of access to health services and technologies or whether people have healthy behaviors or safe neighborhoods, but also in terms of the nature of power relations and control over resources, their implications for social inequalities, and the institutions that challenge or reinforce the distribution of power and resources at local, national, and international levels (Navarro 2002). Individual and medical factors are thus understood as part of larger societal forces that influence health and well-being.

The political economy framework separates this textbook from the dominant approaches to understanding international health described above. Not only will the nuts and bolts of international health be presented, but the textbook will also analyze and explain each topic—from health data to research and development, disease patterns, and cooperative efforts—through a critical, political economy lens which fundamentally alters the way these issues are understood.

Other international health textbooks mention the role of social and political factors but they typically remain unintegrated with the main approach; here we will make links among factors that are often considered separately and ask tough questions that do not necessarily yield straightforward or rapid solutions. Not only, then, do we intend for the *Textbook of International Health* to provide students with a comprehensive understanding of the different aspects of international health; more importantly, we offer a framework for critically analyzing international health issues, one that we hope you can take with you and apply throughout your careers.

This *Textbook of International Health* has four main aims:

1. to convey an understanding of international health in terms of the interaction of global, national, regional, and local forces, processes, and conditions;
2. to provide grounding in the epidemiologic, economic, political, ethical, historical, environmental, and social underpinnings of health and disease patterns within and among countries and populations;
3. to show the consequences of these patterns at global, societal, and community levels; and
4. to present a range of international, national, and local approaches to improving health and effecting change, based on scientific and social knowledge and experience, health systems development, social and political movements, and public policy making.

In sum, we view international health in an integrative manner, focusing on the interrelationships among local, regional, national, and international factors that influence health and on the development of effective interventions, institutions, and policies that will address these factors.

Throughout this text, we speak of "industrialized" (or developed or rich) countries and "developing" (or underdeveloped or poor) countries as if these were real, and mutually exclusive, categories. As we will discuss in Chapter 4 and elsewhere, levels of national well-being and social and economic development cannot be measured solely by per capita gross national product (GNP): various countries with high per capita GNPs have not undergone balanced social and economic growth, whereas certain countries with low per capita GNPs are extremely well-developed socially. This is because accumulated wealth may not be well distributed and does not necessarily lead to social investment in the well-being of the population. At the same time, poorer countries may use considerably less wealth in ways that enhance population health and welfare by more equitably distributing resources.

Outline of Chapters

The first section of the textbook (Chapters 2–7) provides the basic tools for understanding international health. Chapter 2 explores the historical antecedents of international health, analyzing the forces and developments that shaped international health patterns in the past, some of which continue to influence the field's ideas, institutions, and practices. Chapter 3 profiles the range of agencies, actors, and activities that have characterized and affected international health from World War II to the present, critically examining the role, motivations, and impact of international health aid and of the most important international health players, including international financial institutions, bilateral agencies, foundations, and social movements. Chapter 4 presents the book's political economy of health and development framework, providing a theoretical and practical basis for understanding and addressing the challenges of international health and drawing from the arena of health and human rights as a stimulus for action. Chapter 5 outlines how mortality and morbidity are measured and statistics produced, how and why health data are or are not collected, and what the gaps in information are that must be filled in order to address international health problems adequately. Chapter 6 provides an overview epidemiologic profile of health and disease patterns across the world, contesting traditional dichotomies of infectious and chronic diseases to explore the causes of premature death and disability under conditions of marginalization, modernization, and the combined effects of marginalization and modernization. Chapter 7 focuses on the societal determinants of health, premature death, and disability/disease—at household, community, national, and global levels—*and* how they intertwine with, and are underscored by, social inequalities in health, both within and across societies.

The next section of the textbook (Chapters 8–12) analyzes international health and its ongoing challenges from a series of key lenses—the priority areas and building blocks for understanding and improving international health efforts. In Chapter 8 we examine the issue of health under crisis conditions: ecological disasters, humanitarian emergencies, and war and militarization. Chapter 9 explores the impact of neoliberal globalization on health, particularly in underdeveloped countries, and the effect of work and working conditions on health. Chapter 10 reviews health concerns arising from the natural and built environments and their effects on air, water, and places, as well as the economic and social determinants of these problems, and a range of current and potential solutions to them. Chapter 11 covers health economics, health financing, and the economics of health, explaining, analyzing, and critiquing the main tools of these fields. Chapter 12 offers a comparative analysis of a range of health systems and health reforms, and lays out the elements and policies that make for effective health systems.

The final section of the book (Chapters 13 and 14) turns to the making of healthy policies across the world—and the roles and responsibilities of those working in the field locally, internationally, and transnationally. Chapter 13 provides a set of examples of countries and cities that have effectively improved health, sometimes under trying circumstances. These efforts are contrasted with the disease-control approaches that still characterize mainstream international health. Chapter 14 focuses on the practice of international health: how to foster bona fide cooperation, how to understand, navigate, contribute to, and ethically engage in the field, and possible alternatives to mainstream approaches to international health. The brevity of this final section of the book should be taken as a sign of its importance—or rather *your* importance collectively—as leaders, specialists, and activists in shaping international health into the future. In that sense, the subsequent chapters of the *Textbook of International Health* remain to be written, based on the aspirations and contributions of coming generations.

NOTE

1. For example, in 1998, the National Council of International Health, based in Washington, DC, changed its name to the Global Health Council.

REFERENCES

Almeida Filho N and Paim JS. 1999. La crisis de la salud pública y el movimiento de la salud colectiva en Latinoamérica. *Cuadernos Médicos Sociales* 75:5–30.

Bashford A, Editor. 2006. *Medicine at the Border: Disease, Globalization, and Security, 1850 to the Present*. Basingstoke and New York: Palgrave Macmillan.

Birn A-E. 2006. Introduction: Canada, Latin America, and international health. *Canadian Journal of Public Health* 97(6):I-1.

Buchanan A and DeCamp M. 2006. Responsibility for global health. *Theoretical Medicine* 27(1):95–114.

Holtz TH, Holmes SM, Stonington S, and Eisenberg L. 2006. Health is still social: Contemporary examples in the age of the genome. *PLoS Medicine* 3(10): e419–e422.

Institute of Medicine. 1997. *America's Vital Interest in Global Health: Protecting Our People, Enhancing Our Economy, and Advancing Our International Interests.* Washington, DC: National Academies Press.

Kickbusch I. 2002. Influence and opportunity: Reflections on the US role in global public health. *Health Affairs* 21(6):131–141.

Koivusalo M. 2006. The impact of economic globalisation on health. *Theoretical Medicine and Bioethics* 27(1):13–34.

Krieger N and Birn A-E. 1998. A vision of social justice as the foundation of public health: Commemorating 150 years of the Spirit of 1848. *American Journal of Public Health* 88(11):1603–1606.

Lantz PM, Lichtenstein RL, and Pollack HA. 2007. Health policy approaches to population health: The limits of medicalization. *Health Affairs* 26(5):1253–1257.

Lexchin J. 2007. The secret things belong unto the Lord our God: Secrecy in the pharmaceutical arena. *Medicine and Law* 26(3):417–430.

Merson MH, Black RE, and Mills AJ. 2006. Introduction. In Merson MH, Black RE, and Mills AJ, Editors. *International Public Health: Diseases, Programs, Systems and Policies, Second Edition.* Sudbury, MA: Jones and Bartlett Publishers.

Navarro V. 1998. Whose globalization? *American Journal of Public Health* 88:742–743.

———, Editor. 2002. *The Political Economy of Social Inequalities: Consequences for Health and Quality of Life.* Amityville, NY: Baywood Publishing Company.

Nixon S and Forman L. 2008. Exploring synergies between human rights and public health ethics: A whole greater than the sum of its parts. *BMC International Health and Human Rights* 8(2):1–9.

Nunes ED. 1996. Saúde coletiva: Revisitando a sua história e os cursos de pós-graduação. *Ciência & Saúde Coletiva* 1(1):55–69.

Pappas G, Hyder AA, and Akhter M. 2003. Globalization: Toward a new framework for public health. *Social Theory and Health* 1(2):91–107.

Pillay Y and Mahlati P. 2008. Health-worker salaries and incomes in sub-Saharan Africa—Comment. *The Lancet* 371:632–634.

Preamble to the Constitution of the World Health Organization as adopted by the International Health Conference, New York, June 19–July 22, 1946; signed on July 22 1946 by the representatives of 61 States (Official Records of the World Health Organization, no. 2, p. 100) and entered into force on April 7, 1948.

Public Health Agency of Canada. 2004. What is the population health approach? http://www.phac-aspc.gc.ca/ph-sp/approach-approche/appr-eng.php. Accessed March 17, 2008.

Puliyel JM and Madhavi Y. 2008. Vaccines: Policy for public good or private profit? *Indian Journal of Medical Research* 127(1):1–3.

Sreenivasan G and Benatar SR. 2006. Challenges for global health in the 21st century: Some upstream considerations. *Theoretical Medicine and Bioethics* 27(1):3–11.

WHO Commission on Social Determinants of Health. 2008. *Closing the Gap in a Generation: Health Equity through Action on the Social Determinants of Health.* Final report of the Commission on Social Determinants of Health. Geneva: WHO.

Winslow C-EA. 1920. The untilled fields of public health. *Science* 51:23–33.

Yach D and Bettcher D. 1998a. The globalization of public health, I: Threats and opportunities. *American Journal of Public Health* 88(5):735–738.

———. 1998b. The globalization of public health, II: The convergence of self-interest and altruism. *American Journal of Public Health* 88(5):738–741.

2

The Historical Origins of Modern International Health

Key Questions:

- When and why did governments, wealthy interests, and the public become concerned with the spread of disease across borders and territories?
- How were these concerns addressed?
- What motivated the rise of international health agencies, and what influenced their development?

Now that you have a sense of what constitutes the international health field and what are its principal goals and dilemmas, it is worth pausing to ask how concern with international health arose historically. Central issues include the following: what part was played by international (as opposed to local or national) factors in shaping patterns and perceptions of sickness and disease; how did these factors interact with the social experience of ill health; and how did the larger economic and political context affect the emergence, spread, consequences, and fight against (mostly) epidemic diseases.

This chapter explores the main antecedents of modern international health, beginning with the 300-year-long waves of Eurasian plague. Next we examine the rise of imperialism and the slave trade and their health consequences. We then turn to the Industrial Revolution of the 19th century, the rise of the sanitary reform movement, and their implications for international health. We will also touch upon the so-called demographic and epidemiologic transitions and the constellation of factors that have led to the worldwide decline in mortality and increase in life expectancy over the past century. The final section of the chapter traces the appearance and development of a new set of international health institutions—both inter-governmental and nongovernmental—from the mid-19th to the mid-20th centuries.

In Chapter 3 we will examine the institutional development of international health from World War II (1939–1945) to the present.

Given that there are so many pressing health needs today, it may seem unexpected to find an entire chapter of this textbook dedicated to the early history of international health. Nonetheless, as we will see, contemporary patterns, priorities, and practices of international health have been shaped by past experience, making this historical introduction an essential tool in understanding the field's challenges, pitfalls, and prospects.

ANTECEDENTS OF MODERN INTERNATIONAL HEALTH: BLACK DEATH, COLONIAL CONQUEST, AND THE ATLANTIC SLAVE TRADE

Although the modern system of international health—involving disease surveillance, sanitary regulation, international organizations, information exchange, and cross-border activities—did not emerge until the 19th century, some of its features were present long before. Preoccupation with public health started several thousand years ago in ancient Chinese, Egyptian, Persian, Hindu, Greco-Roman, Ethiopian, Moorish, Mesoamerican (Maya, Aztec, Toltec), and other civilizations. All of these societies developed means of communication, theories of disease causation, and specific tools to address health problems. Each had sophisticated engineering capacity (as evidenced in the palaces, pyramids, and temples they left behind) and often developed elaborate systems of water supply (e.g., Artesian wells and aqueducts), irrigation, garbage disposal, and drainage. Observational and empirical skills enabled the development of botanical remedies and surgical techniques, oftentimes disbursed in combination with supernatural practices. This knowledge mostly remained within particular societies but was also passed from one to another through war, conquest, trade, and exploration. Until the Middle Ages, however, health concerns and disease outbreaks rarely extended beyond limited regions, except in the case of military incursions (e.g., as per Thucydides's account of plague during the Peloponnesian war in 5th century BCE), and the occasional ailing trader.

Plague and the Beginnings of Health Regulation

For the most part, scientific ideas, technologies, and practices in medieval Europe trailed those of other societies, particularly the Islamic world. European healing involved a combination of local wisdom—knowledge of medicinal herbs passed down from generation to generation and among popular practitioners, especially midwives who apprenticed with other wise women—and a budding hierarchy of town-based practitioners, including apothecaries, barber-surgeons, and, later in the Middle Ages, university-trained physicians.

But changes were afoot that would test Europe's sanitary backwardness. As rival leaders fought for power, and merchants became interested in the riches and resources of far away places, travel and commerce gradually increased. The congested towns of late medieval Europe had far lower standards of water supply, sanitation, and hygiene than ancient civilizations. As such, they were excellent candidates for outbreaks of epidemic disease.

It may be said that the Middle Ages were bracketed by two great outbreaks of plague. The first pandemic, also known as the Plague of Justinian, struck in 542 CE and decimated populations from Asia to Ireland. The second was the great Black Death of the 14th century, the most destructive epidemic in the history of mankind. Mortality from AIDS (in total numbers and proportionally) pales by comparison.

Starting from wild rodents in the plains of Central Asia, the plague reached the Black Sea in 1346, and by 1348 it had spread eastward to the British Isles and westward to China, northward to Russia, and southward to India. The entire social, economic, political, and ecclesiastical structure of Europe was shaken to its foundations. Europe alone lost more than 25 million people, and throughout the Eastern Mediterranean, India, and China, tens of millions more died, causing similar devastation. Contemporaries had little conception of the origins of the disease, ascribing it to a conjunction of the planets or to a variety of cosmic, meteorological, and divine causes. Many doctors fled the cities, and aristocrats and wealthy merchants took refuge in their country estates. Scapegoats were sought, and many blamed Jews, who suffered greatly as a result. All told, perhaps one-third of the population perished.

Although its cause was unknown, plague's suspected spread through human contact led to the earliest attempts at international disease control. In the belief that plague was introduced by ships, the city-state of Venice in 1348 adopted a 40-day detention period for entering vessels (soon copied by Genoa, Marseille, and other major ports) after which the disease was believed to remit. This practice of *quarantine*—from the Italian word for forty—was minimally effective in stopping plague. Quarantine's stricter counterpart, the *cordon sanitaire*—a protective belt barring entry of people or goods to cities or entire regions—would also be used frequently in succeeding centuries. Venice established the first *lazaretto* in 1403, a quarantine station to hold and disinfect humans and cargo. Its island location was emulated by other cities.

Because the Black Death's initial appearance preceded the formation of nation-states, sanitary efforts were adopted and implemented by municipal authorities, one at a time, rather than by (nonexistent) national governments. Thus, although the disease traveled from place to place, it was dealt with locally, in terms of measures to dispose of and fumigate the bodies and belongings of the dead, as well as through the use of quarantine. Quarantine was imposed on ships and persons suspected of disease, thus protecting those within city limits (walls). While word of disease spread through rumor and travelers, there was no official system of notification or cooperation between city-states. Following the first plague pandemic, many cities established plague boards, or even permanent public health boards, charged with imposing the necessary measures at times of outbreak. Ironically, this precursor to international health authority was local and unilateral rather than cooperative and international.

The appearance of disease was understood by some in cosmological terms, or considered the wrath of God in punishment for sin. Others believed that plague derived from a mix of foul air (*mal'aria*) and personal shortcomings (explaining why not everyone got sick). Still others held that it was transmitted from person to person. In 1546, the Veronese physician-scholar Girolamo Fracastoro revived ancient notions of contagion in his tract on plague transmission, theorizing that "seeds of disease" could be spread either through direct contact or by disseminating into the atmosphere. Fracastoro's theory, reconciling person-to-person transmission with the concept of bad air, also served to justify harsh quarantine measures.

It was during the Middle Ages that hospitals became established in Europe. Stimulated in part by ideas of contagion, these institutions were at the time the only places that specialized in the care of the sick. Religious orders dedicated to healing were created in this period, partly to meet the needs of returning crusaders. Some institutions, such as St. Bartholemew's (St. Bart's) in London, founded in 1123, still function today. From about the 13th century on, secular hospitals were also founded in many municipalities.

While the virulence of plague lessened somewhat in the late 14th and 15th centuries, subsequent visitations of the Black Death worsened. In 1630–1631 plague killed one quarter of the population in Bologna, one-third in Venice, almost half in Milan, and almost two-thirds in Verona. A scant generation later, half of the inhabitants of Rome, Naples, and Genoa succumbed to the plague of 1656–1657. Such was the plague's grip on both imagination and collective experience that Daniel Defoe's fictional first-person account of London's great (and last, as it turned out) plague of 1665 (which he experienced only as a small child) was received as a definitive eyewitness account of the shared dread of a dozen generations. Defoe recounted the experience of the well-off, who escaped the plague far more often than the poor in this way:

[T]he richer sort of people, especially the nobility and gentry from the west part of the city, thronged out of town with their families and servants in an unusual manner... [on] the Broad Street where I lived; indeed, nothing was to be seen but waggons [sic] and carts, with goods, women, servants, children, and coaches filled with people of the better sort and horsemen attending them, and all hurrying away (Defoe 1722).

Plague, of course, was not the only deadly epidemic ailment of the Middle Ages and early modern period. Smallpox, diphtheria, measles, influenza, tuberculosis, scabies, erysipelas, anthrax, and trachoma were also rife (Rosen 1958). Mass hysteria in a climate of superstition led to outbreaks of dancing mania (St. Vitus' Dance). Ergotism, arising from fungal contamination of rye, killed or crippled large numbers of people in dozens of epidemics between the 9th and 15th centuries. It is possible that leprosy, present in Europe for centuries, became epidemic in the 13th and 14th centuries. After the Black Death, which killed many people who were confined in leprosaria, the disease was never again important in Europe.

Despite strict sanitary enforcement during plague years, concepts of cleanliness and sanitation took hold slowly in Europe's cities. Through increasingly forceful legislation and public awareness, marshaled by the printing press and town criers, urban centers began to approach the hygienic standards reached by the Roman Empire more than a millennium earlier. Although plague boards disbanded in the 17th century, many towns took over control of street cleaning, disposal of dead bodies and carcasses, public baths, and water maintenance. By the 18th century cities began to employ, fitfully, a new environmental engineering approach to epidemic disease, which emphasized preventive actions including improved ventilation, drainage of stagnant water, street cleaning, reinterment, cleaner wells, fumigation, and the burial of garbage (Riley 1987).

Even before the plague fully retreated, a new economic system began to develop that would irrevocably shape worldwide patterns of disease and eventually lead to international health measures and institutions.

The Rise of European Imperialism

During the Middle Ages, classical scientific and medical knowledge was retained by Islamic scholars, who established learned settlements in Spain, Portugal, Sicily, and throughout the Middle East and North Africa. Contacts with the Muslim world opened new vistas to European eyes. Commodities of high value, mostly from the East, were in great demand, but the traditional routes of passage for such goods went through the Mediterranean and the Italian city-states. Partly as a continuation of the Christian–Muslim rivalry, partly for riches and adventure, and aided by technical improvements in navigation and seamanship, western Europeans of the early 15th century embarked on a series of conquests by sea. The Iberian countries were early entrants, and Portugal, by virtue of its maritime traditions, large fleet, and well-established coastal trade, was first.

Beginning in 1415, the Portuguese attacked Muslim settlements in nearby North Africa, and instead of plundering and retreating, they established permanent garrisons. In some ways the early 15th century voyages may be considered extensions of the Crusades. The influence of Islam had expanded rapidly during the preceding centuries (to the Balkans, western Asia, Egypt, East Africa, India, and what is now Indonesia); spreading Christianity was a powerful stimulus to the conquistadores of Portugal and Spain. Royal power and material and territorial greed went hand in hand with proselytizing aims, brutally carried out under the Spanish Inquisition starting in 1478. The long struggle to push out the Moorish Kingdom of Granada was finally accomplished in 1492 under united Spain's Catholic monarchs, Ferdinand and Isabela, the same year their sponsored voyage of Columbus arrived in the Caribbean. The excitement generated by discoveries of islands—not to mention gold, minerals, and precious objects—in the western Atlantic, thought to be a gateway to China, can only be imagined.

The Portuguese arrived in India in 1498 and loaded the first of many cargoes of spices for the return voyage to Lisbon, challenging Italy for this trade. The English and Dutch in the 17th century challenged Iberian dominance and extended European influence to the farthest reaches of the world through the establishment of colonies under European political control. The colonial era lasted to the 1960s, with few colonies remaining beyond the 1970s.

Dire health consequences accompanied every phase and every locale of imperial expansion centuries before industrialization's urban misery put public health on domestic political agendas. The Spanish invasion and colonization of what is now Latin America and the Caribbean had a devastating demographic impact on indigenous populations. The Spanish Bishop Bartolomé de las Casas reported that the indigenous population of the Antilles when Columbus arrived in 1492 was 3,770,000; by 1518 only 15,600 had escaped slavery, disease, and death (Guerra 1993). Although such precise numbers are undoubtedly inaccurate, similar scenarios were then in progress, or were soon to occur, in other parts of the western hemisphere. Most infamously, smallpox is believed to have been spread throughout Mesoamerica through distribution of infested blankets by the forces of Spanish conquistador Hernán Cortés, though mortality from forced labor was likely higher. All told, between one-third and one-half of indigenous inhabitants were killed in the late 15th and early 16th centuries by the military, economic, and social aspects of the conquest (Berlinguer 1992; Crosby 1993; McCaa 1995; Cook 1998).

While pre-Columbian societies in Mesoamerica experienced high death rates from violence, occasional famine, and infectious diseases (Alchon 1997, 2003), the conquest stood out because of the magnitude of death as well as the enormous mortality differential between invaders and invaded. Spanish invaders used this differential to military and cultural advantage, trumpeting the presumed constitutional superiority of the invaders (now understood to have been immune due to previous exposure to microorganisms). In subsequent centuries, corresponding devastation was wrought by British, French, Belgian, and other European invasions and occupations across North America, Africa, Asia, and the Pacific.

Medical practitioners joined these colonial ventures, initially hired by conquistadores to protect military forces. As region after region came under European control, physicians began to be integrated into colonial authority structures, treating colonists, setting rules for medical practice, and, sometimes in competition with the viceroy and Church, implementing emergency measures during epidemics (Lanning 1985; Hernández Sáenz 1997).

Given the paucity of therapeutic measures in the European medical armamentarium, the Spaniards were eager to learn from indigenous healing knowledge and the local pharmacopeia and began to sponsor catalogs of this knowledge. The earliest and most important of these was the *Codex Badianus* of 1552, an illustrated compendium of hundreds of medicinal herbs. Written in Nahuatl by Martín de la Cruz and translated into Latin by Juan Badiano (both Aztec men who had been trained in a Franciscan academy in Mexico City), it was produced for the Spanish emperor.

The colonial Spanish and Portuguese administrations supported the founding of medical faculties in leading colonial cities, such as Lima (Peru) and Salvador da Bahia (Brazil), greatly abetted by the Catholic Church, and built hundreds of hospitals across the continent, segregating care for colonists and native populations. A new hierarchy of medical practitioners was established, with titled physicians serving urban elites, Catholic hospitals providing charity care, and traditional healers and midwives—who melded indigenous and European-Galenic beliefs and practices—attending the majority of the population (Foster 1987). Religious missionaries—first Catholic, later, especially in Africa and Asia, joined by Protestant denominations—played a large role in building and running leprosaria and hospitals, intertwining medical and religious proselytization (Worboys 2001).

By the late renaissance, the diminishing authority of the Church in Europe and increasing imperial needs led to greater patronage for science, generating new military, transport, and agricultural technologies. There were also important developments in chemistry, astronomy, physics, botany, and medicine, some of which renewed ideas and technologies that were thousands of years old. Such was the case of smallpox prevention, long practiced by Chinese and Ayurvedic healers who observed that previous contact with smallpox conferred protection. Inoculation—prepared by grinding up smallpox pustules and administering the powdered material in a wad of cotton fibers placed inside the nose—was effective but caused substantial mortality. When English surgeon Edward Jenner—observing milkmaids (circa 1796)—found that vaccination with cowpox (generally not deadly to humans) could prevent smallpox in humans, he helped transform smallpox prevention into a far safer endeavor. In 1803 Charles IV, the Bourbon king of Spain, having lost a child to smallpox, sponsored an extraordinary expedition throughout the Spanish Empire in the Americas and the Philippines. The small Balmis-Salvany group left Spain in late 1803, arrived in Puerto Rico in 1804, and then traveled on to what are today Venezuela, Panama, Colombia, Ecuador, Peru, Chile, and Bolivia, delivering smallpox vaccine throughout these territories on foot, horseback, and along waterways. Because there was no means of preserving the vaccine, it was administered live—arm to arm—preserved in the bodies of 21 Spanish orphans, with instructions for preparation passed along (Rigau-Pérez 2004). This first mass health campaign was a distant prelude to the World Health Organization's smallpox eradication campaign, conducted almost 300 years later (see Chapters 3 and 13).

Notwithstanding this expedition, throughout the colonial period and beyond, disease and death were rife among Mestizos, and especially indigenous and African-descended populations, owing to a variety of factors: conflict; slavery or indentured servitude; dangerous work in mines, building sites, and plantations; dispossession from land, cultural heritage, and livelihoods; crowded living conditions in towns; food shortages; trade and travel (with accompanying maladies); ecological alterations (canalization, railroads, exploitation of forests) facilitating mosquito breeding sites and malaria; and so on. To be sure, colonists also suffered widely from infectious and childhood disease, but occupational mortality and early death among Mestizo laborers, African slaves, and indigenous groups, coupled with staggeringly high infant mortality rates (Crosby 1972; Kiple 1989; Gaspar and Clark Hine 1996; Florentino and de Góes 1999), meant that these groups on average lived far shorter and sicklier lives than Iberian elites.

The exchange of specific diseases is a subject of continual review and argument. Diseases that accompanied the Europeans are believed to have been influenza, typhus, smallpox, measles, cholera, and yellow fever. Certain kinds of malaria parasites may have already been present in the Americas, but the deadly tertian (*falciparum*) malaria came from Africa via European ships. Other ailments, such as hookworm, may also have arrived in the Americas via the slave trade. The filarial worm *Wuchereria bancrofti*, a causative agent of elephantiasis, was endemic in the region of Charleston, South Carolina, from the 17th century until about 1920. This mosquito-transmitted human parasite was probably introduced from Barbados, which in turn received it from Africa (Savitt 1977). Many believe that syphilis was introduced to Europe by early Iberian explorers who acquired it in the New World.

Though imbalanced in magnitude, the fatal impact of conquest was to prove double-edged, with initial waves of European soldiers and settlers often felled by endemic diseases to which they had scant resistance. Nowhere was this truer than in West Africa, the "white man's grave" (Curtin 1989). The Portuguese had established slaving stations along the coast as early as the 15th century, but their small disease-ridden outposts did not last. Dysentery (then called bloody flux, among other names) and malaria were rampant. Many early European groups attempting to colonize Africa were decimated by disease (Curtin 1998). The Niger expedition of 1841 illustrates the extreme susceptibility of Europeans vis-à-vis Africans. One hundred and forty-five Europeans and 158 Africans participated in this mission along the Niger River to "civilize" Africans through Christianity (sponsored by the British government, under pressure from abolitionists, as an alternative to slavery). Forty-two Europeans, but not one African, died of malaria, with all but fifteen taken ill (Temperley 1991).

Similar events occurred in the New World. Of 10,000 French colonists who landed in Guiana in 1765, 8,000 were dead within a few months, and the colony failed to develop despite the fact that France sent more persons there than to Canada (Gourou 1980).

Still, the hope of obtaining riches outweighed the fear of sickness and death in the minds of many Europeans, especially those who profited from these exploits without leaving Europe. Gold from the Gold Coast, ivory from the Ivory Coast—to say nothing of palm oil and, above all, slaves—provided the stimulus for continued expeditions to the coasts of Africa by adventurers, soldiers, and mercenaries.

The Slave Trade

Labor was central to the imperial project—to extract profitable raw materials, minerals, and agricultural products. As discussed above, indigenous populations in many places were wiped out by conquest and disruption; others were found "unsuitable" for labor. At the same time the supply of voluntary migrants and European indentured servants and criminals was hard to control in vast territories and was not available in sufficient numbers to meet the greed of elites and the growing labor needs in the colonies. The British became adept at transferring forced laborers from one part of its Empire to another (explaining the large populations of Indian ancestry in places as distinct as Trinidad, Fiji, and South Africa). But this was not sufficient.

As the colonial system developed in the 16th century, a heinous and sordid industry arose—the capture, sale, transfer, and condemnation to slavery of millions of human beings. Slavery was not a new phenomenon, having been common in antiquity, but it was never before practiced on a worldwide scale. Whether racism arose out of slavery or slavery out of racism, the two were deeply intertwined (Jordan 1968). Europeans selected Africans to be slaves due to a combination of factors: a visible physiological characteristic—dark skin color—enabling control and vigilance over escapees; perception of Africans' easy physical adaptation to tropical climates (see ahead) where most agricultural labor was needed (on plantations growing coffee, cotton, rice, sugar, and tobacco); and dispersion of social groups and limited weaponry in much of Africa, which facilitated capture.

The Atlantic route between Africa and the Americas accounted for most of the slave trade. Between 1502 and 1870, an estimated 11.4 million Africans were captured, shipped, and forced to become slave laborers. Between 4 and 5 million were sent to each of Brazil and the Caribbean and another half a million each to the United States and to Spanish South America. Almost 12% to 15% of those captured died in the "middle passage" before reaching American shores (Curtin 1968).

The slave trade was a source of enormous profit for those who invested in it, purportedly including England's Queen Elizabeth I. By the middle of the 18th century, the city of Liverpool alone had 87 ships engaged in the transport of slaves from West Africa to the Caribbean and southern United States. English adventurer Lovett Cameron observed:

> a gang of fifty-two women tied together in three lots; some had children in their arms, others were far advanced in pregnancy, and all were laden. They were covered with weals and scars. To obtain these fifty-two women, at least ten villages had been destroyed, each with a population of one to two hundred, or about 1,500 in all…. In

chained gangs the unfortunate slaves are driven by the lash from the interior to the barracoons [slave barracks] on the beach; there the sea-air, insufficient diet and dread of their approaching fate, produce the most fatal diseases; dysentery and fever release them from their sufferings.... On a short march, of six hundred slaves...one hundred and twenty-five expired on the road. The mortality on these rapid marches is seldom less than twenty per cent (Scott 1939, pp. 988–989).

The slave trade continued for over three centuries. Even after the importation of slaves was banned by most countries in the early 19th century, the practice of slavery was not abolished in the United States until 1865 and in Brazil until 1888.

Slavery was a premature death knell for hundreds of millions of people. Such bondage entailed extremely long days of hard physical labor, poor nutrition, crowded and inadequate housing, harsh physical punishment, and extreme emotional hardship. Pregnant women and nursing mothers were not spared heavy field work. Slave life expectancy in the United States before the Civil War was 21 years, approximately half that of whites. This was largely due to astronomical rates of infant mortality—half of all babies born into slavery died before turning one year old, compared to one-fourth of non-slave infants. For those slaves who survived into adulthood, few lived past 50. Slaves in Brazil, the Caribbean, and elsewhere faced similar conditions (Postell 1951; Campbell 1984; Amantino 2007).

HEALTH, THE TROPICS, AND THE IMPERIAL SYSTEM

As long as profits were being made, imperial authorities paid little attention to the health of slaves. By the 1800s, however, many other health concerns surfaced, particularly ailments associated with the climates and habitats of many European colonies. It is important to understand "the tropics" as a conceptual, and not merely a physical, space nestled in the middle latitudes of the globe. A geographic distinction is sometimes made between the hot, humid tropics, the dry savannas, and the alpine zones. In the medical literature, it was mainly the hot, wet regions that were taken to represent the tropics in their most essential form. Calling a part of the globe "the tropics" became a way for imperial powers to define something culturally alien to, as well as environmentally distinct from, Europe and the other parts of the temperate world. The idea of the tropics was, in origin and essence, the perception and the experience of white men (and women) venturing into an unfamiliar world in which climate, vegetation, disease, and people all appeared to be different, and in which the familiar forms of temperate life were threatened, overturned, or inverted (Arnold 1997; Harrison 1999).

This "invention" of the tropics and of tropical medicine also shaped a series of racialized explanations regarding susceptibility to disease, suitability for work, and underdevelopment (Gorgas 1909; Arnold 1996; Harrison 1996; Peard 1999; Deacon

2000). Acclimatization arguments inevitably favored the colonizer—whether providing an argument for why so many Europeans perished in their initial encounters with hot climes despite supposed racial superiority; rationalizing the use of "brown labor" that could better tolerate hot, humid weather; or justifying the exploitation of regions and peoples deemed unable to escape their medico-geographic state of underdevelopment.

Notwithstanding tropical medicine's assumption that place shaped disease, many ailments labeled "tropical"—leprosy and malaria, for example—were previously endemic in temperate or cold regions. As of the 18th century, they were disappearing thanks to improvements in nutrition, housing, and sanitation, not due to any climatic change (though global warming may greatly extend mosquito habitats in the future—see Chapter 10). Yet even today, this inaccurate conception of tropical diseases as those only found in, highly prevalent in, or especially hard to control in tropical and subtropical regions retains its salience in medical quarters. Past and present, tropical medicine's definition (Warren 1990) leaves out the interaction of political and economic factors (production, organization of labor, class relations, political context) with ecological conditions.

Whether or not diseases were tropical in nature or provenance, the "Columbian exchange" between Europe and the lands it invaded (in tropical, semi-tropical, and temperate latitudes) resulted in circulation of flora, fauna, microbes, and people, all with health implications. Early travelers carried cultivated plants from one continent to another: rice, bananas, yams, taro, and sugar from Asia; coffee and oil palm from Africa; and maize, cassava, peanuts, tomatoes, papayas, pineapples, and potatoes from the New World. These foods were distributed and added to diets throughout the world, improving nutrition in some cases, and resulting in heavy, single-crop reliance (as in the case of potatoes in Ireland) in others. European demands for these and other products stimulated development of estates or plantations, with labor needs met either by the importation of slaves or, after the slave trade was abolished, large-scale hiring of contract workers, resulting in further untoward health consequences.

The rubber industry offers a good example of the effects of these imperial imperatives. When the mid-19th century process of vulcanizing rubber turned rubber trees from novelty to commodity (replacing leather belts in factories and later used for tires, military, and many other products), rubber plantations were in high demand. In the 1850s, the Royal Botanical Garden sent a British agent to smuggle thousands of seedlings of the rubber tree (*Hevea brasiliensis*), native to South American rainforests, out of imperial Brazil (which was seeking to protect its share of the lucrative rubber trade). Grown in London hothouses, they served as the basis for commercial plantings of natural rubber trees in the British Empire, designed to give Britain greater control over this lucrative and useful industry. Conditions on the Malay Peninsula—Britain's possession—were ideal for this tree, and the plantations were prepared in the 1890s (Manderson 1996). However, the local population was sparse, and Chinese workers were deemed difficult to manage. No longer able to transfer slaves, Britain turned to its new source of labor, contract workers from southern India, which it controlled as of the early 19th century (Guilmoto 1993). With thousands of Tamils from the Madras region already working on Malayan coffee and sugar estates, the British began to transfer tens of thousands more each year. Almost immediately, there were severe malaria, hookworm, and other health problems on the rubber estates (Darling et al. 1920), causing many of them to be abandoned and helping motivate Britain's interest in malaria control.

Imperialism shaped and was shaped by patterns of malaria infection (Cohen 1983). Rapid development, the building of cities and clearing of forests, and inadequate drainage and sewage disposal exacerbated malaria infection rates throughout the colonial world, starting in the Americas, from the 16th century onward. During this period, various French, British, Belgian, and Dutch attempts to establish permanent settlements in Africa and Asia were delayed by the malaria problem, while a number of existing settlements were forced to relocate due to the high death toll from malaria.

In the early 1600s, Jesuits in South America learned of an indigenous cure for malaria. It consisted of an alkaloid that occurs in the bark of *Cinchona officinalis*, a tree native to Peru. By the middle of the 17th century, the fame of this "Jesuit bark" or *Lignum febrium* had spread throughout Europe, where it rapidly gained favor as a specific treatment for agues and fevers. The great demand for cinchona bark almost led to the disappearance of the trees in Peru, Bolivia, and Ecuador. Growing wild in the forests, they were searched out and cut down by bark collectors without regard for the future. Several attempts at estate cultivation of the trees met with indifferent success until the Dutch finally established profitable plantations in Java. Careful selection, grafting, and cultivation resulted in growth of high-quality trees rich in quinine, as cinchona became known in the 19th century. The Dutch had a virtual monopoly of quinine production until World War II when the supply was cut off, creating an incentive for development of synthetic antimalarials, such as chloroquine. The spread of chloroquine-resistant malaria in recent years has renewed demand for quinine and the Chinese remedy artemisinin.

Tropical Medicine

Although towns in Europe and the Americas had seen the retreat of malaria and other ailments after implementing environmental and sanitary measures starting in the 18th century (Dobson 1997; Knaut 1997; Rodríguez and Rodríguez de Romo 1999), scientific attention to these questions did not come to a crescendo until the 19th century, when various factors lent greater urgency to the matter and facilitated detailed study: malaria's threat to European colonization and to the productivity of plantation workers, as described earlier; the rise of bacteriology; and imperial patronage of scientific work. Malaria research was thus crucial to the establishment of the field of tropical medical research.

One key player was British physician-parasitologist Patrick Manson. After medical training, Manson was posted as medical officer to the Chinese Imperial Maritime Customs on Formosa (now Taiwan), charged with ship and crew inspection. He spent several more decades working at missionary hospitals on mainland China and Hong Kong. Closely observing "tropical" diseases, Manson elaborated a model of disease transmission—hypothesizing a link between parasite and mosquito vector—initially based on his observations of filariasis and later of malaria in 1898. Manson's work drew from French military medical officer Charles Laveran's 1880 discovery of the malaria parasite while he was posted in the French colony of Algeria. Manson's studies would enable Ronald Ross, a surgeon with the Indian Medical Service who himself had had a bout with malaria, to describe the life cycle of malaria parasites in mosquitoes and demonstrate the role played by mosquitoes in bird malaria, which earned him the 1902 Nobel Prize (Laveran won it in 1907). (Italian entomologist Giovanni Grassi later specified the role of the *Anopheles* mosquito in the transmission of the disease among humans.) When Manson returned to London in the 1890s, he became medical advisor to the Colonial Office, persuading Britain's Colonial Secretary to establish schools of tropical medicine in London (where he worked) and Liverpool (where Ross later worked) in support of imperial needs (Haynes 2001).

Despite numerous advances in the scientific understanding of malaria and methods for its control (e.g., insecticides, drug prophylaxis), today it continues to plague sub-Saharan Africa and other developing regions, with almost 1 million annual deaths (mostly among young children and pregnant women). As we will see in subsequent chapters, malaria and other vector-borne diseases—as well as a range of chronic and infectious diseases not necessarily associated with the tropics—remain rampant in many former colonies. Valiant clinical research notwithstanding, addressing premature death and disability entails understanding the historical roots of political and economic exploitation, which greatly contribute to the impact of malaria.

To reinforce this point, we turn to the relation of imperialism to trypanosomiasis (sleeping sickness) in Africa, which is discussed in greater detail in Chapter 14. The parasite, transmitted by biting tsetse flies, has prevented introduction of large domesticated animals for food protein, labor, or transportation in many areas of the continent. There is little doubt that the commercial and agricultural activities of Europeans acted to spread this pathogen to new areas of Africa (Lyons 1992). Until the late 19th century, for example, sleeping sickness was not recorded in East Africa. Its probable introduction by the ruthless expedition led by Englishman Henry Morton Stanley from the Congo area to the East African lake region (1874–1877) resulted in an enormous outbreak among residents of Uganda from 1900 to 1908. Today 250,000 to 300,000 people are infected by trypanosomiasis each year, with Uganda at the center of the affected region (WHO 2008).

The few examples cited here only hint at the multitude of health-related effects set in motion by worldwide exploration, colonization, and commerce since the 15th century. Very significant demographic changes have occurred, with massive forced and voluntary migration of populations from India, Asia, and Europe to virtually every spot on the globe. The establishment of colonial regimes imposed the cultures and social institutions of the ruling country, which both destroyed and blended with preexisting local norms. This is true of languages, legal systems, and medicine, including concepts of causality and treatment, and patterns of medical organization and practice.

In sum, the system of imperialism entailed far more than a set of ecological encounters. Long before the emergence of the modern science of public health, health concerns accompanied the colonial enterprise of invasion, occupation, and commercial exploitation. Conquest itself bequeathed ominous health effects: new biological exposures were not unidirectional, but the intensity of devastation on native populations and slaves was unparalleled.

Box 2–1 Motives for Imperial Health

- Protecting soldiers and settlers
- Safeguarding commerce
- Ensuring productivity of workers
- Improving colonial relations and staving off unrest
- "Civilizing" colonial populations

INDUSTRIALIZATION AND THE EMERGENCE OF MODERN PUBLIC HEALTH

At the height of the imperial grab for colonies, and largely bankrolled through the riches generated by colonial exploits, Europe began to undergo a massive transformation.

The period of European industrialization from 1750 to the beginning of the 20th century was characterized by a complex of interlocking developments in the political and economic order, and in the realm of social relations and scholarly inquiry. Advances in science and technology both contributed to capitalist industrialization and, in large part, were stimulated by it. Most European countries went in several steps from collections of fiefdoms to larger nation-states. Revolutionary movements in France, North America, and elsewhere generated and disseminated ideas of the right to political freedom, even while the largest colonial empires in history were being assembled.

The transition from feudalism to capitalism entailed vast social and demographic shifts, fundamentally altering the way people lived and died. Between 1750 and 1900 the world's human population doubled, from about 800 million to 1.7 billion, following centuries of stagnating and sometimes falling populations in times of food shortages. The feudal era's social divisions among monarchs and noblemen, a small artisan class, and the vast peasantry were eventually replaced by new classes of merchants and industrialists (the bourgeoisie) and workers (the proletariat) under the capitalist economic system. Industrial processes, based on a new organization of production (first in home-based cottage industries under "proto-industrialization"), and drawing from advances in engineering and chemistry, flourished. Agriculture became more efficient and less labor-intensive. Unprecedented volumes of raw materials and consumer goods crisscrossed the world.

The health of the population became more important with the rise of the state and of the capitalist system. There were new political obligations to citizens, and worker health maintained productivity and loyalty. Moreover, trade needed to remain disease-free to circulate smoothly without interruption. Health also became a question of moral and social order, as indicated in Bavarian Johann Peter Frank's 1790 academic address "The People's Misery—Mother of all Disease" and his seminal, multivolume *A System of Complete Medical Police* published between 1779 and 1827, the first known comprehensive public health treatise. But then, as today, understanding of the connections between poor social conditions and ill health did not automatically translate into social reform.

Box 2–2 The Demographic Transition

Over the last several centuries, many populations have experienced important demographic changes. The so-called demographic transition, a term devised by F.W. Notestein in 1945, describes the changes in birth and death rates that historically accompanied the shift from a "traditional" to a "modern" society, based on the experience of western European countries: in brief, after nutritional and sanitary improvements take place, declines in mortality, especially infant mortality, ensue. Mortality declines are followed, after some lag, by a reduction in fertility, as illustrated in Figure 2–1. In Notestein's classical description, a stage of high birth and death rates and little or no population growth gives way to a transitional stage of falling death rates, sustained high birth rates, and rapid population growth, and then to a new stationary stage in which birth and death rates and population growth are relatively low. Demographic transitions can lead the age structure of the population to change dramatically, with proportionately fewer children, many more older people, and a substantial increase in median age and life expectancy.

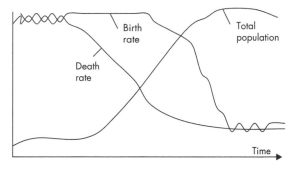

Figure 2–1 The demographic transition. *Source*: Based on Notestein (1945).

(continued)

Box 2–2 Continued

However, it is important to bear in mind that although a singular process of demographic transition is widely referred to in international health, this is a description based on observations of certain European population patterns rather than a generalizable theory. Not only have many countries followed patterns distinct from those described by Notestein, the demographic transition does not include any explanation of *how* changes take place or by what kinds of mechanisms. For example, despite extensive study, there are no definitive answers as to how fertility declines took place in the past (Coale and Watkins 1986). The range of reasons postulated include the following:

1. shift from subsistence agriculture to factory work as smaller family size was needed to maintain household revenues (and child labor was increasingly restricted);
2. higher marginal cost of each additional child in urban settings;
3. decline of multifamily and multigenerational households that facilitated child care;
4. larger numbers of women educated and working in the paid labor force;
5. development of social security systems replaced family responsibility for elder care;
6. long workdays/shift work resulted in less leisure time;
7. contraceptive technologies (e.g., condoms developed in 1840s);
8. women's networks relayed knowledge regarding pregnancy prevention; and
9. infant mortality declines (and greater child survival) were associated with greater birth spacing and lower fertility.

There is a great deal of argument over whether industrialized countries are a template or road map for corresponding changes bound to come in currently developing countries. Most observers consider this unlikely, because development of low income countries in the second half of the 20th century has not always been characterized by the same positive changes in social and health status as experienced in most late 19th and early 20th-century Western settings. This may be due in part to comparatively worse economic conditions and growing inequalities, including uneven allocation of resources such as education and sanitation in many developing countries (Hertz, Hebert, and Landon 1994).

Moreover, even in European countries, transitions did not necessarily follow a smooth or universal pattern. Many rapidly industrializing cities of the early 19th century—for example, Manchester, England and Liège, Belgium—saw mortality increases rather than declines due to miserable urban living and working conditions. As well, in various places, mortality declines have not necessarily been followed by fertility declines due to cultural preferences, social necessity, or state incentives for large family sizes. As discussed in Chapter 3, during the Cold War, large-scale family planning efforts led by the United States sought to decrease fertility rates in developing countries as a means of improving maternal and child health and enabling economic development. Because the United States and other Western powers perceived growing developing country populations as a breeding ground for communism, defusing population pressure and jump-starting demographic transitions became highly politicized.

Industrial Revolution in England

The term "industrial revolution" is now commonly used to denote the period from about 1750 to 1850 during which factories and power-driven machinery were first employed for mass production of articles of commerce. A constellation of basic social and economic changes of considerable significance to health accompanied the development of the factory system, which was itself made possible by rapid advances in technology during the 18th century and accelerated urbanization of the 19th century. The textile industry played the leading role in early industrialization in northern Europe, with the flying shuttle, spinning machines, and, above all, intricate power looms making possible the production of vast amounts of cotton cloth. Early textile machinery was operated by water power, restricting the placement of the mills, but after James Watt's invention of the steam engine in 1781, factories could be located at almost any site, limited only by supplies of labor, coal, and materials.

The need for factory workers produced a whole new category of specialized wage laborers derived largely from impoverished farmers, apprentices, and destitute women and children. Many factory owners displayed an indifference to the welfare of the workers comparable to that of slave traders. Safety devices were minimal and small children, sometimes literally chained to the machines, toiled from dawn to dusk in dusty, noisy, unheated, and unventilated workrooms.

This was an era of rapid economic growth, but the gains were not shared across the population. The new factories generated enormous wealth for their owners, who bought raw materials at rock bottom prices from the countryside and colonies, and paid their workers the lowest wages they could get away with, even as they invested heavily in changing technology. It would take over a century of struggle before workers would be protected by welfare states through economic security, workplace safety, and social services.

In the first half of the 19th century industrial cities were bursting at their seams, with populations doubling, tripling, or more within a generation. Laborers flocked to factory towns from the countryside, unable to survive as pastoralists after new laws banned collective farming. Urban housing was constructed as quickly and cheaply as possible, packing dozens of people into windowless rooms. City planning was nonexistent and sanitation neglected. The smoke from innumerable factories and coal fires filled the air and blackened buildings and lungs alike. Despite improvements in agricultural production, nutrition was poor. Rickets became common in children rarely exposed to sunshine, and contagious diseases such as tuberculosis, diphtheria, and louse-borne typhus took a great toll. The first cholera pandemic to strike western Europe took thousands of lives in the early 1830s and quickly extended to North America via shipping. Occupational injuries and deaths were common, as were diseases arising from unrestricted industrial use of lead, mercury, phosphorus, and other toxic substances.

Workers began to organize collective efforts to better their conditions, joined by certain middle-class social reformers who were outraged at the shocking conditions in city slums, factories, and mines. But these efforts faced formidable foes in industrial owners and their political partners. By the mid-19th century, the resistance of moneyed interests to sanitary and industrial reform was no longer tenable.

Edwin Chadwick and Friedrich Engels

The movement for sanitary reform in Britain engendered heated debates over the role of the state and of private interests in the protection of public health and welfare. The two most prominent figures in these debates were Edwin Chadwick and Friedrich Engels. Both published studies in the 1840s on the horrendous living conditions of urban industrial workers, but their analyses diverged.

Chadwick, a lawyer and lifetime civil servant, cut his administrative teeth as the head of the Poor Law Commission, charged with updating welfare policy dating from Elizabethan times. He was author of the new Poor Law of 1834, which compelled the destitute to enter urban "hellhole" workhouses instead of receiving welfare support in their home parishes. According to esteemed British historian Eric Hobsbawm, the Poor Law "created more embittered unhappiness than any other statute of modern British history" (Hobsbawm 1968, p. 82). A few years later, the Commission was asked to extend its work beyond "relief" of the indigent poor to the saving of welfare funds by preventing illness (which, it was believed, led to destitution). This resulted in Chadwick's 1842 *Report on an Inquiry into the Sanitary Condition of the Labouring Population of Great Britain*. Chadwick pointed out that the majority of children of the working class died before their fifth birthday and showed how mortality varied by social and economic class (Hamlin 1998). He also made a key point about public health measures:

> The great preventives, drainage, street and house cleansing by means of supplies of water and improved sewerage, and especially the introduction of cheaper and more efficient modes of removing all noxious refuse from the towns, are operations for which aid must be sought from the science of the Civil Engineer, not from the physician, who has done his work when he has pointed out the disease that results from the neglect of proper administrative measures, and has alleviated the sufferings of the victims (Chadwick 1842, p. 396).

When Chadwick turned his attention to sanitary reform, his belief in the miasmatic origins of disease—putrid air arising from festering filth—shaped his reforms. Chadwick's zeal was for clean water, sewage, and public sanitation, measures which he believed would prevent most diseases and premature death. As the sanitary movement spread, towns implemented proper disposal of waste, urban sewage systems, and supplies of pure water, with dramatic improvements in population health. However, Chadwick rejected improved working conditions, wages, and food as remedies for pauperism. The notion that poverty itself was the cause of illness was, for Chadwick, unthinkable. He believed that the poor were immoral and unclean, but he also held that noxious environmental conditions—not individual moral failings—were the cause of disease and poverty.

Friedrich Engels was the son of a wealthy German manufacturer who was sent to Manchester, England to work in one of his father's textile factories. His father had hoped that this experience would rid him of his radical political interests; instead, Engels spent much of his time examining the living and occupational environments of industrial workers. In *The Condition of the Working Class in England* (Engels 1845), Engels documented social conditions as dismal as those in Chadwick's report, but he developed a fundamentally distinct explanatory framework. Engels attributed the cause of misery and ill health to the exploitation of the industrial working class under the capitalist economic system:

> When one individual inflicts bodily injury upon another, such injury that death results, we call the deed manslaughter; when the assailant knew in advance that the injury would be fatal, we call this deed murder. But when society places hundreds of prole-tarians in such a position that they inevitably meet a too early and an unnatural death, one which is quite as much a death by violence as that by the sword or bullet, when it deprives thousands of the necessaries of life, places them under conditions in which they *cannot* live—forces them, through the strong arm of the law, to remain in such conditions until that death ensues which is the inevitable consequence—knows that these thousands of victims must perish, and yet permits these conditions to remain, its deed is murder just as surely as the deed of the single individual; disguised, malicious murder, murder against which none can defend himself, which does not seem what it is because no man sees the murderer, because the death of the victim seems a natural one, since the offence is more one of omission than of commission. But murder it remains (Engels 1845, p. 27).

Moreover, he believed political action was necessary to redress these conditions. Shortly after publishing his book, Engels began working with German philosopher Karl Marx. In 1848, Marx and Engels issued *The Communist Manifesto*, calling for revolutionary overthrow of the exploitative capitalist system.

While Britain did not undergo a communist revolution, a combination of sanitary (later public health) reforms and militant class struggles from the mid-19th to early 20th century resulted in marked improvements in social conditions, moderate income redistribution, and increases in life expectancy, although intractable social inequalities in health (as we will see in Chapter 7) remained.

Chadwick's 1842 report eventually formed the basis of the Public Health Act of 1848 that established the General Board of Health and authorized the post of Medical Officer of Health to local boards. The first Medical Officer of Health of London, John Simon, wrote, "Sanitary neglect is mistaken parsimony. Fever and cholera are costly items to count against the cheapness of filthy residences and ditch-drawn drinking water: widowhood and orphanage make it expensive to sanction unventilated work places and needlessly fatal occupations..." (Simon 1890, cited in Rosen 1958, p. 202).

The year 1849 marked the publication of a slender pamphlet, *On the Mode of Communication of Cholera*, by John Snow, a work expanded and augmented in 1854 and destined to become a classic of epidemiological reasoning. Snow deduced the mode of transmission of cholera as being through contaminated drinking water at London's Broad Street pump. He showed how water drawn from the lower Thames, after passage through London, was far more likely to transmit cholera than was water taken from localities upstream of the city. At the same time, however, Snow explicitly disavowed a class analysis of contaminated water patterns, instead proposing an atomistic "risk factor" approach.

Within a few decades important advances had been made in: knowledge of waterborne disease transmission; sanitary engineering innovations enabling piped water supply, sewage, and drainage systems; and development of water purification techniques of filtration, chemical treatment, and chlorination. The only wanting ingredients for urban public health were political struggle and political will, neither of which Snow himself embraced.

Sanitary Reform in Other Countries

The appalling conditions in England at the turn of the 19th century were not unique to that country but occurred also wherever industrial centers developed, often prompting similar responses. Consensus over the nature, funding, and reach of public health measures was far from automatic. Public health became embroiled in the political and social struggles of the day, at times offering a justification for an activist state, at times suffering from a backlash against such intervention, and at times, paradoxically, serving purely private interests (Baldwin 1999).

France occupied a premier position in social and political thought in the 19th century and had employed revolutionary means to overthrow the despotic *ancien régime*, but child labor legislation and public health measures were not immediate. Though the ideas of Louis-René Villermé regarding the moral and physical status of factory workers and the relationship between neighborhood poverty and ill health were pathbreaking (see Chapter 5 for details) (LaBerge 1992), it was action in the streets and legislative reform that led to political change.

Across Europe and throughout the world, an unfurling of social movements, culminating in a series of 1848 uprisings, showed widespread resistance to the Industrial Revolution and the concentration of wealth and power that it generated. The people of Berlin, Paris, Vienna, Palermo, Milan, Naples, Parma, Rome, Warsaw, Prague, Dakar, Budapest, and other cities rose up in protest against miserable living and working conditions; in India, the Second Sikh War demonstrated continued protest against British colonial rule. Where the protests were not brutally repressed, they resulted in concrete gains including for public health. For example, the uprising in Paris led to the abdication of France's last king, Louis-Philippe, and the founding of the Second Republic, which created a public health advisory committee and established a network of local public health councils. By the 1880s, France was developing one of the world's foremost protectionist systems for mothers and children.

Box 2–3 The McKeown Thesis

How might we explain the modern decline of mortality featured in demographic transitions? According to the writings of English social medicine analyst Thomas McKeown, who based his ideas on death patterns in England and Wales, there were four possible avenues for mortality improvements:

1. spontaneous change in the virulence of microorganisms;
2. medical measures;
3. public health measures (state policies); and
4. improvements in standard of living.

McKeown's much-cited studies (McKeown and Record 1962; McKeown 1976) concluded that improved nutrition (and immunological resistance)—stemming from economic growth and a rising standard of living—was the key explanatory factor, with medicine deemed largely irrelevant since effective interventions appeared only after mortality rates had already fallen substantially. Figure 2–2 uses McKeown's tuberculosis graphic to illustrate the irrelevance of medical factors in the disease's mortality decline. This provocative thesis has stimulated numerous national and local level mortality studies that challenge McKeown's dismissal of the role of human agency in terms of social policy efforts, public health measures—such as sanitation and housing improvements (Szreter 1988)—and political change (Burström 2003), and reveal an enormous complexity of factors and experiences (Corsini and Viazzo 1997; Wolleswinkel-van den Bosch et al. 2000; Haines 2001), including an "urban penalty" of increased mortality in northern Europe during the early phases of industrialization (Kearns 1988).

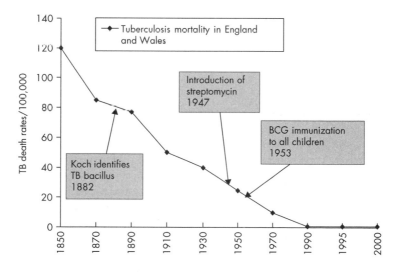

Figure 2–2 Tuberculosis mortality and medical interventions.
Source: Based on McKeown, Record, and Turner (1975).

(*continued*)

Box 2–3 Continued

James Riley has shown that countries have historically chosen one or more of six strategies to reduce mortality: better income distribution; improved diet; public health; medicine; changes in household behavior; and increased education—with no single factor universally successful (Riley 2001).

Because European analyses focus on the era that preceded the expanded armamentarium of antibiotics, vaccines, and vector-control measures in the wake of World War II, some observers have speculated that falls in postwar mortality in developing countries might have derived more from technical and medical interventions than was the case in Europe (Frenk et al. 1989). However, since these improvements in mortality were coterminous with improvements in social and political conditions (including decolonization), education, income and its distribution, and medical and public health measures, it is nearly impossible to untangle the separate effects of each factor. Amidst these complexities, as we shall discuss in Chapters 4 and 7, political, social, and economic determinants of health have clearly played a far larger role in mortality declines than have medical and behavioral changes.

In Prussia (before Germany was unified), agitation for similar legislation was led by the famous medical scientist Rudolf Virchow, the founder of social medicine, who, when asked in 1848 to investigate the cause of a typhus epidemic in Silesia, pinpointed lack of democracy as the culprit, forever marking the fields of medicine and public health as fundamentally political (see Chapter 4). In 1873 a Reich Health Office was set up and Munich health officer Max von Pettenkofer delivered his well-known orations on "The Value of Health to a City," in which he reiterated Johann Peter Frank's ideas regarding the sanitary order and added observations on nutrition, housing, bathing, customs and habits, and political and social conditions. Pettenkofer exemplified the growing mood toward social responsibility in these words:

In every large community there are always many people who have not the means to procure for themselves the things that are absolutely necessary to a healthy life. Those who have more than they need, must contribute to supply these wants, in their own interest. It is not a matter of indifference if, in a city, the dwellings of the poor become infested with typhoid and cholera but is a threat to the health of the richest people also. This is true for all contagious or communicable diseases. Whenever causes of disease cannot be removed or kept away from the individual, the citizens must stand together and accept taxation according to their ability. When a city provides good sewerage, good water supplies, good and clean streets, good institutions for food control, slaughter houses and other indispensable and vital necessities, it creates institutions from which all benefit, both rich and poor. The rich have to pay the bill and the poor cannot contribute anything; yet the rich draw considerable advantages from the fact that such institutions benefit the poor also. A city must consider itself a family, so to say. Care must be taken of everybody in the house, also of those who do not or cannot contribute toward its support (Pettenkofer 1941, p. 48).

The cities of North America had the advantages of relative newness (such as wider streets than those of medieval cities), but by the middle of the 19th century the crush of immigration had rendered the larger urban centers of the East Coast as noxious as their European counterparts. New York City, for instance, grew from about 75,000 people in 1800 to more than half a million by 1850. Local boards of health had been established in some of the larger eastern cities before 1800, but these were ineffective in stemming the tide of disease. From early colonial times, North America had been swept by epidemics of smallpox, yellow fever, typhoid, and typhus; tuberculosis, malaria, and other communicable diseases were firmly entrenched. The cholera pandemics of the 1830s and 1840s struck the Americas with full force, even coming to California along with the gold fever of the '49ers.

Using Chadwick's 1842 report as a model, John Griscom in 1845 published *The Sanitary Condition of the Laboring Population of New York*, followed five years later by Lemuel Shattuck's *Report of the Sanitary Commission of Massachusetts*, neither of which resulted in prompt legislative or sanitary actions. The gradual awakening of interest in such matters resulted in the U.S. National Sanitary Conventions of the late 1850s. A National Board of Health was established by an Act of Congress in 1879 but disbanded four years later, devolving public health into a primarily local concern for many decades to come.

In Latin American countries, most independent as of the early 19th century, the sanitary authorities that had periodically mobilized to combat epidemic outbreaks during almost four centuries of colonial rule were transformed into permanent health and hygiene boards and departments in the late 19th century. Infused with the new ideas and practices of the day, national health agencies sought to centralize power, implement modern public health measures, and increase the purview of the state over social welfare, but their efforts catered mostly to urban elites.

In colonial settings, meanwhile, these measures were not systematically applied outside colonists' enclaves and sites of commercial importance—only in "model" colonies, such as Ceylon (Jones 2004), did the new public health yield organized local measures.

Approaching 1900, these developments were undergirded by the increasing scientific and technical potential of public health and medicine. Spawned by the germ theory of disease transmission, and the bacteriological and parasitological findings by the likes of Louis Pasteur, Robert Koch, Carlos Finlay, and Patrick Manson, public health's new capacity included laboratory-based verification of disease and a small but growing armamentarium of disease-control measures, such as diphtheria antitoxin treatment deriving from work by Emile Roux, Emil von Behring, and others. This powerful explanatory framework and the accompanying interventions began to displace public health's environmentally oriented activities. The "new" public health thus found itself at the vortex of clashing constituencies—scientific experts striving to assert their status, reformers seeking to improve the social order, liberal industrialists eager for steady economic growth, and bureaucrats looking to increase their purview, as well as socialists, feminists, and laborites fighting for better working and living conditions.

Almost simultaneous in their unfolding, various "local" public health concerns—
spurred by the industrial and bacteriological revolutions—generated ideas, legislation, techniques, and explanatory schemes that would be employed in the debates
and actions of a new, far wider, domain, that of "international health."

Box 2–4 The Epidemiologic Transition

This term, proposed by Abdel Omran, refers to changes in mortality from infectious to noncommunicable causes, accompanying the process of development (Omran 1971). According to Omran,
the pattern of major diseases and causes of death shifts from the age of "pestilence and famine" to
"receding pandemics" to "degenerative and human-made diseases" (Fig. 2–3). In Western Europe
and North America, the transition is postulated to have taken approximately 100 years. In Japan
and Eastern Europe the transition started later but evolved more rapidly ("the accelerated model").
Elsewhere the transition is believed to be proceeding in various phases, some nearing completion,
some not ("the contemporary delayed model"). Some authors have combined the demographic and
epidemiologic transitions into a single "health transition" (Frenk et al. 1991).

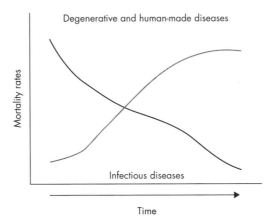

Figure 2–3 Epidemiologic transition. *Source*: Based on Omran (1971).

A number of health analysts have argued that the epidemiologic transition is so flawed that it
should be discarded. For example, Omran did not take into account the role of warfare and violence,
the interaction of food insecurity with contagious ailments, or increased industrial, urban, and trade-
related deaths that shape and have shaped transitions in causes of death.
    According to Julio Frenk and colleagues (Frenk et al. 1989):

· the eras are not necessarily sequential, since two or more may overlap;
· the evolutionary changes in the patterns of morbidity and mortality are reversible, giving rise to
  what could be called a "countertransition";

(continued)

Box 2–4 Continued

• there is, in consequence, a new model of epidemiologic transition, typical of countries where the changes do not fully take place and where different types of diseases coexist in the same population; and

• the coexistence of pre- and posttransitional diseases is associated with inequalities between social classes.

Working and marginalized classes not only experience higher death and disability rates, but some ailments, such as infections or nutritional disorders, may be entirely absent among elite classes.

Moreover, as discussed in Chapter 4, a countertransition has occurred in the former Soviet Union, where infant mortality rates have risen and male life expectancy, in Russia in particular, has dropped to levels of the 1960s due to deteriorating social protection and conditions and increases in economic inequality. AIDS has also had a great demographic impact, particularly in sub-Saharan Africa.

In sum, recent experiences with a range of infectious diseases—some of which, such as TB, AIDS, and avian influenza, are closely linked to development and globalization processes—challenge Omran's ideas about epidemiologic transitions, past and present. The notion of a uniform epidemiologic transition only reinforces the stereotype that people in developing countries only die of infectious diseases and people in industrialized countries only die of noncommunicable diseases, and that the latter pattern is "more advanced" than the former. Most importantly this model fails to recognize differences in causes of death within populations, reflecting larger societal inequalities. These issues are discussed further in Chapters 6 and 7.

THE MAKING OF INTERNATIONAL HEALTH IN THE AMERICAS

By the mid-19th century, medicine and public health were established as major ingredients in the colonization of peoples around the world, far more nefarious activities than their sometime portrayal as the humanitarian component of decidedly unphilanthropic military and political ventures. Indeed, the "assumption that imperialism, whatever its other faults, at least led to an improvement in the health of the indigenous populations" (Farley 1988, p. 189) belies the intent of colonial public health measures: to protect the well-being of the imperial military; to make "the tropics" habitable by European settlers; to improve the productivity of local workers; to subjugate conquered populations; and to reinforce the political and social stratification between colonizer and colonized (MacLeod and Lewis 1988; Bashford 2004).

Colonizers' belief in the "civilizing" function of medicine upon native peoples, their adherence to the notion that infectious diseases originated in the "primitive and dangerous world" of the tropics, their fascination with questions of acclimatization and racial difference (Lorcin 1999), and the hiding of diseased settlers in order to perpetuate the myth that Europeans possessed superior immunity meant that the role of public health in human well-being was a low-order consideration.

By the 19th century, intense economic competition between empires, together with increasing frequency of shipborne disease outbreaks, brought colonial health to the fore. The appearance, beginning in the 1830s, of terrifying worldwide outbreaks of cholera, which violently killed by dehydration via multiple orifices, would bridge the distance between colonial and metropolitan health. Cholera's importance in Europe was intimately tied to industrialization—the rise of commerce and faster transport, together with the urban squalor accompanying factory life, all facilitated the spread and severity of this dreaded ailment (Evans 1987). Cholera was also perceived as a disease from "the tropics," given its increasing appearance in South and East Asian locales. The political and epidemiological implications of colonial health problems thus began to be understood in new ways: for their impact on trade, profits, and citizens in "home" countries.

But these concerns transcended the responsibilities of particular colonies. Even as individual imperial powers undertook incipient efforts to carry out surveillance activities and control disease outbreaks, the scale of interchange between, among, and beyond empires demanded a new level of cooperation and communication.

Large-scale immigration and the explosion of materials extraction, manufacturing, circulation, and marketing of goods—in turn enabled by a revolution in transportation (steamships and railroads) and transport routes, such as the opening of the Suez Canal in 1868—heightened the threat of epidemic disease throughout the world, not just between colony and "mother country." No longer were outbreaks of plague, yellow fever, cholera, or other epidemic diseases solely the concern of localities, binational disputes, or colonial powers; the now globalized commercial system meant that a real or threatened epidemic in one part of the world could impede production, trade, and sales elsewhere (Chandavarkar 1992). A new global economic interdependence magnified the potential dangers of disease and made its control a far more politically complicated matter.

The expansion of social, scientific, and economic relations between countries enabled public health problems to be identified and understood with greater consistency and facilitated the worldwide diffusion and implementation of standard public health measures. But nations were slow to cooperate in health matters, jealously guarding national sovereignty over information and decision making.

In the Americas, international sanitary cooperation was somewhat easier, with the United States as its beacon. Not impeded by age-old rivalries, commercially ambitious, and politically and economically influential in Latin America, the United States was strongly motivated to provide regional leadership in public health. As the world's foremost immigrant destination between 1890 and 1920, the United States also became a potential importer of transmissible disease and, to protect itself, unilaterally began a world epidemic monitoring and notification center. In the late 1870s, the U.S. Marine Hospital Service started publishing epidemic outbreak news in its weekly bulletins, as reported by a global network of informants. An 1893 U.S. Presidential Act obliged all immigrants and cargo ships to present certificates of health signed by the U.S. consul and a medical officer in the departing port, and the Marine Hospital Service stationed a number of its officers in key ports in the United States (most famously Ellis Island in New York) and around the world to inspect ships and passengers for disease and to enforce quarantine (Birn 1997).

These concerns accelerated when the United States acquired colonies in the Caribbean and the Pacific after its 1898 war with Spain (Anderson 2006). U.S. forces invading Cuba had suffered disastrous troop losses due to yellow fever and other infectious diseases. Like other colonial powers before it, the United States took on public health activities to protect its troops and colonists from "tropical" diseases (Cirillo 2004). But it was construction of the Panama Canal that most alerted the United States to the importance of international health.

The Panama Canal

Desire to construct a canal in the Central American isthmus was ignited in the 16th century, when a Spanish conquistador discovered that only a narrow land strip separated the two oceans. Although Spanish Emperor Charles I backed the building of a canal, the project was deemed impossible and abandoned until the 1870s when French naval officers undertook a new feasibility survey. Years of complex planning and negotiations finally led to groundbreaking in 1880. After 8 years of effort, US$300 million in expenditure, the hiring of tens of thousands of workers, principally from France and Jamaica, and almost 20,000 deaths from malaria and yellow fever, the Compagnie Universelle du Canal Interocéanique de Panama went bankrupt and abandoned its efforts in 1888.

Almost no planning or funds had been allocated by the company for hygiene and sanitation, even though the region was a well-known bed of yellow fever, a feared and deadly ailment—especially to the previously unexposed. Yellow fever had been afflicting ports from Buenos Aires to Halifax since the 18th century. Still, at the start of the French effort, the cause and means of transmission of the two great diseases were not fully established. Despite keen U.S. interest to take over the building and control of a canal, the French still held the concession. By the time negotiations with the French and Panamanian authorities were concluded in 1904, the U.S. military had had its own disastrous encounter with malaria and yellow fever in Cuba. The U.S. war with Spain provided further military impetus for a canal. The United States had another advantage at hand, which ultimately enabled its completion of the Panama Canal in 1914.

To understand the events in Panama we must turn to Havana, where Cuban physician Carlos Finlay had proposed that yellow fever was transmitted through the bite of a mosquito, as announced in 1881 (López Sánchez 1987). Few people believed him, and it would be well over a decade before Ronald Ross would demonstrate the mosquito transmission of malaria. After an outbreak of yellow fever at the U.S. military garrison in Havana, the American Yellow Fever Commission, headed by Walter Reed, conducted experiments using mosquitoes fed on patients and then on uninfected volunteers (Stepan 1978; Bean 1982). The commission fully confirmed

Finlay's observation and announced at the Pan American Medical Congress in Havana in 1901 that the mosquito *Stegomyia fasciata* (now called *Aedes aegypti*) is the sole vector of yellow fever. The hardy *Aedes* mosquito could last for long periods aboard ships, making it a menace to commerce.

U.S. Army surgeon and Chief Sanitary Officer for the Department of Cuba William C. Gorgas, in charge of sanitation in Havana as of 1898, established a series of ordinances that resulted, within a few years, in a dramatic decline in yellow fever within the city. These rules included the abolition, or protection by screening, of all domestic water containers likely to breed mosquitoes; daily inspection of houses and yards by an army of sanitarians; the imposition of a stiff fine on property owners found to have mosquito larvae on their premises; and the reporting and isolation of every suspected case of yellow fever (Fig. 2–4).

When the United States took over the Canal Zone in 1904, Gorgas was appointed to head the medical department of what may have been the most fever-ridden place on earth. By 1905 more than 4,000 men were employed in mosquito extermination alone. Two brigades were formed—the *Stegomyia* brigade to work primarily around houses and settlements, and the *Anopheles* brigade to clear jungles, drain and oil swamps, and work to reduce the recently confirmed vector of malaria (Fig. 2–5). Piped water supplies were constructed to eliminate the barrels that had formerly produced clouds of mosquitoes. Houses were screened and bed nets provided to the canal workers. Quinine was issued both as a prophylactic against malaria and as a cure, and persons with fevers were isolated behind mosquito-proof screening. As the engineers blasted and dredged, the war waged against *Aedes* and *Anopheles* by

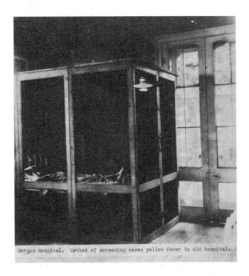

Figure 2–4 Yellow fever patient segregated in a screened cubicle in the Gorgas Hospital, Ancon, Canal Zone. Courtesy of the U.S. National Library of Medicine.

the sanitarians gradually brought yellow fever and malaria under control (Gorgas 1915). Although hailed for enabling completion of the Panama Canal, these sanitary efforts overlooked—and the U.S. occupation of Panama exacerbated—more pressing endemic problems for local populations, such as malnutrition, diarrhea, and tuberculosis (McBride 2002).

Ironically, though the building of the Canal required malaria and yellow fever control, its very completion raised the peril of new epidemics due to shorter shipping routes to and from Asia. Commercial concerns had long affected political relations between South American countries. The meat and hide economies of Argentina and Uruguay were particularly intent on keeping out yellow fever from Brazil, which might interrupt their profitable exports. An 1887 Sanitary Convention signed by Brazil, Argentina, and Uruguay detailed quarantine periods for ships bearing cholera, yellow fever, and plague and was in effect for 5 years before breaking apart. The following year the Andean countries of Bolivia, Chile, Ecuador, and Peru signed the Lima Convention of 1888 (Moll 1940). But these efforts were short-lived and circumscribed due to mutual mistrust and poor enforcement.

In December 1902, representatives of seven American governments met at an International Sanitary Convention in Washington, DC, at the behest of the Conference of the American States (Bustamante 1952). Together, they founded the International Sanitary Bureau (it became the Pan American Sanitary Bureau [PASB] in 1923 and Pan American Health Organization [PAHO] in 1958).

The United States was the prime mover behind the founding of this first international health organization, which was initially run out of the U.S. Public Health Service and headed until 1947 by a succession of United States Surgeon-Generals.

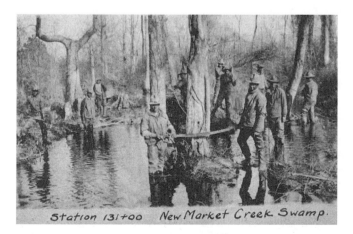

Figure 2–5 Caribbean laborers felling trees for swamp drainage and canal construction at New Market Creek Swamp, Panama, Circa 1910. Courtesy of the U.S. National Library of Medicine.

In short order, most Latin American republics joined the bureau and were represented at its quadrennial conferences. The United States was particularly concerned that Latin American countries participate in the drafting of, and thus comply with, enforceable sanitary treaties. The PASB's early years were devoted to the establishment of region-wide protocols on the reporting and control of epidemic diseases, including yellow fever, plague, and cholera, culminating in a 1924 Sanitary Code, the first Pan American treaty to be signed by all 21 PASB member countries. In its leadership and shaping of activities, the Bureau reflected U.S. hegemonic interests in Latin America, which covered investments in oil, fruticulture, mining and metallurgy, real estate, railroads, banking, and other industries. Under the Monroe Doctrine of 1823, the United States had occupied ports and countries across the region whenever it sensed its interests were threatened. Yet even as its agenda remained focused on sanitary and commercial concerns into the 1930s, the Bureau began to engage in other activities, sponsoring a widely disseminated public health journal, addressing—after being pushed by Latin American members—maternal and child health concerns, and organizing an incipient system of technical cooperation (Birn 2002; Cueto 2004). After World War II, the PASB would officially become the Americas Office of the World Health Organization.

THE INTERNATIONALIZATION OF HEALTH IN THE EUROPEAN EMPIRE AND BEYOND

Well before the yellow fever problem motivated the organization of the PASB, another ailment had emerged as a worldwide menace, shaping an even larger effort. Cholera had been endemic for centuries in the Ganges River basin, but in 1818 it spread to Southeast Asia, China, Japan, East Africa, the eastern Mediterranean (Syria and Palestine), and southern Russia. Less than a decade later another wave, originating in India in 1826, swept Russia, where hundreds of thousands died, and into the major cities of Europe, from which it reached the British Isles in 1831. Within a year, transatlantic ships brought cholera to New York, New Orleans, Montreal, and other seaports. It spread to the American interior, reaching the Pacific Coast and Mexico in 1833. The Middle East was not spared, and Muslim pilgrims returning from the Hajj in Mecca were blamed for carrying cholera to Egypt and the countries of northern Africa. In 1882 the Ottoman Empire set up a quarantine station in the Red Sea specifically to prevent spread of infectious diseases through the Hajj. The station lasted until 1956.

Cholera's frequent recurrence and continuing havoc were intense stimuli for investigators. In 1854 the Italian researcher Filippo Pacini had discovered (and named) the cholera *vibrio* in the stools and intestines of cholera patients and cited it as the cause of the illness. Thirty years later, German bacteriologist Robert Koch, in imperial service, showed that cholera in Calcutta was caused by the same organism.

A flood of discoveries emanated from the world's laboratories in the latter half of the 19th century, identifying the causal agent and basic means of transmission of almost every major bacterial and parasitic disease of humans and domestic animals. From about 1850 to 1910, theories of miasma and vague conceptions of communicability of disease gave way to experimentally based laboratory data regarding the genesis of infectious disease and its effects upon the body. The extreme intellectual ferment provoked by Charles Darwin's theories provided a further stimulus to biological studies after about 1860. Knowledge of physiology, nutrition, biochemistry, and many other aspects of medical science also advanced during this period together with deepened understanding of endocrine and metabolic conditions.

Although some important work on disease control had been done in the 18th century (for instance, James Lind's demonstration of the prevention of scurvy through citrus consumption and Edward Jenner's work on vaccination), the rise of microbiology awaited the chemical and technological underpinning provided by the Industrial Revolution. Refinements in microscope design produced the lenses of the 1880s, close forerunners to those in use today. The chemistry of dye manufacture, developed for the textile industry, was incorporated into histology and bacteriology. Entomological studies, as discussed earlier, also brought key contributions. Little by little, the basis of modern medical laboratory and clinical practice was hammered together.

New knowledge and techniques fostered and were fostered by extensive institutional developments. The Pasteur Institute was founded in the late 1880s with an outpouring of funds donated by a citizenry anxious to help in the development of Louis Pasteur's antirabies vaccine. The institute quickly flourished in research and teaching realms. Starting in Saigon (now Ho Chi Minh City) in 1891, Pasteur Institutes were also established in several dozen countries in France's colonial empire in Africa, Asia, and the Caribbean, as well as in Europe and the Middle East (Moulin 1996; Pelis 2006). In these outlying laboratories, pioneering work was done on plague by Yersin, on malaria by Laveran, and on the Bacille Calmette-Guérin (BCG) by Albert Calmette.

But these developments did not inevitably lead to international action. The repeated pandemics of cholera compelled governments to develop feasible steps to control transmission. The idea of the *cordon sanitaire*, enforced by quarantine regulations and sometimes by military force, had existed since the 14th century, but as international commerce grew, these blockades were increasingly seen by maritime nations as obstacles to trade.

By the mid-1800s the pressure had become intense for some sort of international agreement. Accordingly, an International Sanitary Conference was organized in Paris in 1851 representing 12 states: Austria, France, Great Britain, Greece, the Papal States, Portugal, Russia, Sardinia, Spain, Tuscany, and the Two Sicilies. International health was not the only topic for such conferences at the time. During the same year the "Great Exhibition" in London, the first World's Fair, celebrated trade and manufacturing, while the First International Congress on Statistics was held in Brussels, followed by a demography and hygiene congress in 1852, ophthalmology in 1857, and veterinary medicine in 1863. By the 1880s, international conferences (and exchange of journals and correspondence) were taking place in virtually every scholarly and professional domain, marking the rise of international exchange of ideas, standards, challenges, and breakthroughs. During the same era, the first international nongovernmental agency, the Red Cross, was founded by Jean-Henri Dunant, a Swiss national inspired by the terrible suffering of war victims (Hutchinson 1996). The founding document of the Red Cross, which promoted neutral humanitarian assistance to wounded combatants and entered into force in 1865, has come to be known as the original Geneva Convention (see Chapters 3 and 8 for further details).

The International Sanitary Conferences, most often convened by France and attended by Europe's leading imperial powers plus Russia and Turkey (the main foreposts [especially via new railroad lines] of disease), met eleven times over more than half a century before coming to agreement that an international health organization was needed.

Despite John Snow's studies just a few years earlier, the learned men of Europe, debating for 6 months at the First International Sanitary Conference, could not agree on whether cholera was or was not contagious. The marathon 1851 conference eventually produced a lengthy convention dealing mainly with the quarantine of ships against plague, cholera, and yellow fever, but it came to naught as only France, Portugal, and Sardinia ratified the document, whereupon the latter two then revoked their acceptance. A similar convention was generated by the second (1859) conference, which was never ratified by anyone. One of the reasons that these early conferences ended in frustration was that participating countries were represented by diplomats defending national interests rather than by scientists. But even among scientists there was no consensus concerning the causes and transmission of the diseases in question. A third conference, held in Constantinople in 1866, reviewed voluminous evidence regarding the cause of cholera, including the works of Snow and Pettenkofer, and concluded that the disease was transmitted through what we would today call the "fecal-oral" route. At the fourth International Sanitary Conference in Vienna (1874) a proposal was made to establish a permanent International Commission on Epidemics but was rejected (Howard-Jones 1975; Bynum 1993).

Britain remained opposed to any form of regulation of its extensive trade, ready to condemn the Hajj for the 1865 cholera pandemic (Afkhami 1999) but not the transmission of disease along commercial routes. The British government went so far as to reverse its quarantine and isolation policies in India before the opening of the Suez Canal in 1868, so that the reduced transport time for trade to and from its most profitable colony would not be inconvenienced by disease-control measures (Watts 1997).

Britain's refusal to endorse cholera conventions, and its negotiation of side deals that exempted it (Maglen 2002), stemmed not only from commercial self-interest.

Britain had its own system of "intercolonial" (de facto international) health structures of information-gathering, research, and conferences, essentially precluding the need for participation in a supranational effort with potential rivals.

The first involvement of the United States in the International Sanitary Conferences was its hosting, on its own initiative, the fifth conference in 1881. With the presence of seven Latin American countries plus China, Japan, Liberia, and the usual European participants (represented by diplomats posted in Washington and by special medical delegates from a handful of European countries), the conference aimed to obtain international approval for the U.S.'s 1879 law to inspect and regulate sea vessels en route to the United States to prevent "the introduction of contagious or infectious diseases from foreign countries." While some delegates expressed interest in a system of disease notification, the U.S. proposal was struck down. As mentioned above, the United States developed a system of epidemic informants on its own.

The sanitary conferences took a new turn in the 1890s when they were punctuated by pandemics of cholera, resulting in international conventions in 1892 and 1893 (on cholera control along the Suez Canal and in Europe), in 1894 (specifically on the sanitary control of the Mecca pilgrimage), in 1897 (on plague), and in 1903 (replacing the previous conventions) (International Sanitary Convention of Paris 1903; Textes juxtaposés 1897).

Another product of the 1903 agreement was a conference 4 years later in Rome that set up L'Office Internationale d'Hygiène Publique (OIHP), known informally to English speakers as the "Paris Office." Opening its doors in 1909, the Paris Office was charged "to collect and bring to the knowledge of the participating states the facts and documents of a general character which relate to public health and especially as regards infectious diseases, notably cholera, plague, and yellow fever, as well as the measures to combat these diseases" (Rome Agreement Establishing the Office International d'Hygiène Publique, December 9, 1907).

A formal internationalism in health had finally been established. The Paris Office, with a permanent staff of barely half a dozen people, worked diligently but could hardly keep up with its stated mission. Nevertheless, progress was made—for example, studies on the most effective methods of ship crew and passenger inspection, the de-ratting of ships, an international agreement to control sexually transmitted diseases in seamen, standardization of some biological products, and a study of hospital organization. The permanent committee representing each of the member states did not meet at all in the wartime years of 1914–1919, as conditions in Europe deteriorated dramatically. During this period the great influenza epidemic of 1918–1919 killed an estimated 50 million people worldwide, and the deprivations of World War I led to outbreaks of diseases such as typhus that infected millions of people in war-torn Europe. The conditions of war revealed the limits to international cooperation: the OIHP could not intervene to decry or address disease, and war secrecy impeded early and effective communication regarding the outbreak of

> **Box 2–5** International Health Imperatives
>
> · Charity
> · Missionary work
> · War relief
> · Philanthropy
> · Diplomacy
> · Economic development
> · Paternalism/colonialism
> · Sharing of expertise (and technology transfer)
> · Transnational training
> · Data collection/disease surveillance; standardization

influenza among troops, especially the half million Americans who were mobilized amidst the epidemic.

The Rockefeller Foundation

With prerogatives of bureaucratization, standardization, epidemic disease control, and trade protectionism beginning to be addressed through nascent multinational institutions, international health entered a new phase, one that combined tropical medicine concerns with country-to-country (or-colony) "cooperation" from metropolitan powers to underdeveloped settings. In addition to controlling disease outbreaks, cooperation offered the potential to stimulate development and economic growth; stabilize colonies and emerging nation-states by helping them meet the social demands of their populations; improve diplomatic relations; expand consumer markets; and encourage the transfer and internationalizing of scientific, bureaucratic, and cultural values. At the same time, local elites—through participation in international health activities—could be linked to the world's great powers. International health thus offered the promise of generating goodwill and economic development in place of gunboat diplomacy and colonial repression, all the while supporting the expansion of global capitalism.

It was precisely at this time that a new kind of player emerged on the international health scene, a player that was probably the first to employ the term "international health" and was to have an enormous bearing on the field. The Rockefeller Foundation (RF) was founded in 1913 by oil mogul-turned-philanthropist John D. Rockefeller to promote "the well-being of mankind throughout the world." After uncovering the important part played by public health campaigns in the economic advancement of the U.S. South, the RF created an International Health Board to promote health and social development, befriending dozens of governments around the world by helping modernize their institutions and preparing vast regions for investment and increased productivity (Fig. 2–6). Between its founding in 1913, and its dismantling in 1951, the International Health Board (renamed International Health Division in 1927) carried out scores of hookworm, yellow fever, and malaria

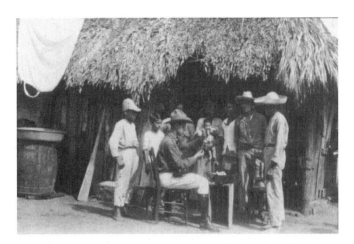

Figure 2–6 House-to-house administration of antihelminthics, Rockefeller Foundation International Health Board's Cooperative Hookworm Campaign in Rural Mexico, 1920s. Courtesy of the Rockefeller Archive Center.

campaigns (as well as efforts to control tuberculosis, yaws, rabies, influenza, schistosomiasis, malnutrition, and other health problems) in more than 90 countries and colonies around the globe, sponsored thousands of public health fellows to pursue graduate study, and founded several dozen schools of public health in North America and across the world (Fee 1987; Cueto 1994; Farley 2004).

The 17D yellow fever vaccine (considered by many to be the best vaccine ever made) was developed in RF laboratories in 1936, resulting in a Nobel Prize for Max Theiler and the protection of commerce and lives. In the late 1930s the introduced African mosquito *Anopheles gambiae* was responsible for an immense outbreak of malignant tertian malaria in Brazil, with more than 100,000 cases and 14,000 deaths in 1938 alone. RF money and workers, together with the Brazilian government, eventually eradicated *A. gambiae* from that country after years of effort, demonstrating the effectiveness of vector control under particular conditions (introduced species, or on islands, as in Sardinia) (Stapleton 2004).

The new international health as pioneered by the RF was neither narrowly self-interested (in economic and political terms) nor passively diffusionist. Instead, the RF actively sought national partnerships to spread its public health gospel, interacting with political and professional authorities and local populations. The RF's philanthropic status, its purported independence from both government and business interests, and its limited accountability enabled its success. Its work patterns included rapid demonstrations of specific disease-control methods based on proven techniques, a missionary zeal in its own officers, facilitating national commitment to public health through considerable cofinancing obligations, and using fellowships to mold a cadre of public health leaders. It also carefully avoided disease campaigns that might be costly, overly complex, time consuming, or distracting from its technically oriented public health model (Birn 2006). As we will see in Chapter 3, these strategies continue to influence the operating policies and practice of international health today.

The First International Health Offices

A conference in London in 1920 recommended the establishment of a health section of the newly created League of Nations to include the Paris Office, but this plan was aborted by the United States and France. Since the United States had declined to join the League of Nations, it refused to permit the OIHP (of which it was a member) to be absorbed by the League. France, meanwhile, preferred to retain the Paris Office. Nevertheless a health section of the League of Nations was established, building on the successful postwar Epidemic Commission, formed to control outbreaks of typhus, cholera, smallpox, and other diseases in eastern and southern Europe (Goodman 1971). With minimal official U.S. participation, the League of Nations Health Organization (LNHO) convened health experts and institutionalized international health, providing a collective response initially to Europe's public health needs, eventually expanding its mission and reaching South, East, and West (Balinska 1995; Weindling 1995; Zylberman 2004). The LNHO played a vital coordinating function for an array of activities far beyond disease control (Borowy 2005), its wide charter allowing "active opportunism" under Polish hygienist Ludwik Rajchman's universally recognized leadership. This institution-building success took two key forms: first, the establishment of international institutions that played a strategic role in planning and marshaling expertise to address world health problems, and second, the cultivation of a cooperative spirit that began to make health an international priority.

Where there had been none a scant 20 years before, now three official international health organizations functioned more or less separately: the Pan American Sanitary Bureau in Washington, the OIHP (Paris Office), and the LNHO in Geneva (Weindling 1995). Further international health engagement was provided by the League (now Federation) of Red Cross Societies and the Comité International de la Croix-Rouge (which competed and feuded with each other), the war relief agency Save the Children (founded in Britain in 1919, with an international counterpart

---

Box 2–6 Early International Health Organizations, Location, and Year of Founding

- Pan American Sanitary Bureau, Washington, DC, 1902
- Office International d'Hygiène Publique, Paris, 1907
- Rockefeller Foundation (International Health Commission/Board/Division), New York, 1913
- Save the Children, London, 1919 (Geneva, 1920)
- League of Nations Health Organization, Geneva, 1923

established in Geneva in 1920), and several other organizations of worldwide scope (Weindling 1997).

The LNHO, drawing in part on social medicine precepts, had a multinational staff and set of advisors who pursued an ambitious agenda of epidemiologic surveillance, expert scientific research, health commissions, standardization, and interchange of health personnel. Its activities were far broader and more ambitious than the OIHP's mandate of previous decades. In matters of epidemics and outbreaks, and gathering epidemiological information, the office collaborated with the OIHP. It pioneered in the collection, standardization, and dissemination of vital and health statistics from around the world. In 1926 the LNHO started publication of the *Weekly Epidemiological Record*, which has been continued to the present day by the World Health Organization. Considering itself a worldwide organization, the LNHO organized a branch in Singapore in 1925 to gather information on health conditions in Asia, and it held conferences in South Africa and South America. It established many scientific and technical commissions to set standards for drugs and vaccines; to study general subjects such as medical education, public health reorganization, housing, the operations of medical facilities, and the health impact of the worldwide economic depression; and to report not only on major infectious diseases (e.g., syphilis, tuberculosis, malaria) but also on nutrition, the social causes of infant mortality, opiates, traffic in women, rural hygiene, health insurance, cancer, and heart disease. Health personnel were sent to other countries for training and consultation and to establish international networks of professionals.

In the 1930s, operations of the OIHP and the LNHO were marked by international bickering, the chaos of the worldwide economic depression, and tensions in Europe, with resultant wavering support and a worsening shortage of funds. Communication was carried out by (sea) mail, telegrams, and, where possible, by telephone or two-way radio. Obtaining timely information about disease outbreaks in remote areas was a continuing challenge (Howard-Jones 1978).

The OIHP was the agency with official jurisdiction over international agreements in the health field and served, in principle, as an advisory council to the LNHO. This arrangement permitted the United States, as a nonmember of the League of Nations, to keep a window open to the LNHO, and various U.S. experts served as staff or consultants to the LNHO (Dubin 1995). The period between the wars saw for the first time the interactions of official governmental and intergovernmental agencies with private and voluntary organizations. An important American connection was through the Rockefeller Foundation, which exerted considerable influence by providing advice and essential funding for many LNHO activities. Both the Paris and Geneva offices diminished operations with the advent of World War II.

The outbreak of World War II suspended many cooperative international health efforts, although others continued, with a military focus. For example, U.S. authorities tested and administered the widespread use of the insecticide DDT against louse-borne typhus and to destroy malaria mosquito vectors in the Pacific military theater, around military bases, and in areas of strategic military importance, such as rubber-growing regions of Brazil. As well, the accelerated production processes of newly developed sulfonamides (to prevent wound infections) and the antibacterial wonder drug penicillin were distributed to Allied soldiers in the latter years of the war. During this time period, the U.S. government also launched a large-scale cooperative sanitary effort throughout Latin America to improve diplomatic relations and forge alliances to fend off German influence in the region, as well as to assert its role in the projected postwar development and rebuilding. But other international health concerns dwindled; the research and standardization efforts of the LNHO and the public health projects of the RF (outside the Americas) had to be suspended because of the war, only to be, as we shall see, resurrected under a new guise in the postwar period.

CONCLUSION

Learning Points:

- International health was (and is) intertwined with social, political, and economic factors.
- The rise of imperialism, industrialization, global capitalism, and commerce played a critical role in shaping worldwide patterns of health and disease and spurring the formation of international health measures and institutions.
- International health institutions were formed for a variety of complex motives, far beyond shared health needs.

In this chapter we have touched upon a range of human activities, preoccupations, interactions, and developments over hundreds of years, all of which have left their imprint upon world health as we find it today. This is why the study of history has the same relevance for students of international health as does the study of evolution for students of biology: it explains why the world looks the way it does and what forces continue to shape its operation and development. As William Faulkner said, "History is not dead. It is not even past."

The historical events covered in this chapter remind us how embedded international health remains in questions of *power* and *influence*, notwithstanding the proliferation of humanitarian, philanthropic, multinational, and development institutions seemingly aimed at generating and sharing technical international health measures. In sum, this chapter and the next serve not simply to lay out the background of international health but to present three key underpinnings of the field that allow us to understand how and why it operates as it does, and how the field and its actions may be shaped in the future. First, as we have seen, international health needs to be understood within a larger context of power and influence. That is to say, medicine and health are not neutral domains but fields that are framed socially and culturally—

in temporal and spatial terms—and politically, in terms of local, regional, international, social, economic, ideological, and institutional struggles for power.

The second point has to do with international health as a form of development and how it operates historically and contemporaneously. Here the central questions have to do with the *hows* of the field. What are the incentives for developing countries to participate? How are the specific mechanisms of the field, such as disease campaigns and fellowships, implemented? And how do these activities result in what economists call "path dependence"?

Third, attention must be paid to the processes of negotiation that have shaped and continue to characterize international health efforts. Here the role and interplay of local actors, international networks, and health agencies can be understood as a complex dance involving multiple partners who participate in the institutions, ideologies, politics, and practices of public health internationally.

REFERENCES

Afkhami AA. 1999. Defending the guarded domain: Epidemics and the emergence of an international sanitary policy in Iran. *Comparative Studies of South Asia, Africa, and the Middle East* 19(1):122–136.

Alchon SA. 1997. The great killers in Precolumbian America: A hemispheric perspective. *Latin American Population History Bulletin* 27.

———. 2003. *A Pest in the Land: New World Epidemics in a Global Perspective.* Albuquerque, NM: University of New Mexico Press.

Amantino M. 2007. As condições físicas e de saúde dos escravos fugitivos anunciados no Jornal do Commercio (RJ) em 1850. *História, Ciencias, Saúde—Manguinhos* 14 (4):1377–1399.

Anderson W. 2006. *Colonial Pathologies: American Tropical Medicine, Race, and Hygiene in the Philippines.* Durham, NC: Duke University Press.

Arnold D. 1997. The place of "the tropics" in Western medical ideas since 1750. *Tropical Medicine and International Health* 2(4):303–313.

———, Editor. 1996. *Warm Climates and Western Medicine: The Emergence of Tropical Medicine, 1500–1900.* Clio Medica 35. Wellcome Institute Series in the History of Medicine. Amsterdam: Rodopi.

Baldwin P. 1999. *Contagion and the State in Europe 1830–1930.* New York: Cambridge University Press.

Balinska M. 1995. *Une vie pour l'humanitaire: Ludwik Rajchman, 1881–1965.* Paris: Editions la Découverte.

Bashford A. 2004. *Imperial Hygiene: A Critical History of Colonialism, Nationalism and Public Health.* Houndmills and New York: Palgrave Macmillan.

Bean WB. 1982. *Walter Reed: A Biography.* Charlottesville, VA: University Press of Virginia.

Berlinguer G. 1992. The interchange of disease and health between the Old and New Worlds. *American Journal of Public Health* 82(10):1407–1413.

Birn A-E. 1997. Six seconds per eyelid: The medical inspection of immigrants at Ellis Island, 1892–1914. *Dynamis* 17:281–316.

———. 2002. "No more surprising than a broken pitcher?" Maternal and child health in the early years of the Pan American Health Sanitary Bureau. *Canadian Bulletin of Medical History* 19(1):17–46.

————. 2006. *Marriage of Convenience: Rockefeller International Health and Revolutionary Mexico*. Rochester: University of Rochester Press.

Borowy I. 2005. World Health in a Book—the League of Nations International Health Yearbooks 1925–30. In Borowy I and Gruner W, Editors. *Facing Illness in Troubled Times. Health in Europe in the Interwar Years, 1918–1939*. Frankfurt am Main: Peter Lang.

Burström B. 2003. Social differentials in the decline of infant mortality in Sweden in the twentieth century: The impact of politics and policy. *International Journal of Health Services* 33:723–741.

Bustamante M. 1952. Los primeros cincuenta años de la Oficina Sanitaria Panamericana. *Boletín de la Oficina Sanitaria Panamericana* 33(6):471–531.

Bynum W. 1993. Policing hearts of darkness: Aspects of the international sanitary conferences. *History and Philosophy of the Life Sciences* 15:421–434.

Campbell J. 1984. Work, pregnancy, and infant mortality among Southern slaves. *Journal of Interdisciplinary History* 14:793–812.

Chadwick E. 1842. *Report to Her Majesty's Principal Secretary of State for the Home Department, from the Poor Law Commissioners, on an Inquiry into the Sanitary Condition of the Labouring Population of Great Britain*. London: W. Clowes and sons for H.M.S.O.

Chandavarkar R. 1992. Plague, panic and epidemic politics in India, 1896–1914. In Ranger T and Slack P, Editors. *Epidemics and Ideas: Essays on the Historical Perception of Pestilence*. Cambridge: Cambridge University Press.

Cirillo VJ. 2004. *Bullets and Bacilli: The Spanish-American War and Military Medicine*. New Brunswick, NJ: Rutgers University Press.

Coale AJ and Watkins SC, Editors. 1986. *The Decline of Fertility in Europe*. Princeton, NJ: Princeton University Press.

Cohen WB. 1983. Malaria and French imperialism. *Journal of African History* 24:23–36.

Cook ND. 1998. *Born to Die: Disease and New World Conquest, 1492–1650*. Cambridge: Cambridge University Press.

Corsini CA and Viazzo PP, Editors. 1997. *The Decline of Infant and Child Mortality: The European Experience: 1750–1990*. Cambridge, MA: Kluwer Law International.

Crosby A. 1972. *The Columbian Exchange: The Biological and Social Consequences of 1492*. Westport, CT: Greenwood Press.

————. 1993. *Ecological Imperialism: The Biological Expansion of Europe, 900–1900*. Cambridge: Cambridge University Press.

Cueto M. 2004. *El Valor de la Salud: Historia de la Organización Panamericana de la Salud*. Washington, DC: Organización Panamericana de la Salud.

————, Editor. 1994. *Missionaries of Science: The Rockefeller Foundation and Latin America*. Bloomington, IN: Indiana University Press.

Curtin PD. 1968. Epidemiology and the slave trade. *Political Science Quarterly* 83(2):190–216.

————. 1989. *Death by Migration: Europe's Encounter with the Tropical World in the Nineteenth Century*. New York: Cambridge University Press.

————. 1998. *Disease and Empire: The Health of European Troops in the Conquest of Africa*. Cambridge: Cambridge University Press.

Darling ST, Barber MA, Hacker HP, and Goldsmith R. 1920. *Hookworm and Malaria Research in Malaya, Java, and the Fiji Islands: Report of the Uncinariasis Commission to the Orient, 1915–1917*. New York: Rockefeller Foundation, International Health Board.

Deacon H. 2000. Racism and medical science in South Africa's Cape Colony in the mid- to late nineteenth century. *Osiris* 15:190–206.

Defoe D. 1722. A Journal of the Plague Year. http://etext.library.adelaide.edu.au/d/defoe/daniel/d31j/part1.html. Accessed February 10, 2008.

Dobson MJ. 1997. *Contours of Death and Disease in Early Modern England.* Cambridge Studies in Population, Economy, and Society in Past Time. Cambridge: Cambridge University Press.

Dubin MD. 1995. The League of Nations Health Organization. In Weindling P, Editor. *International Health Organisations and Movements, 1918–1939.* Cambridge: Cambridge University Press.

Engels F. 1845. *The Condition of the Working Class in England.* Translated by Institute of Marxism-Leninism. 1969 edition. Moscow: Panther Books.

Evans R. 1987. *Death in Hamburg: Society and Politics in the Cholera Years 1830–1910.* New York: Oxford University Press.

Farley J. 1988. Bilharzia: A problem of "Native Health," 1900–1950. In Arnold D, Editor. *Imperial Medicine and Indigenous Societies.* Manchester and New York: Manchester University Press.

———. 2004. *To Cast Out Disease: A History of the International Health Division of the Rockefeller Foundation, 1913–1951.* New York: Oxford University Press.

Fee E. 1987. *Disease and Discovery: A History of the Johns Hopkins School of Hygiene and Public Health, 1916–1939.* Baltimore, MD: Johns Hopkins University Press.

Florentino M. and de Góes JR. 1999. Crianças Escravas, Crianças dos Escravos. In Mary Del Priore, Editor. *História das Crianças no Brasil.* São Paulo: Contexto.

Foster GM. 1987. On the origin of humoral medicine in Latin America. *Medical Anthropology Quarterly* 1(4):355–393.

Frenk J, Bobadilla JL, Sepúlveda J, and López-Cervantes M. 1989. Health transition in middle-income countries: New challenges for health care. *Health Policy and Planning* 4(1):29–39.

Frenk J, Bobadilla JL, Stern C, Frejka T, and Lozano R. 1991. Elements for a theory of the health transition. *Health Transition Review* 1(1):21–38.

Gaspar DB and Clark Hine D. 1996. *More Than Chattel: Black Women and Slavery in the Americas.* Bloomington, IN: Indiana University Press.

Goodman N. 1971. *International Health Organisations and their Work.* Edinburgh: Churchill Livingstone.

Gorgas WC. 1909. The conquest of the tropics for the white race. *Journal of the American Medical Association* 52(25):1967–1969.

———. 1915. *Sanitation in Panama.* New York: Appleton.

Gourou P. 1980. *The Tropical World: Its Social and Economic Conditions and its Future Status, Fifth Edition.* Translated by Beaver SH. London: Longmans.

Guerra F. 1993. The European-American exchange. *History and Philosophy of the Life Sciences* 15(3):313–327.

Guilmoto CZ. 1993. The Tamil migration cycle 1830–1950. *Economic and Political Weekly* 28(3–4):111–120.

Haines M. 2001. The urban mortality transition in the United States, 1800–1940. *Annales de Démographie Historique* 1:33–64.

Hamlin C. 1998. *Public Health and Social Justice in the Age of Chadwick: Britain, 1800–1854.* New York: Cambridge University Press.

Harrison M. 1996. "The Tender Frame of Man": Disease, climate and racial difference in India and the West Indies, 1760–1860. *Bulletin of the History of Medicine* 70(1):68–93.

Harrison M. 1999. *Climates and Constitutions: Health, Race, Environment and British Imperialism in India, 1600–1850.* Oxford: Oxford University Press.

Haynes DM. 2001. *Imperial Medicine: Patrick Manson and the Conquest of Tropical Disease.* Philadelphia, PA: University of Pennsylvania Press.

Hernández Sáenz LM. 1997. *Learning to Heal: The Medical Profession in Colonial Mexico, 1767–1831.* New York: Peter Lang.

Hertz E, Hebert JR, and Landon J. 1994. Social and environmental factors and life expectancy, infant mortality, and maternal mortality rates: Results of a cross-national comparison. *Social Science and Medicine* 39(1):105–114.

Hobsbawm E. 1968. *Industry and Empire: An Economic History of Britain Since 1750.* London: Weidenfeld & Nicolson.

Howard-Jones N. 1975. *The Scientific Background of the International Sanitary Conferences, 1851–1938.* Geneva: World Health Organization.

———. 1978. *International Public Health Between the Two World Wars—the Organizational Problems.* Geneva: World Health Organization.

Hutchinson JF. 1996. *Champions of Charity: War and the Rise of the Red Cross.* Boulder, CO: Westview Press.

International Sanitary Convention of Paris. 1903. Paper read at 11th International Sanitary Conference, Paris.

Jones M. 2004. *Health Policy in Britain's Model Colony: Ceylon, 1900–1948.* New Delhi: Orient Longman.

Jordan W. 1968. *White Over Black: American Attitudes Toward the Negro, 1550–1812.* Chapel Hill, NC: University of North Carolina Press.

Kearns G. 1988. The urban penalty and the population history of England. In Brändstrom A and Tedebrand LG, Editors. *Society, Health and Population during the Demographic Transition.* Stockholm, Sweden: Almqvist and Wiksell International.

Kiple KF. 1989. The nutritional link with slave infant and child mortality in Brazil. *Hispanic American Historical Review* 69(4):677–690.

Knaut AL. 1997. Yellow fever and the late colonial public health response in the port of Veracruz. *Hispanic American Historical Review* 77(4):619–644.

LaBerge AF. 1992. *Mission and Method: The Early Nineteenth-Century French Public Health Movement.* Cambridge: Cambridge University Press.

Lanning JT. 1985. *The Royal Protomedicato: The Regulation of the Medical Profession in the Spanish Empire.* Durham, NC: Duke University Press.

López Sánchez J. 1987. *Finlay: El hombre y la verdad científica.* La Habana: Editorial Científico-Técnica.

Lorcin PME. 1999. Imperialism, colonial identity, and race in Algeria, 1830–1870: The role of the French Medical Corps. *Isis* 90(4):653–679.

Lyons M. 1992. *The Colonial Disease: A Social History of Sleeping Sickness in Northern Zaire, 1900–1940.* Cambridge: Cambridge University Press.

MacLeod R and Lewis M. 1988. *Disease, Medicine, and Empire: Perspectives on Western Medicine and the Experience of European Expansion.* London: Routledge.

Maglen K. 2002. "The first line of defence": British quarantine and the port sanitary authorities in the nineteenth century. *Social History of Medicine* 15(3):413–428.

Manderson L. 1996. *Sickness and the State: Health and Illness in Colonial Malaya, 1870–1940.* Cambridge: Cambridge University Press.

McBride D. 2002. *Missions for Science: U.S. Technology and Medicine in America's African World.* New Brunswick, NJ: Rutgers University Press.

McCaa R. 1995. Spanish and Nahuatl views on smallpox and demographic catastrophe in the conquest of Mexico. *Journal of Interdisciplinary History* 25(3):397–431.

McKeown T. 1976. *The Modern Rise of Population*. London: Edward Arnold.

McKeown T and Record RG. 1962. Reasons for the decline of mortality in England and Wales during the nineteenth century. *Population Studies* 16(2):94–122.

McKeown T, Record R, and Turner R. 1975. An interpretation of the decline of mortality in England and Wales during the twentieth century. *Population Studies* 29(3):391–422.

Moll A. 1940. The Pan American Sanitary Bureau: Its origin, development and achievements: A review of inter-American cooperation in public health, medicine, and allied fields. *Boletín de la Oficina Sanitaria Panamericana* 19(12):1219–1234.

Moulin AM. 1996. Tropical without the tropics: The turning point of Pastorian medicine in North Africa. In Arnold D, Editor. *Warm Climates and Western Medicine: The Emergence of Tropical Medicine, 1500–1900*. Amsterdam: Rodopi.

Notestein FW. 1945. Population—the long view. In Schultz T, Editor. *Food for the World*. Chicago, IL: University of Chicago Press.

Omran AR. 1971. The epidemiologic transition: A theory of the epidemiology of population change. *Milbank Memorial Fund Quarterly* 49(4):509–538.

Peard J. 1999. *Race, Place, and Medicine: The Idea of the Tropics in Nineteenth-Century Brazil*. Durham, NC: Duke University Press.

Pelis K. 2006. *Charles Nicolle, Pasteur's Imperial Missionary: Typhus and Tunisia*. Rochester: University of Rochester Press.

Pettenkofer MJ von. 1941. *The Value of Health to a City, Two Lectures Delivered in 1873*. Translated by HE. Sigerist. Baltimore, MD: Johns Hopkins University Press.

Postell W. 1951. *The Health of Slaves on Southern Plantations*. Baton Rouge: Louisiana State University Press.

Rigau-Pérez JG. 2004. La real expedición filantrópica de la vacuna de viruela: Monarquía y modernidad en 1803. *Puerto Rico Health Sciences Journal* 23(3):223–231.

Riley J. 1987. *The Eighteenth-Century Campaign to Avoid Disease*. Basingstoke: The Macmillan Press Ltd.

———. 2001. *Rising Life Expectancy: A Global History*. New York: Cambridge University Press.

Rodríguez ME and Rodríguez de Romo AC. 1999. Asistencia médica e higiene ambiental en la Ciudad de México, Siglos XVI-XVIII. *Gaceta Médica de México* 135(2):189–198.

Rosen G. 1958. *A History of Public Health*. New York: M.D. Publications.

Savitt TL. 1977. Filariasis in the United States. *Journal of the History of Medicine and Allied Sciences* 32(2):140–150.

Scott HH. 1939. *A History of Tropical Medicine, Based on the Fitzpatrick Lectures Delivered before the Royal College of Physicians of London, 1937–38*. Baltimore, MD: Williams and Wilkins.

Simon J. 1890. *English Sanitary Institutions, Reviewed in the Course of Development, and in Some of their Political and Social Relations*. London: Cassell.

Stapleton DH. 2004. Lessons of history? Anti-malaria strategies of the International Health Board and the Rockefeller Foundation from the 1920s to the era of DDT. *Public Health Reports* 119(2):206–215.

Stepan, NL. 1978. The interplay between socio-economic factors and medical research: Yellow fever research, Cuba and the United States. *Social Studies of Science* 8(4):397–423.

Szreter, S. 1988. The importance of social intervention in Britain's mortality decline c.
     1850–1914: A reinterpretation of the role of public health. *Social History of Medicine*
     1(1):1–37.
Temperley H. 1991. *White Dreams, Black Africa: The Antislavery Expedition to the Niger,*
     1841–1842. New Haven, CT: Yale University Press.
Textes juxtaposés. 1897. Conventions Sanitaires Internationales de Venise
     1892-Dresde 1893-Paris 1894-Venise 1897. Bruxelles: Hayez, Imprimeur
     de la Chambre de representatives.
Warren KS. 1990. Tropical medicine or tropical health: The Heath Clark lectures, 1988.
     Reviews of Infectious Diseases 12(1):142–156.
Watts S. 1997. *Epidemics and History: Disease, Power and Imperialism*. New Haven, CT:
     Yale University Press.
Weindling P. 1997. Philanthropy and world health: The Rockefeller Foundation and the
     League of Nations Health Organisation. *Minerva* 35(3):269–281.
———, Editor. 1995. *International Health Organisations and Movements, 1918–1939*.
     Cambridge: Cambridge University Press.
WHO. 2008. Control of neglected tropical diseases. http://www.who.int/neglected_diseases/
     en/. Accessed January 31, 2008.
Wolleswinkel-van den Bosch JH, van Poppel FWA, Looman CWN, and Mackenbach JP.
     2000. Determinants of infant and early childhood mortality levels and their decline in
     the Netherlands in the late nineteenth century. *International Journal of Epidemiology*
     29(6):1031–1040.
Worboys M. 2001. The colonial world as mission and mandate: Leprosy and empire
     1900–1940. *Osiris* 15 (Nature and Empire: Science and the Colonial
     Enterprise):207–218.
Zylberman P. 2004. Fewer parallels than antitheses: René Sand and Andrija Stampar on
     social medicine, 1919–1955. *Social History of Medicine* 17(1):77–92.

3

International Health Agencies, Activities, and Other Actors

WHAT IS INTERNATIONAL HEALTH?

This chapter explores the evolution of the principal international health agencies and their activities since the mid-20th century, describes the range and roles of other international health activities and actors, and lays out a set of current challenges facing international health.

Key Questions:

- What shapes the organization of international health?
- How have the various agencies and actors in international health and their activities evolved over the past half-century?

There is a dizzying array of organizations and people operating in the international health arena. Some, such as the International Committee of the Red Cross, first appeared over a century ago. Many others were established more recently, and new agencies and partnerships continue to appear on the international health stage. But not all of these offices and actors have equal significance. Three key sets of organizations were established in the wake of World War II (1939–1945) which have profoundly shaped international health ideas, activities, and developments: (1) the World Health Organization (WHO) and other United Nations (UN) agencies; (2) the World Bank and related multilateral financial institutions; and (3) bilateral aid and development organizations based in industrialized countries (mostly in former colonial powers).

Numerous other entities are involved in international health, including business interests—for example, the pharmaceutical and insurance industries—private philanthropies, and countless nongovernmental organizations (NGOs) based in virtually

Sidebar 3-1 Definitions

Organization—a group or organized structure of people working together with the aim of achieving collective goals.

Agency—an organization with a defined purpose, often administratively related to or subsumed under a larger governmental or intergovernmental structure.

Multilateral—denoting the involvement of three or more nations (i.e., a multilateral agency).

Bilateral—denoting the involvement of two nations (i.e., a bilateral agency).

International—relating to activities or relations between two or more nations; also connoting interaction that reaches beyond national boundaries.

Program—an umbrella structure (often overseen by an agency or organization) involving several related projects, generally with a particular purpose.

Project—an endeavor with a defined time-frame and resources, designed to reach a specific goal.

NGO (Nongovernmental organization)—not-for-profit civic entity or network that is not directly related to government structures and focuses on a particular issue or purpose.

INGO (International nongovernmental organization)—NGO that works internationally or transnationally.

PPP (Public–private partnership)—collaborative entity involving both public and private sector organizations.

Foundation—a tax-exempt nonprofit organization, usually supported by a philanthropic endowment.

Function—role, actions, and activities (of a particular organization).

Fund—a sum of money collected and set aside for a particular purpose, and/or the entity that administers it.

every country, as well as joint initiatives on the part of several agencies. Two of the most influential international health players appeared on the scene since the last edition of this book was published in 1999: the Bill and Melinda Gates Foundation; and the Global Fund to Fight AIDS, Tuberculosis and Malaria. Bolstered by the voices of experts, business leaders, politicians, and even celebrities, they have helped place international health on the global political agenda. As we shall see, most of the aforementioned agencies share an approach to health based on "North-to-South" aid derived from donor agendas and cost-effective technical control of the issues they deem priorities.

Indeed, the term "international health" is a bit of a misnomer. The vast majority of international health work is not shared among nations as equivalents, but rather reflects the prevailing international political and economic order, whereby international assistance is "provided" by wealthy, industrialized countries and "received" by poor, underdeveloped countries. Yet high-income countries have their health needs addressed domestically through their own democratically established institutions. They do not have foreigners interfering or "helping" them organize health services; for example, there are no Zambian agencies providing health care to Swiss citizens in NGO-run clinics. As such, it is essential to understand that international assistance reflects geopolitical relations and reproduces dominant imbalances of power and resources.

Still, large multilateral, bilateral, private, and nongovernmental entities are not the only international health actors. Many other health organizations, with far smaller budgets but often sizeable memberships, have emerged in recent decades. Based in both industrialized and underdeveloped settings, these include community action NGOs, human rights organizations, activist and advocacy movements, as well as organizations promoting alternative models of health and welfare provision. Many of these groups agree on the importance of local priority-setting and advocate an integrated social, political, and technical approach to health and health care in the context of economic redistribution and meeting human needs. For example, the People's Health Movement (PHM), founded in Bangladesh in 2000, operates via grassroots and international campaigns on the right to health and health care, women's health, and through activism and advocacy, on issues of global health governance and accountability. Social justice actors insist that the ultimate aim of international health is for sovereign states to be in a position—economically and politically—to provide services to meet their own people's needs (or, in the interim, to receive aid without prescriptions as to how and on what it should be spent).

With the political and human welfare stakes of international health so high, it is essential to understand the diverse range of players and activities and their basic structures, influences, and parameters (Lee, Buse, and Fustukian 2002). Here we present a panorama of organizations and actors involved in international health: those with a direct mandate for health; those that provide public health and health care services through public and private channels; and those that influence the determinants of health, including international financial and trade agencies as well as social justice and health organizations (see Table 3–1). We pay closest attention to those agencies which, past and present, have had the greatest bearing on international health policy making and practice, including the WHO, the World Bank, bilateral agencies, and foundations.

THE EVOLUTION OF INTERNATIONAL HEALTH AFTER WORLD WAR II

By the 1930s, international health activities were being carried out by a delimited set of agencies—OIHP, LNHO, PASB, and RF (see Chapter 2)—largely focused on the health dimensions of migration, trade, and commercial stability, but with burgeoning cooperative activities relating to standardization, epidemic control, and public health policy. While fragile, these agencies drew legitimacy from the growing public health armamentarium in fields such as bacteriology and parasitology. At the same time, some of these efforts were influenced by social medicine movements aimed at improving living and working conditions.

International health agencies and activities were also shaped by the larger political context. For several centuries until just 50 years ago, the world—and international health—was characterized by large imperial blocks: rival powers in Europe, North America, and Australasia; colonized regions (Africa, the Caribbean, South Pacific, much of Asia); and regions that were economically dominated by imperial powers, but either had gained independence or were never colonized (Latin America and parts of Asia). Each imperial power had its own health office, charged with control of epidemics, medical care organization, and infrastructure, often bolstered by "tropical health" research institutes and the activities of religious missionaries. Both the world political order and the organization of international health would undergo profound changes in the aftermath of World War II.

The first half of the 20th century was a wretched time for most of the world's people. World War I and the Russian Civil War left much of Europe devastated. The 1918 influenza pandemic killed some 50 million people, almost half of whom were already facing famine in Assam and other parts of colonial India. The economic turmoil, hyperinflation, depression, and unemployment of the 1930s were followed by the rise of fascism and the world's most brutal war to defeat it. By the 1940s, many leaders within and outside the United States had learned a painful lesson from U.S. isolationism during the interwar years and realized that, for any major power, such a policy was ultimately self-defeating.

The intense collaboration undertaken to defeat the Axis Powers during World War II and to rebuild after the war, helped U.S. and Western European planners envision a future of international economic and political stability through new institutions and policies. Immediate attention was given to the reconstruction of industries and economies ravaged by the war and assuring monetary stability and realistic exchange rates in order to promote orderly international investment and commerce. Thus, the new postwar institutions initially emphasized the recovery of Europe, the formulation of trade policies, and currency stabilization; but they soon turned to issues of international cooperation, health, and social development.

Box 3–1 Eras of International Health Activity

- Meeting and Greeting, 1851–1902: early meetings and agreements on the need to share information on epidemic outbreaks and enforce quarantine during the imperial era
- Institution-Building, 1902–1939: first international health agencies established; sanitary treaties signed; incipient international health research/education; disease campaigns
- Bureaucratization and Professionalization, 1946–1970: permanent health organizations founded; large scale training of personnel; global disease campaigns in the context of the Cold War
- Contested Success, 1970–1985: vertical campaigns (i.e., smallpox) versus horizontal health and social infrastructure efforts (e.g., primary health care)
- Evidence and Evaluation, 1985–present: demand for measurable successes and "evidence-based" interventions; reinforcement of technical and cost-effective disease control efforts; renewal of alternate paradigm stressing social justice, infrastructure, human rights

Source: Adapted from Birn (2009).

The Role of the UN

In 1944, a year before the end of World War II, the U.S. government organized the UN Monetary and Financial Conference in Bretton Woods, New Hampshire, inviting representatives from 43 countries to attend. While more than half of the countries were from underdeveloped regions, their bargaining power was negligible and they wielded minimal influence over the decisions made.

The main outcomes of the conference were the establishment of the International Monetary Fund (IMF), to focus on macroeconomic policy and, eventually, provide loans conditional on adoption of anti-inflationary and international payment policies (particularly for underdeveloped countries), and the International Bank for Reconstruction and Development (IBRD), more commonly called the World Bank, to provide loans for particular development projects in areas such as infrastructure and agriculture. An international trade organization was planned but failed to achieve ratification at the time.

The origin of the UN system stems from the "Declaration by United Nations" of January 1, 1942, when representatives of 26 nations pledged to continue fighting against the Axis Powers. In 1944, representatives of China, the Soviet Union, the United Kingdom, and the United States developed plans for the UN, culminating in the creation of the UN Charter by representatives of 50 countries who met in San Francisco from April to June 1945.

When the charter of the UN came into force in 1945, it recommended the establishment of a specialized health agency with wide powers. An international health conference, convened in New York in 1946, produced the Constitution of the WHO (discussed ahead), which was ratified by 26 UN member states (a majority) on April 7, 1948. This date is commemorated annually as World Health Day. Between 1946 and 1948 an Interim Commission began the work of the WHO. Based on certain new ideas and democratic organizing principles, the WHO also drew personnel and practices from existing international health agencies, including the LNHO and RF. As of 1943, the UN Relief and Rehabilitation Administration (UNRRA) had been organized to provide food, shelter, and other aid to displaced persons and refugees; UNRRA's health division, which coordinated with the remnants of the prewar international health agencies, was also an important influence on the WHO.

During this period, international health was not only institutionalized at the WHO. Extensive colonial medical and health systems were replaced by powerful bilateral development agencies and in the case of the British Commonwealth, the Colombo Plan. Although some organizations, such as the Rockefeller Foundation, greatly reduced their role in international health in the 1950s, new entities were formed and other previously prominent players later resurfaced.

Many supporters of UN agencies viewed international cooperation idealistically— as a means of preventing war and freeing humanity from widespread misery; sadly the UN's mandate would prove less sanguine. Moreover, the powers that established the UN machinery harbored no such optimistic illusions. From the start, the

UN was designed to maintain the international balance of power, under the control of a handful of large countries.

From the Colonial Legacy in Health to the Cold War

Relations among the imperial blocks changed fundamentally after World War II, as explicit colonialism was replaced with a less politically volatile and less costly (to the imperial powers) division of world power. Decolonization came first in Asia, beginning with the retreat of Japanese armies. By 1950 British rule over India, Pakistan, Burma, and Sri Lanka, and French colonization of Laos and Cambodia, had essentially ended. In the ensuing decades dozens of African colonies achieved independence, many after bitter and bloody struggles. These new countries—most denuded of resources and facing enormous population needs—were generally superimposed on the borders of former colonies, which had been established with little regard for historical, cultural, and political affinities. From the start, many recently independent nation-states were tugged at from above by former colonial powers and by the demands of intergovernmental organizations; from below by their own citizens with varying ethnic, religious, and political allegiances; and by neighboring countries. With weakened self-government, a skeletal civil service, shortage of trained staff in all fields, and few resources, the new countries assumed the responsibility of providing services to their populations.

A complex of affiliations among sovereign nations emerged, marked by a mix of hope, economic growth, destructive civil wars, occasional solidarity, paternalistic "development," and continued political and economic hegemony. Indeed, former colonial powers (most notably the British in India) learned that it was far cheaper and more efficient to have national elites serve as political and economic intermediaries in the continued exploitation of labor and resources. Dominant powers (countries in Europe and North America, Japan, and Australia) individually and collectively cultivated new kinds of arrangements with emerging countries—the Commonwealth, La Francophonie, and so on, as well as through regional associations and multilateral agencies—that nonetheless preserved the prior imbalances of power. Occasionally, developing country-led alliances based on oil (OPEC) and/or regional and political affinities managed to challenge these arrangements, forming separate relationships of power (most notably the nonaligned movement).

As the imperial system gave way to a new political and economic order, the international health field and its key institutions were shaped by two factors: (1) the context of the Cold War—the political and ideological contest between Western capitalism and Soviet communism—which lasted from 1946 to 1991; and (2) the paradigm of economic development, which was perceived as the sole path of progress for countries in Asia, Africa, and Latin America. The Cold War competition for allies led both Western (U.S.-led) and Eastern (Soviet-led) bloc countries to employ strategic forms of military aid, health and infrastructure support, and training under the guise of development assistance. The development prerogative emphasized modernization, state-building (including support for education, roads, hospitals, etc.), and industrialization. The dominant approach of the international health field, with its biomedical bias, focus on disease eradication rather than holistic well-being, and agenda-setting by the powerful, became institutionalized during this era.

Although this development model was pervasive, alternative paradigms did emerge. The 1955 Bandung (Indonesia) Conference gathered leaders from the newly decolonized nations of Africa and Asia who sought to challenge neocolonialism and structure developing country cooperation "on the basis of mutual interest and respect for national sovereignty" (Group of 77 2007). Seven years later, the non-aligned movement (countries not aligned with the United States or the USSR) was created, and in 1964 the Group of 77 (now 130 countries) was formed—the largest intergovernmental organization of developing states within the UN. The G-77 has since articulated and advocated for the collective economic needs of developing countries, including fair terms of trade. This concern was institutionalized at the UN through the General Assembly's Conference on Trade and Development (UNCTAD). In the 1970s, UNCTAD gave voice to the principal project of southern, underdeveloped countries—the formation of a New International Economic Order (NIEO), an effort adopted in principle by the UN General Assembly in 1974 (though with extreme reservations by developed countries). The NIEO and its accompanying Charter of Economic Rights and Duties of States call for full and permanent sovereignty over natural resources and economic activities, including the right to nationalize foreign-owned property, to form primary producer cartels, and to establish price supports for developing country commodity exports. Though heavily resisted by powerful countries, the NIEO has helped shape ideas and efforts around social and economic justice, including, as we shall see, an international movement for primary health care (PHC) (Centre Tricontinental, Gresea, and Editions Syllepse 2007).

In sum, notwithstanding hopes on the part of many for a new world based on *bona fide* cooperation, the Cold War led Western and Eastern blocs to compete for power and influence throughout the developing world. International health became a pawn in this chess game, with multilateral institutions and the largest bilateral agencies calling many—but not all—of the shots.

CURRENT SNAPSHOT OF INTERNATIONAL HEALTH ACTORS, AGENCIES, AND PROGRAMS

Key Questions:

- Who are the major players in international health?
- What political, economic, and ideological rationales guide their policies and activities?

International health agencies and actors may be characterized according to their sources of funding, their influence over the local, regional, and global agenda, their relationship to other global agencies and priorities, their accountability and breadth of membership, their aims, motivations and values, their arena of activity, and their approach to improving health and well-being. Other important features include technical capacity, political legitimacy, whether staff is voluntary or paid, and historical trajectory (see Table 3–1). Here we classify them according to source of funding, mission, scope of activities, and their role and influence in the field. We include actors that operate in the health services sector and those that affect various social determinants of health, including economic and social policy.

Table 3–1 Typology of International Health Actors, Agencies, and Programs

Type	Examples
Multilateral International Agencies	World Health Organization (WHO), UN Agencies
International Financial and Economic Institutions	World Bank, International Monetary Fund (IMF), World Trade Organization (WTO)
Bilateral Aid and Development Agencies	European Community Humanitarian Aid (ECHO), United States Agency for International Development (USAID), Canadian International Development Agency (CIDA)
South-to-South Aid	Ministerio de relaciones exteriores (Cuba), Bolivarian Alternative for the Americas (ALBA), India-Brazil-South Africa (IBSA) trilateral agreement
Contract Providers and Consulting Agencies	Management Sciences for Health, John Snow, Health Systems Trust
Technical Agencies	Royal Netherlands TB Association, Centers for Disease Control and Prevention (CDC), European Centre for Disease Prevention and Control
Regional Cooperative Organizations	Organization for Economic Cooperation and Development (OECD), Southern African Development Community (SADC), African Union, European Union (EU)
Foundations	
The Old Guard	Rockefeller Foundation, Ford Foundation, Wellcome Trust
The New Guard	Bill and Melinda Gates Foundation, William J. Clinton Foundation
Corporate Foundations	Shell, Levi Strauss, ExxonMobil
Developing Country Foundations	Aga Khan Foundation, Carso Health Institute
Public–Private Partnerships (PPPs)	Global Fund to Fight AIDS, Tuberculosis and Malaria, GAVI Alliance, Stop TB Partnership
Business Interests	PepsiCo, Big Pharma, Merck, insurance companies

(continued)

Table 3–1 Continued

Type	Examples
Missionaries and Religious Agencies and Charities	World Vision, Diakonia, Mennonite Central Committee, Hadassah, Islamic Relief Worldwide
Nongovernmental Organizations (NGOs)	
Large Humanitarian NGOs	Save the Children, CARE
Relief Groups	National Societies of the Red Cross & Red Crescent, International Rescue Committee
Social Rights/Service Provision NGOs	Oxfam, Médecins Sans Frontières (MSF), Partners In Health, Doctors for Global Health
Human Rights and Health Groups	Physicians for Human Rights, Amnesty International, Dignitas International
Developing Country NGOs	BRAC, Urmul Trust, Grameen Bank, Jamkhed Comprehensive Rural Health Project
International Health and Development Think Tanks	Center for Global Development, Overseas Development Institute
Advocacy Groups/Campaigns	Equinet, Treatment Action Campaign, Global AIDS Alliance, Focus on the Global South
Social and Political Movements	People's Health Movement (PHM), International Labor Rights Forum, World Social Forum
University and Hospital Collaborations	Harvard Initiative for Global Health, Emory Global Health Institute, Latin American School of Medicine (ELAM), Aga Khan University
Research Institutions	National Institutes of Health, Institut Pasteur, Medical Research Council, Fundação Oswaldo Cruz, ICDDR,B
Research Alliances	Council on Health Research for Development (COHRED), Global Forum for Health Research
Professional Membership Organizations	Global Health Council, ALAMES, World Federation of Public Health Associations
Smaller-Scale and Individual Efforts	Kiva, GlobalGiving

Multilateral Agencies with a Health Focus

These largely UN-aligned agencies, with membership of most countries, are aimed at aid, cooperation, the provision of technical assistance, and the setting of international norms and standards. Funded multilaterally, with differential donation levels based on national capacity and interest, many of these agencies are governed through quasi-democratic decision-making processes, though larger donors often hold more sway. Several multilateral agencies are focused exclusively or largely on public health (most notably the WHO and UNAIDS), while others—such as the UNEP and ILO—have different mandates, though their work bears significantly on health. Table 3–2 lists a selection of UN organizations.

A number of autonomous specialized agencies are also linked to the UN through specific agreements (see Table 3–3). These organizations help set standards, formulate

Table 3–2 Selected UN Organizations

Organization	Function
UN Development Programme (UNDP)	The UN's largest source of grants for sustainable human development
	Facilitates technical cooperation
UN Children's Fund (UNICEF)	Lead UN organization working for the survival, protection, and development of children
	Programs focus on immunization, primary health care, nutrition, maternal health, and basic education
UN Environment Programme (UNEP)	Encourages sound environmental practices
UN High Commissioner for Refugees (UNHCR)	Protects the security and well-being of refugees
World Food Programme (WFP)	Largest international food aid organization for emergency relief; also operates as part of development programs
UN Population Fund (UNFPA)	Provides population assistance to developing countries
UN Human Settlements Programme (UN-HABITAT)	Assists people living in health-threatening housing conditions
UN Conference on Trade and Development (UNCTAD)	Promotes fair international trade, particularly by addressing concerns of developing countries
UNAIDS	Coordinates the UN's efforts to battle HIV/AIDS
UN Office of the High Commissioner for Human Rights (OHCHR)	Promotes and protects the rights established in the UN Charter and in international human rights laws and treaties

Table 3–3 Selected Autonomous UN Specialized Agencies

Agency	Function
World Health Organization (WHO)	See Box 3–2
International Labour Organization (ILO)	Sets and monitors employment standards
Food and Agriculture Organization (FAO)	Helps raise levels of nutrition, improve agricultural productivity and food security, and better the conditions of rural populations
UN Educational, Scientific, and Cultural Organization (UNESCO)	Promotes education, cultural development, protection of the world's natural and cultural heritage, and press freedom and communication
International Fund for Agricultural Development (IFAD)	Mobilizes financial resources for better food production and nutrition among the poor in developing countries
UN Industrial Development Organization (UNIDO)	Promotes the industrial advancement of developing countries through technical assistance, advisory services, and training

policies, and provide technical assistance in their areas of expertise. The World Bank is among these UN specialized agencies.

While most UN agencies operate independently from one another, their in-country activities are meant to be complementary and they occasionally share in large initiatives. To promote international development, the UN declared the 1960s to be the Development Decade, and since then every decade has had a designated UN theme. One of the most salient to health was the International Decade for Clean Drinking Water in the 1980s. Although 1.2 billion people gained access to water by 1990, the goal of universal access to safe water and sanitation was not met; currently over 1 billion people have inadequate access to safe water and 2.6 billion lack appropriate sanitation (UNESCO 2007; WHO 2006b).

The UN has also sponsored or cosponsored numerous large international conferences relating to health, many of which are listed in Table 3–4. These conferences generate resolutions, declarations, and programs of action that can have significant bearing on social and economic policy. Though these documents are typically approved by most participating countries, the UN has no power of implementation or enforcement, leaving compliance as a matter of domestic politics.

UN conferences have achieved varying results. For example, the 1992 Conference on Environment and Development was co-opted by wealthy-country interests who prevented commitment to enforceable laws and allowed transnational corporations to adopt voluntary codes of conduct not subject to public regulation or control. The 1994 Population and Development Conference was important in shifting the focus from controlling reproduction in developing country populations to reproductive rights and to the health of the whole woman (not just her reproductive apparatus). The Beijing Women's Conference of 1995 similarly produced an extremely thorough declaration on women's rights—incorporating issues of poverty eradication, sexuality and reproduction, fair pay for work, the effects of armed conflict, racial and ethnic discrimination, natural resource management, and the special needs of girls—but its long-term record on progress in gender justice is ambivalent (Molyneux and Razavi 2005).

Similarly equivocal, the World Food Summit of 1996, while lauded for setting a goal of halving the level of chronic undernourishment, was also criticized for adopting the goal of "food security" (which focuses on short-term hunger alleviation and the use of agri-technologies such as GMOs and monocultures) rather than "food sovereignty"—the "right of peoples, communities, and countries to define their own agricultural, labor, fishing, food, and land policies which are ecologically, socially, economically and culturally appropriate to their unique circumstances" (La Via Campesina 2002).

More recently, the Millennium Declaration and the Millennium Development Goals (MDGs) were adopted in 2000 by nearly all UN member states with the aim of improving various dimensions of human well-being by the year 2015 (UN Millennium Project 2006). As will be discussed further in Chapter 4, these

Table 3–4 Major UN Conferences and Summits Relating to Health

Subject/Short Title	Year	Site
Application of Science and Technology for the Benefit of Less-Developed Areas	1963	Geneva
Human Environment	1972	Stockholm
Women (1st)	1975	Mexico City
Human Settlements (Habitat I)	1976	Vancouver
Discrimination Against Indigenous Peoples of the Americas	1977	Geneva
Primary Health Care	1978	Alma-Ata
Science and Technology for Development	1979	Vienna
Women (2nd)	1980	Copenhagen
Least Developed Countries	1981	Paris
Population (4th)	1984	Mexico City
Promotion of International Cooperation in the Peaceful Uses of Nuclear Energy	1987	Geneva
World Summit for Children	1990	New York
Environment and Development (Rio Summit; Earth Summit)	1992	Rio de Janeiro
Population and Development (5th)	1994	Cairo
Women (4th)	1995	Beijing
World Food Summit	1996	Rome
Global Warming	1997	Kyoto
Establishment of an International Criminal Court	1998	Rome
Fighting Landmines	1999	Maputo
Millennium Summit	2000	New York
World Conference against Racism and Related Intolerance	2001	South Africa
Problem of HIV/AIDS	2001	New York
Aging	2002	Madrid
Financing for Development	2002	Monterrey
Permanent Forum on Indigenous Issues	2004	New York
Global Road Safety Crisis	2004	New York
Disarmament	2005	Geneva
International Migration and Development	2006	New York
World Water Forum (4th)	2006	Mexico City
Convention to Combat Desertification	2007	Madrid

Source: UN (2007).

worthy goals—several focused directly on health—are not accompanied by strategies for addressing the underlying conditions of poverty and underdevelopment, and are thus unlikely to be reached, especially in Africa.

The World Health Organization

The WHO is generally considered the flagship international health organization. Founded as an independent agency within the UN, the WHO's membership grew rapidly as newly independent states joined the organization: it now includes 193 countries (all except Taiwan, which used to be a member but was replaced in the UN system by China in 1971[1]).

Functions

The mission of the WHO is spelled out in Article 1 of its Constitution: "the attainment by all peoples of the highest possible level of health." Its specific functions, listed in article 2 (and Box 3–2), are no less ambitious.

Box 3–2 Functions of the WHO

- To act as the directing and coordinating authority on international health work;
- to assist governments in strengthening health services and emergency aid;
- to promote maternal and child health and welfare;
- to foster activities in the mental health field;
- to promote the improvement of nutrition, housing, sanitation, recreation; and of economic, working, and environmental conditions;
- to study and report on public health and medical care;
- to promote research and health training;
- to advance work to eradicate epidemic, endemic, and other diseases, and to prevent injuries;
- to propose conventions, agreements, and regulations, and make recommendations regarding international health matters;
- to standardize diagnostic procedures and revise as necessary international nomenclatures of diseases, causes of death, and public health practices; and
- to develop, establish, and promote international standards with respect to food, biologicals, pharmaceuticals, and similar products.

The work of the WHO is divided into two major categories: central technical services and services to governments. The central services include epidemiologic intelligence, development of international agreements concerned with health, standardization of vaccines and pharmaceuticals, and dissemination of knowledge through meetings of experts and technical reports. At the request of member countries, the WHO provides services through its six regional offices (see Table 3–5) and coordinates inter-regional and intraregional projects. The WHO headquarters in Geneva also coordinates the work of several hundred WHO collaborating centers, laboratories, and institutes throughout the world that provide expert advice and services. Among the most important is the Institute of Nutrition of Central America

Table 3-5 WHO Regional Offices

Region	Headquarters
Europe (EURO)	Copenhagen
Eastern Mediterranean (EMRO)	Cairo
Africa (AFRO)	Brazzaville
Southeast Asia (SEARO)	New Delhi
Western Pacific (WPRO)	Manila
The Americas (PAHO)[a]	Washington

[a] Founded in 1902 as the International Sanitary Bureau, then the Pan American Sanitary Bureau (PASB), it maintains more independence than the other regional offices.

and Panama (INCAP), founded in 1949 in Guatemala. Currently, the WHO has an international staff of 8,000 at headquarters, the regional offices, and 147 country offices. The WHO also establishes commissions specific to health topics—such as the 2000–2002 Commission on Macroeconomics and Health (discussed in Chapter 11), the 2003–2006 Commission on Intellectual Property Rights, Innovation and Public Health (see below), and the 2005–2008 Commission on Social Determinants of Health (discussed in Chapter 7).

Governance

Policy priorities and annual budgets are determined at the parliament-like World Health Assemblies (WHAs) held each May in Geneva, attended by delegates of all member governments, observers from affiliated NGOs, inter-governmental organizations (IGOs), and other agencies, and the 34-member WHO executive board (EB). Members of the EB are representatives of their national governments—balanced among the WHO regions—and serve 3-year terms.

　　The EB, which meets at least semi-annually, is responsible for preparing the agenda for the WHA, working on budgets, and facilitating the daily work of the WHO. The WHO is led by the Director-General (DG), who is elected by the WHA every 5 years and is subject to the authority of the EB. The current DG, Dr. Margaret Chan from the People's Republic of China, was elected in November 2006.

　　The EB may authorize the DG to take action toward combating epidemics, provide health relief to victims of a calamity, and undertake studies and research on urgent matters. It is important to note that the WHO can only intervene in countries when requested and that all resolutions *urge* but never *oblige* member states to act. WHO members are required to provide routine reports on domestic health conditions, and, according to the new 2005 International Health Regulations, must notify WHO headquarters in the case of important epidemic outbreaks (see Chapter 5 for details).

　　WHO country representatives (known as WRs) are assigned to a specific country (or cover several small adjacent countries) and typically work closely with national health authorities and other agencies and donors, assisting governments in reviewing health needs and resources, and planning, coordinating, implementing, and evaluating national health programs and policies.

Budget

The WHO operates with a fixed budget comprised of required member state contributions (made on a sliding scale based on national population and GNP) as well as extrabudgetary funds that are voluntarily donated by member states. The 2008–2009 budget is US$4.227 billion for the biennial period (i.e., approximately US$2 billion/year), an increase of 14% from 2006–2007. Many projects are paid for jointly by the WHO's regular budget, by the country concerned, and by funds from UN and private partners, as well as bilateral sources (WHO 2007b).

Extrabudgetary funding arrangements arose during the global malaria campaign of the 1950s (see below), when certain countries sought to donate more than their assessed quota to support the undertaking. After the World Bank expanded its involvement in international health in the late 1980s, large member states (most notably the United States) reduced their fixed contributions to the WHO, leaving its budget frozen.

With the decline in fixed budgetary contributions, the WHO began to rely more heavily on extrabudgetary contributions that are not subject to regulation and priority setting by the WHA. In essence, this has provided "donors" with the power to determine how their extrabudgetary funds are allocated and has led to funding instability and insecurity, as well as undemocratic policy-making processes. Moreover, unlike the 1950s–1970s, the WHO today is no longer the hub of most international health activity. Its current budget comprises less than 10% of total international health spending compared to a 1970s peak of approximately two-thirds of spending (Kates, Morrison, and Lief 2006).

Major Activities

The WHO's earliest efforts, even before it was formally established in 1948, involved the control of postwar epidemics in the Mediterranean region, most notably stemming a cholera epidemic in Egypt. It soon began other activities, including a campaign to control yaws through penicillin, the administration of BCG vaccine to children (against tuberculosis), and a large-scale fellowships program, which trained some 50,000 health workers in the WHO's first two decades (see Table 3–6).

Notwithstanding the dreams of health cooperation, Cold War tensions soon surfaced: Soviet bloc countries started pulling out of the WHO in early 1949 (returning only in 1957), claiming that the organization did little to address their own enormous postwar needs. These tensions spurred the WHO to demonstrate its commitment to improving conditions in underdeveloped countries.

VERTICAL DISEASE CAMPAIGNS In 1955, prodded by successes in malaria control in Latin America, the WHO launched the Global Malaria Eradication Campaign

Table 3-6 Major WHO Activities

Years	Activity
1946–1948 (Interim Commission)	Control of post-World War II epidemics
1947–1970s	Fellowships program, sponsoring more than 50,000 doctors, nurses, sanitary engineers, and other health workers for training fellowships
1950s	Mass BCG immunization to protect children from tuberculosis
1952–1970	Yaws campaign (with UNICEF): treated 300 million people in 50 countries, resulting in 95% reduced global prevalence
1955–1969	Global Malaria Eradication Campaign
1963	Codex Alimentarius created
1967–1980	Smallpox Eradication Campaign
1974–	Expanded Program on Immunization (EPI) launched, focusing on six diseases: diphtheria, pertussis, tetanus, measles, poliomyelitis, and tuberculosis
1975–	Special Program for Research and Training in Tropical Diseases started
1977–	Essential Drugs Program started with publication of first *Model List of Essential Medicines*; Health for All declaration
1978	Alma-Ata International Conference on Primary Health Care (with UNICEF)
1981	International Code of Marketing of Breast Milk Substitutes
1982–	Selective Primary Health Care/Child Survival Programs launched
1986–	Global Program on AIDS established
1986	Ottawa Charter for Health Promotion
1988–	Global Polio Eradication Initiative launched (with Rotary International, CDC, and UNICEF)
1990s–	Rise of public–private partnerships, e.g., Roll Back Malaria (1998–); Stop TB Partnership (2000–); GAVI Alliance (2000–)
1995–	Launch of DOTS program for TB control, reaching 30 million people
2000–2002	Commission on Macroeconomics and Health
2001–	Measles Initiative started (in partnership with the American Red Cross,UNICEF, CDC)
2003	Framework Convention on Tobacco Control adopted by World Health Assembly
2003–2005	3 by 5 Initiative, which aimed to get 3 million people on antiretroviral treatment by 2005 (not achieved)
2003–2006	Commission on Intellectual Property Rights, Innovation and Public Health
2005–2008	Commission on Social Determinants of Health
2007 (1951, 1969)	Implementation of new International Health Regulations (and previous revision years)

Source: Adapted from *WHO in 60 years: A Chronology of Public Health Milestones*, Geneva, WHO (2008).

aimed at eliminating the malaria vector, the *Anopheles* mosquito, through massive spraying of the powerful insecticide DDT, which had been developed during World War II. Malaria was then, as now, a major killer of children, especially in Africa (see Chapters 6 and 13 for details).

The malaria campaign was backed by the United States (which provided over 85% of the budget) and other major donors, who viewed it as a means of both fostering economic development and combating communism. The campaign followed military-style phases (planning, preparation, attack, consolidation, maintenance) to achieve malaria eradication, relying heavily on DDT rather than on the previous mixed approach of drainage, spraying, and chemotherapy. Within a decade, some three dozen countries in temperate zones in Europe and the Americas, as well as in warmer endemic areas in the eastern Mediterranean, Asia, and the Pacific, were freed from malaria. Yet by excluding sub-Saharan Africa—the world's most malarious region—from the global campaign (because malaria was deemed impossible to eradicate there) (Dobson, Malowany, and Snow 2000), the WHO set itself up for failure.

Moreover, problems of insecticide resistance to DDT, coupled with the campaign's indifference to basic health infrastructure, political concerns regarding the vertical structure of the campaign, and environmental resistance to the widespread application of DDT, led the WHO to abandon the eradication campaign in the late 1960s in favor of a control program (Packard 1998). The failure of its malaria campaign put pressure on the WHO to ensure success in its next endeavor.

WHO authorities found the ideal candidate in smallpox, a viral disease leading to blindness, facial pockmarks, and death of up to one quarter of people afflicted (see Chapter 13 for details on the campaign). With no animal reservoir and an easy-to-use vaccination technique (freeze-dried vaccine, jet injectors, and later bifurcated needles), smallpox eradication was feasible, albeit at a steep price, especially for "recipient" national governments. Starting in 1967, massive vaccination campaigns were carried out throughout the world by large teams of vaccinators who required minimal training. Ironically, at the launch of the campaign, smallpox incidence and mortality had already been declining for many decades thanks to widespread use of the vaccine; outside India and a few other settings, smallpox was not a significant health priority. The last known case of smallpox occurred in 1977 and in 1980 smallpox was the first disease to be declared completely eradicated.

The smallpox campaign, first proposed by the USSR when it rejoined the WHO in the late 1950s, has been touted as evidence of Cold War cooperation (Henderson 1998), and for three decades it has been hailed as the quintessential global health success—the pride of local health officers and international officials alike. However, the campaign was enormously costly to the (endemic) developing countries, who footed two-thirds of the bill. Still, it has saved money subsequently since smallpox vaccination is no longer carried out (although bioterrorist threats in recent years have raised questions, especially in the United States, about whether frontline health and military personnel should undergo vaccination). The smallpox campaign's technical approach disregarded—and was implemented at the expense of—far more pressing health needs, including water and sanitation, safe housing, education, and occupational health. Moreover, the campaign caused divisions between international and national authorities and experts, as well as within countries, particularly India (Bhattacharya 2006). The campaign was also dangerously coercive in some places in South Asia, leading to resentment of public health activities, and jeopardizing the ability of subsequent endeavors to reach certain populations (Greenough 1995). Given these circumstances, some have asked whether the end justified the means (Birn 2009).

The Expanded Program on Immunization (EPI)   The WHO began the EPI in 1974, to cover six diseases (diphtheria, pertussis, tetanus, measles, poliomyelitis, and tuberculosis) for which proven vaccines were available. At the time only about 4% of people living in developing countries had been fully immunized against all six diseases. The program has evolved in close collaboration with UNICEF, which continues to furnish the vaccines and much of the supplies and equipment. Private funders, such as Save the Children, provide additional funding and logistical assistance. The goal of the EPI is universal coverage, ideally in the context of primary care or maternal and child health programs. Although vaccine coverage has more than tripled since 1980 for some diseases, it is estimated that more than 2 million deaths each year are vaccine-preventable—including the deaths of 1.4 million children under the age of 5 years (UNICEF 2005). While the EPI and other initiatives continue to work to improve "cold chain" technologies and thermostability for regions where refrigeration is difficult, the PHC underpinnings of vaccine campaigns have received little attention. Indeed, stagnating vaccination rates have motivated new vaccine campaigns against measles, and, most notably, against polio. Spearheaded in 1988 by Rotary International, the joint polio effort has now become the most expensive international health campaign ever, costing billions of dollars.

Essential Drugs Program   In 1977 the WHO established an action program specifying some 200 to 500 "essential drugs," including vaccines, salts, nutrients, and vitamins, to satisfy the baseline pharmaceutical needs of almost any population, with variations for diseases of local importance in different areas. Since its founding, the program has sought to ensure that essential medications are available and affordable to those most in need. The 15th *WHO Model List of Essential Medicines*, published in March 2007 (WHO 2007c), was expanded to include health technologies and traditional medicines. The list has helped numerous governments to develop pharmacopoeias, avoid dangerous drug combinations, and reduce reliance on expensive imports. However, the WHO has no control over global pharmaceutical marketing, regulations, and research practices: its 2006 Commission on Intellectual Property Rights can only recommend, exhort, and monitor. It has to rely on incentives, goodwill, and public–private initiatives to stimulate research and increase access to medicines rather than on more effective regulatory mechanisms (WHO 2006b).

More recent WHO initiatives, such as the Framework Convention on Tobacco Control, will be discussed in subsequent chapters.

Box 3-3 Primary Health Care and its Fates

In narrowly addressing one ailment at a time using technical tools, the malaria and smallpox campaigns represented vertical approaches to disease control. In contrast, horizontal (also known as upstream) approaches emphasize strengthening health systems and infrastructure, and integrating technical and social aspects of public health to improve overall well-being. While there was broad-based and longtime support for addressing such underlying health needs, they were not formally articulated as a priority until the late 1970s, when the WHO's primary health care (PHC) approach emerged out of a decade of advocacy and struggle. In September 1978, WHO (together with UNICEF) convened hundreds of high-level government and NGO representatives at the International Conference on Primary Health Care in Alma-Ata, USSR—its most prominent conference to date. The *Alma-Ata Declaration*, signed by 175 countries, called for health needs to be addressed as a fundamental human right through integrated social and health measures tailored to local conditions, and by tackling the underlying economic, political, and social causes and context of ill health (see Chapter 12 for more details). Drawing from the principles of the NIEO, this joint call for "urgent and effective national and international action to develop and implement primary health care throughout the world" in order to achieve "health for all by the year 2000" (WHO 1978) represented an explicit alternative to international health's (and WHO's) existing reductionist disease-control modus operandi. The Alma-Ata conference and declaration entailed complex political negotiations at all levels. Using China's experience with barefoot doctors as an example, the declaration reflected the demands of health activists and developing countries, in part mirroring Cold War rivalries over the path the international health field would pursue.

Selective Primary Health Care and Child Survival

The heart of the Alma-Ata strategy—a commitment to addressing the roots of leading health problems, including food supply, basic sanitation, and social and economic inequality, from a community-based, primary-care approach—generated enormous discursive currency, but in practice it was quickly fragmented and criticized for being overtly political (Werner and Sanders 1997). In the wake of Alma-Ata, the Rockefeller Foundation sponsored a conference on *"selective* primary health care"—a technical approach based on vaccines and vector control—to replace the broad view of PHC, which was deemed overly ambitious and insufficiently cost-effective (Walsh and Warren 1979; Warren 1988). Selective PHC's (SPHC) promise of producing results led UNICEF, the WHO, and various bilateral agencies to work for several decades on a far narrower agenda than that envisioned by the *Alma-Ata Declaration*.

In 1984, a Task Force for Child Survival was established by representatives from the WHO, UNICEF, the World Bank, UNDP, and the Rockefeller Foundation to promote effective efforts at reducing morbidity and mortality among children. One prominent program was UNICEF's GOBI (Growth monitoring, Oral rehydration, Breast feeding, and Immunization) initiative—in its augmented form GOBI-FFF (incorporating Food supplementation, Female literacy, and Family planning). Child Survival and other SPHC programs had mixed success (child mortality declined much faster in settings where community-based PHC was adopted). Notably, SPHC programs failed to address long-term nutritional security and sanitation, focusing on ignorance and behavior change while overlooking the underlying causes of child mortality (Kent 1991). Another move away from PHC's emphasis on the structural determinants of health was the WHO's Global AIDS Program, established in 1986. The program defended the human rights of people with AIDS, but focused narrowly on providing information on disease transmission and behavior change, consistent with larger trends to assign individual responsibility and culpability for disease, rather than addressing the economic and social

(continued)

Box 3–3 Continued

context of HIV/AIDS. By this time there was no doubt that the United States and other wealthy interests deemed PHC and its call for a NIEO to be subversive, even revolutionary. PHC was all but abandoned. As we shall see in subsequent chapters, however, PHC and the Alma-Ata principles have inspired new movements in recent years.

By the early 1990s the international health tempest over top-down technological fixes versus locally controlled and integrated approaches left the WHO divided and under barrage. Extrabudgetary funds rose to over half of WHO's total budget and in 1990 World Bank health project loans surpassed WHO's budget.

The ideological tensions over PHC led WHO's largest donor, the United States, to withdraw much of its support. Formally, the excuse was that the WHO was inefficient, autocratic, and poorly managed (an accusation that might be leveled at virtually any bureaucracy). In reality, the opposite was true, at least in regards to PHC. PHC's public provision of primary care through social and economic redistribution was not only efficient and participatory, it threatened the dominant economic paradigms that had reemerged in the 1980s: deregulation, privatization, and government downsizing. With its budget in crisis, the WHO was no longer marshalling the bulk of the field's resources. Its mission was dispersed among other UN agencies, and it became "frustrated by turf wars" (Silver 1998, p. 728). A massive shift from public WHO programs to private influences transpired, through a multiplicity of alliances, partnerships, and initiatives that persist to the present (Brown, Cueto, and Fee 2006). As discussed ahead, these partnerships shrewdly draw on WHO for legitimacy, but many are controlled by actors who are not appropriate decision-making authorities and who have no public accountability. This development has also yielded enormous competition for private funds with little policy coherence.

In the 1980s, as WHO's primordial place in international health was being challenged, a new set of actors was already poised to take on a larger role.

International Financial and Economic Institutions

International financial and economic institutions (IFIs)—most notably, the World Bank, the IMF, and the WTO—are involved in setting macroeconomic policy and establishing and overseeing trade rules, as well as providing sector-specific grants and loans (employing incentives and conditionalities). These activities directly affect the delivery of health and other social services and indirectly influence health through policies relating to the labor market, employment, living, and social conditions.

In contrast to other multilateral agencies, IFIs are not democratically run: wealthier countries exert considerable power over decision-making processes and priority-setting. Yet IFI policies and programs have enormous global repercussions and have in recent decades played an instrumental role in imposing structural adjustment policies on developing countries. These policies emphasize the primacy of free markets, national and international deregulation, privatization of public assets and services, and a reduced role of the state (the genesis and implications of these neoliberal policies will be explored further in Chapters 4 and 9).

The World Bank

The World Bank Group includes two lending institutions for development and a tripartite investment arm, each with discrete roles:

- The IBRD provides 15 to 20 year loans to middle-income and "credit-worthy poor countries." To be eligible for IBRD loans, countries must fall below an annual income threshold (in 2007) of US$6,055 per capita. Interest rates are below commercial bank levels.
- The International Development Association (IDA) provides low-interest loans and grants to countries with annual income (in 2007) of less than US$1,065 per capita. As of 2007, US$3.5 billion was committed in support of up to 81 countries. Typically, IDA credits mature in 35 to 40 years, followed by a 10-year grace period before repayment of the principal.
- The International Finance Corporation promotes private investment in developing countries, with investments guaranteed by the Multilateral Investment Guarantee Agency, and disputes resolved through the International Center for the Settlement of Investment Disputes.

Bank personnel are grouped into four networks—the Human Development Network, the Poverty Reduction and Economic Management Network, the Environment and Socially Sustainable Network, and the Finance, Private Sector and Infrastructure Network—and six geographic regions: Africa, East Asia and the Pacific, Europe and Central Asia, Latin America and the Caribbean, the Middle East and North Africa, and South Asia.

Prior to 1980, World Bank loans supported mainly classic "bricks and mortar" infrastructure development projects. In the 1980s the Bank agreed to lend money directly to health projects, creating a Health, Nutrition and Population branch (HNP) from smaller precursor programs in nutrition and population control. Beginning with a loan to Tunisia in 1981 for health systems development, the Bank lent hundreds of millions of dollars for projects involving health financing, hospitals, pharmaceuticals, and nutrition, mostly in rural areas. Lending rapidly increased over the next decade (Ruger 2005). This new involvement was motivated by the perceived inefficiency of the WHO and the UN bureaucracy. Yet these same institutions are far more democratic than the IFIs, where decision-making and funding priorities are governed by a handful of large donors (see Table 3–7). The World Bank was also a partner in structural adjustment programs (SAPs), discussed ahead.

Under the World Bank's aegis, international health policy has emphasized efficiency, investment, and the predominance of the market. As the practical dilemmas of providing PHC to billions of people became more evident, the Bank turned to

Table 3–7 Voting Power as a Function of Shareholding

World Bank	United States	16.4% of votes
	Japan	7.9%
	Germany	4.5%
	United Kingdom	4.3%
	France	4.3%
	Five Country Total	37.4%
	Note: China, India, Russia, and Canada each have 2.8% of votes	
IMF	Similar pattern, with the United States holding 16.8% of votes	

Sources: World Bank Corporate Secretary. 2008. International Bank for Reconstruction and Development, Subscriptions, and Voting Power of Member Countries; and International Monetary Fund. 2008. IMF Members' Quotas and Voting Power, and IMF Board of Governors. Accessed September 5, 2008, from http://siteresources.worldbank.org/BODINT/Resources/278027-1215524804501/IBRDCountryVotingTable.pdf; and http://www.imf.org/external/np/sec/memdir/members.htm.

questions of financing and organizing health systems, to the chagrin of many public health advocates. Many detailed studies published by the Bank in the 1980s and early 1990s paved the way for its highly influential 1993 *World Development Report: Investing in Health*, which emphasized user fees, private sector competition, and cost-effectiveness as governing principles for the health sector (see Chapter 11).

By the mid-1990s the World Bank became the world's largest external funder of health, securing over US$1 billion in health-related loans annually (Ruger 2005). In the mid-1990s, total lending for all sectors was over US$20 billion annually, about US$16 billion of which were IBRD loans and US$6 billion IDA credits. The largest recipient of IBRD/IDA funding is India, which received US$3.7 billion in loans in 2006–2007 for 67 projects—with over US$2 billion for health projects. From 1970 through 2007 the HNP sector of the Bank lent US$27 billion to over 100 countries for some 850 projects and programs (with another US$5 billion for health activities carried out by other parts of the Bank) (World Bank 2007e).

Lately, the World Bank's position as preeminent international health financier has been partially displaced—due to the appearance of new players and initiatives, such as the Global Fund, the U.S. President's Emergency Plan for AIDS Relief (PEPFAR), and the Gates Foundation, but also owing to the failure of its prescriptions (Levine and Buse 2006). Nevertheless, in 2007, HNP issued a new 10-year strategy establishing health system strengthening as its top priority, despite having admitted that the prior strategy had not been systematically evaluated. Analysts have expressed alarm at this strategy, given the World Bank's role in furthering market-oriented policies that have deteriorated access to care for the poor and reduced health care "to a set of tradeable commodities" (McCoy 2007, p. 1500). The Italian office of Global Health Watch announced grave concern at this attempt "to institutionalize the role that the WB has de facto carried out in the last two decades, i.e. a 'global super health ministry'" (Maciocco and Italian Global Health Watch 2008, p. 47).

Other Development Banks

In addition to the World Bank Group, regional level lending is conducted by the Inter-American Development Bank (IDB), the Asian Development Bank, the African Development Bank, the Islamic Development Bank, and the European Bank for Reconstruction and Development. As well, the Caribbean Development Bank, the East African Development Bank, the Development Bank of Southern Africa, the West African Development Bank, and the Central American Bank for Economic Integration are funded by developing countries and provide loans to member states. While each of these banks has less capital than the World Bank, they all provide loans and grants in various fields, including health-related projects, and offer regional training and research programs.

The International Monetary Fund

Created in 1945, the IMF is charged with maintaining the stability of the international monetary system—the balance of payments (the financial flows for imports and exports, credit, and debit among countries) and the exchange rate system—to ensure economic growth and trade. It provides member countries with advice on how to avoid crises, technical assistance and training, and temporary financing when they are low on foreign exchange. With such promises of protection, most countries became members of the IMF (joined by the former Soviet republics in the 1990s), and its current membership stands at 185 countries with loans outstanding to 26 countries (IMF 2007a).

The IMF was relatively inactive during the early postwar years, as the various countries sorted out issues of liquidity and currency convertibility. After vigorous negotiations, access to IMF support in the form of loans was made conditional on adoption of certain anti-inflationary and international payments policies, particularly so for underdeveloped countries.

How and why conditionalities are controversial requires a bit of background. Sovereign governments cannot become bankrupt, and their assets and collateral cannot be seized by foreigners to satisfy debts. But governments can default on their obligations, causing problems within the country (e.g., leading government credit ratings to drop so that the cost of borrowing money to fund public infrastructure increases) and, especially, in international markets. In the early 1980s a deep economic crisis caused by rising oil prices and soaring interest rates left numerous developing countries with mounting debt. Mexico's 1982 announcement that it would renounce its foreign debt came as a bombshell to the international financial community (see Chapter 4 for details).

In accordance with its charter, the IMF swung into action to "stabilize" economies by rescheduling debt and providing short-term finance to restrain immediate balance-of-payment problems. Where additional money was needed, the World Bank joined the IMF in providing structural adjustment loans (SALs, better known as SAPs), defined by the bank as "non-project lending to support programs of policy and institutional change necessary to modify the structure of the economy so that it can maintain both its growth rate and the viability of balance of payments in the medium term" (Greenaway and Morrisey 1993, p. 242; Breman and Shelton 2007).

The IMF/IBRD loans are purportedly designed to help countries stabilize their economies, lower inflation, restore external balance, and survive a temporary economic crisis. The lenders impose conditionalities, saying in effect, "we will help you reorganize your debt and reschedule payments on your loans, but in order to get our money we insist that you do certain things." Conditionalities are time-specific targets negotiated (though more often compelled by the IFIs) between the IMF/IBRD and the borrowing government. The first conditions are to increase economic efficiency by imposing discipline and austerity on the government's operations, concurrent with trade liberalization. Typical strategies are to:

- decrease imports and increase exports;
- decrease consumption and increase production;
- decrease government expenditures;
- decrease subsidies to "inefficient" state-run businesses; and
- attain a more realistic foreign exchange rate.

The deregulation of foreign exchange usually leads to significant devaluation of local currency. With less domestic consumption and reduced trade barriers and tariffs, more goods can be exported to pay for essential imports, at least in theory. But devaluation also causes extreme pain to populations who suddenly wake up to find that their money has lost half or more of its value and they can no longer afford to buy food or pay for shelter.

A second set of conditions implemented through SAPs and subsequent strategies involves reform to government institutions and policies, including reducing the number of people employed by the government to provide social services, and privatization through selling off state-owned enterprises. The private sector, through purportedly open competition, is called upon to take on more of the functions previously performed by the state, resulting in loss of democratic control and accountability. Privatization hurts the population because services that were previously provided for publicly (water, sanitation, education, health, etc.) must now be paid for out of pocket, even as the real value of wages declines. As well, two essential public health functions are weakened—prevention and health promotion—because they are far less profitable than curative and medicalized health services.

As will be discussed in Chapter 9, SAPs and other loan conditionalities have imposed tremendous hardship on dozens of countries, undermining health and social development by reducing public education, health, and other social-sector spending, and often jeopardizing future economic security. Rather than stabilizing economies, the policies imposed have wreaked havoc by abolishing controls on financial flows and encouraging reliance on a single commodity for export earnings, leaving economies vulnerable to overnight crashes, as prices of copper, coffee, or cotton plummet. Moreover, the combination of unfair lending practices and the IMF's debt control measures have locked countries into "debt bondage," which is near impossible to escape (Toussaint et al. 2003).

Perhaps the highest profile critic of the IMF has been the Venezuelan President Hugo Chávez. In 2007, having paid off its debt to the IMF and the World Bank, Venezuela announced its intention to leave the fund (also terminating its membership in the World Bank), citing the inordinate power of the U.S. Federal Reserve and Treasury in IMF decision making, the negative historical legacy of IMF actions and activities (including supporting the effort to oust Chávez through a military coup), and discriminatory practices against the Venezuelan economy. In December 2007, Venezuela, together with the support of Brazil, Argentina, Bolivia, Ecuador, Uruguay, and Paraguay, created a "Bank of the South" (Banco del Sur) as an alternative to the IFIs. This South American development bank, with US$7 billion in capital, plans to focus on infrastructure and social development programs, rejecting the privatization pressures and conditionalities of IFI loans.

Cuba's longtime leader Fidel Castro similarly observed that Cuba's survival and ability to thrive despite the economic hardships incurred from losing Soviet trade advantages in the early 1990s, was due to its great privilege of *not* belonging to the IMF. By contrast, Argentina, which religiously followed IFI prescriptions through the 1990s, saw its economy teetering on the edge of collapse at the end 2001. The country's currency lost nearly 70% of its value, GDP dropped by 11% in one year, and the official poverty rate went from 38% to 53% of the population in the space of 6 months (Fiszbein, Giovagnoli, and Aduriz 2002). Argentina's impoverishment has been a boon to foreign investors and transnational corporations, who have bought up assets at cut-rate prices.

Box 3–4 International Health Aid in Nicaragua

Some of the problems relating to the political uses, duplication, and fragmentation of international health aid are evident in the situation of Nicaragua. During the long Somoza dictatorships of the mid-20th century, the United States dominated foreign aid, and the health and well-being of the population was abysmal: less than 30% had access to health care services, and Nicaragua remained the third poorest country in Latin America. Following the leftist Sandinista revolution of 1979, USAID, the IMF, the World Bank, and the Inter-American Development Bank pulled out of Nicaragua for political reasons. Several smaller Scandinavian aid agencies stepped in to provide aid.

Despite large-scale U.S. funding of contra rebels against the Sandinista government in the 1980s, the Sandinista redistributive and social welfare efforts had an enormous impact in just a few years, with improvements in education, literacy, and access to health care. Infant mortality, for example, went from 120 deaths/1,000 live births to 60/1,000. Still, the epidemiological effects of warfare exacerbated many health problems, including malaria in rebel areas, deaths and injuries from mines and rebel attacks, and war-induced shortages of basic necessities (Garfield and Taboada 1984).

(continued)

Box 3–4 Continued

Since the Sandinistas were elected out of office in 1990, warfare has subsided, but health and social conditions have deteriorated markedly. In the 1990s, structural adjustment programs were imposed on Nicaragua, with international financial agencies pressuring the Ministry of Health and other social sectors to privatize/decentralize. In these years overseas development assistance climbed to constitute between 25% and 50% of health spending. Because the Ministry had lost so much funding and personnel, foreign aid personnel posted to Managua became de facto division chiefs, running, for example, the maternal and child health office, the epidemiological surveillance unit, and so on.

Meanwhile health indicators quickly worsened with malnutrition mounting and infant mortality climbing back up to 83 deaths/1,000 live births in 1993 (Birn, Zimmerman, and Garfield 2000).

In recent years, donor funds—from Germany, Spain, the World Bank, IDB, and others—have fluctuated between US$700 million and US$1.2 billion, funding fully one-third of the national budget. While Nicaragua is one of just 20 countries to have had some of their debts "forgiven" through the Heavily Indebted Poor Country (HIPC) Initiative, this has come at the expense of quid pro quo financial reforms and social sector spending cuts. Indeed more than 50% of Nicaragua's bilateral aid goes to debt servicing.

Poverty Reduction and SWAps

Dissatisfaction with the minimal impact of many projects and the disruption programs cause to host countries has stimulated the development of a new approach to lending, variously called the sector-wide approach (SWAp), sector investment program (SIP), or sector expenditure program (SEP). Of all sectors, health has been at the forefront of this approach because of the urgency of problems, the large number of donor agencies and interest groups working in the sector, and the trend toward health sector reform (see Table 3–8).

The sector-wide approach aims to ease the host government's burden of coordinating the proliferation of donor activities and the accompanying reporting requirements. In meetings with donors, technical agencies, and NGOs, the various agencies accept responsibility for different aspects of the programs within the government's overall health sector strategy. The donor agencies in effect transform themselves into a consortium of health partners that agree to use common procedures for planning, implementation, monitoring, and reporting.

Rather than fund and implement specific projects run by a fragmented set of development agents, SWAps are an attempt to coordinate various actors on a particular issue or within a particular region in order to reduce duplication of service provision and develop a single, sustainable coherent vision (Cassels 1997). Ideally, SWAps are government-led and rely on local knowledge and methodologies (HLSP Institute 2005).

While SWAps have numerous advantages—among them giving greater priority-setting control to recipient countries—few donors participate (only nine countries had full SWAp programs as of 2004) precisely because they are unwilling to cede control.

Over the last decade, the IMF and World Bank have sought to address some of the criticisms aimed at SAPs. In 1996 they jointly inaugurated the Heavily Indebted Poor

Table 3-8 Recent IFI Development Strategies

	Poverty Reduction Strategy Papers (PRSPs)	Sector-Wide Approaches (SWAps) in Health	Heavily Indebted Poor Countries Initiative (HIPC)	Multilateral Debt Relief Initiative (MDRI)	Policy Support Instrument (PSI)
Main Actors	World Bank, IMF	IFIs, WHO, other health & development actors, national governments	World Bank, IMF	IMF, World Bank, IDB, African Development Fund	IMF
Year Started	1999	1997	1996	2006	2005
Countries Involved	Over 70 full reports as of 2008 Required from all countries wishing to borrow from the World Bank/IMF	9 countries as of 2004, several dozen more in various stages of preparation	33 countries as of 2008, with 8 additional eligible countries	40 countries eligible, 18 of which have received debt relief	5 countries as of 2007
Main Features	Demonstrate how governments will achieve poverty reduction and macroeconomic growth through 3-year programs, as "defined" by countries with participation from domestic and foreign stakeholders	National governments coordinate actors and funds in order to reduce duplication of service	Debt reduction for countries meeting the HIPC profile (and which have completed a PRSP); countries must adhere to certain policy conditions	Cancels 100% of debt from participating institutions for countries that have reached HIPC completion point (to help them achieve the MDGs)	Support for countries that no longer want or need IMF loans but seek its ongoing "advice, monitoring and endorsement of their economic policies" (IMF 2007b)

Sources: IMF (2008); World Bank (2007b, 2007d).

Countries (HIPC) Initiative aimed at making the external debt of some of the world's poorest and most indebted countries "sustainable," and thus protecting the integrity of IFIs. Though hailed for fairly and constructively addressing developing country debt, debt servicing increased 25% in HIPC countries during the first 3 years of the program and HIPC covers less than 10% of world debt. Moreover, according to critics, this initiative does not cancel debt but rather augments undemocratic, outsider control of economic policies, and the continued exploitation of local resources (Katz 2005).

The IFIs also joined the SWAp effort in 1997. In 1999 the World Bank and IMF jointly launched the Poverty Reduction Strategy Papers (PRSPs), whereby governments themselves design "pro-poor" efforts through consultation with domestic and international development stakeholders. These plans must subsequently be endorsed by the IMF and World Bank boards (Gwatkin, Wagstaff, and Yazbeck 2005, IMF 2008).

Yet to date the rhetoric is more promising than the reality. The HIPC Initiative, PRSPs, and SWAps are impeded by:

- short time frames that weaken long-term planning strategies;
- the strong influence of donors in determining priority setting, thus undermining local decision-making and planning capacities;
- conditionalities imposed by donors that are detrimental to overall health system development (Pettifor, Thomas, and Telatin 2001; Welch 2001; WHO 2004; Wamala, Kawachi, and Mpepo 2007).

The World Trade Organization

The World Trade Organization (WTO) was founded in 1995 as a permanent replacement for the General Agreement on Tariffs and Trade (GATT), started after World War II. The end of the Cold War, during which the goal of free trade was balanced against geopolitical concerns, gave way to this more powerful entity. The WTO administers trade agreements and negotiations, monitors and enforces trade policies, and resolves trade disputes among its 153 members. Over 90% of global commerce is governed by the WTO, which ostensibly promotes *laissez-faire* free trade, open markets, global competition, and nondiscrimination through eliminating import tariffs, lowering subsidies, and homogenizing rules and trade concessions. Of course this official view is one-sided—over the past decade the WTO has forced open the economies of poor countries, while rich countries have held on to tariffs and subsidies. Indeed, as historically borne out, "free" trade overwhelmingly favors rich countries at the expense of poor countries and, within countries, the rich at the expense of the poor.

Proponents of the WTO (those with large financial and business interests) claim that its policies have led to increased economic growth in developing countries, which according to the WTO could reduce poverty for as many as 144 million people by 2015. Critics (including unions and many civil society organizations) denounce the WTO for being an undemocratic, unelected international authority and blame its trade rules for causing enormous losses to local industries and jobs, for privileging multinational corporations over human lives, and for challenging and/or overruling national laws, regulations, and political processes. WTO policies have also led to continued destruction of the agricultural base of underdeveloped countries and impeded the development of an industrial base. Developing countries are pushed to concentrate on export earnings, based on one or two primary products used in manufacturing in other countries. Because of increased competition under the WTO by commodity exporters, exporting countries are vulnerable to significant changes in earnings.

The WTO and its policies affect international health through the Agreement on Trade-Related Aspects of Intellectual Property Rights (TRIPS), the application of sanitary/phytosanitary measures, and the General Agreement on Trade and Services (GATS), all discussed in Chapter 9.

Critiques of the IFIs

Over time, the IFIs have played an increasingly active role in developing country economies overall and in particular sectors, such as health. One set of critiques of the IFIs ties colossal and immovable poverty and immiseration in developing countries to IFI policies advocating deep cuts in social sector spending, privatization, unfettered trade, deregulation, and the ratcheting down of social rights. Another decries the undemocratic decision-making structures at the World Bank and IMF, which give far larger voting power to large donors (and pro-business interests) than to other members, constituting a form of neocolonialism. Several social movements, including Jubilee 2000 and 50 Years is Enough, call for the immediate dismantling of these institutions. We will discuss the implications of IFI policies in later chapters.

Bilateral Aid and Development Agencies

Key Questions:

- What motivates development assistance? Who benefits?
- What are the respective roles of donors and recipients?
- What is the impact of development assistance on health?

In addition to the programs and projects supported through multilateral organizations, most high-income countries maintain separate official development aid organizations to fund bilateral projects (i.e., those involving one donor and one recipient government). The greater part of official development assistance (ODA) comes from the members of the Organization of Economic Cooperation and Development (OECD), made up of various industrialized countries plus a smaller group of emerging economies. ODA is big business, with annual flows in the range of US$100 billion in recent years. At the OECD's Development Assistance Committee (DAC) meetings, representatives of the donors (22 countries plus the

European Commission) review and compare their respective national contributions to both bilateral ("foreign aid") and multilateral aid programs.

Bilateral donor agencies are official arms of the governments of many former (or current) colonial powers in Western Europe, North America, and the Pacific. Typically subsidiary to or dependent on foreign affairs and trade ministries, bilateral agencies sponsor a range of health and development activities in developing countries, usually through counterpart government channels. Collectively the largest source of development funding, these agencies are often in charge of channeling national contributions to multilateral and international financial agencies. Countries are targeted for health development assistance for strategic reasons, due to conflict situations, to address a particularly heavy burden of disease, and based upon historical and political ties. ODA makes up a significant percentage of smaller recipient governmental health expenditures, although larger recipient countries receive greater absolute amounts of aid.

Bilateral agencies—most established after World War II—are diverse in scope and focus (see Table 3–9). Some have a large personnel component actively involved in projects. Most sponsor, oversee, and assess rather than implement, usually operating through contracts with intermediary organizations including universities, research organizations, for-profit companies, and NGOs. Donor country motivations and policies regarding ODA vary widely. For instance, bilateral ODA may be limited to certain sectors, or even to specific activities that would not have been the first priority of the recipient country's government and people.

Typically the procurement of goods and equipment (or the use of airlines and other services) is "tied aid" (also known as phantom aid), restricted to spending in the donor country. The same holds true for the hiring of technical personnel to design or implement projects.

Indeed, most aid flows back to the donor country—approximately 90% in the case of the United States and France in recent years (ActionAid International 2005)—making it more of a domestic subsidy to the private sector than foreign assistance per se. According to the UNDP, "such arrangements cost developing countries up to 20 percent more than buying the same goods on the open market…the tied aid tax costs Africa alone $1.6 billion a year" (UNDP 2005, p. 2). The United Kingdom *ties* a somewhat smaller proportion of its foreign aid to domestic industry than other OECD donors. Nonetheless the United Kingdom, like the United States, Canada, and other donors, sells billions of dollars of military equipment to developing countries, often as an implicit quid pro quo for aid (Oxfam International 2004; McKee 2007; Wintour and Leigh 2007).

U.S. Bilateral Assistance

The United States is the largest bilateral donor in the world (totaling almost US$24 billion in aid in 2006) but lags far behind virtually every OECD country in the percentage of GDP dedicated to ODA (see Fig. 3–3). Its flagship development office, the U.S. Agency for International Development (USAID) was founded in 1961 from a U.S. State Department predecessor office, the International Cooperation Administration.

Table 3–9 Selected Bilateral Agency Budgets and Priorities

Agency	Budget	Priorities
UK Department for International Development (DFID)	£5.3 billion budget for 2007–2008	Poverty alleviation Commits support over multiple years, earning DFID high marks for effectiveness
Agence Française de Développement (AFD)	€3.5 billion for 2007	Works on poverty reduction, finances economic growth, and protects Global Public Goods, all within the framework of the MDGs
German Organization for Technical Cooperation (GTZ)	€1.06 billion for 2007	Works in a consulting role with developing countries, focusing on rural and economic development
Japanese International Cooperation Agency (JICA)	US$1.5 billion for 2007	Long-standing focus on supporting government and economic development; now shifting toward health and postconflict activities
Swedish International Development Cooperation Agency (SIDA)	SKR 15.5 billion for 2008	Rights-based approaches for poverty alleviation
USAID	US$36 billion for 2008	Economic growth, agriculture and trade Global health Democracy, conflict prevention and humanitarian assistance

Sources: Agency Web sites and Lane and Glassman (2007).

USAID carries out a variety of programs relating to child nutrition and child survival, health care financing, environmental health (sanitation), infectious diseases, and HIV/AIDS control.

Notwithstanding this array of activities, USAID's mission is to "Create a more secure, democratic, and prosperous world for the benefit of the American people and the international community" (USAID 2006). With this primary focus on advancing U.S. security and economic interests, much of USAID's work supports U.S. overseas business development and "democracy-building" activities, often aimed at opening developing countries to investment and trade (Ollila 2005a).

From 1965, USAID has prioritized population control (also known as family planning) among its international health activities. This has entailed expanding fertility control services through aid to government programs, NGOs, and the private sector, as well as supporting policy making, evaluation, biomedical research on contraception, and demographic research and data collection. To carry out these functions, the agency has provided over US$9.8 billion in population assistance to developing countries. Currently US$1.5 billion is spent each year by donor countries—led by the United States—on population aid, today far overshadowed by programs aimed at HIV and other priority diseases (Population Action International 2005).

While population aid has addressed certain important questions of birth spacing, women's reproductive health, and infant mortality, during the Cold War, the U.S.'s (and its allies') aims of reducing the size of developing country populations in order to defuse revolutionary, potentially pro-Soviet, pressures led many sterilization and contraceptive efforts to be coercive and insensitive. Population aid was also embroiled in controversies around "reproductive freedom" and abortion. Some programs were accused of following the cultural agenda of Western feminists regarding family size preferences. At the UN population conference held in Mexico City in 1984, the U.S. government announced a policy prohibiting support to organizations that provided or offered information on abortion (the "gag rule"). At the landmark 1994 Cairo population conference, feminists from around the world worked together to widen the scope of reproductive health, influencing the policies of many countries, including the United States. However, in 2001, following the election of a conservative government influenced by fundamentalist religious values, the U.S. government reimposed the gag rule, limiting contraceptive services to millions of women around the world. U.S. funding for HIV/AIDS, anchored by so-called faith-based approaches that emphasize abstinence and other fundamentalist precepts, has also come under fire. Brazil, for example, rejected US$40 million to combat AIDS because USAID required recipients to have an explicit policy opposing prostitution.

In recent years, various large-scale international (health) aid initiatives have been created directly out of the U.S. Department of State, indicating their close ties to U.S. foreign policy. Indeed, critics charge that the United States has increasingly prioritized the provision of aid based on relevance to U.S. national security (Hirvonen 2005). These aid initiatives include PEPFAR (see Box 3–5), the President's Malaria Initiative to increase funding for mosquito nets, indoor insecticide spraying, and antimalarial drugs, and the Millennium Challenge Corporation, founded in 2004 with a multibillion dollar budget to support "good governance, economic freedom" (providing grants that favor pro-growth private sector efforts in countries selected according to development, governance, and political criteria).

U.S. foreign aid has also become increasingly militarized, with the Pentagon controlling almost one-fourth of U.S. development assistance—US$5.5 billion in 2005 (Center for Global Development 2008). This is an extremely worrisome trend in that it justifies militarism, conflates peaceful with military goals, and may further jeopardize those who have suffered under military occupation or violence (see Chapter 8).

Box 3–5 PEPFAR

In 2003, U.S. President George W. Bush launched PEPFAR (the President's Emergency Plan for AIDS Relief), one of the highest profile bilateral health programs of recent years. PEPFAR is based in the U.S. Department of State, with collaboration from USAID, the Departments of Defense, Commerce, Labor, and Human Services, and the Peace Corps. With US$15 billion allocated for the initial 5-year initiative (and renewal legislation committing another US$37 billion for 2009–2013), PEPFAR

(continued)

Box 3–5 Continued

tripled the U.S.'s existing commitment to combat HIV/AIDS internationally. Focusing on 15 countries selected on the basis of political and strategic importance and HIV prevalence, the original plan aimed to provide treatment to two million people infected with HIV and prevent seven million new infections (now increased to 12 million with the renewal), with palliative care for 10 million other people with HIV/AIDS. Midterm assessments found that over 822,000 people (including 285,000 pregnant women), received antiretroviral treatment (ARVs), over 18 million were reached through HIV counseling and training sessions, and 2 million orphans received care (AVERT 2007). In its first 4 years, PEPFAR increased the number of people in Africa on ARVs from 50,000 to 1.2 million.

While PEPFAR has greatly expanded U.S. efforts against AIDS, the program has been criticized on a number of grounds by government and civil society reports. It has overlooked numerous countries with high or growing HIV prevalence and large numbers of sex workers and injection drug users. It has created almost no public health infrastructure, relying on temporary foreign and national health workers, many of whom have been hired away from other needed health activities (Institute of Medicine 2007). In focusing exclusively on HIV/AIDS, PEPFAR ignores other more pressing health needs, including sanitation, nutrition, maternal and child health, and basic health services (Salaam-Blyther 2007).

The original PEPFAR budget rules stipulated that at least one-third of prevention funding had to go toward abstinence (i.e., delayed onset of sexual debut) and "be faithful" (reduced number of concomitant partners) programs. While this requirement was removed in 2008, a report must now be sent to the U.S. Congress if in any host country less than 50% of funding is spent on abstinence and fidelity programs. Not only does this "faith-based" approach stifle prevention efforts, often through arcane funding rules, it is particularly insensitive to the needs and status of women and girls (Center for Public Integrity 2006). Moreover, abstinence programs show no evidence of preventing the spread of HIV (Institute of Medicine 2007). PEPFAR only supports condom distribution for "high-risk" groups (excluding young or married people, unless one partner tests positive for HIV) (Salaam-Blyther 2007). The program does not fund harm reduction programs for injection drug users and refuses to provide support to organizations that work with sex workers.

Although it was initially feared that PEPFAR would pay full prices for ARVs, to date the program has paid discounted rates negotiated by the Clinton Foundation. However, because PEPFAR relies on U.S. Food and Drug Administration (FDA) criteria for pharmaceutical approvals rather than WHO criteria, generic ARVs manufactured in developing countries at far lower prices were initially overlooked. This resulted in U.S. pharmaceutical profits having been prioritized over maximizing the number of people reached by ARVs. Under pressure from the WHO and countries receiving PEPFAR assistance, the FDA has begun a special approval process for generic drugs used by PEPFAR outside the United States; from 2005 to 2007 generics went from 11% to 57% of PEPFAR spending on drug procurement.

Still, PEPFAR has been unduly influenced by ideology rather than scientific evidence, limiting the potential impact of this initiative (Editorial 2006). Moreover, its one-disease focus has caused funding inequities, whereby diarrhea, malnutrition, respiratory diseases, and other ailments associated with extreme misery have been overlooked.

OECD Donor Comparisons

In 2006, OECD members provided US$103.9 billion in aid. Since 1990, although per capita income in the OECD countries has increased by US$6,000, development assistance from those same countries has in fact dropped by US$1 per capita (see Fig. 3–1). As shown in Figures 3–2 and 3–3 the U.S. government is the largest donor in dollar terms, but not as a percentage of GDP (OECD 2006b). In 2005 the United States spent US$27.5 billion in aid, of which US$3.5 billion went to Iraq, US$1.5 billion to the antidrug program in Afghanistan and US$4 billion to countries in sub-Saharan Africa. The only countries to meet or exceed the UN target of providing 0.7% of GNI in aid were Denmark, Luxembourg, the Netherlands, Norway, and Sweden (see Fig. 3–3).

Just 4.5% of OECD ODA is allocated to health (OECD 2006a), far shy of the 40% of all bilateral aid that goes to debt relief, emergencies, interest, administration, and technical intermediaries, rather than to actual development efforts (UNCTAD 2004). The debt–aid relationship is especially problematic for the poorest countries. Between 1970 and 2002, African countries borrowed US$540 billion, repaid US$550 billion and were still left with a debt of US$295 billion (UNCTAD 2004). In 2001, US$51 billion was provided in development aid, but debtor countries repaid more than sevenfold that amount (US$382 billion) in debt payments. In some countries, four times more is spent on debt repayments than on health and education combined. In total, "for every dollar received in aid, three go back to rich countries to service the debt," making debt "itself a major impediment to development" (Katz 2005, p. 179).

Although (health and) development aid purports to enable economies to thrive, bilateral agencies do virtually nothing to improve the terms of trade or pricing policies for export commodities, which are the key source of revenue for most developing countries. For example, in a typical year, coffee-producing countries earn just US$5.5 billion of the US$70 billion generated from the global retail sale of coffee, incredibly low returns for primary producers (UNCTAD 2004). If bilateral aid agencies helped to raise and stabilize commodity earnings for developing countries, they could potentially achieve far greater health and development gains than through assistance to in-country projects.

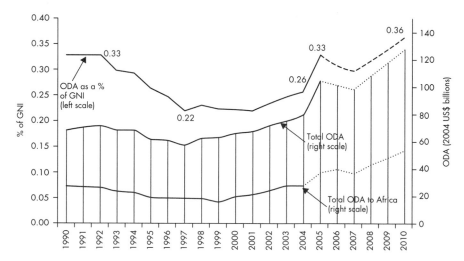

Figure 3–1 DAC members net ODA 1990–2004 and DAC Secretariat simulation of net ODA to 2006 and 2010. Credit Line: OECD Journal on Development: Development Cooperation—2006 Report—Efforts and Policies of the Members of the Development Assistance Committee Volume 8 Issue 1, © OECD 2007.

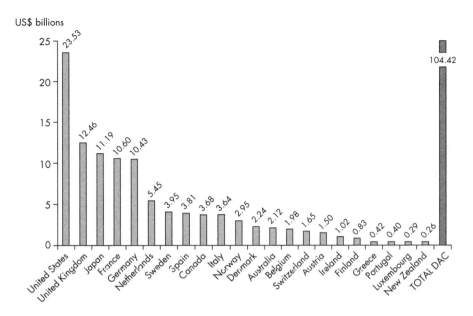

Figure 3–2 Net ODA in 2006: Amounts. Credit Line: Figure 1. DAC Members' Net Official Development Assistance in 2006, Net ODA in 2006—amounts (p. 9), FINAL ODA FLOWS IN 2006, Room Document 2, DAC Senior Level Meeting, 11–12 December 2007, © OECD 2007.

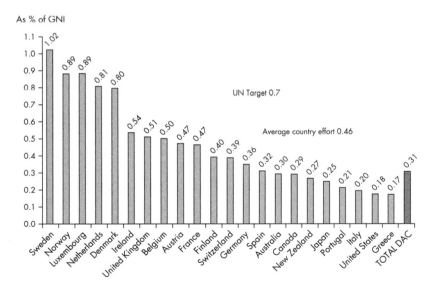

Figure 3–3 Net ODA in 2006 as a percentage of GNI. Credit Line: Figure 1. DAC Members' Net Official Development Assistance in 2006, Net ODA in 2006—as a percentage of GNI (p. 9), FINAL ODA FLOWS IN 2006, Room Document 2, DAC Senior Level Meeting, 11–12 December 2007, © OECD 2007.

South-to-South Aid

A growing number of developing and emerging countries are engaged in government-to-government health cooperation. Donors outside the DAC group with 2006 disbursements of over US$5 billion include Taiwan, the Czech Republic, Iceland, Israel, Korea, Kuwait, Latvia, Lithuania, Saudi Arabia, the Slovak Republic, and Thailand. Various countries, for example, China, Turkey, Venezuela, Cuba, and Brazil, are both aid donors and recipients. Perhaps most notably, beginning in the early 1960s, Cuba has sent medical missions to over 100 countries in Asia, Africa, and Latin America to aid in disaster relief, provide medical services in under-resourced areas, and offer health systems policy advice. Cuba also trains thousands of foreign doctors. Historically, the Soviet Union and other Soviet bloc countries were also deeply involved in health infrastructure-building efforts in developing countries and training foreign medical professionals, most notably at Patrice Lumumba Moscow Friendship University.

Venezuela has recently undertaken aid activities, primarily to other Latin American countries, in the form of debt relief and the provision of subsidized petroleum products. Venezuela also supplies subsidized household heating oil to marginalized populations in the United States. As well, in 2007 Venezuela donated US$4.6 million to the UN FAO for food security and drought prevention activities in Mali and Burkina Faso, the first time ever that a Latin American government funded an external FAO project (FAO 2007).

China has also increased its development assistance, particularly in the area of food aid. The US$5 billion China–Africa development fund provides loans and credits to Africa, together with US$1.27 billion in cancelled debts (Tull 2006). For some countries (such as the Sudan, Zimbabwe, and Cambodia) where—due to human rights violations, conflict, and governance concerns—major IFIs and OECD nations will not invest or send aid, China has become the major aid partner (IRIN 2006; Perlez 2006; Nyiri 2006).

Much smaller than Chinese development aid, Brazilian international assistance (US$15 million between 1998 and 2004) prioritizes South-to-South cooperation and mutual solidarity. Approximately one-third of Brazil's development aid is directed toward Latin American countries (Paraguay in particular), one-third to Portuguese-speaking African nations (Angola, São Tome and Principe, Mozambique), and 22% to East Timor. Aid is concentrated on education, agriculture, health (including supporting generic drug programs), alternative energies, and environmental issues. Brazil recently cancelled the outstanding bilateral debts of Mozambique, Tanzania, Mauritania, and Guinea-Bissau (Schlager 2007).

Other types of South-to-South cooperation are also materializing. South Africa provides aid to Mali and the Democratic Republic of the Congo (DRC), and in turn receives aid in the form of ophthalmologists from Tunisia to eliminate its cataract backlog. The Bolivarian Alternative for the Americas (ALBA) is a regional group that includes Bolivia, Venezuela, Cuba, and Nicaragua. Member states contribute funds, goods, and services to be used by other members (Wilpert 2007).

In 2003 the IBSA trilateral agreement among Brazil, India, and South Africa was formed "to promote South–South dialogue, cooperation and common positions on issues of international importance" (http://www.ibsa-trilateral.org/), including social development, information exchange, and economic cooperation. The IBSA working group on health focuses on epidemiological surveillance, sanitary regulations, traditional medicines, and intellectual property rights.

Contract Providers and Consulting Firms

Among the entities working in international health project planning and implementation are technical assistance and consulting firms. Some of these are mainline NGOs or have an NGO-like character, although most, for example, Abt Associates, John Snow Inc., Macro International, and Family Health International, operate on a for-profit basis. Large nonprofits include Management Sciences for Health (MSH), PATH (Program for Appropriate Technology in Health), University Research Council (South Africa), HLSP, and JHPIEGO. Many are based in industrialized countries—often concentrated in and around Washington, DC, London, Geneva, Seattle, and other cities with large donor agencies and have satellite offices in the countries where they are working. Similar organizations run projects in Africa and elsewhere, for example the African Medical Research Foundation (AMREF), based in Kenya, and the South African-based Health Systems Trust (HST). A large number of individual consultants in all areas of international health are employed on a subcontracted basis by such companies, which themselves receive contracts from bilateral and multilateral agencies. Other consultants work on short- or long-term contracts with development banks.

Although consulting firms, together with growing numbers of nonhealth specialist for-profit contractors (such as those operating in Iraq and Afghanistan as part of "rebuilding" efforts), are intermediaries rather than agenda-setters per se, they often play an instrumental role in project evaluation and in determining which programs are deemed successful by donors.

Technical Agencies

Some national disease-control agencies, notably the U.S. Centers for Disease Control and Prevention (CDC), the European Centre for Disease Prevention and Control (ECDC), and various European surveillance networks (such as Euro TB), are involved in providing technical assistance and capacity-building support to government disease-control programs in a variety of settings. The CDC also assists with international surveillance and cooperation efforts (e.g., TB control in Southern Africa and the former Soviet Union, malaria control, etc.), as well as outbreak investigations around the globe. Many para-statal organizations, including the European Medicines Agency (EMEA), the European Environment Agency, the Royal Netherlands TB Association, and the European Food Safety Authority play an essential part in global health by setting standards and maintaining networks with other international health agencies. While these are small efforts in the overall scope of international health work, they can serve a vital role in identifying disease outbreaks and supporting local efforts to stem them (e.g., CDC's role in identifying the neuropathy outbreak in Cuba in the early 1990s).

Regional Cooperative Organizations

Regional political and economic organizations have potentially powerful effects on health through specific trade rules, policy frameworks, and mutual priority-setting, as well as through direct aid programs. The G-8 (the United States, Canada, France, Germany, Italy, Japan, Russia, and the United Kingdom) wields enormous influence on the global economy and global health priority setting. G-8 nations account for 48% of the global economy and 49% of global trade, exercise shareholder control over the IMF and World Bank, have four-fifths of permanent seats on the UN Security Council, and provide 75% of all annual ODA. Member states played a key role in setting the Millennium Development Goals and backing the Global Fund to Fight HIV/AIDS, Tuberculosis and Malaria as part of their articulated support for enabling the world's poor and developing countries to participate in and benefit from the global economy. However, the G-8's commitment to a market-driven global economy has also worsened health conditions for the poor and exploited (Schrecker, Labonte, and Sanders 2007).

The European Union (EU) consists of 27 states that together contribute a substantial portion of global development aid (roughly half currently, with projected growth to two-thirds of global aid by 2010). Although many G-8 members are also part of the EU, the latter's social, economic, and aid policies often stand in contrast to the former's, reflecting the values of various EU member states that emphasize egalitarian and socially just public policies.

Several trade-based regional organizations founded in the 1990s also influence health and health care policy. NAFTA (the North American Free Trade Agreement) and Mercosur (a trade agreement involving Brazil, Argentina, Uruguay, and Paraguay, and, pending full ratification, Venezuela) govern commercial policies among member countries, including reductions in state subsidies, elimination of barriers to trade, and openness to private investors from other member nations. Controversial health-related outcomes of NAFTA include the proliferation of U.S.-owned factories operating in Mexico with less stringent occupational health rights policies than those of the United States and Canada, and the deterioration of small-scale agriculture. The Southern African Development Community (SADC) and the African Union, meanwhile, have designed a framework for mutual health assistance and guidelines for donors regarding health aid to Africa.

Foundations

Diverse philanthropic foundations have long been active in international health work. Funded through the donations or bequests of wealthy individuals or of companies, these organizations operate according to particular missions often as specified by their founders (see Table 3–10). Unlike government entities, which are subject to public scrutiny, philanthropies are accountable only to their self-selected boards, and decision making is often in the hands of a few executives and program officers. In North America and some other settings, foundations are not subject to taxation and thus are indirectly subsidized by a public that has no role in decision making regarding how and on what priorities these monies are spent. The majority of international health philanthropies are based in the United States and to a smaller extent in Europe and Asia, but there are also newer health philanthropies appearing elsewhere. While many foundations state altruistic aims, such as the Rockefeller Foundation's (RF) motto, "For the well-being of mankind around the world," the particular conceptions of how to meet those aims can be contested. The RF in the early 20th century, like the Gates Foundation today, had an inordinate influence over the international health agenda, at least in part because it could mobilize quickly and allocate substantial sums to large or innovative efforts. From a social justice perspective that sees health as a right rather than the object of charity, however, philanthropic actors have little legitimacy to influence or decide upon public health policy.

The largest donation of private funds to the UN was made in 1997 by television and communications executive Ted Turner, who announced a personal gift of US$1 billion to support a variety of areas, including health. But outright gifts are not what most donors have in mind.

The Old Guard

As seen in Chapter 2, the RF was instrumental in the institutionalization of international health and public health training. Between its founding in 1913, and the restructuring of its International Health Division in the early 1950s, it operated public health and disease control programs in almost 100 countries, shaping health research, ideas, institutions, and practices across the world. As well, the Foundation sponsored the training of over 13,000 fellows, mostly in the United States and founded 25 schools of public health across the world. It pioneered influential approaches to health and development, including agricultural technologies to increase food output (the so-called Green Revolution) and population and reproductive control efforts (later established separately as the Population Council). It advised and shaped the design and work of both the LNHO and the WHO.

Having made some US$2 billion (unadjusted) in grants since 1913, and with current assets of US$4.1 billion, the RF mostly allocates its resources to the arts, community development, and other sectors, but health remains an interest. For instance, it was instrumental in developing the public–private partnership (PPPs) arrangement in international health and launched a major health equity initiative in the 1990s.

In addition to the large foundations listed in Table 3–10, many smaller foundations have interests in global health. For example, the Milbank Memorial Fund is primarily a research institute, which supports the application of social and behavioral sciences to public health and preventive medicine.

Table 3-10 Endowments and Priorities of Selected Foundations

Foundation	Endowment/2007 Grants	Health-Related Priorities
Bill and Melinda Gates Foundation	US$38.7 billion/1.2 billion plus ≈US$31 billion pledge from Warren Buffett (1.8 billion in 2008)	• Infectious diseases, vaccines, HIV/AIDS, and TB • Reproductive and child health
Wellcome Trust	£15.1 billion	• Biomedical research • Fellowships and research in developing countries
Ford Foundation	US$13.7 billion	• Education, economic development, food production • Population and family planning
William and Flora Hewlett Foundation	US$9.3 billion	• Population and reproductive health
W.K. Kellogg Foundation	US$8.4 billion	• Educational programs in health, agriculture, and education in Latin America and Africa
John D. and Catherine T. MacArthur Foundation	US$7 billion/267 million	• Population and reproductive health
David and Lucille Packard Foundation	US$6.4 billion/300 million for 2008	• Population and reproductive health
Rockefeller Foundation	US$4.1 billion/22 million	• Public health (historically) • Equity in health • Poverty alleviation
Kresge Foundation	US$3.9 billion	• Capital construction grants in health and education • Health-related services
Aga Khan Foundation	US$153 million	• Health, education, information technology, and rural development
William J. Clinton Foundation	Raises over US$100 million per year/ US$10 billion in commitments since 2004	• HIV/AIDS • Health systems infrastructure
Nuffield Foundation	£14.8 million	• Health care policy • Fellowships and research in developing countries
Friedrich Ebert Stiftung Foundation	€11 million (annual grant-giving)	• Development cooperation

Sources: Foundation Web sites; and http://www.imf.org/external/pubs/ft/fandd/2007/12/bloom.htm.

The New Guard

The Bill and Melinda Gates Foundation, established in 2000 by Bill Gates (Microsoft founder and for many years the world's richest man) together with his wife, is the largest and one of the newer philanthropies involved in international health. The current endowment stands at US$38.7 billion, supplemented in 2006 by a US$31 billion donation from investor Warren Buffett, spread out over time. With recent annual spending of over US$3 billion—approximately 60% of which goes to global health programs (the remainder to educational and local efforts in the Pacific Northwest of the United States)—the Gates Foundation's global health budget has surpassed that of the WHO in some recent years. Its sheer size—and the renown of its founder—have turned the Gates Foundation into a leading global health player virtually overnight.

According to its Web site, the Gates Foundation aims to reduce inequality through the development and application of technologies. The foundation makes large grants and has a relatively small bureaucratic infrastructure, though this has changed in recent years with the establishment of an office in India. Its most prominent efforts involve support for vaccine development (through a US$1.5 billion donation to the GAVI Alliance and US$258 million to the Malaria Vaccine Initiative) and funding to develop tools to combat HIV/AIDS (for example through topical microbicides) and malaria. As exemplified in its Grand Challenges in Global Health initiative, created in 2003, the Gates Foundation takes a technological and reductionist approach to global health, viewing the determinants of health in narrow terms (Birn 2005; Brown 2007) (see Chapter 13 for further analysis).

In recent years the Gates Foundation has been accused of investing its endowment in polluting industries and profiteering pharmaceutical companies (Piller, Sanders, and Dixon 2007), ultimately causing more harm to health than good. The Gates Foundation and Microsoft are also under attack for their stance on protecting intellectual property rights (and pharmaceutical earnings) over the need for affordable life-saving medicines (Médecins Sans Frontières 2007). Given that the head of the Gates global health program is a former executive and current board member of the pharmaceutical giant GlaxoSmithKline, the conflict of interest between corporate profits and public health is palpable but rarely articulated, since critics fear offending the powerful foundation.

Because the Gates Foundation operates according to a challenge grant strategy—and with programs designed to achieve positive evaluations through delimited goals—it has had enormous influence on global health in the space of just a few years. When the Gates Foundation supports an initiative, many other bilateral, multilateral, public, and private donors are often keen to join or match its funding in order to be associated with a successful, high-profile activity. As discussed in the PPP section ahead, this gives enormous public policy-making powers to a private actor which is not democratically accountable.

The William J. Clinton Foundation, founded by the former U.S. President in 2001, has also turned its attention to global health, with a particular focus on HIV/AIDS and developing health systems infrastructure. The foundation acts as a "hub" for other health and development actors, who channel funds through it. It has also succeeded in getting pharmaceutical companies to reduce the prices of some drugs, notably ARVs. Due to the high profile of its founder, the foundation has garnered media attention and engaged well-known and highly influential global public and private sector actors with issues of global health. However, Clinton and his foundation walk a fine line between negotiating lower (but still profitable) prices for Big Pharma drugs sold to developing countries and threatening trade sanctions against developing countries that produce and sell generics.

Corporate Foundations

Various corporations also run small foundations, often as corporate public relations and marketing efforts, or even as a means of purveying their own products. The two largest each spent US$10 million in 2005: the BristolMyers Squibb Foundation and the Merck Company Foundation, focused on vaccines and HIV/AIDS treatment. Examples of "corporate philanthropy" include: the ExxonMobil and Levi Strauss Foundations, which work in the area of HIV/AIDS; the Shell Foundation, which focuses on health care provision and immunization; the Eli Lilly and Company Foundation, prioritizing women's health and TB control; and the Nestlé Foundation, which since 1968 has funded research and activities related to public health and nutrition in developing countries—this despite its unethical marketing of baby formula to women in developing countries (see Chapter 9). Corporate foundations, which usually enjoy tax-free status, are often active in areas where their workers, factories, and markets are located.

Developing Country Foundations

The Aga Khan Foundation (AKF) is a private, nondenominational development agency operating in low-income countries of Asia and Africa. The foundation was established in 1967 by H.H. the Aga Khan, 49th Imam of the Shia Imami Ismaili Muslims, and incorporated in Switzerland, with branch offices in Pakistan, India, Bangladesh, Kenya, and elsewhere. More than 200 educational and 160 health institutions, as well as large international workshops and conferences, have been supported by AKF.

The proliferation of billionaires in developing countries is sparking new foundations. Mexican telecom billionaire Carlos Slim (now the world's richest man) founded the Carso Health Institute in 2007 to support health-related activities in Latin America. With a start-up endowment of US$500 million (slated to grow to US$10 billion for health and education), the new institute plans to combine in-house research with program design, financing, and implementation.

Business Interests

The private sector has long operated international health activities, most notably to protect the health of the labor force, prevent the interruption of commerce due to epidemics, and establish international markets for health-related goods and services, including private health insurance, medicines, and equipment. Past and present, businesses have pressed bilateral and multilateral agencies to support health-oriented development and aid efforts, either with the aim of promoting particular businesses (i.e., U.S. agri-business supporting food aid) or of opening markets and increasing worker productivity. It is essential to note that such activities—unjust as they may seem—are entirely consistent with the primary legal obligation of companies: to generate profits. As such, business involvement in international health is not a matter of largesse but rather one of moneymaking.

Today a wide range of businesses are involved in international health, sometimes through their philanthropic arms—which allow for tax breaks and help generate profits (e.g., by donating a certain amount of drugs, additional quantities of which must subsequently be purchased)—but more typically through marketing and sales. Those involved include purveyors of health technology and equipment, as well as insurance companies attracted to the market for private sector coverage among the elites and middle-classes of developing and developed countries.

Private health insurance penetration has grown rapidly in recent years, particularly in developing countries. In 2001, Brazil, Chile, Namibia, Zimbabwe, South Africa, the United States, and Uruguay financed "more than 20% of their health care via private health insurance" (Sekhri and Savedoff 2006, p. 357). The private health care market in the latter three reached approximately 40% of the total. This pattern is becoming more pronounced over time (see Table 3–11), jeopardizing the public provision of care (see Chapters 11 and 12).

The multi billion dollar pharmaceutical industry, too, has enormous implications for international access to medicines, through the setting of prices, patent control, generic production, and drug development policies (Table 3–12).

Box 3–6 Role of "Big Pharma" in International Health

Big Pharma is big business, with the top 20 companies generating over US$300 billion in sales in 2004 and spending close to US$49 billion on research and development. From 1995 to 2002, it was the most profitable industry in the United States. Mergers and acquisitions have led to a significant concentration in the sector with the top 10 companies increasing their market share from a third in 1992 to over 50% in 2004: "globalisation has created a new breed of corporate giant which rivals the size of some national economies and has wider reach than some intergovernmental organizations" (Buse and Lee 2005, pp. 12–13).

Like other corporate interests, pharmaceutical companies are obliged to make profits for shareholders; this fiduciary responsibility is in conflict with serving the health needs of the world. Emboldened by enormous economic power and reach, pharmaceutical companies have increasingly flouted the law to increase profits (Buse and Lee 2005).

Pharmaceutical companies' profit-making imperative makes them far less interested in the vast needs of the majority of developing country populations (with limited ability to pay for drugs) than in developing and selling medicines to patients with deeper pockets. In 1968 the International Federation of Pharmaceutical Manufacturers & Associations (IFPMA) was created as a "nonprofit NGO" representing the pharmaceutical industry. While its mission promises to foster research innovation, access to medicine, and adherence to its marketing code, the IFPMA's main activity is to ensure "adequate and effective" intellectual property protections and to limit regulation of the industry.

In recent years, pharmaceutical companies have sought to ensure patent protection through WTO rules and lawsuits against governments violating intellectual property (see Chapter 9). Because of their ruthless campaign against the production of generic drugs (especially to treat

(continued)

Box 3–6 Continued

HIV/AIDS) in South Africa and other countries, drug companies have become known as one of the most nefarious international health players. In light of concerns that patent protection would limit access to affordable medicines, the Doha Declaration of 2001 stated that the WTO's TRIPS Agreement should not interfere with national public health needs. But in practice the provisions are weak and the procedures incredibly complicated and difficult. In 2004, the Canadian government passed bill C-9, which would allow Canada to produce low-cost generic drugs for export to countries lacking production capacity. This was the first such action by any government, but implementation of the bill has been extremely slow.

Certain pharmaceutical companies garner attention for making donations or offering discount drug stocks in disaster situations. Sometimes these drugs are near or past expiry or have been replaced with better alternatives. Most famously, starting in 1987, Merck has donated Mectizan to treat onchocerciasis (river blindness) free of charge to hundreds of millions of people exposed to the disease (and more recently, to treat lymphatic filariasis). But the story of Merck's self-proclaimed generosity is less than inspiring. When Mectizan was developed from Merck's existing dog deworming drug, the company first tried to sell the drug at market and below-market rates, then to strong-arm the WHO and U.S. Congress into purchasing and distributing it. Only after these strategies failed did Merck consider a donation—as a last resort, not as a model of philanthropy. Indeed, Merck has yet to offer any other needed drug nor have other pharmaceutical companies stepped up to the plate.

A growing number of companies have global health offices or company foundations that run "wellness" programs or donate to health behavior campaigns. In the case of snack food and soft drink giant PepsiCo, these efforts are accompanied by

Table 3–11 Private Health Insurance Penetration in 2006

Country	Private Expenditure on Health as Percentage of Total Expenditure on Health Care	Private Health Insurance Expenditure as Percentage of Private Expenditure on Health Care	Private Health Insurance Expenditure as Percentage of Total Health Care
Brazil	52.1	33.9	17.7
Chile	47.3	45.1	21.3
Namibia	35.6	79.5	28.3
South Africa	56.5	68.9	45.1
United States	54.2	66.4	36.0
Uruguay	56.5	68.9	38.9
Zimbabwe	47.4	29.1	13.8
China[a]	58.0	6.3	3.6
India	80.4	0.8	0.6

[a] The estimates do not include expenditures of Hong Kong and Macao Special Administrative Regions.

Source: World Health Organization, National Health Accounts by country. http://www.who.int/nha/country/en/index.html. Accessed September 5, 2008.

Table 3–12 Leading Pharmaceutical Companies by Revenues and Profits

Company	2007 Revenues (US$ billions)	2007 Profits (US$ billions) (Rank, by profits)	Approximate Percentage of 2006 Sales/Market in Developing Countries
Johnson & Johnson	61.1	10.6 (2)	20%
Pfizer	48.4	8.1 (4)	17% (includes Japan)
GlaxoSmithKline	45.4	10.4 (3)	15%
Roche Group	40.3	8.1 (5)	15%
Sanofi-Aventis	40.0	7.2 (6)	22% (all but United States and Europe)
Novartis	39.8	11.9 (1)	
AstraZeneca	29.6	5.6 (7)	14%
Abbott Laboratories	26.0	3.6 (9)	
Merck	24.2	3.3 (10)	40%
Wyeth	22.4	4.6 (8)	
Bristol-Myers Squibb	20.0	2.2 (12)	
Eli Lilly	18.6	3.0 (11)	

Sources: *Fortune* 2008 Global 500 issue, 158 (2) July 21, 2008, p. F-24: and company Web sites/annual reports.

marketing of products with "essentially healthy ingredients or offer[ing] improved health benefits" (PepsiCo 2008), a clearly self-interested move in the face of wide criticism of the unhealthy chemical, sugar, and fat content of convenience foods. Others, including agricultural feed supplier Cargill and fruit giant Dole, have formed partnerships with development agencies to create an image of corporate social responsibility, even as their infinitely larger for-profit endeavors carry on business as usual. As we will see in Chapter 9, multinational corporations and their subsidiaries influence the determinants of health across the world through environmental and occupational contamination, low wage levels, poor working conditions, and regulatory incompliance.

Through the World Economic Forum (an annual forum that gives the top corporate interests privileged access to and influence over government leaders), and other such meetings, businesses have become major donors to the Global Fund and the Stop TB and Roll Back Malaria Partnerships, and sit on their boards. Portrayed as humanitarian philanthropy, business involvement in these partnerships nonetheless remains consistent with the fiduciary responsibilities of corporations to make money for their shareholders.

Public–Private Partnerships

Philanthropic and business interests have had long involvement with international health organizations, but it was not until the mid-1990s that public–private partnerships (PPPs) were formalized as a central modality of international health (WHO 1993; Buse and Walt 2000). While portrayed as an opportunity to expand funding and visibility of international health efforts, these "collaborations" between the private sector and public agencies (both multilateral and national) have given the business sector a major role in public health policy making.

There are now several dozen large-scale global PPPs in existence, with the WHO involved in nearly 100 PPPs. PPP budgets range from millions to many billions of dollars. These include the Stop TB Partnership, Roll Back Malaria, the International AIDS Vaccine Initiative, and the Global Alliance for Improved Nutrition. While some global health PPPs have spurred research and development and facilitated the supply of medicines, on the whole, they bring most of the same problems as health donors writ large: imposition of outside agendas, poor harmonization with stakeholders and national governments, underfunding, and vilification of the public sector (Buse and Harmer 2007). Almost by definition, narrowly-targeted PPPs entrench vertical programs (there is no PPP for primary health care!), jeopardizing health systems development and impeding integrated approaches. WHO's mandated responsibility for world health is superseded in some PPPs, which relegate it to the margins. In others, there are so many partners (in the case of Roll Back Malaria, over 80) that management and governance problems are insuperable (Maciocco and Italian Global Health Watch 2008).

Such concerns are compounded by the contradictions between the profit-making mandates of corporations and the WHO's commitment to health as a human right. These partnerships have marshaled billions of dollars to international health, but have led to extensive commercialization and enormous private sector influence on international health policy making. The net result is that most PPPs channel public money into the private sector, not the other way around (Richter 2004; Ollila 2005b).

The largest PPP, the Global Fund to Fight AIDS, Tuberculosis and Malaria, was established as an independent Swiss foundation in 2002. It raises money, reviews proposals, and disburses grants and contracts, rather than implementing programs directly. Designed to bypass the "bureaucratic encumbrances" of UN agencies, the Global Fund's governing board is split 50/50 between representatives of donor countries, philanthropic agencies, and the private sector on one hand, and developing countries and NGOs on the other. As of late 2008, the Global Fund had approved US$14.4 billion to fund programs in 140 countries, with almost US$7 billion distributed. The Global Fund disburses approximately two-thirds of all donor monies to combat tuberculosis, half for malaria, and one-fourth for HIV/AIDS. Its disbursements focus on vertical programs to deliver therapeutics, with 58% spent on HIV/AIDS, 24% on malaria, 17% on TB, and just 1% on health systems (http://www.theglobalfund.org). Despite its grand declared ambitions, the Global Fund's performance has not only been disappointing (in treatment coverage terms), but has had "wider harmful consequences due, for instance, to competitive recruitment of staff in privileged areas of intervention and consequent neglect of other sectors" (Maciocco and Italian Global Health Watch 2008, p. 47).

Incredibly, the WHO and UNAIDS have no vote on the board of the Global Fund (and many other PPPs). Moreover, these partnerships offer "business opportunities"—lucrative contracts—as key features of their work, illustrating how international health is being captured by business interests.

Another visible PPP is the GAVI Alliance (formerly the Global Alliance for Vaccines and Immunization), based in Geneva, which focuses on increasing children's access to vaccines in developing countries through the development of new vaccines and the distribution of existing ones. A partnership of philanthropic foundations, UNICEF, the WHO, the World Bank, private businesses, and NGOs, the GAVI Alliance builds on WHO's Expanded Program on Immunization (EPI), but WHO plays only a marginal role. With a vertical focus on global immunization coverage carried out through external funds, partnerships with local governments, and promotion of research into new vaccines, GAVI runs the risk of repeating the same results as EPI—high infant mortality rates and childhood deaths even in countries with apparently high vaccination coverage (Greenwood et al. 1987; Ollila 2005a). GAVI has also been critiqued for placing too much emphasis on new and novel vaccines (often developed by its pharmaceutical partners) rather then ensuring that basic vaccination is universally carried out (Heaton and Keith 2002), and for being heavily "top-down," paying scant attention to local needs and conditions (Muraskin 2005).

Table 3-14 indicates the extent to which WHO's work is overshadowed by PPPs. Indeed, WHO's ability to tackle major international health problems is inhibited by the PPP model. For example, in 2003 WHO and UNAIDS launched an effort to provide 3 million people living with AIDS in developing and transition countries with ARVs by 2005 (the 3 by 5 Initiative). Despite the recognized importance of improving ARV accessibility, WHO's larger member government contributors refrained from voting for larger dues for this effort, since many of them had contributed to PPPs instead. As a result, the target was not met by the end of 2005 (at the time 1.3 million people were receiving treatment), and 3 by 5 and Beyond now aims at almost universal access by 2010 (WHO 2006a). This failure has further undermined WHO's authority and ability to function. The WHO's EB has belatedly recognized the numerous problems posed by PPPs, such as fragmentation of health care, low cost-effectiveness, and insufficient accountability (WHO 2008).

In sum PPPs—whether in health or other domains—are narrowly focused, duplicative of existing efforts and one another, and insufficiently subject to public safeguards that would prevent conflicts of interest between corporate and public objectives (Richter 2004; Ollila 2005b; Utting and Zammit 2006). Moreover, PPPs in health:

- Allow private interests to set/influence/compromise the public health agenda and provide legitimacy to corporations' activities through association with UN agencies.

- Sacrifice broad public health goals of preventing disease, protecting and promoting health, and tackling the underlying social and economic determinants of avoidable disease and death.
- Favor short-term, vertical approaches, profit-making on technological interventions, and privatization of essential public services rather than horizontal, comprehensive, and sustainable public services.

According to the PHM, the sole solution to the problem of undue corporate interests in global health is "economic justice, including an adequate tax base, both nationally and internationally, to cover all public services, as well as proper funding

Table 3-13 Selected Religious Agencies—Spending and Activities

Religious Agency	Annual Spending	Details
Mennonite Central Committee	US$43.8 million in goods; US$11.7 million in food aid	• 1,000 staff in 56 countries
Lutheran World Relief	US$35 million in 2007	• Works in 35 countries
Adventist Development and Relief Agency	US$92 million in 2006	• Works in 125 countries
American Friends Service Committee	US$43.3 million	• Works for peace, economic and social justice, humanitarian assistance, and protection of immigrant and prisoner rights
World Vision	US$946 million in 2006	• 23,000 staff in 100 countries
		• 4.7 million donors in United States
Catholic Relief Services	US$597 million in 2007	• Works in 98 countries
Comité Catholique contre la Faim et pour le Développement	€33 million in 2007	• 500 projects in 80 countries
		• Food sovereignty, natural resource protection, the rights of women, children, and the poor
Hadassah		• Jewish women's organization supporting hospitals and biomedical research in Israel
Muslim Aid	£19.6 million in 2007	• Active in 50 countries
		• Emergency relief, water and sanitation, poverty alleviation
Islamic Relief Worldwide	£40 million	• Activities in 20 countries
		• Education, emergency relief, health and nutrition, income generation, and sanitation
American Jewish World Service	US$24.7 million	• Supports grassroots efforts to end violence, poverty, and inequality
		• Advocacy and volunteer work

Source: Agency Web sites.

of public institutions such as WHO through regular budgets so that it may fulfill its international responsibilities unimpeded by corporate interests" (People's Health Movement 2005, p. 4).

The extent of private involvement in global health is also evidenced by the recent formation of the H-8—WHO, UNICEF, UNFPA, UNAIDS, the World Bank, the GAVI Alliance, the Global Fund, and the Gates Foundation—which now hold meetings, like the G-8, in which private entities wield equivalent decision-making powers to public agencies.

Missionaries and Religious Agencies and Charities

Religious missions have sponsored health-related activities for hundreds of years, operating leprosaria, hospitals, and orphanages in Asia, Africa, and Latin America. Historically, a variety of Christian medical missions were associated with repressive colonial regimes and used health activities to proselytize religious beliefs. The relative importance of mission hospitals has declined in many countries, but a resurgence is taking place in sub-Saharan Africa, with some missions broadening activities to include community development and agricultural work. Religious missions are funded primarily through contributions from members/congregations/headquarters in Europe and North America but may also receive support from development agencies.

Today most religious health aid is centralized in multimillion dollar charitable agencies—World Vision, American Friends Service Committee, Adventist Development and Relief Agency, Catholic Relief Services, France's Comité Catholique contre la Faim et pour le Développement, and so on (see Table 3–13 for a listing of prominent religious agencies)—emphasizing humanitarian relief and, in some cases, espousing social justice. Smaller groups include Helps International. Diakonia (made up of five Swedish churches) and Norwegian Church Aid advocate for economic justice and human rights in their work, as part of the Scandinavian tradition of antiimperialist missions. In these latter groups, religion (and religious conversion) may be portrayed more as background inspiration than overt goal.

Combined efforts include Caritas International, a confederation of 162 Catholic development, social service, and relief agencies that work in 200 countries; ACT (Action by Churches Together), an alliance of scores of Protestant and Orthodox churches (all members of the World Council of Churches and the Lutheran World Federation) that provide emergency relief in 34 countries; the Church World Service, which encompass 35 Protestant, Anglican, and Orthodox denominations; and Coopération Internationale pour le Développement et la Solidarité, an alliance of 15 European and North American Catholic development organizations. International health alliances also form across religions. The Global AIDS Interfaith Alliance provides community-based HIV services in low-income countries through partnerships with religious organizations.

While fewer in number than Christian organizations, Jewish and Islamic agencies also sponsor international health and relief work, typically aimed at people of the same faith. United Jewish Agency federations exist in numerous North American and European cities; and many Islamic communities have Waqf boards that set aside land and goods for charitable purposes. Among the largest non-Christian religious agencies are Islamic Relief Worldwide and American Jewish World Service.

Small Christian missions with explicitly religious aims still operate today. The Mission Doctors Association sends Catholic doctors from the Unites States to serve at mission hospitals and clinics overseas, and the Aloha Medical Mission is active in Asia. FAME sees medical aid as a path to evangelism. Over 100 organizations belong to the Mission Exchange (formerly the Evangelical Foreign Missions Association), which carries out related activities. Some "faith-based" organizations such as Christian Connections for International Health, based in the United States, have been criticized for infusing fundamentalist values (sexual abstinence, prohibition on abortion) into their work, for refusing to hire gay men and lesbians, and for blocking the implementation of harm reduction initiatives.

Another growing development is the spread of Pentecostal and other evangelical churches across Latin America, Africa, the former Soviet Union, and Asia. In some settings church healing is replacing the role of traditional healers, whose rising fees and sometime connection with international health players is viewed with suspicion (Pfeiffer 2005).

NGOs

Nongovernmental organizations (NGOs), previously known as private voluntary organizations (PVOs), are neither public nor profit-making. NGOs are diverse, ranging from local grassroots efforts to small or large international NGOs (INGOs) that work transnationally sending resources and personnel from one (usually developed) to another (usually developing) country. NGOs are involved in expert consultation, training, direct service delivery, advocacy, contract work, and many other activities. Networks of NGOs, such as InterAction (the American Council for Voluntary International Action) or the International Council of Voluntary Agencies, which build alliances and exchange information, also form formidable advocacy groups.

Within the "aid community," NGOs, foundations, and donor government agencies may work in conjunction or compete unproductively. Some groups receive contributions from the general public, foundations, and government agencies and are bound by the funder's mandate. In the field of population and family planning activities, for example, USAID has allocated hundreds of millions of dollars to NGOs including the International Planned Parenthood Federation, the Pathfinder Fund, the Population Council, Family Health International, and EngenderHealth. All have been constrained by the Mexico City policy preventing support to organizations that endorse abortion.

NGOs are funded by a variety of sources. Some obtain resources through direct appeals to the public. Religiously based NGOs have obvious constituencies, and secular organizations use a variety of channels to solicit funds. Some NGOs (most notably BRAC, based in Bangladesh) generate income from the sale of products or services. Increasingly, INGOs receive contracts from their home government's bilateral development agencies to implement particular projects or to provide humanitarian relief.

The proliferation of NGOs since the 1980s has been viewed by some as a sign of vibrant civil society: in many settings, they have arisen to meet needs that are not addressed by governments; elsewhere, they operate in parallel or competition with public agencies, purveying otherwise "public goods." According to the *Human Development Report* of 2002, there were almost 40,000 international NGOs, with over 2,000 involved in the health sphere (Anheier, Glasius and Kaldor 2001 cited in UNDP 2002). This is likely an underestimate, given that most countries do not have an official count of NGOs. Moreover, it does not include many local NGOs, many of which play a key part in bringing cooperative health efforts to fruition.

However, NGOs, especially INGOs, are not necessarily a neutral "third way" that transcends the public and private sectors. They are often unaccountable, undemocratic, and—to the extent to which they exist because appropriate, democratically determined structures for public service have been destroyed—may be a dangerous development. INGOs can fragment health systems and other social services, cause chaos and undercut local decision making, exacerbate inequality, drain resources and staff from health systems, and generate unproductive hierarchies among health workers and between outsiders and nationals (Pfeiffer 2003). Moreover, many INGOs now promote the same approach as the donor governments that fund them (Mercer 2002).

Indian novelist-activist Arundhati Roy lucidly argues:

> As the state [has] abdicated its traditional role, NGOs [have] moved in to work in these areas. But their available funds are a minute fraction of the cut in public spending. Most wealthy NGOs are financed and patronised by aid and development agencies, funded by western governments, the World Bank, the United Nations and multinational corporations. Though they may not be the same agencies, they are certainly part of the same political formation that oversees the neoliberal project and demands the slash in government spending (Roy 2004).

Indeed, by the mid-1990s, NGOs had reportedly displaced governments as the primary recipients and conduits of aid for humanitarian relief and emergency assistance. It is estimated that about one-third of development financing now goes to NGOs, which has led to competition for these funds. Such contracting to NGOs can facilitate work in the field where the funding agency lacks experience, personnel, and equipment; may permit a more rapid, flexible, and informal response; can circumvent government bureaucracies; and may present a more acceptable face to the public and to donor countries. At their best, committed NGOs can deliver imaginative, appropriate, and meaningful humanitarian assistance. At their worst, NGOs can become, or are created as, inefficient routine contract service providers with little innovation or dedication to the public welfare, dislodging and discrediting the public provision of services.

There are almost as many types of NGOs as there are NGOs. Here we group them according to size, aim, and mode of operation. Most of the organizations we outline here have a primary, but not exclusive, focus on health; arguably all of their activities affect health—and the determinants of health—on some dimension.

Large Humanitarian NGOs

Large humanitarian organizations, often with national donor or operating affiliates, work in multiple settings, on multiple issues, with enormous budgets. The International Committee of the Red Cross (ICRC), the first such entity, was established in 1863 by Jean-Henri Dunant—who witnessed the bloody Battle of Solferino and provided help to its victims—with the aim of assisting people wounded and displaced by warfare. Operating with a budget of almost US$800 million, ICRC is engaged in international health issues through some 80 projects, including war-related efforts, postwar infrastructural redevelopment, promotion of international law and human rights, and protection of people affected by conflict and detention.

The International Save the Children Alliance, which was founded by English socialite and children's rights advocate Eglantyne Jebb in 1919 to help starving children in Eastern Europe in the wake of World War I, today operates (together with several dozen national affiliates) around the world with a budget of over US$1 billion in areas such as emergency relief, nutrition and sanitation, HIV/AIDS prevention, reproductive health, education, and children's rights.

U.S.-based CARE, founded in 1945 to provide relief to World War II survivors, today operates humanitarian projects aimed at fighting poverty through projects particularly aimed at helping women via education, sanitation, health, and economic support. It operates in over 40 countries with a budget of US$590 million in 2006.

Catholic Relief Services (CRS) founded in 1943 by the U.S. Catholic Bishops, also provides large-scale (its 2007 budget was US$600 million) relief and development support to poor people in almost 100 countries. Its mission is explicitly religious, and thus it may also be considered a religious charitable group.

Relief Groups

As witnessed in the public and institutional response to the 2004 Asian tsunami, the Pakistan earthquake of 2005, and many other "natural disasters," relief aid is among the most active and publicly supported aspects of international health. The 186 national societies affiliated with the International Federation of Red Cross and Red Crescent Societies (IFRC) constitute by far the largest of these efforts and are active in emergency relief and the provision of medical services in the countries in which they are based as well as abroad. In conflict situations, the Red Cross often takes on the role of caring for and protecting people within the conflict zone, while protection and care of war refugees is largely left to the UNHCR. Individual and public donations to relief efforts often coincide with media coverage of crises, though many agencies are effective at fund-raising year round. The International Rescue Committee (IRC), whose founding was urged by Albert Einstein in 1933, began by rescuing people suffering under German fascism. Today, with a budget of approximately US$250 million, the IRC provides emergency relief and support to refugees in Africa, Central and South Asia, and elsewhere, in settings where people are uprooted by war and ethnic persecution. More modestly sized NGOs, for example Merlin, based in the United Kingdom, and Project Hope and International Relief Teams, both of the United States, provide emergency medical care, training, and health and sanitation infrastructure support. Although these efforts sometimes include funding for long-term rebuilding and conflict/disaster prevention, short-term and immediate relief take priority.

Social Rights/Service Provision NGOs

These agencies, some large, others with more limited budgets, sometimes operate in similar arenas as humanitarian and relief agencies but have explicitly political and social rights missions. Oxfam International, one of the largest such organizations, with a 2007 budget of over US$700 million, funds small-scale development projects, emergency relief, and campaigns for social/economic justice.

Médecins Sans Frontières (MSF, founded in France in 1971), with 2007 expenditures of approximately €580 million, is a humanitarian medical aid agency that operates in some of the neediest/resource-poor places in the world. MSF has made the witnessing and reporting of atrocities—particularly those conveniently ignored by dominant political actors—central to its mission, as recognized by the Nobel Prize committee in 1999. MSF also carries out policy and advocacy work, for example in its Essential Drugs Campaign and Drugs for Neglected Diseases Initiative. Somewhat smaller, Médecins du Monde (Doctors of the World) carries out similar activities.

Boston-based Partners In Health (PIH) has drawn attention to the possibility— and indeed the human right—of providing first-rate medical care to people with multidrug resistant TB and other ailments deemed "untreatable" in marginalized settings in Peru, Russia, Rwanda, and Haiti. PIH has successfully demonstrated that HAART (highly active antiretroviral therapy) can be delivered in resource-poor circumstances. These efforts have also helped drive down the cost of ARVs worldwide.

Other groups, such as Physicians for Peace, focus on international peace-building through medical education, clinical care, or medical donations.

There are also several groups with clear political, social justice, and health aims, such as Doctors for Global Health (DGH), working in a small number of places where their projects can be locally sustained. Similarly, Health Alliance International explicitly links its efforts to increase access to quality health care among disadvantaged populations to underlying structural and policy changes, most notably in Mozambique.

Human Rights and Health Groups

This diverse group of NGOs puts human rights at the forefront of their approach to international health. They include small professionally based groups that run direct health cooperation projects, small think tanks and advocacy groups that carry out research on health and human rights, such as the Center for Social and Economic Rights, and large human rights organizations. For example, Amnesty International and Human Rights Watch have established health programs as part of their larger mandate. Most of these groups are experienced in using media outlets to raise awareness and provoke political responses. Dignitas International, which provides services with dignity to people living with HIV/AIDS, puts human rights at the center of its activities. Physicians for Social Responsibility, founded to prevent the use and spread of nuclear weapons, now also focuses on environmental conditions, and Physicians for Human Rights, drawing attention to the role of U.S. policies in impeding the realization of health of peoples around the world, has effectively used physicians as advocates.

Health and human rights efforts are also advanced by the Hesperian Foundation, a nonprofit community health and advocacy publisher. Its book, *Where There is No Doctor* was first issued in 1977. This PHC handbook, and many other manuals, have since been translated into dozens of languages and are used all over the world.

Developing Country NGOs

There are literally tens of thousands of NGOs working locally in diverse settings across the world. Here we include them as international health actors because many of these groups interact with other international health players as service deliverers, grantees, and contributors to the larger policy agenda. The largest and most well-known of these is BRAC, which began as a donor-funded war relief effort following the Bangladesh independence struggle in the early 1970s and has been transformed into a self-funded development effort reaching 100 million people through poverty alleviation, employment generation, and maternal and child health efforts. BRAC has been praised for improving health equity, as evidenced through better growth in girls (Khatun, Stenlund, and Hörnell 2004), but it is also under attack for (unethically) promoting the sale of its own products (Kelly 2008).

The Grameen Bank, also based in Bangladesh, has provided microcredit for over 30 years, reaching over 7 million people. By providing small loans, primarily to women, the Grameen Bank attempts to alleviate poverty through small-scale economic growth. The Bank has created the Grameen Family, which consists of educational facilities, utility service providers, and businesses. The Bank's founder, Mohammed Yunus, was awarded the Nobel Peace Prize in 2006 and his model of microcredit and microenterprise has been adopted throughout the world. Recently, the Grameen Foundation has begun funding programs in the United States, focusing on underemployed urban populations. The counterpart of economic self-sufficiency—social services and infrastructure—remains unaddressed by this model, and both BRAC and Grameen have been critiqued for failing to reach the poorest populations (Develtere and Huybrechts 2002).

On a much smaller scale, the Urmul Trust, founded in 1972 in Rajasthan, India, articulates its mission as leading "the poor towards self-reliance by making available to them a package of development services that they themselves decide on, design, implement, and eventually finance" (http://www.judypat.com/india/urmul.htm). It began as a milk cooperative that went from producing 200 L/day to 1 million L/day and soon expanded into health and education outreach to women and girls. Following a 1987 drought, the Urmul Trust's participants collectively adapted themselves into a weaving cooperative that has followed in the successful footsteps of its predecessor.

Other grassroots NGOs will be covered elsewhere in the book.

International Health and Development Think Tanks

Think tanks engage in extensive research and advocacy activities in an effort to improve access to health services and push for the effectiveness and accountability of donor development aid, including health aid. These organizations, for example the Center for Global Development in Washington and the Overseas Development Institute in London, often have close connections to multilateral and bilateral agencies and to politicians, and can have significant influence on decision making. The U.S.-based Treatment Action Group is a research and policy think tank fighting for better treatment, a vaccine, and a cure for HIV and TB. The modestly sized yet highly effective Center for Policy Analysis on Trade and Health (CPATH) addresses public health concerns in international trade agreements and relies on the internet as a forum for advocacy.

Advocacy Groups/Campaigns

Some grassroots efforts, such as the Third World Network, Equinet (the Regional Network on Equity in Health in Southern Africa), and Focus on the Global South, also have advocacy and research components. These groups produce publications and coordinate seminars and presentations to represent developing countries' interests, engage in activism campaigns, and build research and advocacy capacity. In South Africa, the Treatment Action Campaign (TAC) has lobbied government and industry for equitable access to affordable treatment and prevention programs for HIV/AIDS and is an oft-cited example of NGOs having a crucial impact on policy. PHM, discussed ahead, is also an effective advocacy group and social movement.

A high profile advocacy coalition based in the United Kingdom and the United States, DATA (Debt, AIDS, Trade, Africa, formed in 2002) harnesses the celebrity of its founder, Irish rock star Bono, to raise awareness around poverty and ill health in Africa. DATA (and its sister campaign, ONE: Make Poverty History) attempts to engage citizens in wealthy countries to pressure their governments on issues related to global health and trade and to buy goods from companies that donate part of the proceeds to the Global Fund.

A number of issue-based NGOs have arisen in recent decades. To cite just two: the International Baby Food Action Network has mobilized around adherence to the WHO's International Code of Marketing of Breast Milk Substitutes, and the Global AIDS Alliance focuses on advocacy regarding all aspects of the AIDS pandemic.

Social and Political Movements

While not international health players in the strictest sense, these transnational movements, including the World Social Forum and anti-WTO and anti-G-8 activism, draw attention to the untoward health and social consequences of global economic policies. Their efforts have been instrumental in raising awareness and resistance to international financial and trade policy. Perhaps most famously, the Multilateral Agreement on Investments (MAI)—which would have removed virtually any impediment to foreign investment—was derailed in the late 1990s by a multicountry campaign led by the Council of Canadians (see Chapter 9).

The People's Health Movement (PHM), founded in 2000 in Bangladesh, is an international network of health workers and activists who carry out research and advocacy work, host biannual conferences, and undertake political actions. Its People's Health Charter, calling for a resurrection of "health for all" has been endorsed by thousands of people and organizations across the world, and PHM played an instrumental role in the establishment of the WHO's Commission on Social Determinants of Health in 2005.

Countless other national and solidarity groups, trade unions, and people's movements of all kinds have enormous bearing on local health, but also have considerable international resonance in that their ideas and actions are shared from place to place. Their explicitly political activities—for land reform (e.g., Brazil's Movimento dos Trabalhadores Rurais Sem Terra (MST), with over 1.5 million landless members); for keeping water in public hands (e.g., Bolivia's Coalition in Defense of Water and Life); for labor rights (e.g., International Labor Rights Forum)—do more for health by fighting for water, land, workplace, and other rights than dozens of international health programs.

University and Hospital Collaborations

In recent decades, university-based researchers and hospitals have become increasingly involved in international health, either carrying out donor-funded research or establishing collaborations between researchers in developed and developing countries. Though international health training has typically been funded by WHO, foundations, governments, and other large donors, universities are also involved in educational programs for health personnel. Hospital exchanges often provision equipment, short-term in-country training programs, and intensive "donation" of medical services, for instance cataract operations, surgery for children, etc.

Some developing countries also have extensive scholarship programs. The Latin American School of Medicine (ELAM), based in Havana, provides free medical education for students from developing countries, with the understanding that those students will practice in underserved areas in their home countries. In April 2007, a sister school—the Alejandro Prospero Reverend School of Medicine—opened in Venezuela.

In the United States, the Center for Global Health and Economic Development at Columbia University is a key partner in the Millennium Villages Initiative (linked to the MDGs) and focuses on improvements in the larger determinants of global health. The Harvard Initiative for Global Health has international training programs and participates in global health research and cooperation. The Francois-Xavier Bagnoud Center for Health and Human Rights, also at Harvard, was the first academic unit with an explicit focus on health and human rights. Johns Hopkins University's Center for Clinical Global Health Education trains health professionals and provides medical care in developing countries; its Center for Global Health offers training courses and fellowships, and helps form partnerships among public health schools. Emory University, University of Washington, University of Iowa, University of Toronto, and many other universities have similar training initiatives.

The WHO Collaborating Center on Global Change and Health, based at the London School of Hygiene and Tropical Medicine (LSHTM), acts as a hub within the LSHTM and communicates innovations and research findings to the WHO. The Aga Khan University, based in Pakistan, trains medical and public health practitioners and maintains hospitals in Karachi and Nairobi. In the Americas, Mexico's Instituto Nacional de Salud Pública and Brazil's Fundação Oswaldo Cruz (FIOCRUZ) undertake research on local and global health issues and offer postgraduate training in public health.

Research Institutions

Some nationally run institutions play a large role in global health research. The Fogarty International Center (part of the U.S. National Institutes of Health) provides grants and runs training programs for health researchers around the world. France's Institut Pasteur, and its network of national affiliates in former French colonies, and Britain's Medical Research Council play similar roles. In Brazil, the FIOCRUZ engages in research and development of medical interventions and public health innovations. The International Centre for Diarrhoeal Disease Research, Bangladesh (ICDDR,B)—building on its predecessor, the Cholera Research Laboratory (founded in 1960)—was established by the Bangladesh government in 1978, and is supported by numerous bilateral and multilateral agencies and private foundations. In addition to carrying out community-based and hospital care and research—which has expanded to include child health and HIV/AIDS—ICDDR,B has trained approximately 15,000 health professionals.

A few governments, most notably Canada, through its International Development Research Centre (IDRC), and ECHO, the humanitarian assistance arm of the European Union, based in Brussels, have small development research arms that provide funding for collaborative research.

Research Alliances

Members of the Council on Health Research for Development (COHRED)—established in 1993 and based in Switzerland—undertake global health research with an explicit focus on equity and social justice issues and giving voice to partners from the global South. COHRED has partnered with numerous multilateral and bilateral agencies to run the annual forums for global health research, which seek to strengthen global research capacity and coherence. The Global Forum for Health Research—also based in Switzerland—has since its founding in 1998 used research and advocacy to draw attention to global health issues, including the "10/90 gap" whereby only 10% of health sciences research dollars address the health problems of 90% of the world's population. Each year, the Global Forum hosts an international health research conference with attendance of many key players in international health.

Professional Membership Organizations

Many people who work with international health agencies also belong to professional organizations. Membership in these organizations include public health and medical personnel, academics, policy actors, field workers, and activists who are involved in research, advocacy, running programs, and communication with the public. The advocacy-oriented U.S.-based Global Health Council (GHC) is the largest such entity and includes individual and organizational members. It also holds annual conferences and training events and maintains regular contact with its members through publications. The Canadian Society for International Health (CSIH) plays a similar role and also carries out cooperative projects.

Various professional public health and medical associations are engaged in global health work. The New Delhi and Philadelphia-based International Clinical Epidemiology Network, which aims at improving the health of disadvantaged populations through research and training, has over 1,500 member-professionals. The American Public Health Association (APHA), founded in 1872, early on served as a regional public health association for U.S., Canadian, Mexican, and Cuban health professionals, but since the 1950s it has been involved in international health mainly through collaboration with U.S. government agencies, such as USAID, and NGOs.

The European-based International Association of Health Policy (IAHP) and the Latin American Social Medicine Association (ALAMES) are international networks of academics, health workers, and activists who promote scientific analysis of public health issues and offer a forum for international comparisons and political debate on health policy issues. These groups also engage in research and advocacy from the perspective of health as a social and political right.

Many countries have national public health associations, such as the Public Health Association of South Africa (WHO 2007a). These include the Bangladesh Public Health Association, the Ethiopian Public Health Association, the Mexican Society for Public Health, and the Turkish Public Health Association. There are also two global public health associations that partner with the WHO: the World Federation of Public Health Associations; and the International Association of National Public Health Institutes.

Smaller-Scale and Individual Efforts

Although near impossible to count, numerous doctor and nurse groups and civic organizations are involved in international health cooperation on a small scale, sometimes as "flying doctors," whose commitment is minimal. Medical Expeditions International and International Health Service organize such volunteer stints.

Microcredit networks such as Kiva and GlobalGiving, connect individuals in industrialized countries with developing country residents seeking loans or donations.

On a different front, secular and church-based efforts collect and send medicines and health supplies to countries facing embargoes (e.g., the longstanding U.S. embargo against Cuba). Those who take part in global health exchanges, work, and advocacy on a small or individual basis are often moved to join organizations so that their actions will have greater collective bearing.

WHAT IS (OR SHOULD BE) THE ROLE OF INTERNATIONAL HEALTH AGENCIES AND OTHER ACTORS

Key Questions:

• How is the international health field shaped by agencies, actors, and movements?
• What are the strengths and limitations of the approaches of key global health actors?

Not including NGOs, over 100 major organizations are involved in global health aid, "a much higher degree of proliferation than in any other sector" (World Bank 2007a). The varied players and activities that we have covered thus far—from grassroots movements, to bilateral and multilateral agencies, to pharmaceutical multinationals—have competing, overlapping, and, only rarely, shared approaches to international health. Some US$14 billion was spent in the global health arena in 2004 (Kates, Morrison, and Lief 2006) (less than half of which likely made it to developing countries). Since then, upwards of US$20 billion is estimated to have been spent annually in international health. Given that much of this donor money is accompanied by substantial matching donations at the country level, international health activities constitute a sizeable—if insufficient, according to many—component of health-related spending across the world.

Notwithstanding the vast array of actors and agencies involved in international health, the legitimacy of many of them may be questioned. As discussed above, few major health agencies are democratically run or representative, and they rarely offer sustainable or reliable (over the long-term) services. If they serve as stop-gap measures on the way to a world in which all countries have the resources and freedom to make their own decisions about health systems and the determinants of health, they may well play a legitimate—and vital—role. But the very proliferation of international actors appears to be more a reflection (or even reinforcement) of the increasing inequalities within and between countries, than an indication of the forging of sustainable health services by independent nations.

Of course, various organizations work to achieve such ends, but power is not shared equally among health actors. A handful of large bilateral agencies, multilateral financial agencies, and foundations finance and influence the field's practices and paradigms to a great extent (see Table 3–14). The biggest killers—diarrhea, respiratory disease, and heart disease—which have complex social and economic roots, receive far less attention (and international health funding) than a few cases of a disease (e.g., SARS) transmitted via air travel. While HIV, malaria, and TB have recently garnered significant new resources, many other health problems, including mental illnesses, injuries, and chronic diseases, are largely neglected by these actors. Despite the massive infusion of dollars to global health in recent years, the interventions that are a focus of this funding are unlikely to address the health needs of most of the 3 billion plus people who survive on less than US$2 per day (Garrett 2007), nor of those with high priority diseases like AIDS, malaria, and tuberculosis, but whose marginalization makes targeted programs insufficient to meet their needs; nor of those who suffer ill health and debility from causes that are not global priorities.

Because donor agencies increasingly follow corporate-style governance objectives that prioritize short-term, *efficient*, activities to demonstrate success, they tend to favor narrowly targeted, measurable interventions that are promoted as cost-effective over the short term. Numerous analysts have critiqued this approach for not addressing the underlying political, economic, and social determinants of health or the need to strengthen infrastructure and PHC in many recipient countries (Birn 2005; Cohen 2006; Garrett 2007).

The organization of international health today is marked both by historical legacies and new developments. The reductionist, technological approach to public health was developed in the early 20th century and consolidated during the Cold War. The competition between communism and capitalism proved fruitful for the

Table 3-14 Largest Current International Health Funders

Organization	Donors	Funds Pledged/Spent/Committed to Health
President's Emergency Plan for AIDS Relief (PEPFAR)	U.S. Government	US$15 billion (2003–2008) US$37 billion (2009–2013)
Global Fund to Fight AIDS, Tuberculosis and Malaria	Governments, Foundations, Corporations	US$11.3 billion committed since inception in 2002
Bill and Melinda Gates Foundation	Bill and Melinda Gates Warren Buffett	US$38.7 billion endowment, includes 1.8 billion from Buffett in 2008 US$16.5 billion granted since 2000
World Health Organization	Governments	US$4.2 billion (2008–2009, 2-year budget)
GAVI Alliance	Gates Foundation, Governments, NGOs, Private Businesses, Multilateral agencies	US$3.7 billion pledged as of April 2007 US$2.2 billion committed between 2000 and 2006
World Bank	Governments	US$2.8 billion (2007 budget)
OECD ODA (health, population, and sanitation)	22 DAC countries	US$12.4 billion (2006) (largest donor was United States at US$5 billion, followed by Japan at US$1.6 billion, Germany at US$1 billion, the United Kingdom at US$0.7 billion, and France at US$0.5 billion)
European Commission (health, population, and sanitation)	EU countries	US$1.3 billion (2006)

Sources: Adapted from Cohen (2006); Garrett (2007); and http://stats.oecd.org/wbos/default. aspx?DatasetCode=ODA_SECTOR.

developing countries that learned to play the superpowers against one another, benefiting from investments in social infrastructure. There was ability in certain settings to develop successful import substitution models and redistributive social welfare states. In most places, these advancements remained skewed toward elites who won local struggles over power and resources.

By the 1980s, the priority given to public sector spending was overturned by an ideology—known as neoliberalism—and its corresponding set of policies aimed at reducing social spending, privatizing state activities, and suspending regulations on business and the protection of the public (see Chapter 4). This shift affected both domestic policy making and the international aid arena. The Soviet Union, facing its own political and economic crises, no longer provided a counterbalance to what became known as the Washington Consensus. Invariably, neoliberal policies have affected both health and the activities of international health cooperation. Accompanying this change, the WHO's role was displaced by multilateral, financial, and bilateral agencies, PPPs, and large philanthropies.

Undoubtedly, the direct work of international health actors has far less impact on health status across the world than do the combination of international economics and domestic politics (i.e., how redistributive each country is in terms of providing access to health, education, and other social services, in ensuring fair working and living conditions, etc.). Health is subject to the enormous structural influences of international economic practices (commodity prices, terms of trade, multinational business) and World Bank and IMF loans and policies (and those of regional banks and private creditors) on national production patterns, wage levels, social infrastructure, and redistributive policies.

While the goals and projects of leading institutions have changed in concert with the broader political and social context—the Cold War, and then the dissolution of the Soviet empire, tensions between welfare state policies and neoliberal social and economic policies, the emergence of new ailments (HIV/AIDS), and the resurgence of old (TB, malaria)—there is a durability to their missions and modus operandi.

Just a few international players marshal considerable resources and have significant influence over national and international health priorities (see Fig. 3–4). These agencies not only have an inordinate role in shaping the major global and local

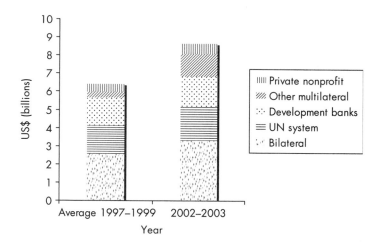

Figure 3–4 Development assistance for health by source, 1997–2003. *Note*: The category of other multilateral includes the European Union and the Global Fund to Fight AIDS, Tuberculosis and Malaria.
Source: Michaud, CM. 2003. "Development Assistance for Health (DAH): Recent Trends and Resource Allocation." Paper prepared for the Second Consultation of the Commission on Macroeconomics and Health, World Health Organization, Geneva, October 29–30. Also see (Gottret and Schieber 2006, p. 134).

approaches to health—oriented to technical disease-control interventions over short timelines, they also reinforce dominant ideologies that view health as a function of individual and medical factors.

Because of aid stipulations that require recipient governments to allocate substantial matching funds to donor programs, national needs and decision making inevitably become subsidiary to the priorities of donors. Funding criteria may require that discrete targets are met in a specified period of time, and therefore donors may select interventions that can provide these aims more readily (see Box 3–7).

Box 3–7 Rockefeller Foundation Principles of International Health Cooperation

1. Agenda-setting from above: international health activities are donor-driven, with the agenda of cooperation formulated and overseen by the international agency, whether through direct in-country activities or the awarding of grants.
2. Budget incentives: activities are only partially funded by donor agencies; matching fund mechanisms require recipient entities to commit substantial financial, human, and physical resources to the cooperative endeavor.
3. Technobiological paradigm: activities are structured in disease-control terms based upon: (a) biological and individual behavioral understandings of disease; and (b) technical tools applied to a wide range of settings.
4. A priori parameters of success: activities are bound geographically, through time limits, by disease and intervention, and/or according to clear exit strategies in order to demonstrate efficiency and ensure visible, positive outcomes.
5. Consensus via transnational professionals: activities hinge on transnational professionals—who are trained abroad (often alongside donor agency staff) and involved in international networks—easing the local translation of cooperative endeavors.
6. Reality check for successful implementation: adaptation to local conditions, as needed.

Source: Adapted from Birn (2006, p. 270).

Some have noted that critiquing the international health arena is akin to criticizing one's own mother. Yet, as we may all recall from moments in our own childhood (or in parenthood), even the best parents stand to improve on their abilities, and so can the international health field.

The international health system and health aid have been critiqued on a number of grounds:

- political and economic interests—rather than health needs—drive health aid;
- underlying global and local determinants of ill health are not addressed by health aid;
- bureaucratic institutions act to preserve and expand their power;
- ideologically-driven policies promote a market ethos;
- political interests upstage health outcomes;
- annual evaluations mean narrow objectives;
- little aid reaches the neediest;

- health "cooperation" is not cooperative (but reflects donor agendas);
- poverty alleviation and social justice principles are much touted but little practiced;
- aid tends to exacerbate inequalities; and
- global health threats to commerce and industrialized countries (e.g., Avian influenza, SARS) and fears of bioterrorism shape health aid more than needs-based rationales.

It is not even certain whether international health aid—as currently configured—is worth pursuing. For instance, PPPs arose during the WHO's funding crisis of the early 1990s—a crisis created by the willful reduction of U.S. support, which made the private sector appear as the only untapped source of funds. However, the insistence by donors for greater control over programs and policy making meant that industry was "invited" as a full partner in decision-making processes concerning what are, in fact, public issues. This proliferation of private, less than democratic, health aid has diverted attention away from the corporate sector's role in, for example, maintaining inequitable trade arrangements that jeopardize the livelihoods of millions of developing country workers and farmers (Ncayiyana 2007).

The Global Fund, despite its enormous resources and potential impact, has taken a narrow business-like approach to grant-making: applicant countries must propose technical, measurable-in-the-short-term approaches to AIDS, TB and malaria rather than address underlying determinants of all three ailments. Together with the Gates Foundation, the Fund has been accused of diverting local health workers from PHC roles, and overlooking related problems stemming from poverty and inequality, including nutrition, transportation, and housing (Piller and Smith 2007).

A recent Global Fund evaluation found that countries with weaker health systems and where many donors were involved received relatively low evaluation scores on their grants. Interestingly, while grants made to governments rather than NGOs generally had weaker scores, countries that "have or have had socialist governments received higher scores" (Radelet and Siddiqi 2007, p. 1811), suggesting the importance of existing infrastructure and social redistribution as key factors in the success of Global Fund programs. Indeed, it took 5 years for the Global Fund to begin to direct significant grant funding to health system strengthening, but it has yet to consider the role of other social and economic determinants of disease.

Just because an organization is removed from government structures does not necessarily enhance its ability to redress inequities in power. As discussed above, many NGOs operate as sub-contractors for—and are thus accountable to—large bilateral, private, and multilateral actors, inevitably, if inadvertently, reflecting their interests and approaches. Rather than representing an engaged public, NGOs are increasingly displacing social movements. The ostensibly apolitical stance of NGOs and humanitarian organizations—through which these agencies stay out of political discussions regarding the contexts within which they work and instead focus purely on "humanitarian aid"—leaves them open to criticism. Historically, the Red Cross was accused of rationalizing war for aiding war wounded and war victims without taking a stance against war per se (Hutchinson 1996).

While many global health actors articulate noble intentions, by no means does this certify that money is well spent or reaches its target. There is currently no framework of accountability for global health, and no mechanisms to ensure that actors do not duplicate some services at the expense of others (Cohen 2006). Some see recipient government corruption as a major impediment to service provision, and consequently do not direct funding through national ministries. Others perceive inefficiencies on the part of donor governments and agencies, which siphon off aid funds to corrupt contractors or spend excessive sums on administration and consultant salaries. Without global accountability mechanisms, significant amounts of donor funding is unlikely to reach its target populations (Garrett 2007).

More importantly, global health problems stem largely from political and economic priorities across and within countries. For example, in the 1980s and early 1990s, Israel and Egypt were the largest beneficiaries of U.S. government assistance, reflecting their strategic importance to the United States. Even today Israel, categorized as a high-income country, receives more donor aid than some of the world's poorest countries—US$115 per capita compared to US$40 per capita in Burkino Faso (Hirvonen 2005).

To the extent that health aid from resources in the North/West originates from exploitation of countries of the South/East, health aid simply perpetuates larger economic forces. Underdeveloped countries put far more money into international agencies and projects than they receive back. Accordingly, fundamental to the reform of global health is the reform of commodity pricing and terms of trade that condemn more than half the world's population to poverty.

CONCLUSIONS

Learning Points:

- There has been a proliferation of international health actors in recent years, including PPPs and large and small NGOs, leading to fragmented and unrepresentative decision making and activities.
- While multilateral institutions, especially the World Bank, and the U.S. government, continue to play an important role in international health activities, the role of foundations and private sector interests has soared, exacerbating undemocratic agenda-setting.
- International health aid lacks an accountability framework, and continues to reflect donor-driven, technologically-oriented priorities.

International health (agencies and actors) face(s) persistent dilemmas. Should it (they) pursue horizontal approaches to health aimed at providing permanent and universal infrastructure and integration with other sectors or should it (they) carry out vertical (top-down) efforts that are fast and straightforward? Should it emphasize underlying causes of ill health or immediate problems? Or both? Are PPPs an effective marshalling of private-sector funding or a manipulation of democratic processes? How can the international health field address duplication of efforts, competition for resources, and lack of coordination? Who is responsible for improving international governance and accountability—institutions themselves or elected bodies?

Of course these dichotomies may be oversimplified and much depends on particular situations. But why not think outside the box and consider the possibility of developing government-to-developing government cooperation? After all—as various Latin American and African countries have discovered—there is much horizontal learning that takes place under such circumstances.

What remains certain is that without a better alignment of global health priorities and understandings of the underlying determinants of premature death and disability, global health initiatives—no matter how well funded—are unlikely to achieve long-term health improvement.

Before contemplating what might be done to improve global health, we must first deepen our understanding of the patterns of health across the world, and their social, political, and economic determinants.

NOTE

1. The issue of Taiwan's renewed membership in the WHO has been raised frequently since then.

REFERENCES

ActionAid International. 2005. Real Aid: An agenda for making aid work. http://www. actionaid.org/docs/real_aid.pdf. Accessed February 5, 2007.

AVERT. 2007. What is PEPFAR? 2007. http://www.avert.org/pepfar.htm. Accessed May 29, 2007.

Bhattacharya S. 2006. *Expunging Variola: The Control and Eradication of Smallpox in India, 1947–1977.* Hyderabad, India: Orient Longman.

Birn A-E. 2005. Gates's grandest challenge: Transcending technology as public health ideology. *Lancet* 266(9484):514–519.

———. 2006. *Marriage of Convenience: Rockefeller International Health and Revolutionary Mexico.* Rochester: University of Rochester Press.

———. 2009. The stages of international (global) health: Histories of success or successes of history? *Global Public Health* 4(1):50–68.

Birn A-E, Zimmerman S, and Garfield R. 2000. To decentralize or not to decentralize, is that the question? Nicaraguan health policy under structural adjustment in the 1990s. *International Journal of Health Services* 30(1):111–128.

Breman A and Shelton C. 2007. Structural adjustment programs and health. In Kawachi I and Wamala S, Editors. *Globalization and Health.* New York: Oxford University Press.

Brown H. 2007. Great expectations. *British Medical Journal* 334(7599):874–876.

Brown T, Cueto M, and Fee E. 2006. The World Health Organization and the transition from "international" to "global" public health. *American Journal of Public Health* 96(1):62–72.

Buse K and Harmer A. 2007. Seven habits of highly effective global public-private health partnerships: Practice and potential. *Social Science and Medicine* 64(2):259–271.

Buse K and Lee K. 2005. Business and Global Health Governance: Discussion Paper No. 5. Geneva: World Health Organization.

Buse K and Walt G. 2000. Global public-private partnerships: Part I—A new development in health? *Bulletin of the World Health Organisation* 78(4):549–561.

Cassels A. 1997. *A Guide to Sector-Wide Approaches for Health Development: Concepts, Issues and Working Arrangements.* Geneva: World Health Organization.

Center for Global Development. 2008. The Pentagon as a development agency? Q&A with Stewart Patrick. http://www.cgdev.org/content/general/detail/15359. Accessed February 20, 2008.

Center for Public Integrity. 2006. Bush's AIDS initiative: Too little choice, too much ideology. Divine Intervention: US AIDS Policy Abroad. http://projects.publicintegrity.org/aids/. Accessed May 5, 2007.

Centre Tricontinental, Gresea, and Editions Syllepse. 2007. Coalitions d'Etats du Sud: Retour de l'esprit de Bandung? Points de vue du Sud. *Alternatives du Sud.* 14(3).

Cohen J. 2006. Global health: The new world of global health. *Science* 311(5758):162–167.

Develtere P and Huybrechts A. 2002. *Evidence on the Social and Economic Impact of Grameen Bank and BRAC on the Poor in Bangladesh.* Leuven, Belgium: Higher Institute of Labour Studies, Catholic University of Leuven.

Dobson MJ, Malowany M, and Snow RW. 2000. Malaria control in East Africa: The Kampala Conference and the Pare-Taveta Scheme: A meeting of common and high ground. *Parassitologia* 40(1–2):149–166.

Editorial. 2006. HIV prevention policy needs an urgent cure. *Lancet* 367(9518):1213.

FAO. 2007. Venezuela donates US$4.6 million for agricultural development in Mali and Burkina Faso. http://www.fao.org/newsroom/en/news/2007/1000496/index.html. Accessed May 30, 2007.

Fiszbein A, Giovagnoli PI, and Aduriz I. 2002. Argentina's crisis and its impact on household welfare. *CEPAL Review* 79:143–158.

Garfield R and Taboada E. 1984. Health services reforms in revolutionary Nicaragua. *American Journal of Public Health* 74(10):1138–1144.

Garrett L. 2007. The challenge of global health. *Foreign Affairs* 86(1):14–38.

Gottret P and Schieber G. 2006. *Health Financing Revisited: A Practitioner's Guide.* Washington, DC: World Bank.

Greenaway D and Morrisey O. 1993. Structural adjustment and liberalisation in developing countries: What lessons have we learned? *Kyklos* 46(2):241–261.

Greenough P. 1995. Intimidation, coercion and resistance in the final stages of the South Asian Smallpox Eradication Campaign, 1973–1975. *Social Science and Medicine* 41(5):633–645.

Greenwood, BM, Greenwood AM, Bradley AK, Tulloch S, Hayes R, and Oldfield FSJ. 1987. Deaths in infancy and early childhood in a well-vaccinated, rural, West African population. *Annals of Tropical Paediatrics* 7(2):91–99.

Group of 77 at the United Nations, Nairobi Chapter. 2007. Historical background. http://www.unon.org/g77/history.html. Accessed November 15, 2007.

Gwatkin DR, Wagstaff A, and Yazbeck AS, Editors. 2005. *Reaching the Poor with Health, Nutrition, and Population Services: What Works, What Doesn't, and Why.* Washington, DC: World Bank.

Heaton A and Keith R. 2002. *A Long Way to Go: A Critique of GAVI's Initial Impact.* London: Save the Children UK.

Henderson D. 1998. Smallpox eradication: A Cold War victory. *World Health Forum* 19(2):113–119.

Hirvonen P. 2005. Stingy Samaritans: Why recent increases in development aid fail to help the poor. http://www.globalpolicy.org/socecon/develop/oda/2005/08stingysamaritans. pdf. Accessed October 31, 2007.

HLSP Institute. 2005. *Sector Wide Approaches: A Resource Document for UNFPA Staff.* HLSP Institute: London.

Hutchinson JF. 1996. *Champions of Charity: War and the Rise of the Red Cross.* Boulder, CO: Westview.

IMF. 2007a. Review of the Fund's income position for FY 2007 and FY 2008. http://www. imf.org/external/np/pp/2007/eng/040907.pdf. Accessed February 1, 2008.

———. 2007b. The Policy Support Instrument: A Factsheet. http://www.imf.org/external/ np/exr/facts/psi.htm. Accessed November 4, 2007.

———. 2008. Poverty Reduction Strategy Papers (PRSP): A Factsheet. http://www.imf. org/external/np/exr/facts/prsp.htm. Accessed September 3, 2008.

Institute of Medicine (IOM), and Committee for the Evaluation of the President's Emergency Plan for AIDS Relief (PEPFAR) Implementation. 2007. *PEPFAR Implementation: Progress and Promise.* Washington, DC: The National Academies Press.

IRIN (Integrated Regional Information Networks). 2006. China to double aid to Africa. http://www.worldpress.org/Africa/2554.cfm. Accessed May 30, 2007.

Kates J, Morrison JS, and Lief E. 2006. Global health funding: A glass half full? *Lancet* 368(9531):187–188.

Katz A. 2005. The Sachs report: Investing in health for economic development—or increasing the size of the crumbs from the rich man's table? *International Journal of Health Services* 35(1):171–188.

Kelly A. 2008. Growing discontent. *The Guardian*, February 20, 2008.

Kent G. 1991. *The Politics of Children's Survival.* New York: Praeger Publishers.

Khatun M, Stenlund H, and Hörnell A. 2004. BRAC initiative towards promoting gender and social equity in health: A longitudinal study of child growth in Matlab, Bangladesh. *Public Health Nutrition* 7(8):1071–1079.

Lane C and Glassman A. 2007. Bigger and better? Scaling up and innovation in health aid. *Health Affairs* 26(4):935–948.

La Via Campesina. 2002. Declaration NGO forum FAO summit Rome +5. http://www. viacampesina.org/main_en/index.php?option=com_content&task=view&id=418&Item id=38. Accessed October 12, 2007.

Lee K, Buse K, and Fustukian S, Editors. 2002. *Health Policy in a Globalising World.* Cambridge: Cambridge University Press.

Levine R and Buse K. 2006. The World Bank's new health sector strategy: Building on key assets. *Journal of the Royal Society of Medicine* 99:569–572.

Maciocco G and Italian Global Health Watch. 2008. From Alma Ata to the Global Fund: The history of international health policy. *Social Medicine* 3(1):36–48.

McCoy D. 2007. The World Bank's new health strategy: Reason for alarm? *Lancet* 369(9572):1499–1501.

McKee M. 2007. A UK global health strategy: The next steps. *British Medical Journal* 335(7611):110.

Médecins Sans Frontières. 2007. G8 declaration on innovation and intellectual property will directly harm access to medicines across the developing world. http://www.msf. org.hk/public/contents/news?ha=&wc=0&hb=&hc=&revision%5fid=28030&item%5 fid=27009. Accessed January 22, 2008.

Mercer C. 2002. NGOs, civil society and democratization: A critical review of the literature. *Progress in Development Studies* 2(1):5–22.

Molyneux M and Razavi S. 2005. Beijing plus ten: An ambivalent record on gender justice. *Development and Change* 36(6):983–1010.

Muraskin W. 2005. *Crusade to Immunize the World's Children: The Origins of the Bill and Melinda Gates Children's Vaccine Program and the Birth of the Global Alliance for Vaccines and Immunization.* Los Angeles, CA: USC Marshall Global Bio Business Initiative.

Ncayiyana DJ. 2007. Combating poverty: The charade of development aid. *British Medical Journal* 335(7633):1272–1273.

Nyiri P. 2006. The yellow man's burden: Chinese migrants on a civilizing mission. *The China Journal* 56:83–106.

OECD. 2006a. *OECD Factbook: Economic, Environmental and Social Statistics.* Paris: OECD Publications.

———. 2006b. Development Aid at a Glance: Statistics by region. http://www.oecd.org/dataoecd/59/5/37781218.pdf. Accessed May 4, 2007.

Ollila E. 2005a. Global health priorities—priorities of the wealthy? *Globalization and Health* 1(6):1-5.

———. 2005b. Restructuring global health policy making: The role of global public-private partnerships. In Mackintosh M and Koivusalo M, Editors. *Commercialization of Health Care: Global and Local Dynamics and Policy Responses.* Basingstoke, UK: Palgrave Macmillan.

Oxfam International. 2004. Guns or Growth? Assessing the impact of arms sales on sustainable development. http://www.oxfam.org/files/Guns_or_Growth_0.pdf. Accessed May 1, 2007.

Packard RM. 1998. "No other logical choice": Global malaria eradication and the politics of international health in the postwar era. *Parassitologia* 40(1–2):217–230.

People's Health Movement. 2005. A statement prepared for "Making Partnerships Work for Health," World Health Organization, October 26–28, 2005. http://www.phmovement. org/cms/en/node/117. Accessed May 3, 2007.

PepsiCo. 2008. PepsiCo's health and wellness philosophy. http://www.pepsico.com/PEP_Citizenship/HealthWellness/philosophy/index.cfm. Accessed February 11, 2008.

Perlez J. 2006. China competes with West in aid to its neighbors. *New York Times*, September 18.

Pettifor A, Thomas B, and Telatin M. 2001. HIPC: Flogging a dead process: Jubilee Plus. http://www.jubileeusa.org/fileadmin/user_upload/Resources/Policy_Archive/deadHIPC. pdf. Accessed May 12, 2007.

Pfeiffer J. 2003. International NGOs and primary health care in Mozambique: The need for a new model of collaboration. *Social Science and Medicine* 56(4):725–738.

———. 2005. Commodity fetichismo, the Holy Spirit, and the turn to Pentecostal and African Independent Churches in central Mozambique. *Culture, Medicine and Psychiatry* 29:255–283.

Piller C, Sanders E, and Dixon R. 2007. Dark clouds over the good works of Gates Foundation. *Los Angeles Times*, January 7.

Piller C and Smith D. 2007. Unintended victims of Gates Foundation generosity. *Los Angeles Times*, December 16.

Population Action International. 2005. 2005 Update: Trends in international development assistance for reproductive health and population. http://216.146.209.72/Publications/ Reports/Progress_and_Promises/Interactive/pandp/2005update.htm. Accessed October 10, 2007.

Radelet S and Siddiqi B. 2007. Global Fund grant programmes: An analysis of evaluation scores. *Lancet* 369(9575):1807–1813.

Richter J. 2004. *Public-Private Partnerships and International Health Policy-Making: How can Public Interests be Safeguarded?* Helsinki: Ministry for Foreign Affairs of Finland.

Roy A. 2004. Help that hinders. *Le Monde Diplomatique*, November. http://mondediplo. com/2004/11/16roy. Accessed February 14, 2008.

Ruger JP. 2005. The changing role of the World Bank in global health. *American Journal of Public Health* 95(2):60–70.

Salaam-Blyther T. 2007. *PEPFAR: From Emergency to Sustainability. CRS Report for Congress*. Washington, DC: Congressional Research Service.

Schlager C. 2007. *Challenges for International Development Co-operation: The Case of Brazil*. Berlin: Friedrich Ebert Stiftung.

Schrecker T, Labonte R, and Sanders D. 2007. Breaking faith with Africa: The G8 and population health after Gleneagles. In Cooper A, Kirton J, and Schrecker T, Editors. *Governing Global Health*. Burlington, VT: Ashgate.

Sekhri N and Savedoff W. 2006. Regulating private health insurance to serve the public interest: Policy issues for developing countries. *International Journal of Health Planning and Management* 21(4):357–392.

Silver GA. 1998. International health services need an interorganizational policy. *American Journal of Public Health* 88(5):727–729.

Toussaint E, Diouf M, Mata GT, Desgain S, Peter J, and Millet D. 2003. *La dette: Tragédie, illusion et arnaque*. Liège, Belgium: CADTM, CNCD, CONGAD.

Tull D. 2006. China's engagement in Africa: Scope, significance and consequences. *Journal of Modern African Studies* 44(3):459–479.

UN. 2007. Past conferences and general assembly special sessions 2007. http://www. un.org/events/conferences.htm. Accessed October 12, 2007.

UN Millennium Project. 2006. Goals, targets and indicators. http://www.unmillenniumproject. org/goals/gti.htm#goal1. Accessed March 23, 2007.

UNCTAD. 2004. *Least Developed Countries Report 2004*. New York: United Nations.

———. 2005. More aid vital to eradicating extreme poverty, says UNDP Report. http:// www.un.lv/uploaded_files/PR2.pdf. Accessed May 11, 2007.

UNDP. 2002. *Human Development Report 2002: Deepening Democracy in a Fragmented World*. New York: Oxford University Press for the United Nations Development Programme.

UNESCO. 2007. 1972–2006: From Stockholm to Mexico. http://www.unesco.org/water/ wwap/milestones/index.shtml. Accessed May 29, 2007.

UNICEF. 2005. *Progress for Children: A Report Card on Immunization, Number 3*. New York: UNICEF.

USAID. 2006. USAID Policy: Mission organization and structure. http://www.usaid.gov/ policy/par06/highlights_002.html. Accessed May 20, 2007.

Utting P and Zammit A. 2006. *Beyond Pragmatism. Appraising UN-Business Partnerships. Markets, Business and Regulation Programme Paper Number 1*. Geneva: United Nations Research Institute for Social Development.

Walsh J and Warren K. 1979. Selective primary health care: An interim strategy for disease control in developing countries. *New England Journal of Medicine* 301(18):967–974.

Wamala S, Kawachi I, and Mpepo BP. 2007. Poverty Reduction Strategy Papers: Bold new approach to poverty eradication or old wine in new bottles? In Kawachi I and Wamala S, Editors. *Globalization and Health*. New York: Oxford University Press.

Warren KS. 1988. The evolution of selective primary health care. *Social Science and Medicine* 26(8):891–898.

Welch C. 2001. Structural adjustment programs and poverty reduction strategy. *Foreign Policy in Focus* 5(14). http://www.fpif.org/briefs/vol5/v5n14sap.html. Accessed May 13, 2007.

Werner D and Sanders D. 1997. *Questioning the Solution: The Politics of Health Care and Child Survival*. Palo Alto, CA: HealthWrights.

WHO. 1978. *Declaration of Alma-Ata. International Conference on Primary Health Care*. Alma-Ata, USSR.

———. 1993. Resolution WHA46.17 Health development in a changing world—a call for collective action. Forty-sixth World Health Assembly. Geneva, May 3–14. Geneva: World Health Organization.

———. 2004. *The World Health Report 2004: Changing History*. Geneva: World Health Organization.

———. 2006a. *Progress on Global Access to HIV Antiretroviral Therapy: A Report on "3 by 5" and Beyond*. Geneva: World Health Organization.

———. 2006b. *The World Health Report 2006: Working Together for Health*. Geneva: World Health Organization.

———. 2007a. Knowledge Management for Public Health (KM4PH). Partners. http://www.who.int/km4ph/partners/en/. Accessed October 10, 2007.

———. 2007b. Programme budget 2008–2009. http://www.who.int/gb/ebwha/pdf_files/AMTSP-PPB/a-mtsp_4en.pdf. Accessed October 18, 2007.

———. 2007c. WHO model list of essential medicines, 15th list. http://www.who.int/medicines/publications/essentialmedicines/en/index.html. Accessed June 27, 2007.

———. 2008. Executive Board, 21–25 January 2008 EB122/19 Partnerships

Wilpert G. 2007. Nicaragua joins Venezuela in regional association and cooperation agreements. http://www.venezuelanalysis.com/news.php?newsno=2190. Accessed May 30, 2007.

Wintour P and Leigh D. 2007. Tories launch challenge over corruption claims in $40m radar sale to Tanzania. *The Guardian*, January 30.

World Bank. 2007a. *Aid Architecture: An Overview of the Main Trends in Official Development Assistance Flows*. Washington, DC: World Bank.

———. 2007b. Board presentations of PRSP documents as of August 31, 2007. http://siteresources.worldbank.org/INTPRS1/Resources/boardlist.pdf. Accessed November 2, 2007.

———. 2007c. Healthy development: The World Bank strategy for health nutrition and population results. http://siteresources.worldbank.org/HEALTHNUTRITIONANDPOPULATION/Resources/281627-1154048816360/HNPStrategyFINALApril302007.pdf. Accessed November 12, 2008.

———. 2007d. HIPC: MDRI. http://siteresources.worldbank.org/INTDEBTDEPT/Resources/Debt_PocketBroch_Spring07.pdf?resourceurlname=Debt_PocketBroch_Spring07.pdf. Accessed October 3, 2007.

———. 2007e. HNP Lending. http://go.worldbank.org/851WC143GO. Accessed November 12, 2008.

4

The Political Economy of Health and Development

UNDERSTANDING HEALTH AND DISEASE

Key Questions:

- What are the underlying causes of health and illness?
- How do the main models of understanding health and disease address these factors?

Imagine you are a middle-aged minibus driver in a highly populated city. Transport, like most industries in your country, is largely unregulated. Vehicle emissions contribute to particularly dangerous pollution levels throughout the year, and road accidents take an enormous toll on the lives of young adults. The pay is low and in order to earn enough to provide for your family, you work upwards of 12 hours per day, 6 days a week, in fierce competition with other private bus drivers. Throughout the day you barely take a break, buying food from street vendors and eating your meals as you drive. Despite your long work hours, you are chronically behind on bills and can only afford an apartment in a dilapidated building that you know to be structurally unsound, without potable water and with unreliable sanitation. Your wages must cover living costs for your family and school fees for your children, as the government only partly subsidizes education. There is no labor union for transit workers, your employer offers no benefits, and your government offers meager social welfare benefits—a worthless pension and no health insurance. Although business is booming throughout your country, with new buildings and companies appearing almost every month, you have not felt the benefits of this economic growth.

One morning, while driving your bus, you experience a brief but frightening episode of shortness of breath and tightness in your chest. You finish your route and decide to see a doctor on your way home. After conducting an EKG and other tests, the doctor diagnoses you with high blood pressure, symptoms of angina, and possible early coronary heart disease. She recommends blood tests to assess cholesterol levels, as these may be high given your sedentary and stressful occupation and weight. After advising you to make dietary and physical activity changes, and prescribing an expensive medication that might lower your risk of a heart attack, the doctor charges you for the consultation. The fee is equivalent to a day's work.

How can we understand and address your (the driver's) health problems?

This chapter presents the main explanations for health and disease patterns, with an in-depth focus on the political economy of health approach. It then explores the role of international development processes and their influence on health since World War II, paying special attention to emerging perspectives and tools, including the human capabilities and health and human rights approaches. The chapter concludes with a discussion of international health aid from a political economy perspective.

MODELS FOR UNDERSTANDING HEALTH AND DISEASE

The relationship between well-being and the contexts in which people are or become healthy or sick is central to understanding the patterns of living and dying across the world. This relationship is taken for granted by many international health actors; sometimes it is explicitly articulated, but often it is overlooked. Here we discuss three basic approaches for explaining how health and illness occur:

- The *biomedical model* views health and illness at the individual level, with the body conceptualized as a machine with constituent parts (i.e., organ systems, genes, and so on) that can be manipulated or repaired. Health is understood primarily in terms of the absence of disease, rather than as an integrated sense of well-being. While the biomedical approach is largely curative, it also includes a preventive armamentarium (such as vaccines, screening, and genetic testing) and considers the role of behavioral determinants of health insofar as they affect so-called risk factors—personal characteristics related to heredity and "lifestyle" that are believed to predispose individuals to disease. Much of the appeal of the biomedical approach stems from the dramatic technological advances in medical treatment over the last century, such as in surgery (including anesthesia and asepsis) and pharmacotherapy. The search for and application of so-called magic bullets—technological fix-it tools—most vividly characterize this model.

  According to the biomedical approach to health, as the bus driver in the example above, you need to heed behavioral change advice and take prescription drugs in order to improve your health.

- The *behavioral model* views health and illness primarily as a consequence of individual or household actions and beliefs; it results either as a reward for healthy living or the (inevitable) outcome of poor lifestyle choices and personal deficiencies. This approach primarily focuses on the regulation or changing of personal conduct and cultural attitudes through education, counseling, and incentives in order to achieve desirable health outcomes. Although social and structural issues are sometimes addressed, this approach primarily views the individual (and sometimes the household or community) as responsible for health. In many cultures, the behavioral model is also filtered through spiritual beliefs, whereby good or ill health may be linked to supernatural phenomena.

According to the behavioral approach to health, you must make different choices regarding the food you eat, avoid stressful situations, take more breaks on the job, work fewer hours, and engage in light physical activity in order to improve your health status.

- The *political economy approach* to understanding health and illness considers the political, social, cultural, and economic contexts in which disease and illness arise, and examines the ways in which societal structures (i.e., political and economic practices and institutions, and class interrelations) interact with the particular conditions that lead to good or ill health. This approach views health as a function and reflection of linked determinants that operate at multiple levels: individual, household, community, workplace, social class,[1] nation, and the global political and economic context. These determinants need to be addressed in order to improve health through, for example, public policy aimed at improving transportation and housing conditions, medical care, social empowerment strategies (gender equity, unionization), and social-class-mediated political involvement aimed at bettering redistribution[2] and overall societal welfare across all social groups. These efforts include, *but are not reduced to,* biomedical technologies and behavior/lifestyle.

According to the political economy approach to health, your health is a result of social, political, and economic structures and relations that constrain your control over stressful situations and work environment, and limit your access to health care, recreation, housing, education, and good nutrition. As such, many of your health problems can only be addressed beyond the behavioral or medical levels, through improved working conditions, social policies, and political mobilization.

It is important to emphasize that these three approaches are not mutually exclusive; in practice, they often overlap and must be understood in conjunction with one another. In a more conducive environment, bus drivers might be able to exert more control over the determinants of their health. This could take the form of a shorter workday with more breaks, forming/joining a union and bargaining for higher wages and better working conditions, or participating in a political process that results in an improved welfare state—that is, government provision or protection of social and economic goods and benefits (such as employment, housing, food, social security, education and health services, maternal and child benefits, etc.) for the collective well-being of the entire society. Stress levels would be lessened if quality housing were subsidized and education provided free of charge. With universal health care coverage, medical practitioners could be consulted before the onset of severe symptoms, and in a less pressured work environment, it would be easier to exercise and eat more nutritious meals.

Because the political economy approach takes into account the proximate biomedical and behavioral factors *and* the larger political, economic, and social context, it has the greatest explanatory capacity of the three models. As we saw in Chapter 2, historical studies show that life expectancy increases in industrializing Europe from the 18th century onwards derived from a mix of social and political factors, such as better nutrition, education, housing conditions, sanitation and public health, maternal and child hygiene, and economic growth (Szreter 1988; Riley 2001). Medical technologies, introduced after mortality declines had already begun, played a marginal role in increasing life expectancy, arguably to the present (McKeown, Record, and Turner 1975; Catalano and Frank 2001). Meanwhile, behavioral changes (such as hand-washing) were heavily mediated by education level, social class, indoor plumbing, and other features of the sociopolitical landscape.

The political economy framework also helps explain why the argument that "wealthier is healthier" (Steckel and Floud 1997) does not bear out—historically or contemporaneously—unless the question of the distribution of increased wealth is taken into account. Indeed, despite soaring economic growth in mid-19th-century English cities (as well as in 20th-century United States, contemporary China, and elsewhere), mortality rates stagnated or even increased (Schofield, Reher, and Bideau 1991; Tapia Granados 2005). Why? Because the benefits of growth were not spread across social classes: industrial laborers faced atrocious living and working conditions, while factory owners accumulated wealth. Not until the late 19th century did these conditions (and the associated mortality) begin to improve in many European countries as part of large-scale social and political struggles to create redistributive welfare states.

More recent mortality declines in underdeveloped settings—postulated to have resulted from either the indirect by-products of economic development or the conscious results of social policy (including diffusion of medical technologies)—require further analysis. Preston estimates that only 20% of life expectancy improvements in these settings is associated with increases in income, leaving deliberate social policy (including improved nutrition, education, and sanitation) as a far more important explanatory factor (Preston 1980). Fogel emphasizes the importance of "technophysio evolution"—that is, the interaction among caloric intake, productivity, and longevity—(Fogel 2004) in developed and underdeveloped settings alike. Others propose that mortality improvements since 1930 have derived largely from vaccines, antibiotics, and other biomedical measures (Cutler, Deaton, and Lleras-Muney 2006), as well as the institutional infrastructure required to enable these developments (Powles 2001). However, there is little data to support such tentative assessments.

While definitive patterns are hard to glean across time and place, the one factor consistently associated with mortality declines in developing countries is a high level of female education (Schultz 1993), which is a clear manifestation of social redistribution. This further bolsters the political economy underpinnings of life expectancy improvement (well beyond the effects of economic development, medical technology, or behavioral changes).

As we shall see in later chapters, a set of low-income settings (e.g., Costa Rica, the Indian state of Kerala, Cuba, Sri Lanka) have managed to reach life expectancy levels similar to far wealthier countries, largely thanks to social–democratic and socialist political systems favoring economic and social redistribution (including, but certainly not limited to, medical technologies and health behaviors) (Halstead, Walsh, and Warren 1985; Cereseto and Waitzkin 1986; UN 1986; Kawachi and Kennedy 2002). This is not to say that biomedical or behavioral factors do not or have not played any role in these health improvements, only that they have a smaller explanatory capacity than the overall political economy approach, which includes medicine and behavior as subsets of the framework.

One way of understanding how these models intersect is by examining the relationship among host (intrinsic, individual factors of the human body and its susceptibility), agent (microbes, toxins, food substances, and other etiologic factors), and environment (broader social and political structures and relations) in determining health and illness. While public health efforts historically prioritized environmental factors as the arena for interventions as per the solid-line circles in Figure 4–1 (i.e., sanitation, food safety, social security, housing, and work hours all aimed at decreasing exposure and improving resistance), the host was never missing from

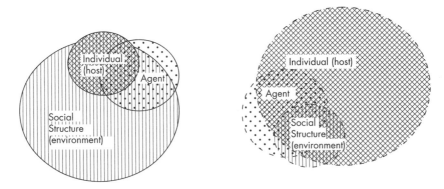

Figure 4–1 Understanding health and illness: the interplay of host, agent, and environment. Solid lines (left): pre-1900 conceptualization; dotted lines (right): post-1970s conceptualization.

this equation. Advice regarding diet, rest, and fresh air was long purveyed by healers, together with herbal and chemical remedies to treat ailments.

By the early 20th century, the rise of the germ theory led to the growing dominance of the medical model, with interventions increasingly focused on the role of the agent in determining illness (i.e., bacteria, viruses, and the corresponding medical interventions such as vaccines, antitoxins, and antibiotics). Of course agent and society overlapped, insofar as improved nutrition, ventilation, neighborhood and work conditions, and so on, also decreased exposure to disease agents, and hygienic measures in the operating room (antisepsis and asepsis) decreased fatal surgical infections. However, societal factors were no longer central to explanations of and interventions against disease.

More recently, as indicated by the dotted line circles (Fig. 4–1), the dominant public (and international) health approach has utilized behavioral and medical models, with the role of broader societal relations and structures de-emphasized. Focus on the individual, in terms of genetic and so-called lifestyle factors (e.g., smoking, narcotics, and alcohol use, interpersonal violence, stress, sedentary lifestyles, diet, etc.), combined with medical interventions (surgery, medications, and other therapeutic measures aimed at attenuating the agent–host interaction), has relegated the social environment to a smaller, subsidiary role (Buchanan 2000).

These shifts are reflective of changes in the accompanying political, economic, and epidemiologic order, particularly in industrializing countries, but also in colonial and other underdeveloped settings. Early 20th century industrialization, with its focus on mechanization and the assembly line, was consistent with the notion of the body as a machine maintained or repaired through technical measures. High rates of infectious disease, previously understood as the result of deleterious social environments, were now conceived of as a problem of microbial invasion (agents of disease) to be addressed through specific pharmaco-therapeutic products.

The consolidation of capitalism[3] by the 1970s (and its near global dominance by the 1990s), combined with the rise of noncommunicable ailments such as cancer and heart disease, brought forth explanations of disease as residing in individual deficiencies that needed to be corrected through personal behavioral change combined with "agent interventions," ranging from beta-blockers to balloon angioplasty, radiation, and chemotherapy (Tesh 1988; Minkler 1999). This behavioral–medical approach further sidestepped the focus on collective structural changes—including regulation of industry, improvement of workplace conditions, wealth redistribution, and pollution abatement—which threatened to interrupt the process of capital accumulation and the extant class power imbalances that enabled a concentration of wealth among an elite class (Navarro 2002). In objective terms, health and disease patterns continued to be subject to the interaction among host, agent, and society, but in health promotion and intervention terms, the behavioral (or lifestyle) and medical approaches—particularly focused on the individual host—became pervasive.

By contrast, Figure 4–2 schematically represents the political economy approach to health, taking into account the micro, meso, and macro, or the individual, household/

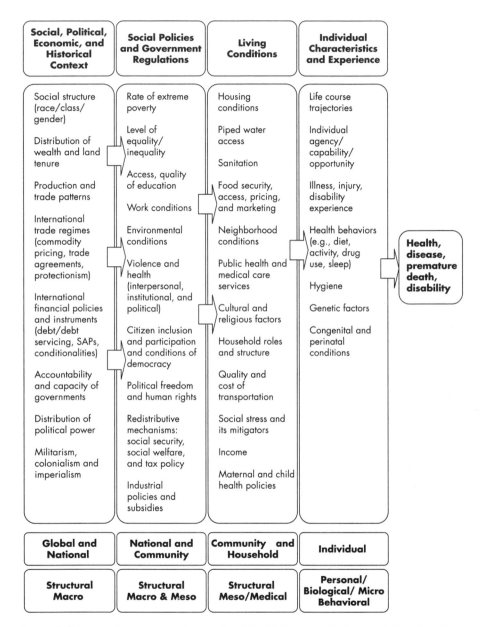

Figure 4-2 Political economy of international health framework. *Source*: Adapted with permission from Gloyd (1987).

community, national, and international determinants of health. Understanding these determinants and the interconnections among them will help us to explain and address the health and disease patterns within, between, and across countries and populations. The following case study illustrates how and why biomedical and behavioral interventions, when employed alone, are unable to improve population health status.

Case Study: Working Conditions, Poverty, and Tuberculosis in South African Mines

The rate of pulmonary tuberculosis (TB)—a long-term ailment of the lungs—is one of the most sensitive indicators of social and political conditions in a society. In an exploration of the history of TB, Randall Packard shows the relationship among working and living conditions, poverty, and tuberculosis in black miners in South Africa in the 20th century as compared to 19th-century British factory workers (Packard 1989). In both countries and eras, TB epidemics surged in conjunction with industrialization. Migration to urban industrial centers in Britain and mining towns in South Africa brought workers in contact with TB for the first time. In both settings, once workers and their families were exposed to TB, they were unable to resist the disease due to persistent poor living and working conditions. The vested economic and political interests of the state and industry in maximizing production relied on exploitation of the working class: these powerful interests were thus opposed to social and labor reforms to improve social conditions.

In Europe, improved housing, working conditions, and nutrition, together with the isolation of the sick in sanatoria, eventually led to declining rates of TB starting in the mid-19th century. In mid-20th century South Africa, there were no comparable broad-based investments in labor or social conditions for the black working class. To the contrary, white workers colluded with the political regime in order to preserve white settler privilege and repress an organized multiracial labor force. As a result, while white South African miners experienced modest improvements in conditions, black workers continued to live in abject poverty. To explain the high mortality rates of TB among the black working class, colonial administrators and national medical officers relied on the biomedical and behavioral models and referred to poor hygiene, supposed racial susceptibility, and an inadequate diet to explain the increase of TB, instead of addressing the underlying conditions that fueled the disease. The use of effective antituberculosis drugs in the 1950s eventually led to a sharp drop in TB deaths among black South Africans, but as new laborers continued to migrate to mining and industrial areas with poor working and living conditions, the incidence of TB cases remained extremely high (Packard 1989).

In recent years, with continued substandard social and working conditions in South Africa, and immune response to TB weakened by other diseases such as HIV/AIDS, tuberculosis rates have soared in rural and urban areas alike. As well, a heavy reliance on health services (as per the biomedical model) that are understaffed and poorly coordinated and the unregulated use of antituberculosis drugs have led to the emergence of extensively drug-resistant TB strains, necessitating longer, more complex treatment.

Over the past few decades a similar phenomenon has taken place in societies as diverse as Peru, the United States, and Russia, where increased homelessness, malnutrition, marginalization, and inadequate health care have caused TB, once close to elimination, to reemerge as a major international health problem. Inadequate health care is certainly part of the story, but TB's resurgence cannot be understood in the absence of larger structural issues.

In sum, an ailment that by the late 19th century was largely preventable through improved housing, nutrition, and other infrastructural factors, and curable by the 20th century through antibiotics, has been turned into a problem of almost insurmountable proportions because the political economy approach was disregarded.

THE POLITICAL ECONOMY OF HEALTH APPROACH

Key Questions:

- How has the political economy approach developed over time?
- How can this approach explain the determinants of illness and help to address them?

Major Tenets

According to the political economy perspective, social structures (namely, observable, patterned relationships between both individuals and groups—i.e., *relations of power*), and the ideology that perpetuates these structures, are largely (though not entirely) determined by economic forces. Economic power roughly correlates with social or political power, and in Karl Marx's terms, relations to the means of production (i.e., whether one is an owner or a worker). As such, business owners have more power than workers, property owners more power than tenants, and so on. As seen in Figure 4–2, a political economy of health approach analyzes the ways in which broad political, economic, and social structures, relations, and interests affect and interact with health conditions in local, national, and international contexts. This approach seeks to understand how power relations influence absolute and relative access to the medical, behavioral, economic, and social determinants of health.

The political economy framework is based on the notion that political and economic factors are intertwined with individual and social factors. The economic structure of a society is assessed by examining the ownership of national resources, the main engines of the economy, and what it buys and sells on international markets. Socially, the approach analyzes the organization of society (its social structure), including class, race, and gender divisions, and the extent to which certain social groups are marginalized. Politically, the approach assesses the organization and distribution of political power at local, national, and international levels, as well as the level of human rights and political freedoms. In sum, a political economy of health approach uncovers how personal, household, social, political, and economic conditions interrelate at various levels to produce particular health circumstances and outcomes.

Key Political Economy of Health Theorists, Past and Present

Philosophers in ancient China, Greece, medieval Europe, and the Middle East recognized that a range of cosmological, geographic, and occupational factors determined health, but it was not until the uneven transition from feudalism to capitalism in Western Europe over the 15th to 18th centuries and the Industrial Revolution of the 19th century that many of these ideas were crystallized. In 1848, social uprisings across the world decried horrendous workplaces, inhumane living conditions, and imperialist repression, providing a landmark for the political economy of health approach. Almost simultaneously, several key thinkers, including social philosopher Friedrich Engels and physician Rudolf Virchow, sought to understand the impact of social, political, and economic conditions on health and illness in the working class.

As mentioned in Chapter 2, Engels's classic study, *The Condition of the Working Class in England,* linked the harsh working and living circumstances of factory workers to specific health problems—including poor diet, alcohol consumption, venereal disease, and chronic mental and physical exhaustion. For example, he documented the direct connection between overcrowding, poor ventilation, and open fires and chronic lung ailments, such as tuberculosis.

In Prussia (present-day Germany), Rudolf Virchow, the founder of modern cellular pathology, became interested in the underlying causes of ill health. In 1848, following a typhus outbreak in Upper Silesia, Virchow was commissioned to conduct a study of the epidemic and to propose policy recommendations on how to avert future outbreaks. To the surprise of the political patrons of the study, Virchow emphasized that the epidemic had been fueled by political and economic factors rather than the more commonly employed disease determinants such as climate, physical constitution, or organic conditions. Calling the epidemic "artificial," Virchow documented high rates of unemployment, inadequate housing conditions, intense overcrowding, and governmental failure to provide adequate supplies of food during famine as the critical factors that contributed to the epidemic. His report concluded that the means of overcoming such misery and preventing future epidemics was "full and unlimited democracy" (Virchow 1848c, p. 307).

Aware of the work of Engels and involved in the radical political movements of his day, Virchow recommended the creation of public health services to respond to medical emergencies and called for improved work conditions, better housing, the establishment of agricultural cooperatives, a more redistributive taxation system, and the decentralization of political authority. Virchow's structural prevention approach—which astonished the commissioners of the report, who expected recommendations geared toward medical intervention—served as a manifesto for the new field of social medicine.

Virchow was one of the first people to demonstrate systematically the political–economic underpinnings of health: notwithstanding his accomplishments as a medical scientist, he understood the limits of scientific advances in the absence of political and social equality. He also noted the special role of physicians in addressing the political economy of health: "medicine is a social science, and politics is nothing else but medicine on a large scale" (Virchow 1848b, p. 33). Moreover, because disease was so often produced by conditions of poverty and deprivation, Virchow deemed physicians to be "the natural advocates of the poor" (Virchow 1848a, p. 4).

The work of these early analysts/activists laid the foundation for a new approach to health and disease. Predictably, because this approach challenged the reigning economic model of exploitative factory-based capitalistic production, it did not elicit a positive response from political or medical authorities in 19th-century Europe. Virchow remained firm in his belief in social medicine and renounced the honorific title of "von" when it became apparent that the government would not implement his recommended social reforms. In spite of rejection by political and economic elites, the ideas of Virchow and Engels were kept alive through generations of labor and reform movements and social medicine adherents who recognized the limitations of the emerging biomedical model of health and disease.

One of the most important 20th century heirs of the social medicine approach was Salvador Allende, a Chilean physician and founder of the Chilean Socialist Party, who was elected President of Chile in 1971 before being assassinated in a U.S.-backed, right-wing military coup aimed at interrupting his government's redistributive reforms. In his 1939 book *The Chilean Socio-Medical Reality* (*La realidad médico-social Chilena*), Allende outlined the relationship between poor social conditions and ill health. Like Virchow, his prescription for better health included social reforms, such as more equal income distribution and better housing (Allende 1939; Tedeschi, Brown, and Fee 2003; Waitzkin 2006). Another Latin American physician—Argentine Ernesto "Che" Guevara, who participated with Fidel Castro in the Cuban Revolution—came to see revolution as an extension of social medicine. He stressed the importance of:

> integrating the doctor or any other health worker into the revolutionary movement, because this work, the work of educating and feeding the children, of educating the army, and the work of redistributing the land from its former absentee landlords to those who sweat every day on that very land without reaping its fruits—is the grandest social medicine effort that has been done in Cuba (Guevara 1960, p. 119).

More than a century after Engels and Virchow, Vicente Navarro, a Catalan doctor and activist who fled the Spanish dictatorship of Generalissimo Francisco Franco and became a professor at Johns Hopkins University in the United States, began writing about the politics of health in the 1970s. Challenging the prevailing notions of ill health in Latin America, Asia, and Africa as a function of inadequate health services, Navarro linked patterns of disease and death to the political and economic conditions of underdevelopment. In books such as *Medicine under Capitalism*

(1976) and *Imperialism, Health and Medicine* (1981), he demonstrates the relationship between health, medical care organization, and the structures of power. Illustrated perhaps most vividly in his writings on the United States, Navarro emphasizes that the structure of health services reproduces the political economy of the country. More recently he has focused on the politics of international health and the role of politics and welfare states as key determinants of health (Navarro 2002; Navarro and Muntaner 2004).

Many others have applied political economy of health arguments to the international health field in order to understand the relationship between biological and socio-political phenomena. Lesley Doyal's classic, *The Political Economy of Health* (Doyal and Pennell 1979), examines the influence of the social, political, and economic organization of societies—particularly the rise of capitalism—in shaping health and illness, and their gendered patterns (Doyal 1995). Debabar Banerji of India, author of *Poverty, Class and Health Culture in India* (1982) and champion of primary health care and the right to health, is at the forefront of "South based" analyses and critiques of multilateral institutions and their role in perpetuating underdevelopment. Further examples include Howard Waitzkin of the United States, author of *The Second Sickness: Contradictions of Capitalist Health Care* (1983) and *At the Front Lines of Medicine* (2001); and Edmundo Granda and Jaime Breilh of Ecuador (Breilh and Granda 1989), who have proposed that social epidemiology derives from critical class theory rather than traditional empiricism. As well, Cristina Laurell of Mexico has written extensively on the political economy of social welfare in Latin America, including the role of class struggle and neoliberal reforms on health (Laurell 1989, 1992, 1995) (see Chapter 13 for discussion of her political endeavors); Saúl Franco of Colombia approaches violence as a social medicine problem (Franco 1999); and Emerson Elías Merhy of Brazil analyzes the world of workers and collective health (Merhy 2000). Various other scholars around the world similarly integrate political economy of health perspectives with active participation in social medicine movements.

Table 4–1 provides a summary of the key questions that run through political economy of health writings. These questions serve as useful analytic tools and

Table 4–1 Key Analytic Questions from the Writings of Vicente Navarro

Components of the Structure, Relations, Interests, and Organization of Society	Key Questions Relating to Local, National, and Global Context
Economic structure	Who owns and controls what? What does a country produce? What does it buy and sell on the international market?
Social structure	Who works in what sector? What are the class/race/gender structures of ownership and labor?
Political structure	Who wields political power? How is power distributed?

differ markedly from standard health analyses, which count the number of doctors, nurses, hospital beds, pharmaceuticals, pieces of equipment, and so on in trying to understand the role, needs, and effectiveness of the health sector. Despite the fact that Virchow illustrated the importance of social and economic conditions on health over 150 years ago, many health analysts still neglect these issues when carrying out national or regional health assessments.

Using the Political Economy of Health Approach to Understand Health Problems

The political economy of health approach remains as relevant today as it was in the 19th century; indeed, given the pervasiveness of a dominant political ideology (neoliberalism) throughout the world, it is even more important. As discussed in Chapter 2, in most societies there has been at least a partial transition from infectious to chronic disease morbidity and mortality together with increases in life expectancy. This shift has occurred largely as a result of economic processes unleashed in two waves: 19th and early 20th century industrialization, mostly in Europe and North America; and post-1945 development processes in much of Asia, Africa, and Latin America (see Fig. 4–3). However, not only is the transition incomplete, it is reversible. Many underdeveloped countries have very high death rates from both communicable and noncommunicable ailments, and various industrialized and developing countries have seen infectious diseases resurge. Furthermore, many diseases—such as inadequately treated TB, hepatitis B, and HIV/AIDS—are both communicable and chronic.

Despite the extensive medical armamentarium targeting particular diseases, life expectancy and the epidemiologic transition remain sensitive to political and economic conditions. For example, although life expectancy has risen in some countries in sub-Saharan Africa, in others it has dropped dramatically (Fig. 4–4). While this is largely due to the high prevalence of HIV/AIDS, attributed by most international health agencies and analysts to unprotected sex, the political economy of health approach offers a far deeper explanation. The sexual transmission of HIV is just the last link in a complex chain of historical events and current circumstances. The legacies of colonization, dictatorial rule, racial discrimination, environmental and human exploitation, debt, and forced economic migration have coalesced to create ideal conditions for the spread of an infectious agent like HIV via work, migration and survival patterns, extreme poverty, and social desperation.

Similarly, in the Russian Federation, life expectancy for males dropped from 70 years in the 1980s to 59 years in the early 2000s—a level lower than India's (UNDP 2006). Why have rates of infectious disease, death from violence, and chronic diseases increased following the collapse of the Soviet Union? As we will see ahead, no such questions can be answered without addressing the severe social, economic, and political upheaval of the 1990s, including massive deindustrialization of the

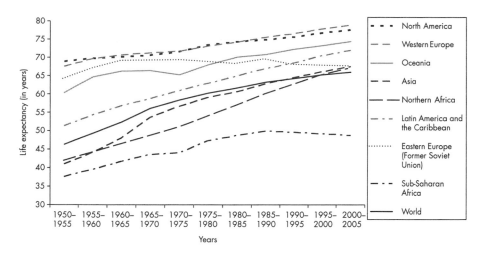

Figure 4–3 Trends in life expectancy by region (5-year averages). *Source:* UN (2006).

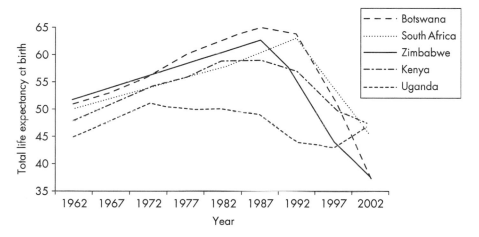

Figure 4–4 Changes in life expectancy, 1962–2002. *Source:* World Bank (2007b).

country (except for the energy sector) and the dismantling of Soviet social security and safety net systems. The effects of "shock therapy" capitalism in the early 1990s and the 1998 devaluation of the ruble and ensuing financial crisis were even more extreme in the Russian Federation than in other former Soviet republics, as witnessed by the differing life expectancy patterns in this period (Fig. 4–5).

The political economy approach also seeks to understand noncommunicable and emerging health problems at a global level. For example, it is estimated that the 110 million people living with diabetes in 2000 will double by 2010 (Shaw et al. 2000); diabetes has become the leading cause of death in Mexico and is poised to outstrip mortality from cancer and heart disease in many settings. Also soaring are

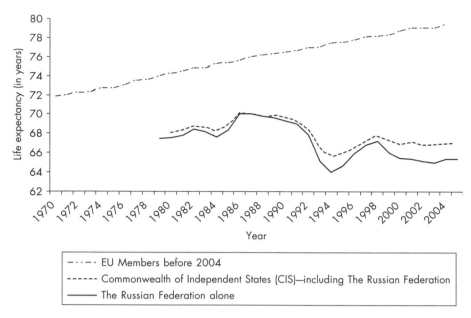

Figure 4–5 Annual life expectancy in EU member states and the Commonwealth of Independent States. *Source*: WHO EURO (2007).

road traffic collisions, causing over 1 million deaths in 2002, with 10 million more injured (Hazen and Ehiri 2006). Most analysts explain increases in noncommunicable mortality using the behavioral approach, arguing, for example, that individuals have largely themselves to blame for their eating habits and exercise levels or for reckless driving. Similarly, the biomedical approach portrays increases in diabetes rates in terms of biological interactions among diet, physical activity, and genetics. Both of these approaches prioritize the individual as the basis of analysis. While there is certainly an individual element in diabetes and road deaths, these ailments must also be understood in terms of global food production, commodity pricing, and marketing, together with transport, trade, industrial, and agri-business policies that have altered dietary and exercise patterns, and worsened road safety, and led millions of people to seek employment in ever-growing cities. Tables 4–2 and 4–3 illustrate these distinctions by comparing political economy to biomedical and behavioral approaches to understanding and addressing the problems of diarrhea and obesity.

In sum, although there has been a general increase in global life expectancy, as seen in the above charts, these gains have not been equally distributed and the ailments contributing to these patterns not equally explained. How can one understand why the life expectancy profiles of some countries have stagnated or dropped over the past few decades? What has been the role of particular diseases

Table 4–2 Causes and Treatment of Diarrhea According to Contrasting Approaches to Health

- Cause of 2.2 million deaths per year, 4% of deaths globally, and 8.5% of deaths in sub-Saharan Africa (WHO 2006b)
- Approximately 4 billion cases worldwide each year
- Primarily affects children under 5; it is the second largest killer of children globally
- Affects nutritional absorption, lowers labor productivity, and increases susceptibility to other diseases

Approach to Health	Determinants/Causal Explanations	Prevention/Treatment
Biomedical	Infectious agents enter the body and cause illness Certain intestinal diseases or other illnesses or disorders Allergic reaction to certain foods or medications Death occurs primarily as a result of dehydration	Vaccine against diarrheal diseases Oral rehydration therapy (ORT) Antibiotic/antiparasitic drugs
Behavioral	Ingesting food or water contaminated with an infectious agent Lack of knowledge/education about infectious agents and treatment Lack of personal hygiene, such as hand-washing Inadequate use of health services	Improve personal hygiene Avoid untreated water and potentially infected food Improve health education regarding causes and treatment of diarrhea
Political economy	Lack of access to safe drinking water Poor basic sanitation Lack of access to primary health care Poverty	Universal access to safe drinking water Improve sanitation and living conditions Universal access to health care Redistribution of wealth and political power

and their determinants? How can we understand the disparities in health status within underdeveloped countries? How do we explain the inequities between blue-collar and white-collar workers within industrialized economies? And why do some very poor countries have health outcomes as good as or better than much wealthier ones?

Not only does the political economy of health lens prompt us to ask these questions, it also seeks to understand *why* these inequities exist and explores what can and should be done about them. This framework's questioning of power relations and the distribution of resources (skills, access to finance, wealth, etc.) is threatening both to those with significant political and economic power and to those comfortably oblivious to national and worldwide poverty and social inequalities (Pogge 2002).

Table 4–3 Causes and Treatment of Obesity According to Contrasting Approaches to Health

- Approximately 400 million adults are obese, projected to increase to 700 million people by 2015 (WHO 2006a); an estimated 22 million children are overweight across the world
- Prevalence higher in developed countries, but obesity rates growing faster in developing countries
- Linked to cardiovascular disease; Type II diabetes; pregnancy complications; colon, endometrial, and other cancers; and early death

Approach to Health	Determinants/Causal Explanations	Prevention/Treatment
Biomedical	Possible genetic predisposition, particularly among aboriginal populations Biological energy imbalance between caloric intake and output Use of certain medications Low birthweight, followed by rapid weight gain	Drugs to curtail food cravings Find gene for obesity; formulate treatment accordingly Drugs to hinder biological reaction to energy imbalance Surgery
Behavioral	Low levels of physical activity Excess consumption overall and of foods high in "empty" calories (processed/prepared with sugars and unhealthy fats and chemicals)	Increase minutes and intensity of daily physical activity Limit energy intake from fats and sugars Increase consumption of fruits, vegetables, whole grains
Political economy	Industrialization of food production Industry subsidies ensuring high availability and lower price per calorie of "junk" (energy dense) foods compared to healthier foods Omnipresent junk food advertisements and food sales in schools, workplaces, parks, and on TV Insufficient time, space, infrastructure, and resources (human, economic, etc.) for healthy food preparation and physical activity Unchecked power of automobile/oil/highway/construction industries Underfunding of public transport/bike lanes/parks	Remove agricultural subsidies favoring overproduction and lower prices for unhealthy (highly processed, chemical-, sugar-, and calorie-laden) food Encourage organic farming, produce, free-grazing livestock Limit advertising for processed, calorie-dense, low-nutrition foods Ensure comprehensive distribution and affordability of healthy food Structure work hours and regulate housing to enable adequate time/conditions for exercise and food preparation Remove subsidies that favor automobile use and highway construction Provide healthy, safe, and culturally appropriate environments for physical activity (e.g., pollution controls, parks, bike lanes, sidewalks)

The World Bank versus Political Economy Approaches to Health

Although the political economy of health framework offers the most integrative approach to addressing health issues—involving technological, behavioral, and structural elements—it has been sidelined by mainstream policy makers as overly ambitious and thus impossible to achieve in the short or medium term (Birdsall 1994; Reich 1994).

For example, in 1993 the World Bank portrayed the "dramatic health improvement" over the 20th century as a triumph of scientific knowledge and accompanying behavioral change (World Bank 1993, p. 6). This argument overlooks the *interaction* of scientific and technological gains *with* improvements in social conditions and the redistribution of economic and political power, central to political economy understandings. In 2006 the Bank's *World Development Report* again asserted that declines in inequalities in life expectancy across countries from the 1960s to the 1980s were due to "the global spread of health technology and to major public health efforts [mostly disease campaigns] in some of the world's highest mortality areas" (World Bank 2006, p. 6). The report attributes the reversal in this trend since 1990 to HIV/AIDS mortality in Africa and mortality increases in the "transition economies" of the former Soviet bloc, without mentioning the role of political and economic conditions. Instead, readers are assured that inequalities in health do "not just reflect different preferences or needs" (ibid, p. 141), but rather derive from "constraints" on individuals that need to be addressed by "boosting people's knowledge about basic health practices and services, expanding their access to affordable care, and enhancing the accountability of providers" (ibid, p. 142). While access to health services is undoubtedly part of the picture, the implication that resolving mortality inequalities is principally a matter of disseminating health technologies and healthy behaviors is not only misleading, it's deadly.

For example, even a limited understanding of the political economy of health approach shows that prevailing behavioral–medical explanations of—and solutions to—AIDS in Africa are untenable. Can HIV prevalence rates in sub-Saharan Africa, which are up to 1000 times higher than in Europe, be explained solely by sexual practices? The world's most comprehensive-ever global sex survey (completed in 2006) shows that individuals in industrialized countries, where HIV prevalence rates are much lower, have a similar number of sexual partners as those in developing regions, including sub-Saharan Africa (Wellings et al. 2006). As such, ascribing high HIV prevalence to Africans' multiple sexual partners is erroneous and prejudicial. Clearly, a more comprehensive explanatory model than individual behavior needs to be pursued, one that includes the part played by chronic malnutrition and coinfections in biological (immunological) vulnerability (Katz 2002). An exclusive focus on sex (and provision of antiretroviral drugs) overlooks the crucial role of societal structures in the host–agent–environment interaction (Stillwaggon 2006).

Likewise, medical or behavioral models alone cannot explain why the health status of people in Eastern Europe and Central Asia deteriorated so rapidly after the collapse of the Soviet Union.

Why is the seemingly obvious role of political economy left out of the World Bank's analyses? The simplest explanation is that it challenges prevailing political and economic forces: biomedical and behavioral approaches are compatible with and reinforce the status quo of the international distribution of power and resources. The behavioral approach seeks the answer to ill health in individual action, and the biomedical approach in technical interventions. For these reasons, global health efforts emphasize technical solutions, such as antiretroviral drugs to treat HIV/AIDS or a vaccine for avian influenza, and behavioral solutions, such as quitting smoking and purchasing bed nets against mosquitoes, instead of attempting to understand and address the underlying determinants and causes of these illnesses and developing measures that address all elements of the host–agent–environment triad. In Chapter 7, we will examine in detail the constellation of social and political determinants of health introduced here.

Imagine you are a middle-aged minibus driver in a highly populated city. The government regulates emissions and traffic safety standards. You are a member of a union and receive benefits and inflation-linked wage increases negotiated by the union. You work 8 hours per day, 5 days a week, and earn paid holidays and sick days. Thanks to national workplace regulations, you have the right to two 15-minute breaks and a 45-minute lunch period daily and are encouraged to participate in neighborhood-sponsored sporting events and physical activities. The transit depots for bus drivers have a lunch program with nutritious food options. With your salary you are able to adequately meet living expenses for your family and can afford a home with consistent supplies of electricity, potable running water, and proper sanitation for all residents. The state fully subsidizes education for your children, as well as medical care.

During one of your yearly medical check-ups, your doctor discusses the potential problems of high blood pressure, high cholesterol, and heart disease given your age and family history. Your doctor recommends that you take greater advantage of healthy meals and exercise programs at your workplace; discusses the possible need for medication should you develop high blood pressure; asks you about your work, community, and home environments in seeking to identify and reduce sources of stress and help prevent future illness; and encourages you to keep politically active.

How have your health problems been understood and addressed?

Reimagining the life and health of this bus driver shows the relevance and importance of stretching beyond the biomedical and behavioral models in order to understand how health is affected by underlying, intermediate, and proximate determinants, as illustrated in the political economy of health framework (Fig. 4–2). The bus driver could be 35 years old or 60, female or male, in Berlin, Bangkok, or Bogotá; the broad determinants of her/his health and illness do not change, although the social, political, and cultural contexts mediate particular responses to agents of disease. Earlier in the chapter we presented a case study of how poor working and social conditions—and concentration of political power among white elites—in South Africa led to high incidence of tuberculosis among black miners. We will now examine what happens when existing social protection measures are dismantled, compromising the underlying, intermediate, and proximate determinants of health. This was the case with the dissolution of the Soviet Union.

Case Study: Decreased Life Expectancy in Russia following the Dissolution of the USSR

When the Soviet Union dissolved in 1991, many economists believed that the establishment of a capitalist economy would generate untold improvements in health and well-being through economic growth. The truth was far more complex: rather than bettering quality of life, a countertransition of sorts occurred. The shift from socialism to market capitalism provoked social disruption, sharp declines in per capita income, and deteriorating health conditions. Mortality rates increased dramatically, particularly among working-age people. Between 1987 and 1994 there was a 50% increase in premature death for Russian males, a slight recovery until 1998, and renewed deterioration since then. Male life expectancy at birth is now below what it was in the 1960s. While women's life expectancy declines are smaller than men's, the pattern is similar; all told there are close to 1 million excess deaths per year beyond expected mortality rates. The rates of injury, death, and disability among men are now similar to those in sub-Saharan Africa, and the former Soviet Union has worse overall health indicators than all regions except South Asia and sub-Saharan Africa (Lopez et al. 2006).

Underscoring these patterns are explosive increases in violent and occupational deaths, suicide, chronic diseases, and a resurgence of formerly rare infectious diseases (Men et al. 2003). For example, a diphtheria epidemic swept through Russia and former Soviet republics from 1991 to 1997, with 140,000 cases and 4,000 deaths (Vitek and Wharton 1998). AIDS, drug-related deaths, and TB, as well, are ravaging the young adult population.

The World Bank has proffered a behavioral analysis of these problems, recommending that Russians "ease back on the bottle, cut down on smoking, watch their diet, and lead healthier lives" (Reuters, Moscow, Dec. 8, 2005 cited in [King, Stuckler, and Hamm 2006, p. 16]). The Bank's rationale for targeting specific "behavioral" factors rather than the changed economic and social context has to do with gender differences in smoking and alcohol consumption which, they argue, partially protect women from these agents of death (World Bank 2005a). Yet while the male–female gap in life expectancy is almost twice as large as in most industrialized countries, Russian women's life expectancy trails behind European figures.

Part of the explanation resides in widening educational (and social class) differentials in mortality. Russia's mortality increases have mainly affected less educated men and women, and the gap in mortality rates between elementary school educated and university educated men and women has grown tenfold between 1980 and 2001. The gender differential in life expectancy among those with university education stayed almost constant over this period but grew among those with less education (Murphy et al. 2006; Lopez et al. 2006). The greater post Soviet mortality increases in less educated men compared to women may derive from women's greater flexibility in a changing economic environment and overall resilience in times of stress.

In sum, the World Bank's behavioral advice ignores the structural influences on population health of free market economics and the breakdown of the social welfare state. Indeed, the rapid rise in mortality rates in the Russian Federation and other former Soviet bloc countries is largely explained by structural factors including the collapse of public infrastructure and social safety nets (including health care), significant declines in living standards and minimum wage, and loss of employment protection.

In contrast, although the collapse of the Soviet Union had a devastating economic impact on Cuba, Cuban health indicators improved in the years following the USSR's dissolution thanks to continued redistribution and protective policies aimed at the entire population (King, Stuckler, and Hamm 2006). Most notably, the substantial caloric reductions caused by Cuba's economic crisis did not affect overall nutritional levels, instead likely reducing mortality from diabetes and cardiovascular diseases (Franco et al. 2007).

Undoubtedly, there are limits to the prevailing biomedical and behavioral models of understanding and addressing national and international patterns of health and disease. Rather than looking to individual characteristics, a political economy approach examines health differences by, *inter alia*, assessing the nature of the welfare state (see Fig. 4–6). Now we turn to the question of "development" and ask how the economic characteristics of particular countries interact with local and global political and social factors in shaping patterns of health and disease.

PHASES AND "MODELS" OF DEVELOPMENT

Key Questions:

- What is the relationship between health and development?
- How and why have models of development changed over time?

What is *development*? Depending on one's perspective, progress, advancement, economic growth, productivity, profitability, striving for equality, better health and education, democracy, commercialization, improved quality of life, economic integration, and other concepts may all come to mind. Defining development in the international context is even more complex given the multiple players involved—big business, foreign affairs ministries, multilateral agencies, technical experts, politicians, and, most importantly, workers and citizens. Although the term development is widely used, it has no universal definition (Shakow and Irwin 2000).

Today we tend to think of development in terms of a range of social and economic activities within and across countries, but historically development ideas and practices have been closely linked to foreign assistance in terms of aid from industrialized countries (principally the United States, Canada, Western Europe, Australia, New Zealand, Japan, and more recently China and Brazil) to certain countries of Asia, Africa, and Latin America. Yet, arguably, the most successful development assistance effort was the United States's rebuilding of postwar Europe and Japan.

Box 4–1 Categorizing Countries: Income and Redistribution

In making comparisons of different countries and their trajectories, politicians, researchers, and advocates often use certain economic categories as short-hand. Terms such as "developed" vs. "developing," "Northern" vs. "Southern," "industrialized" vs. "industrializing," "wealthy" vs. "poor," "haves" vs. "have-nots," or descriptors such as "resource-poor," "low-income," "middle-income," and "high-income" are commonly used to classify countries by different aggregate indicators, such as gross national income (GNI) per capita, literacy levels, or democratic elections. Most of these terms are value-laden and rank countries according to a generalized hierarchy based on stage of "development" or social and economic "advancement," according to capitalist criteria, often defined in terms of income per capita and industrialization level. Moreover, they do not take into account a fundamental social (and health) distinction across the world: the social class divide through which upper class elites in both developed and developing, Northern (minority world) and Southern (majority world) countries wield power over workers. The dominant classes operate both nationally and as part of larger class alliances across countries that further their own interests against those of the working classes, leading to inequitable distribution of power and resources both among and within countries.

Of course, as we will discuss in Chapter 9, global political and economic forces also influence the shape of domestic policies. Power differentials and geopolitical struggles between larger and smaller economies, both historically and contemporaneously, shape class relations and constrain the ability of countries to redistribute resources and overcome the conditions of underdevelopment. During the Cold War, a categorization emerged that has since fallen out of favor: First World (industrialized, capitalist countries); Second World (industrialized/ing communist countries); and Third World (mostly ex-colonies that were "underdeveloped" through unfair commodity price controls, unfavorable trade agreements, and political domination). Though these various classifications can be useful for grouping apparently similar countries and regions together, they oversimplify differences among countries and obscure internal inequalities in standards of living and economic development within each society.

A note on terms: GNI per capita is defined as the total value of goods and services produced in a particular country plus the income received from abroad (including profits, interest, and remittances), minus the income sent abroad (again in terms of profits, interest, and remittances) divided by the total population of the country (GNI is the term used by the World Bank but many countries employ the closely related term gross national product [GNP]). GNI is considered a more comprehensive accounting of income than the more traditional gross domestic product (GDP) (which measures the value of goods and services within a particular country each year without considering ownership of production or transfer of income across borders) yet neither includes any measure of internal distribution of wages, wealth, or consumption. Moreover, GNI does not

(*continued*)

Box 4–1 Continued

		Annual GNI/capita[a]			
		High Income >US$10,725 GNI/capita	Upper-middle Income US$3,466-10,725 GNI/capita	Lower-middle Income US$876-$3,465 GNI/capita	Low Income <US$875 GNI/capita
Nature of Domestic Welfare State[b]	Highly redistributive	Western Europe Korea New Zealand Singapore	Venezuela (formerly partially redistributive) Costa Rica Czech Republic	Cuba	
	Partially redistributive	United States Saudi Arabia (high social spending but guest workers do not receive social welfare benefits)	Argentina Russia (formerly highly redistributive) South Africa Poland Malaysia Turkey	China (formerly highly redistributive) Iran Egypt Brazil (formerly marginally redistributive) Sri Lanka (formerly highly redistributive)	Vietnam (formerly highly redistributive)
	Marginally redistributive		Botswana	Guatemala Thailand Peru	India Mali Nigeria Bangladesh Haiti

Figure 4–6 Political economy-based classification of countries.
[a]World Bank classification for 2005: from http://siteresources.worldbank.org/
DATASTATISTICS/Resources/CLASS.XLS;[b]Classification developed by authors.

incorporate some services that are not marketed (as in the case of unpaid household work by family members), nor any other effects of economic activity such as levels of satisfaction, economic insecurity, or pollution, much less the impact of political systems or social norms.

For example, oil-rich countries such as the United Arab Emirates have very high GNI per capita and are, strictly in terms of income, highly developed countries. However, literacy rates and levels of education are limited (particularly for women), and the majority of the working class ("guest workers") are denied even minimal levels of social benefits. In contrast, Cuba has a relatively low GNI per capita and in standard terms is categorized as a "developing" country, even though it has one of the strongest welfare states in the world, with record literacy and health indicators. As we will see ahead, the UNDP's Human Development Index is an attempt to take into account a variety of social indicators of a country (including level of literacy, sanitation, life expectancy, etc.), but because it does not represent the distribution of these features within the population, its use is limited. Although it may be inaccurate to use blanket terms such as developed versus underdeveloped countries, this text will at times employ them to remain consistent with broad usage. Figure 4–6 offers an alternative way of categorizing countries, which will be used whenever possible.

(continued)

Box 4-1 Continued

Many orthodox (health) economists have argued that GNI per capita and economic growth are the most important determinants of human well-being. Arguing that growth among the well-off eventually trickles down to the poor, these economists believe that levels of health are directly correlated with GNI per capita. Others suggest that the economics of happiness, albeit difficult to measure, offers some insights on development (Graham 2005). However, heterodox political economists, social epidemiologists, and other scholars have found that GNI per capita is only part of the story, and that as countries climb the GNI per capita scale, internal distribution—as determined by political processes (i.e., the nature of the social welfare state)—becomes a far more important determinant of health and human welfare.

The failure of GNI per capita to take inequality into account has led to the development of the GINI coefficient, which assesses the degree of income inequality within a country, used in conjunction with GNI. However, the GINI does not include wealth or the value of nonincome social transfers, due to the high costs and complex logistics of such an undertaking. Moreover, because income data are not accurately measured in many countries, we use the *nature of the welfare state* (a measurement of the extent to which a national government provides social and economic security to its citizens, typically played out through democratic political processes) to assess the degree of social and economic redistribution. Research into the role of the welfare state in determining health outcomes has found that social protection measures play a significant role in improving health, as measured by infant mortality, low birth weight, and life expectancy, with a greater impact for more egalitarian (redistributive) societies (Navarro et al. 2006; Chung and Muntaner 2007).

Although to date this line of research has focused only on high GNI per capita industrialized countries, here we apply it to the rest of the world. As such, in categorizing countries, Figure 4-6 captures the importance of national wealth (as measured by GNI per capita) *and* the internal distributiveness of the welfare state in underpinning social and health status. Under US$1,000 per capita income, the effects of redistribution are minimal (Dagdeviren, van der Hoeven, and Weeks 2001). Above this level, however, the social distribution of national wealth (here defined in terms of the nature of the welfare state) takes on great importance.

Countries at the lowest per capita income level (less than US$1,000 per capita) are the least able to satisfy the needs of the population. Even if the country's wealth were well-distributed, there would be insufficient resources to provide adequately the most basic of human needs: nutrition, safe shelter, clean water, and basic public health services. Above US$1,000 per capita however, the more evenly distributed national wealth is—through education, housing, neighborhood conditions, employment security, wage levels, primary health care, protection of the vulnerable, etc.—the healthier the population (as determined by life expectancy and mortality rates).

This explains why various countries with relatively low per capita incomes have better health outcomes than the United States, despite the latter's very high per capita income level (see Chapter 11 for details).

Post–World War II Development Priorities

As outlined in Chapter 3, the 1944 Bretton Woods conference established a new world economic order to be maintained by a few key institutions—the World Bank, the International Monetary Fund (IMF), and (as of 1947) the General Agreement on Tariffs and Trade to govern multilateral trade. Although the meeting took place before World War II had ended, leading politicians and financiers recognized that a new global system of economic stability was necessary to avert another world war and economic depression. As well, renewed polarization between capitalist and communist camps—suppressed in the name of the fight against fascism—began to shape global aid strategies.

Redeveloping Europe topped economic and political agendas following World War II. At the time, the worldwide misery and economic slowdown of the 1930s

Great Depression were still fresh memories, and measures to prevent a recurrence of depression were a high priority. Europe's rebirth was central to a new, more controlled form of global capitalism under a Keynesian model of government spending to ensure economic stability and mitigate capitalism's ills. In Britain and other European countries, Keynesian fiscal measures coincided with socialist movements favoring a growing welfare state and improved living conditions.

The World Bank was the initial source of funds for Europe's reconstruction, starting with a loan to France for US$250 million (the equivalent of over US$3.3 billion in 2007) for equipment, fuel, and raw materials, accounting for fully one-third of the Bank's loanable funds at the time. Europe's stability was also politically vital as a buffer against Soviet influence. In March 1947, U.S. President Harry Truman announced that the U.S. government would provide substantial military and economic aid (US$400 million in constant dollars) to Greece and Turkey to fight off communist insurgents—the so-called Truman doctrine of "containment" of Soviet expansion. This new policy marked the beginning of the Cold War between Western capitalist countries (under U.S. leadership) and Eastern communist countries (under Soviet leadership). In the United States, support for European economic growth and social welfare state expansion was viewed as a means of lessening the domestic influence of communist political parties in countries such as France and Italy.

In June 1947, U.S. Secretary of State George Marshall proposed the "Marshall Plan" for Europe. In a speech at Harvard University, Marshall warned that:

> The world situation is very serious....Europe's requirements for the next three or four years of foreign food and other essential products—principally from America—are so much greater than her present ability to pay that she must have substantial additional help, or face economic, social and political deterioration...Aside from the demoralizing effect on the world at large and the possibilities of disturbances arising as a result of the desperation of the people concerned, the consequences to the economy of the United States should be apparent to all (Marshall 1947).

U.S. industry soon became a huge beneficiary of aid to Europe—all goods, equipment, and transport vessels were American, launching a long-standing tradition in development assistance.

Officially titled the European Recovery Program, the Marshall Plan gave a staggering US$13.3 billion (well over US$100 billion today) to 17 countries in Europe during the 4 years of the Plan. With U.S. GDP averaging US$260 billion per year in the late 1940s, the Marshall Plan—at over 1.3% of U.S. GDP per year—was arguably the largest aid program ever.

The United States assisted Japan, too, to recover from war devastation, including the two atomic bombs the United States detonated, and to develop a new, demilitarized society. By the early 1950s, the United States had invested more than US$2 billion (in constant dollars) in Japan during its postwar occupation.

U.S. assistance to Japan (together with the U.S. role in the Korean War) was aimed at keeping Soviet influence out of the region. Indeed, it became increasingly evident that the Marshall Plan's actions in Europe and Asia were far less motivated by humanitarian values than by U.S. fears of the growing ambit of Soviet influence.

Development and the "Third World"

Once the United States began to address Europe's and Japan's problems, it turned to the rest of the world. In his famed 1949 inauguration speech, U.S. President Harry Truman discussed the situation of poorer countries, including those newly decolonized, defining them as "underdeveloped areas" (essentially coining this expression and replacing the previous nomenclature of "backward" countries). In Point IV of his speech Truman addressed the problem of underdevelopment in terms of a new arrangement of international relations, with the United States taking the lead in raising the living standard of the "developing" world through the provision of technical skills, knowledge, and equipment:

> More than half the people of the world are living in conditions approaching misery...Their poverty is a handicap and a threat both to them and to more prosperous areas...The material resources which we can afford to use for assistance of other peoples is limited. But our imponderable resources in technical knowledge are constantly growing and are inexhaustible...And, in cooperation with other nations...Our main aim should be to help the free peoples of the world, through their own efforts, to produce more food, more clothing, more materials for housing, and more mechanical power to lighten their burdens...With cooperation of business, private capital, agriculture, and labor in this country, this program can greatly increase the industrial activity in other nations and can raise substantially their standards of living. Such new economic developments should be devised and controlled to the benefit of the peoples of the areas in which they are established (Truman 1949).

As articulated in Truman's speech and developed in the appropriately termed "Point IV aid programs," early postwar definitions of development and underdevelopment centered on industrialization and modernization—considered the vehicles by which people in poorer countries would acquire the means to emulate the consumption patterns of people in richer countries. Western, capitalist, industrialized countries framed themselves as the ideal. Investments in factories, large-scale agricultural projects, and public infrastructure such as roads and dams were encouraged as the means of producing a surplus from which a country could finance consumption and further investment. Accompanying these economic developments was another goal: staving off Soviet influences.

Of course, imperial powers had long invested in colonial industry, commerce, social institutions, and political stability (the latter bolstering the former), and the United Kingdom, France, and other powers renewed their development efforts after World War II. In addition, starting in 1943, the United States spent tens of millions of dollars on a Cooperative Public Health Services program of infrastructure support in Latin America, in large part to secure support for the Allied Powers during wartime. But the new development ideology, termed modernization theory (see ahead), made even bolder claims about the paths to achieve development and its expected success in both economic (standard of living) and political (anticommunism) terms.

First was the "Green Revolution," which, starting with the Rockefeller Foundation's efforts in mid-1940s Mexico, invested in agricultural equipment and technologies, such as crop hybridization, in an effort to increase wheat and rice production and ensure agricultural self-sufficiency. Extended to Brazil, the Philippines, Indonesia, and other countries (and to maize and other crops), the Green Revolution was widely touted for increasing agricultural output, but its effects were uneven and generated severe economic problems among hundreds of thousands of small farmers who could not initially afford to adopt the new methods (Timmer 1988).

Indeed, the emphasis on modernization and industrialization in development processes undermined efforts to improve rural conditions, such as through land reform (redistribution of agrarian lands). While agricultural extension projects occasionally focused on small-scale farming methods, most development efforts saw farming costs increase (e.g., due to tractorization in the 1970s). Moreover, an increasing concentration of land ownership by large landholders and agri-businesses eventually left millions of rural families landless or confined to subsistence farming (Cleaver 1972; Schumacher 1973).

In the first decade of the Point IV plan, U.S. development aid doubled in dollar terms and went from approximately 0.3% to more than 0.5% of GNP. As European economies were rebuilt, they also participated in official development assistance (ODA) efforts, which increased almost fivefold in the 1950s (Fuhrer 1996).

Development strategies became tied to historic, imperial, and regional groupings, such as the Colombo Plan—launched in 1951 in Sri Lanka for the British Commonwealth countries (former British colonies)—focusing on training, technical assistance, and infrastructure, and the Alliance for Progress, started by the United States in 1961 as a "Marshall Plan" for Latin America. Formed in an attempt to prevent the repetition of Cuba's 1959 revolution, the Alliance for Progress initially focused on improving literacy rates, economic growth, and implementing and supporting democratic governance (in rhetoric) but soon included significant military spending. Additionally, between 1949 and 1961, the World Bank lent US$5.1 billion to 56 countries—focusing on economic development, energy, transportation, and infrastructural development (Kapur, Lewis, and Webb 1997).

These efforts had mixed results. New infrastructure was built, though hydropower, highway, and pipeline projects displaced large populations in India, Ghana, Nepal, Argentina, Brazil, Egypt, Nigeria, and numerous other settings (Thomas 2002). Social and health conditions improved in some places, such as Sri Lanka, where there were significant investments in education. Countless consultants and contractors in donor countries benefited greatly due to "tied aid" requirements stipulating that a high proportion of aid monies be spent domestically. Yet many issues vital to the well-being of populations in developing countries, such as land reform, fair systems of commodity pricing, poverty alleviation, and the distribution of economic gains, were overlooked or even exacerbated. For instance, huge investments in dirty industries—such as minerals and metals mining, logging, and oil drilling—proved environmentally devastating and exploitative. The riches extracted from such natural resources were unevenly distributed, and economic development aid often arrived in the form of arms to protect these valuable industries. Moreover, high commitments for capital investment on the part of recipient countries, and high debt repayments, meant that the net financial flows to most developing countries were actually quite limited.

Although Cold War fears had fueled the redevelopment of Europe, these fears did not translate into the same fervor for helping build the economies of Asia (except Japan), Africa, and Latin America. The United States and its allies never allocated to these regions the massive levels of aid spent rebuilding postwar Europe. By the 1960s, U.S. and European development assistance (with the exception of Nordic countries) began to drop and then stagnated in GNP percentage terms, with the trend in the United States also evident in dollar terms, as seen in Figures 4–7 and 4–8.

Moreover, the proliferation in the 1960s of socialist and communist movements in newly liberated countries, and in others that had received development assistance, made strictly economic assistance appear less effective than targeted military aid in

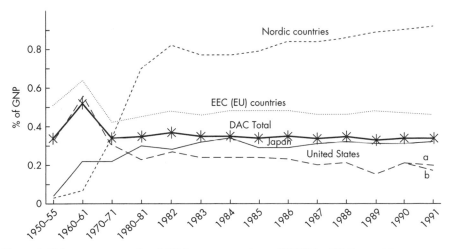

Figure 4–7 Long-term trends of ODA as a percentage of GNP by DAC countries.
[a]Including military debt forgiveness; [b]Excluding military debt forgiveness.
Credit Line: Long-term Trends of ODA as a Percentage of GNP by DAC Countries, The Story of Official Development Assistance: A History of the Development Assistance Committee and the Development Co-Operation Directorate in Dates, Names and Figures, © OECD 1994.

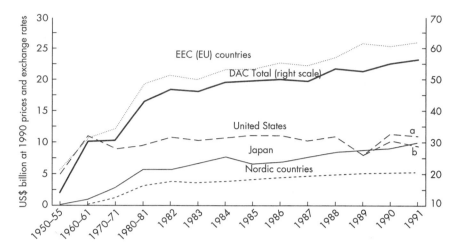

Figure 4–8 Long-term trends of net ODA disbursements by DAC countries in US$ billion (1990).
aIncluding military debt forgiveness; bExcluding military debt forgiveness.
Credit Line: Long-term Trends of ODA as a Percentage of GNP by DAC Countries,
The Story of Official Development Assistance: A History of the Development Assistance
Committee and the Development Co-Operation Directorate in Dates, Names and Figures,
© OECD 1994.

the West's effort to contain communism. Indeed, growing support for brutal pro-Western dictators across Latin America, Africa, and Asia made the underlying political and ideological dimensions of Western development assistance patent. In this period, "development" assistance increasingly emphasized military aid, combined with population control efforts, as the best means of staving off communism. Numerous civil wars erupted, from Vietnam to Angola, and violent military coups, such as the overthrow of the democratically elected Chilean government by U.S.-backed General Augusto Pinochet in 1973, had a devastating effect on countries across the developing world.

Many developing countries did not wish to participate in these ideological turf wars and instead attempted to create a nonaligned movement, beginning with a conference of Asian and African states in Indonesia in 1955 (see Chapter 3), but few escaped the yoke of development and military assistance. Still, Cold War politics had some positive influence on the health status of countries globally. The fight over allies and territory led to Western and Soviet investment in needed infrastructure and social services, including education and public health in many developing nations.

In 1969, Lester B. Pearson, the Prime Minister of Canada at the time, released a report for the World Bank calling for developed nations to join together and set aside 0.7% of GNP for ODA to developing nations. In 1970, the UN General Assembly agreed to the goal of meeting the target of 0.7% of GNP for ODA by 1975, but most countries did not meet this mark. Although absolute aid levels grew initially after Pearson's call, until the mid-2000s average ODA as a percentage of donor GNP remained relatively steady at approximately 0.33% of GNP, with the exception of Scandinavian countries and a handful of others (OECD 2005; UNICEF 2006).

Evolution of Development Theories

Modernization Theory

Cold War politics, particularly the need to form strategic anticommunist alliances, heavily influenced Western development ideologies. Despite extreme diversity in the historical, cultural, political, and economic realities of different countries, modernization theory promoted a linear path from underdevelopment to capitalism. Developed in the 1950s by U.S. economist Walter W. Rostow, its goal was to create a partnership for economic growth and democracy "in association with the *non-Communist politicians and peoples*" (Rostow 1960, p. 164, emphasis added).

Modernization theory maintains that just as Western industrial democracies had started out as "underdeveloped," most developing countries could—and should— follow a parallel path of development through five stages of economic growth. Central to this process was the exchange of traditional cultures and values (including political cultures) of "underdeveloped" or "primitive" countries for modern, technological, and market values: economic openness would replace traditional practices, foster urbanization, and lead to the creation of a middle class.

Modernization theory holds that "traditional societies," such as countries in South Asia, can make the transition to modernity through education, urbanization, and the spread of mass media. Western foreign aid organizations and institutions are considered critical to the achievement of economic growth, increased equality, democracy, stability, and greater national autonomy, simultaneously fending off the threat of communism (Handelman 1996).

Dependency Theory

Many have contested modernization theory as ahistorical, culturally biased (Eurocentric), and inadequately accounting for the colonial legacies of most underdeveloped countries, which would impede them from following the same path to "development" as their European colonizers.

Even before its popularization, modernization theory's economic reasoning was criticized as flawed. In the 1950s, Argentinean economist Raúl Prebisch (and German Hans Singer) argued that as long as developing countries were reliant on primary exports, the terms of trade would continuously decline, making the export of primary goods a less and less satisfactory basis for prosperity. Prebisch became associated with import substitution industrialization (ISI), a policy through which the growth of domestic industries and internal markets replace imports (and trade), thus enabling national social and economic development. During the Great Depression,

Brazil, Mexico, and other Latin American countries had already adopted ISI, with East Asia, Mozambique, and others subsequently implementing this strategy.

ISI, in turn, fostered a more radical challenge to modernization theory. In the 1960s, social scientists in both developing and developed countries argued that "underdevelopment" was not the fault of developing countries' values or cultures but rather stemmed from foreign political and economic domination and exploitation (Handelman 1996). Proponents of dependency theory, such as Paul Baran and André Gunder Frank, rejected the notion that developing countries could follow the same linear path to "development" as had Western industrialized countries. Dependency theory holds that Western colonialism and economic imperialism turned Africa, Asia, and Latin America into sources of cheap resources for the colonial powers, allowing Western countries to develop on the backs of those nations (Gunder Frank 1972).

Dependency theorists maintained that long after developing nations obtained political independence from colonizers, industrialized countries continued to use their political power to perpetuate an international division of capital, resources, and profits. These divisions were between *peripheral* countries, or formerly colonized countries (largely relegated to the production and export of food and raw materials), and the *core* countries, or economically advanced industrialized countries (in which the economically profitable production and export of manufactured goods were concentrated). This international economic division forced peripheral countries to trade, on unfavorable terms, their raw materials and food with core countries for industrial imports.

Frank and others further maintained that elite classes in underdeveloped countries (the *lumpenbourgeoisie*) advanced their own class interests by maintaining this economic division (accompanied by political repression) at the expense of the majority population in their countries, bolstered by the economic and military power of core nations, especially the United States. Accordingly, developing countries, forced to export raw materials and nonindustrial goods, were doomed to economic backwardness. The alternative path supported by dependency theorists emphasized government ownership of industry, agrarian collectivism, and state economic planning, going well beyond Prebisch's ISI.

Dependency theory shifted the focus of research from internal cultural factors to international economic and political arrangements, leading to new fields of inquiry such as international political economy. The theory also helped expand the concept of economic development, broadening its scope from economic growth to the distribution of resources nationally and internationally. Proponents of this theory argue that when rapid economic growth is accompanied by an increased concentration of wealth, it offers little benefit to the majority and can even leave some worse off (Handelman 1996). Under this vision of development, those who stand to gain are, once again, dominant countries and groups.

World Systems Theory

Developed by North American sociologist Immanuel Wallerstein, world systems theory, like dependency theory before it, questions modernization theory's assumption of a linear path to development from "traditional to modern" (Wallerstein 1974). However, world systems theory assumes a capitalist world economy as the basic unit of analysis for modern social change. The theory rejects the concept of "Third World" or "underdevelopment" and states that there is only one world connected by a network of economic exchange relations, a "world system" that is inherently capitalistic. The theory maintains that contemporary economic "backwardness" is not the result of a late start in the race to "develop," but instead stems from the deepening of long-standing economic relationships that commenced in feudal Europe. As the capitalist world economy has expanded, new areas formally external to it have been incorporated into the system, almost always at the periphery (Goldfrank 2000).

The theory builds on the idea of core–periphery relations developed by dependency theorists and introduces the notion of a third category, the *semi-periphery*. The semi-periphery is intermediate in terms of national capital, skills, wage levels, and production processes. It is characterized as a combined phase of development, with trade flowing simultaneously in two directions—export of moderate levels of processed materials to the core and import of simple manufactured goods from the periphery. In Wallerstein's terms, the core, periphery, and semi-periphery cannot exist without one another. Countries categorized as semi-peripheral include Brazil, Korea, and Taiwan (Goldfrank 2000).

Three concepts central to world systems theory are imperialism, hegemony, and class struggle. Imperialism refers to the domination of weak peripheral regions by strong core states. Hegemonic power refers to the notion of uncontestable dominance (even if contested at particular times and places) by core states in production, commerce, finance, military strength, and the values and ideology that underpin it. Class struggle refers to the political conflict over power between workers and elites (owners of significant capital). Similar to dependency theory, world systems theory assumes constant class struggle and shifting alliances within and across state boundaries. States themselves are conceived of as mediating actors within the system of a world economy, and global class struggle as integrated through the market rather than through a single political center or shared political interests (Wallerstein 1974).

Critique of Development Theories
from a Health Perspective

Modernization theory was widely espoused in the international health field, influencing aid policies aimed at assisting countries pass through Rostow's stages of growth. Vicente Navarro has challenged the main tenets of modernization theory, maintaining that "underdevelopment" of health in poorer countries is not due to scarcity of values, capital, or technology from developed countries but rather from their excessive or inappropriate application relative to local needs. He argues that the real problem of supposed "underdevelopment" is actually too much dependency on industrialized (capitalist) models and the subsidization of wealthier countries by resources and commodities from the developing world (Navarro 1981).

The abundance of natural resources in many developing countries could even be detrimental to political, economic, and social development. Known as "the paradox of plenty" (e.g., wealth in natural resources such as petroleum in Iran, Nigeria, Indonesia, Angola, and Venezuela), this argument stresses that (single) commodity dependency leads national and international interests to prioritize its exploitation while social and political institutions are neglected. The illusion of prosperity, accumulated by a small number of local elites and foreign investors, without concomitant redistribution, eventually provokes the deterioration of the economy and civic institutions (Karl 1997).

Navarro also contests the assumption that capital flows from developed to developing countries. To the contrary, he argues that the flow of capital, both financial and human (including health workers), is from developing to developed countries. In terms of health and medicine, Navarro proposes that in developing countries there is not too little but "too much cultural and technological dependency" on a Western biomedical approach and technology, thus diverting limited financial resources away from more needed and appropriate preventive and structural investments that emphasize social and economic redistribution (Navarro 1981).

Financial, Oil, and Debt Crises and the Breakdown of the Postwar Development Model, 1970s–Early 1980s

In the 1970s, a series of energy and financial crises threatened global economic stability. In 1971, U.S. President Richard Nixon abandoned the gold standard backing for the U.S. dollar and the worldwide fixed rate exchange system because the high dollar exchange undermined the competitiveness of U.S. industry. The systems of currency stability, predictable international financial markets, and state interventions that had been set up under the Bretton Woods agreement, while advantageous for welfare state development, were viewed as unsustainable (unprofitable for investors) in the face of growing flows of capital. But underdeveloped countries faced the most severe consequences of the Bretton Woods system breakdown.

In October 1973, members of the Organization of Arab Petroleum Countries decided to cut oil supplies to countries that supported Israel in the Yom Kippur War. The Organization of Petroleum Exporting Countries (OPEC), long frustrated by unchanging oil prices despite rising global inflation, seized on these events and raised the price of crude oil. The quadrupling in the price of oil in early 1974 led to a large stock market decline, then a boom in other commodity prices. The increased circulation of petrodollars (U.S. dollars earned from petroleum sales) initially brought increased access to capital in some (developing) countries while many others (mostly industrialized) experienced the beginnings of economic recession, inflation, public sector deficits, and an increase in unemployment.

The second oil shock began with the lead-up to the Iranian Revolution in 1979, followed the next year by the start of the Iran–Iraq war, both of which severely curtailed oil exports. The real price of crude oil increased from US$8 per barrel in 1971 to US$40 in 1973, and to more than US$60 in 1980 (International Energy Agency 2004). At that time, a world recession took place and interest rates rose sharply.

While countries that were net oil exporters—and the oil companies themselves—benefited from the oil shocks, many underdeveloped countries faced deepening financial problems. Countries in need of revenues to cover the high cost of oil and imports were persuaded to take loans from multilateral and commercial lenders flush with petrodollars (Nasser 2003). Governments that borrowed heavily found themselves increasingly short of foreign exchange to buy imported consumer goods for investment in industry and agriculture. Governments of Britain, the United States, and other industrialized countries sought to combat inflation through tight lending policies, compounding the problems of borrowing countries. The combination of interest rate hikes and large-scale borrowing led to an explosion in the debt of underdeveloped countries.

By the early 1980s a full-blown "debt crisis" had materialized. Total developing country debt increased from US$70.2 billion in 1970 to US$579.6 billion in 1980. Over the same period, service payments on long-term debt from developing countries increased from US$8.2 billion to US$72.1 billion (OECD 2003; World Bank 2003).

Much of this debt was due to irresponsible borrowing and lending practices, almost always carried out at upper levels of government and without stringent accounting practices to determine whether or not the debt would be sustainable in the long term. Borrowing rarely went to improving the economic and social conditions of those bearing the brunt of the financial crisis—the poor and precariously positioned working and middle classes—instead lining the pockets of wealthy elites.

As debt accumulated in the 1980s, it became apparent that some countries were on the verge of defaulting on their loans. In response, foreign investors and commercial interests rapidly withdrew resources and finances from countries vulnerable to a debt crisis. This capital flight, which also involved domestic financiers, further exacerbated and accelerated the financial crisis. Latin America's debt reached US$327 billion by 1982 (World Bank 1991), leading a band of countries across the continent to default on private loans in rapid succession, beginning with Mexico in 1982 (Theberge 1999). By October of 1983, 27 developing countries had defaulted on their loans or were in the process of rescheduling debts (Wellons 1987).

The 1980s are known as the "lost decade" for development. In Latin America, per capita income declined by 7%, consumption by 6%, and investment by 4% between 1980 and 1990. Hyperinflation occurred in much of Latin America, reaching an average of 1,500% in 1990. In sub-Saharan Africa per capita GNP fell nearly 10% during the same period when foreign investment and prices for major agricultural exports declined by 50% (UNDP 1996).

For years on end, and repeated in the late 1990s with the Asian, Russian, and Argentinean debt crises, underdeveloped countries experienced unpredictable economic conditions due to volatile swings in exchange rates, currency devaluations, soaring inflation, and trade imbalances. To this day, many developing nations remain locked in debt and aid arrangements that provide little overall benefit for domestic development: interest and principal payments on debt (outflows from developing countries) occur too soon and are far larger than foreign direct investment (FDI) and ODA (inflows to developing countries). As portrayed in Figures 4–9 and 4–10, overall negative net capital flows total hundreds of billions of dollars. Debt servicing has placed enormous constraints on countries' abilities to invest in public services, such as education, housing, sanitation, and health; in domestic industries; and in environmental, occupational, and consumer protections.

Neoliberalism—Mid-1980s to the Present

Currency liberalization, stagflation, the oil and debt crises, and waning interest in overseas development assistance—particularly as the Soviet Union was facing its own economic and political crises (including the 1980 invasion of Afghanistan) and was no longer perceived as a significant rival on the terrain of developing countries—opened the way for a major shift in development strategies (and overall public policy), that of neoliberal economic policy.

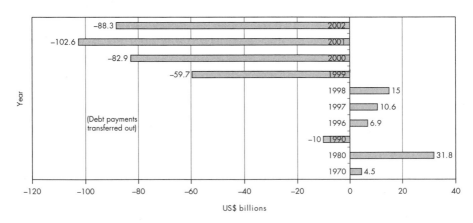

Figure 4–9 Net resource flows on debt from developing countries.
Source: World Bank (2003).

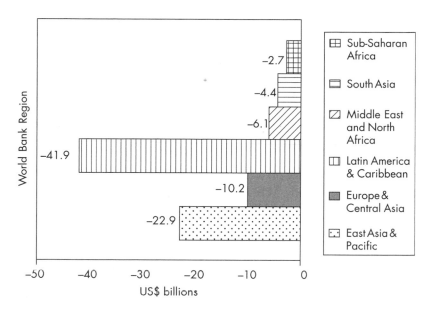

Figure 4-10 Net resource flows on debt from developing countries by region, 2002. *Source*: World Bank (2003).

The term "neoliberalism" refers to a renewal of the European capitalist *laissez-faire* liberalism of the 18th and 19th centuries. Both liberalism and neoliberalism conceive the role of government as protecting corporate and elite interests within a market economy, rather than safeguarding public interests within a welfare state. By the beginning of the 20th century, brutish market liberalism began to be displaced by more social democratic ideologies. Most Western European and American countries, pushed by strident working class mobilization, committed themselves—to differing degrees—to investing in social welfare programs, such as allowances for housing, health care, education, disability, and unemployment. As discussed above, in the wake of the Great Depression, the protective welfare state arrangement was widely accepted as a means to ensure the long-term viability of the capitalist system by attenuating its most harmful effects. The importance of state interventionism to redistribute wealth, regulate industry, and lessen the insecurity of the free market system was further reinforced as an alternative to Soviet communism. With the demise of Cold War rivalries, there emerged a new form of ideological warfare on the redistributive role of the state (justified by widespread economic crisis), and *laissez-faire* economics gained an increasing toehold around the world.

The features of neoliberal economics include:

- belief in the infallibility of the market;
- deregulation of the economy—the market acts as "self-regulator";
- liberalization and expansion of trade and global markets (including in finance);

- monetary measures to control inflation (even if unemployment rises);
- tax cuts and government downsizing;
- reduction of public spending on, and concomitant privatization of, social services;
- privatization of industry;
- strict controls on organized labor;
- abandonment of public health and safety protections; and
- economic growth as the primary aim, with redistribution a distant second (Steger 2002; Shah 2007).

Neoliberal exigencies—both domestic and foreign—influence governments to develop policies that are market-oriented, export-led, subject to fiscal austerity, and characterized by the commercialization and privatization of public sector functions (Bond and Dor 2003). At an international level, a neoliberal model maintains that the state should not intervene in regulating foreign trade or financial markets; the free flow of goods, services, and financial capital is considered to be the best way of guaranteeing an efficient and equitable worldwide distribution of resources (Navarro 2002); and virtually all resources, including minerals, forests, water, and land are opened to private ownership for commercial exploitation in the global market (Jaggar 2002). At a national level, neoliberalism holds that unions and government regulation of wages, working conditions, and public and environmental protection hinder economic growth and job production.

Over the past three decades, there has been enormous pressure on most countries—even those with a well-developed welfare state—to adhere to neoliberal policies, especially in terms of deregulation and privatization of social services. These policies are often pursued with generally baseless arguments that taxes are too high, that the private sector can guarantee more efficient service provision, and that governmental controls impede economic growth.

While neoliberal policies first took hold in Britain and the United States, they soon reached underdeveloped countries, which had become increasingly dependent on international financial institutions after the debt crisis. The IMF and World Bank played a major role in infusing these ideas and practices in underdeveloped countries, arguing that development would come about only with economic growth and a reduction in public expenditure. Key strategies of neoliberalism include the privatization of state assets and services, a reduction in the number of civil servants, and the introduction of user fees for services such as public health care, education, and water.

Box 4–2 Water Privatization

A prime example of the impact of neoliberalism on social services in underdeveloped settings is water privatization. Some of the world's poorest countries, including Benin, Niger, Rwanda, Kenya, and Tanzania, have privatized their water supplies over the past two decades under pressure from the IMF and World Bank (Global Health Watch 2005, pp. 210–212). While the public provision of

(continued)

Box 4–2 Continued

water in many developing countries has long suffered from inadequate resources for the maintenance and extension of water systems to poorer populations, privatization has brought worse problems, jeopardizing safety, quality, and access in the name of profits. Following water privatization in Bolivia and the Philippines, communities were forced to use contaminated water when water service was suspended due to nonpayment. This put them at risk of serious illness. In Argentina, rapidly increasing water prices following privatization—and the cost of service extensions—were borne disproportionately by the urban poor. Nonpayment for water and sanitation is as high as 30% and service cut-offs are common, with women and children bearing the brunt of health and safety consequences (Interagency Task Force on Gender and Water 2004, p. 17). Widespread recognition of the importance of water as a public, nonmarketable good has led to various collective movements to resist privatization. In the late 1990s, the inhabitants of Cochabamba, Bolivia drove out a World Bank-recommended water privatization scheme, and in 2004, an overwhelming majority of Uruguay's population voted for a constitutional amendment to protect water as a natural—and public—resource necessary for life, declaring that access to potable water and sanitation was a fundamental human right.

Critics of neoliberal strategies in the health services sector argue that not only does health service privatization decrease access to care, but it also leads to cost escalations, as inappropriate hospital admissions and unnecessary use of technologies and medicines increase in the drive for profits. Moreover, privatization of health services drains health professionals from the public sector—on which the majority of people in developing countries continue to depend—to the private sector. In sum, privatization policies increase social inequalities (Navarro 2007a), resulting in a similar imbalance of power and resources as under colonialism (Fort, Mercer, and Gish 2004).

Perhaps the most widely known neoliberal policies are Structural Adjustment Programs (SAPs), imposed on numerous developing countries starting in the 1980s in order to meet World Bank and IMF lending conditionalities aimed at balancing trade and domestic budget imbalances. SAPs have affected health through cuts in health care and other social sector services, privatization of public assets, and the introduction of user fees in the public sector. Spending cuts and privatization have resulted in reduced access to, and poorer quality of, health care, education, and other services, disproportionately affecting women and children. The effects of SAPs on health are addressed in Chapter 9.

While the IFIs have more recently sought to correct for the many miseries engendered by SAPs and other neoliberal policies—through Poverty Reduction Strategies, the Heavily Indebted Poor Countries Initiative, and endorsement of the Millennium Development Goals (MDGs) (see below)—many of these efforts have continued previous policies or focused on targets more than strategies. Even the World Bank's own analysts have found that it is near impossible to reach the poorest populations of underdeveloped countries (Gwatkin 2002). The latest antipoverty trend— providing quid pro quo cash transfers to parents who send their children to school or a health clinic, a policy undertaken in settings as varied as Mexico, Brazil, and New York City—has received widespread acclaim. It is no surprise that these conditional transfers have successfully increased school and health clinic attendance: participants are simply responding to monetary incentives. Yet a World Bank study of Ecuador's government cash transfer program showed that parents did not need patronizing conditionalities to ensure that their children were well cared for and attended school (Paxson and Schady 2007). While given hopeful names such as "Progress" and "Opportunities," temporary cash transfer programs are untenable solutions to poverty and underdevelopment as they do not address the long-term corrosion of work and living conditions, wages, and social services, or welfare states writ large, and may result in perverse incentives (Palmer et al. 2004).

In sum, notwithstanding the range of development efforts of the past 60 years, approximately 18 million yearly deaths—one-third of the total deaths per year—are "due to poverty-related causes" (Pogge 2005, p. 719), an enormous indictment of development efforts. Next, we discuss, from a political economy perspective, various means of addressing global health.

THE DEVELOPMENT–HEALTH DIALECTIC AND EMERGING APPROACHES TO GLOBAL HEALTH AND WELL-BEING

Key Question:

• How do the capabilities and the health and human rights approaches compare?

Disease Blocks Development or Development Blocks Disease

Circa 1900 British tropical medicine specialists Patrick Manson and Ronald Ross (working in China and India)—who, respectively, postulated and identified the mosquito vector for malaria—advocated for a greater role for imperial health endeavors because they regarded disease to be the principal factor holding back development (Worboys 1976). They held that a disease-free population would make rubber and fruit plantations, mining, and other industries more profitable and colonized subjects more manageable. The Rockefeller Foundation's large-scale campaigns to combat yellow fever, malaria, hookworm, and other diseases in the early 20th century were similarly based on the belief that diminishing disease rates would increase worker productivity, generate support for government public health efforts, maintain social and political stability, and, ultimately, enable colonies and other so-called backward countries to develop economically and join the world's market economy.

After World War II, the "disease blocks development" paradigm temporarily lost ground to the notion that "development blocks disease." As we have seen, many of the large-scale bilateral development programs held that infrastructural investments could fend off not only communism but also disease. Many underdeveloped countries also recognized the importance of social, political, and economic efforts—including education, housing, health care, and employment security—as a means of improving health, and these ideas were prominent in the Alma-Ata Primary Health Care Declaration of 1978.

But by this time, the pendulum had begun to shift back to the colonial era idea that human disease was impeding economic development, not vice versa; ideas that motivated the World Bank and other financial institutions to become involved in health care financing. U.S. economist Jeffrey Sachs—reviled in the former Soviet bloc as the architect of postcommunist era "shock therapy" and reborn as a health and development guru (Henwood 2006)—likewise justifies spending on health (through medical care and narrowly defined disease-control efforts) as a means of improving economic productivity and growth. As Chair of the WHO's Commission on Macroeconomics and Health (see Chapter 11), he declared:

> The macroeconomic evidence confirms that countries with the weakest conditions of health and education have a much harder time achieving sustained growth than do countries with better conditions of health and education…A typical statistical estimate suggests that each 10 percent improvement in life expectancy at birth…is associated with a rise in economic growth of at least 0.3 to 0.4 percentage points per year, holding other growth factors constant (Sachs 2001, pp. 23–24).

In economists' terms, this amounts to a rather modest contribution to growth. More importantly, as we will see, Sachs's penchant for cost-effective, technical, short-term disease control strategies (the biomedical model), without addressing the concomitant social and political determinants of health (the political economy model), limits the possible gains from health spending by not addressing the potential damage of economic growth without redistribution.

Notwithstanding the prominence accorded to Sachs's position, the view that poor health hinders economic development has been challenged. Various detailed longitudinal analyses demonstrate that higher levels of mortality in underdeveloped countries are more the consequence of poverty than its cause (Acemoglu, Johnson, and Robinson 2003). This does not mean, as discussed earlier, that unfettered economic growth is the salve for ill health. China and India's recent experiences of rapid economic development offer key lessons on the question of which kind of development (i.e., redistributive) effectively blocks disease. As Hsiao and Liu point out, "economic growth does not necessarily translate into better health and better health care for all. Instead, it may increase the disparity in income, nutritional status, health, and health care between the rich and the poor" (Hsiao and Liu 1996, p. 430). Indeed, China's remarkable poverty reduction since 1980 has not translated into diminished social inequalities in health (Reddy 2008).

If disease is not blocking development and development does not necessarily block disease, how else might we gauge human well-being and its determinants?

Development as Freedom

In contrast to the strict neoliberal economic model espoused by many of his colleagues, Amartya Sen, 1998 Nobel Laureate in economics, has been hailed for bringing a humanistic approach to development economics. Building on a generation of economists who abandoned more orthodox paradigms of development to focus on poverty diminution instead of, or alongside, economic growth (Chenery et al. 1974), Sen has proposed that human freedom is both the ultimate goal and the means of achieving development. According to Sen, "Development requires the removal of major sources of unfreedom: poverty as well as tyranny, poor economic opportunities as well as systematic social deprivation, neglect of public facilities as well as intolerance or overactivity of repressive states" (Sen 1999, p. 3).

Sen and Martha Nussbaum have developed a "capabilities approach" to poverty, which focuses on the human ability to realize personal and societal objectives (i.e., what people do), rather than emphasizing what they have or consume. This moves development away from purely material understandings of poverty. Based on philosopher John Rawls' "theory of justice," which conceptualizes individual well-being as the possession of "social primary goods," capabilities are "the substantive freedoms [a person] enjoys to lead the kind of life he or she has reason to value" (Sen 1999, p. 87).

Contrary to many policy makers, Sen and Nussbaum place humans and human agency at the center of development, "both as an end in itself, and as a means to other important capabilities or freedoms" (Stanton 2007, p. 11). The challenges laid out in this humanistic approach render the income per capita measure of welfare emphasized by neoclassical economics grossly inadequate.

Even with its acclaimed human development focus, Sen's approach has been critiqued for omitting an in-depth political and class analysis. Sen addresses political factors, but he does so in a binary fashion, contrasting dictatorships with democracies while overlooking the internal politics of redistribution. For example, Sen would designate Castro's Cuba and Pinochet's Chile as dictatorships. Yet class structure and political impetus distinguished the two societies from one another, with Cuba based on socialist principles of solidarity among the majority of the population and Chile on the privileging of elite class interests against those of the rest of the population (Navarro 2004).

The Human Development Index

Sen's ideas have also shaped the UN's Human Development Index (HDI), which employs the capabilities approach in an "applied measure" of human welfare, and has been called the "godfather" of the UNDP's *Human Development Report* (Malloch Brown 2005).

The HDI is a composite index of levels of literacy and education, life expectancy, and GDP/capita in each country. Developed in 1990 by Mahbub ul Haq, the annual *Human Development Report* has ranked countries by the HDI since 1993. More recently joined by a human poverty index, a gender-related development index, and a gender empowerment index, the use of the HDI has sought to shift development endeavors from focusing purely on economic indicators to expanding the range of human opportunities by removing potential barriers, such as illiteracy, ill health, poor access to sanitation, water, and other basic resources, and lack of civil and political freedoms. Within this framework, health is considered a powerful means of overall economic and social progress in society (Fukuda-Parr 2002).

The HDI has been critiqued for its methodology, the quality of data used, its partial reflection of reality, and its focus on the national rather than global level (Sagar and Najam 1998; Lehohla 2005). Most importantly, the HDI fails to indicate who/what is responsible for inequality and low levels of development or how to resolve these problems. Despite these deficiencies, the HDI remains the sole instrument that allows for an annual comparative snapshot of the world's social and economic conditions.

Millennium Development Goals

These efforts to understand development in human terms helped refocus global attention on addressing the problems of underdevelopment. In 2000, world leaders gathered in New York to sign the UN Millennium Declaration, which called for "collective responsibility to uphold the principles of human dignity, equality and equity at the global level" (UN 2000). The following year, 189 countries (nearly all UN member states) plus all major UN and other international agencies (including the World Bank and IMF) agreed to eight interdependent MDGs, and accompanying measurable targets (see Box 4–3) to be met by 2015. Three of the eight MDGs, eight of the original 16 targets, and 18 of the original 48 indicators relate directly to health, and most others are linked to the underlying determinants of health (UN Millennium Project 2007).

Box 4–3 MDGs and Selected Targets

1. Eradicate extreme poverty and hunger
   Target: Halve the proportion of people living on less than $1 per day and who suffer from hunger
2. Achieve universal primary education
   Target: Ensure that all boys and girls complete a full course of primary schooling
3. Promote gender equality and empower women
   Target: Eliminate gender disparity in primary and secondary education
4. Reduce child mortality
   Target: Reduce by two-thirds the mortality rate among children under five

(continued)

Box 4-3 Continued

5. Improve maternal health
   Target: Reduce by three-quarters the maternal mortality ratio
6. Combat HIV/AIDS, malaria, and other diseases
   Target: Halt and begin to reverse the spread and incidence of these diseases
7. Ensure environmental sustainability
   Targets: Integrate the principles of sustainable development into country policies and programs; reverse loss of environmental resources; improve the lives of at least 100 million slum-dwellers; and halve the proportion of people without sustainable access to safe drinking water and sanitation
8. Develop a global partnership for development
   Targets: Develop a nondiscriminatory trade and financial system that focuses on the needs of the least developed countries; deal comprehensively with the debt problems of developing countries through national and international measures that seek to make debt sustainable; cooperate with the pharmaceutical industry and the private sector to, respectively, provide access to affordable essential drugs, and make available new information and communications technologies.

The Millennium Declaration was the culmination of a process that began in the late 1970s, when World Bank President Robert McNamara invited German Chancellor Willy Brandt to head a commission to resolve and transcend the "North–South" political impasse on development strategies. The commission called for the mutual dependence of industrialized and underdeveloped nations, balancing issues of trade, financial reforms, and economic integration with concerns around the environment, energy use, food and agricultural development, and aid (Brandt 1980; Independent Commission on International Development Issues 1983). Like the Millennium Declaration, the Brandt Commission failed to address inequalities of power within and between countries as both the prime cause of and solution to underdevelopment. Instead it stressed enlightened self-interest and moral appeals for social justice rather than structural change in the global political economy (Navarro 1984). Released just as the debt crisis was unfolding and international financial agencies were turning to SAPs, the Brandt Commission reports were shelved.

While the Millennium Declaration and the setting of MDGs have been lauded for demonstrating a shared global commitment to development and poverty reduction, they have also been critiqued for their narrow definition of poverty, a focus on market-based approaches and debt servicing, the setting of priorities potentially in conflict with domestic needs, and difficulties inherent in monitoring progress.

Sen has found the MDGs insufficiently reflective of the declaration itself (Sen 2004). Alejandro Bendana, founder of the Center for International Studies in Nicaragua, has argued that the emphasis on "good governance" is "taking us away from the [MDGs] because it entails placing the state and society at the service of the market, under the presumption that economic growth alone will deliver development" (Bendana 2004, p. 1). Samir Amin contends, even more powerfully, that far from reflecting global consensus, the MDGs draw from hegemonic (largely Northern) interests in imposing a liberal free-market agenda of capitalist globalization. Accordingly, the social progress aims of the MDGs "cannot be taken seriously" because they are not achievable under—and only serve to legitimize—capitalist globalization (Amin 2006).

Others note that although the MDGs are attractive due to their concrete targets, many of them—especially the health-related targets—are either difficult to measure, or not measurable at all, because most underdeveloped countries do not have reliable statistics (Attaran 2005). Moreover, the MDGs' benchmark approach makes it far harder for the least developed nations to achieve targets as compared to countries that started out with higher development baselines (Easterly 2007). An example of these problems relates to the first goal of eradicating poverty. In employing the proportion of the world's population living on less than US$1/day as the poverty reduction target, the MDGs take a very narrow definition of poverty; for instance, decreasing the proportion of people living on less than US$1/day may bring them to just over the $1 cut-off. As seen in Figure 4–11, from 1990 to 2001, the percentage of people living on less than $1 a day decreased by approximately 8% in underdeveloped countries, but rose by 2% in sub-Saharan Africa. Between 2001 and 2003, excluding China, there was virtually no difference in poverty rates throughout the developing world.

Due to uneven rises in the cost of living in many developing countries since the World Bank set the original $1/day international poverty line, various analysts have proposed raising the standard measurement of poverty to at least US$2/day. This would more adequately account for the cost of obtaining sufficient caloric intake and meeting other basic needs. Of course, any universal poverty line is problematic. For example, $1/day is insufficient for *daily survival* in most Latin American countries (and thus $2/day—or considerably more in urban

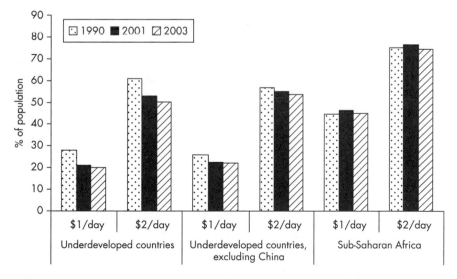

Figure 4–11 World poverty rates, 1990–2003. *Source*: World Bank (2005b, 2007a).

areas—is a better measurement), but in many rural regions in sub-Saharan Africa, $1/day may adequately gauge *extreme poverty* (Reddy and Pogge 2005). A more sensitive $2/day poverty line showed poverty rates in 2003 exceeding 50% across the underdeveloped world and over 75% in sub-Saharan Africa, showing little progress over time (excluding China).

While the proportion of people living on less than $1 and $2/day has declined since 1990 (though with poverty rates falling more slowly than in previous decades [Berry and Serieux 2006]), in absolute numbers many more people now live in poverty than in the 1990 MDG baseline year. Today over 2 billion people—one-third of the world's population—live on less than US$2/day. In sub-Saharan Africa alone, 150 million more people in 2003 lived on less than $2/day compared to 1990, and 100 million more lived on less than $1/day (World Bank 2005b, 2007b). Under mounting pressure from activists and professionals, in 2008 the World Bank finally conceded to raising its global poverty line to $1.25/day. Although the $1.25 yardstick is considerably lower than the measure recommended by many experts, it is enough to show that 1.4 billion people (one quarter of the developing world population)—rather than the previous estimate of 1 billion—lived in extreme poverty in 2005 (Chen and Ravallion 2008).

In September 2005, a 5-year review of the MDGs showed that although progress had been made in achieving some of the goals, many others were marked by setbacks. Kofi Annan, then UN Secretary-General, stated that if current trends continued, many of the poorest countries would not achieve the MDGs. The 2005 report cited three reasons for increased poverty in sub-Saharan Africa—unemployment, a stagnant agricultural sector, and the impact of HIV/AIDS (UN 2005)—problems that the MDG targets can do little to address.

This points to a further, fundamental deficiency of the Millennium Declaration and MDG approach: the failure to address the causes of and solutions to poverty. The Millennium campaign not only bowdlerizes the "urgent struggle to end exploitation" (by failing to recognize exploitation's role in creating and perpetuating poverty), it excludes or thwarts efforts emphasizing successful welfare state and other redistributive measures in either underdeveloped or industrialized settings (Navarro 2007b). Aside from renewed emphasis on the importance of economic growth (despite ample evidence, discussed above, that growth alone does not lead to improvements in health and development), there are no real strategies proposed to realize the shared goals within and across societies or on how to achieve and sustain improvements in human well-being into the future.

By 2007, roughly two-thirds of the way to the target date of 2015 (most indicators use 1990 rates as baseline), the situation appeared even worse than predicted by Annan: the majority of underdeveloped countries, especially those in sub-Saharan Africa, were deemed unlikely to meet their MDG targets by 2015 (UN Millennium Project 2007).

In sum, without bona fide political will and international pressure that take into account the political economy basis of development, the grand ambitions of the

Millennium Declaration and the MDGs may be destined for the rhetorical dustbin, akin to previous development efforts of the 20th century.

Health and Human Rights Approach

"It is my aspiration that health will finally be seen not as a blessing to be wished for, but as a human right to be fought for," Kofi Annan stated in 2002 (WHO 2002, p. 4).

Potentially one of the most powerful instruments for improving global health and addressing its underlying determinants is the health and human rights framework. According to the UN Universal Declaration of Human Rights (UDHR), adopted by the UN General Assembly in 1948, human rights are "those rights which are inherent in our nature and without which we cannot live as human beings." These rights are "inalienable" and "everyone is entitled to all [these] rights...without distinction of any kind, such as race, color, sex, language, religion, political or other opinion, national or social origin, property, birth, or other status" (UN 1948). The UDHR states that these human rights, such as the right to life, to freedom from discrimination, to education, to be recognized everywhere as a person, and to a standard of living adequate for health and well-being, belong equally to all persons.

This is consistent with the WHO Constitution, which declares that the "enjoyment of the highest attainable standard of health is one of the fundamental rights of every human being." Numerous legally binding international and regional human rights treaties (see Table 4–4), signed by all but a handful of countries, codify this right. Furthermore, over two-thirds of all countries have health or health care-related rights enshrined in their constitutions (Kinney and Clark 2004).

During the debates over the UDHR's drafting and role, conflicting views emerged regarding which human rights to prioritize. While Western bloc countries emphasized civil and political rights (CP), Eastern bloc nations concentrated on the rights to health, food, and education (Economic, social, and cultural [ESC] rights), leading to two separate human rights treaties. The dichotomy lasted for decades, despite the UDHR framers' belief that CP and ESC rights were interwoven (Glendon 2001).

The longtime emphasis on CP rights has given way since the end of the Cold War to greater attention to ESC rights, including the rights to food, shelter, and freedom from discrimination in health services (Yamin 2005). This shift creates many new possibilities for using human rights treaties as a legal tool for improving health conditions, country by country and internationally. Many health determinants, from a political economy viewpoint, have been brought under the broad tent of human rights, including access to education, economic and social protection, environmental sustainability, fair employment and labor rights, access to credit, equitable marriage, divorce, and custody laws, political freedom and choice, right to adequate food, physical integrity, water and sanitation, secure housing and living conditions, freedom of religious observance, and social justice writ large.

Table 4–4 Human Rights Instruments as a Baseline for the "Right to Health"

Document/Article	Relation to Health
WHO Constitution (1948)	Obligates member nations to promote health among other human rights as a way of achieving peace among nations
UN Declaration of Human Rights (1948): Article 25	"(1) Everyone has the right to a standard of living adequate for the health and well-being of himself and of his family, including food, clothing, housing, and medical care and necessary social services, and the right to security in the event of unemployment, sickness, disability, widowhood, old age or other lack of livelihood in circumstances beyond his control.
	(2) Motherhood and childhood are entitled to special care and assistance. All children, whether born in or out of wedlock, shall enjoy the same social protection."
International Covenant on Economic, Social, and Cultural Rights (1976): Article 12	Reiterates and expands on the right to health by recognizing "the right of everyone to the enjoyment of the highest attainable standard of physical and mental health"
Convention on the Rights of the Child (1989): Article 24	Obligates "states parties [to] recognize the right of the child to the enjoyment of the highest attainable standard of health"

Source: Gruskin and Tarantola (2005).

The HIV/AIDS epidemic in Africa fueled the creation of the modern health and human rights movement in the early 1990s, particularly under the leadership of Jonathan Mann (Leaning 1998; Tarantola et al. 2006). Mann contextualized HIV/ AIDS as an issue of human rights, not simply one of biological or behavioral origins. In using a human rights framework to address the issue of HIV/AIDS, Mann called attention to the need to address broader structural issues—such as poverty, discrimination, and accessible health care systems—to curb the spread of the epidemic (Mann and Tarantola 1995; Mann 1997). This framework is consistent with a political economy of health approach and also brings structural issues to light when addressing health concerns, rather than relying solely on biomedical and/or behavioral approaches. Pogge and others view shared human rights in terms of a moral obligation to address extreme inequalities in global and regional income through "modest institutional reforms" (Pogge 2007). Of course, meaningful income redistribution entails fundamental political action not only moral justice.

Governmental Obligations

The WHO now recognizes that the promotion of health and the respect, protection, and fulfillment of human rights are inextricably linked (WHO 2007). From a legal perspective, according to the UDHR, the International Covenant on Economic, Social, and Cultural Rights (ICESCR), and the International Covenant on Civil and Political Rights (ICCPR) (together known as the International Bill of Human Rights), governments are obligated to respect, protect, and fulfill the rights set forth in these documents. Respect means that governments should not violate these rights. Protect means

Table 4–5 Pathways to Health and Human Rights

Domains of Health	Governmental Obligations with Respect to Human Rights		
	Respect	Protect	Fulfill
1. Health Outcomes	Government may not violate human rights on the basis of health status, including provision of care and other services and data collection	Government must prevent violation of its citizens' rights by nonstate interests (e.g., private care providers or financers)	Government must take administrative, legislative, judicial and other measures to promote and protect the rights of people, regardless of their health status
2. Health Systems	Same as above, as applied to national health systems	Same as above, as applied to national health systems	Same as above, as applied to national health systems
3. Societal and Environmental Preconditions	Government must not directly violate or neglect the rights of people that affect health	Same as above, as applied to societal and environmental preconditions	Governments must provide known and accessible legal means of promoting redress for rights violations

Source: Adapted from Tarantola and Gruskin (1999).

that governments should prevent violations of these rights by third parties. Fulfill means that governments should take steps to ensure "the full realization" of these rights and creation of conditions that allow people to be healthy (Gruskin and Tarantola 2005). Because the human right to health also "gives rise to entitlements and obligations, it demands effective mechanisms of accountability" (Hunt 2006, p. 604). As shown in Table 4–5, the use of rights-based approaches to guide the formulation of government policies—particularly as related to health systems (UN Human Rights Council 2008)—establishes a framework to account for the stepwise satisfaction of government responsibilities, albeit limited by resource availability (Yamin 2005).

Notwithstanding these developments, scholars and activists critique the health and human rights approach on several grounds. In principle, legal frameworks are more likely to succeed in societies able to translate theoretical rights into concrete measures. First, however, they must agree to these frameworks. The United States—with one of the most extensive judiciaries in the world—is among the few nonratifiers of key human rights treaties including the Convention on the Rights of the Child (CRC) and the ICESCR. But ratification is not enough: the majority of signatories—even those with well-developed judiciaries—have not realized their obligations (e.g., Canada has been intransigent on resolving child poverty despite having signed the CRC). To date, failure to comply with human rights treaty obligations has not been subject to effective enforcement mechanisms.

Box 4–4 Governmental Obligations for Health Under International
Human Rights Law

- Nondiscrimination
- Safeguarding the right to enjoy the benefits of scientific progress
- Reporting under human rights treaties
- Respecting, protecting, and fulfilling human rights

Still, rights to health may be successfully deployed if there are enforceable legal instruments (domestic constitutions or ratified international human rights treaties) *and* effective and willing judiciaries, bolstered by social justice movements, political parties representative of worker and peasant interests, and political systems that do not privilege moneyed interests over others. The social rights jurisprudence emerging in South Africa and various Latin American countries is showing that the right to health is not simply a good set of standards to guide policy, but an increasingly enforceable right in countries of differing levels of economic development (Hogerzeil et al. 2006; Forman 2007). Political mobilization supporting these legal developments is essential, given the potential redistributive implications of the legally enforceable right to health.

Another challenge has to do with the complexity of factors that influence human health—the political economy of health writ large—making it more difficult to specify in legal terms what constitutes the right to health, compared to the right to a fair trial or to education. Nonetheless, the ICESCR defines the right to health as including the underlying determinants of health (e.g., sanitation, shelter), and various UN social rights committees have also made advances in this regard (UN Committee on Economic, Social, and Cultural Rights 2000).

Yet in recent years, the right to health has been distilled to—or misinterpreted as— a "right to health care" by various international and national health actors who argue that improvements in the broad domain of determinants of health may be less easily realized than the right to health care. Not only has "health as a human right" come to signify "health care services as a human right," for some this has been further narrowed to mean access to a particular package of biomedical technologies, such as drugs or surgical sutures (Farmer 2006). Undoubtedly, such technologies are important and useful, but they constitute just one small component of the right to health.

This is not to say that a health and human rights approach is futile, only that in order to operate effectively, it must be accompanied by social justice movements able to effectuate political change and utilize litigation as part of broad social mobilization. The Brazilian landless people's movement (Movimento sem Terra) and the international peasants' organization La Via Campesina are examples of an integrated health and human rights approach—in their struggles for local control over food production and agricultural policy as a human right and as a determinant of livelihood and health. As such, a health and human rights-based approach working in concert with a political economy framework emphasizing the structural determinants of health offers important possibilities for improvements in health.

CONCLUSION: CURRENT ATTENTION TO INTERNATIONAL HEALTH: WHERE DOES A POLITICAL ECONOMY APPROACH FIT IN?

Learning Points:

- Development strategies and aid have been—and are—determined by global political and ideological exigencies. This helps explain why biomedical and behavioral models are far more pervasive than political economy models.
- A political economy approach to international health analyzes the underlying determinants of health and disease patterns in the context of social, political, and economic relations at local, national, and global levels.

In recent years, international health and development has (re)gained considerable prominence as a worldwide concern. Celebrities, billionaire investors, multilateral agencies, and political leaders have all drawn attention to health needs in developing countries and to global inequalities, resulting in new programs and a doubling of health aid almost overnight. The vast majority of international health strategies focus on disease-control measures, based on behavioral and biomedical approaches to health. How and why is it that social justice, political economy, and human rights approaches are left out?

With over US$15 billion approved for spending on global health in 2005 by multinational and bilateral development assistance agencies, international health aid must be understood not only on its own terms, but as a form of foreign policy with goals that go far beyond improved health conditions (Lane and Glassman 2007). Here we examine a selection of foreign policy statements to understand the larger political context of health aid.

Overall, foreign aid policies in the United States and Canada prioritize development, defense, and diplomacy as the main components of national security and international political strategies. The official goals of U.S. foreign aid include strengthening fragile states, promoting "transformational development," providing humanitarian assistance, supporting U.S. geostrategic interests, and mitigating global and transnational ills (Government of the United States of America 2002). Canada—like the United States—has national interests in mind when providing foreign assistance, using overseas aid to safeguard international security and maintain the status quo of the global system. Development aid is justified on the basis of enhancing commerce, advancing the MDGs, and promoting "Canadian values," including Canada's supposed "legitimacy" as a noncolonizer (this despite its appalling legacy of oppressing Aboriginal populations) (Government of Canada 1995, 2005; Canadian International Development Agency 2002).

By contrast, the European Union's development assistance mandate prioritizes principles of solidarity and humanitarian action and is often directed to extremely vulnerable populations, with fewer foreign policy considerations (Commission of the European Communities 2006). USAID's former chief disagrees with this stance, holding that avoidance of foreign policy considerations in development strategies is untenable in an era of "overriding security concerns" (Natsios 2006).

Within this larger foreign policy context, health aid is understood to confer a number of advantages on donor countries. In the case of the United States, these include: protecting the health of its own citizens (narrow self-interest); promoting political stability, economic productivity and growth, and a vibrant civil society (security or enlightened self-interest); and encouraging research, debt relief, and primary care (human rights leadership and diplomatic capital) (Kassalow 2001). Pressing calls for global health to become a vital issue of national interest (U.S. Institute of Medicine 1997) are accompanied by a broad trend of health aid being increasingly shaped by commercial and industrial interests (Ollila 2005).

Britain's chief medical advisor has similarly proposed that the United Kingdom adopt a government-wide foreign health policy strategy in order to "improve global security and health protection, enhance sustainable development, improve trade by promoting health as a commodity, maximize the potential of global public goods, and encourage a human rights approach to health" (Donaldson and Banatvala 2007, p. 857). Like its North American counterparts, this proposal employs largely self-interested criteria for assessing strategies. Moreover, while the United Kingdom has a track record for providing effective, long-term development assistance and debt relief, it cannot escape the contradictions between promoting health and facilitating trade that harms health, including sale of arms; the implications of close political relations with the United States and its unilateral approach (especially from 2000 to 2008) to international problems; and the ethical and policy conundrum regarding whether health is a goal in and of itself, or whether it is a means to other ends (such as improving trade and productivity) (McKee 2007).

In pursuing such goals, a "recipe approach"—employing the same set of techno-medical measures regardless of locale—has flourished. Locally developed ideas and plans are typically considered unwieldy and expensive, and donor priorities dominate aid agendas, regardless of their local relevance. Perhaps most problematically, donor countries and agencies almost never consider key political economy determinants, such as questions of social conditions and resource distribution, in their development assistance strategies.

The Global Health and Foreign Policy Initiative, established at a 2007 meeting of the Ministers of Foreign Affairs of Brazil, France, Indonesia, Norway, Senegal, South Africa, and Thailand, is seeking to highlight health as a foreign policy issue on more geopolitically equitable grounds. These nations called for, *inter alia*, development models that reflect the needs of recipient countries rather than donor interests (Amorim et al. 2007). The absence of major donors at this meeting enabled bold rhetoric on collaborative approaches, fair trade, and health systems as top priorities. Whether global governance and solidarity approaches can be used to counter the self-interested political and economic approaches of large donors remains to be seen.

Although contested, if not ignored, in the international aid world, the political economy of health approach remains invaluable to understanding how complex political, economic, and social forces combine to produce health and ill health within and across societies and how these forces influence the international health field. The tools presented in this chapter—particularly the analytic questions regarding how the distribution of wealth and power influence patterns of health and its multilayered determinants—will serve as a framework for the remainder of the book, both in terms of understanding the challenges of international health and as a means to address them.

NOTES

1. Social classes are broad social groupings indicating societal stratification and hierarchies. Social class may be understood in terms of: one or more measures of socioeconomic status (education, occupation, income); a combination of wealth, power, and prestige (Max Weber's classification); relation to the means of production (according to Karl Marx)—either the class of owners (exploiters) or workers (the exploited) or in an intermediate (contradictory) position as both worker and owner (e.g., administrator, manager, overseer); caste (social position and occupation determined through heredity and racial/ethnic heritage).

2. Redistribution policies seek to even out the spread of wealth (income, property, assets) across a society. Redistribution can be realized through progressive taxation (higher tax rates on the rich), wage controls, and targeted or universal social programs in a capitalist system or, in a socialist system through collective ownership and equitable distribution of societal assets.

3. Capitalism is an economic system in which the means of production are predominantly privately owned; production is operated on a for-profit basis; the "free market" (theoretically created by the sum of rational individual decisions) governs levels and patterns of wages, production, distribution, investment, and prices and availability of goods and services. For more on capitalism's emergence, see Chapter 2.

REFERENCES

Acemoglu D, Johnson S, and Robinson J. 2003. Disease and development in historical perspective. *Journal of the European Economic Association* 1(2–3):397–405.

Allende S. 1939. *La realidad médico-social Chilena: Sintesis.* Santiago, Chile: Ministerio de Salubridad, Previsión y Asistencia Social.

Amin S. 2006. The Millennium Development Goals: A critique from the South. *Monthly Review* 57(10):1–15.

Amorim C, Douste-Blazy P, Wirayuda H, Store JG, Gadio CT, Dlamini-Zuma N, and Pibulsonggram N. 2007. Oslo Ministerial declaration—global health: A pressing foreign policy issue of our time. *Lancet* 396(9570):1373–1378.

Attaran A. 2005. An immeasurable crisis? A criticism of the Millennium Development Goals and why they cannot be measured. *PLoS Med* 2(10):e318.

Banerji D. 1982. *Poverty, Class, and Health Culture in India*. New Delhi: Prachi Prakashan.

Bendana A. 2004. "Good governance" and the MDGs: Contradictory or complementary? Paper read at Institute for Global Network, Information and Studies, Oslo. September 20, 2004.

Berry A and Serieux J. 2006. Riding the elephants: The evolution of world economic growth and income distribution at the end of the 20th century (1980–2000). DESA Working Paper No. 27. New York, NY: UN/DESA.

Birdsall N. 1994. Pragmatism, Robin Hood, and other themes: Good government and social well-being in developing countries. In Chen LC, Kleinman A, and Ware NC, Editors. *Health and Social Change in International Perspective*. Boston, MA: Harvard University Press.

Bond P and Dor G. 2003. Uneven health outcomes and political resistance under residual neoliberalism in Africa. *International Journal of Health Services* 33(3):607–630.

Brandt W. 1980. *North-South: A Program for Survival*. Cambridge, MA: MIT Press.

Breilh J and Granda E. 1989. Epidemiología y contrahegemonía. *Social Science and Medicine* 28(11):1121–1127.

Buchanan D. 2000. *An Ethic for Health Promotion: Rethinking the Sources of Human Well-Being*. New York: Oxford University Press.

Canadian International Development Agency. 2002. *Canada Making a Difference in the World: A Policy Statement on Strengthening Aid Effectiveness*. Hull, QC: Minister of Public Works and Government Services, Canada.

Catalano R and Frank J. 2001. Detecting the effect of medical care on mortality. *Journal of Clinical Epidemiology* 54(8):830–836.

Cereseto S and Waitzkin H. 1986. Economic development, political-economic system, and the physical quality of life. *American Journal of Public Health* 76:661–666.

Chen S and Ravallion M. 2008. The developing world is poorer than we thought, but no less successful in the fight against poverty. Policy Research Working Paper No. WPS 4703. Washington, DC: The World Bank Development Research Group.

Chenery H, Ahluwalia MS, Bell CLG, Duloy JH, and Jolly R. 1974. *Redistribution with Growth*. London: Oxford University Press.

Chung H-J and Muntaner C. 2007. Welfare state matters: A typological multilevel analysis of wealthy countries. *Health Policy* 80(2):328–339.

Cleaver HM Jr 1972. The contradictions of the green revolution. *The American Economic Review* 62(2):177–186.

Commission of the European Communities. 2006. European Commission Directorate-General for Humanitarian Aid—ECHO operational strategy. Brussels: ECHO.

Cutler DM, Deaton AS, and Lleras-Muney A. 2006. The determinants of mortality. *Journal of Economic Perspectives* 20(3):97–120.

Dagdeviren H, van der Hoeven R, and Weeks J. 2001. *Redistribution Matters: Growth for Poverty Reduction*. Geneva: International Labour Organization.

Donaldson L and Banatvala N. 2007. Health is global: Proposals for a UK government-wide strategy. *Lancet* 369(9564):857–861.

Doyal L. 1995. *What Makes Women Sick: Gender and the Political Economy of Health*. London: Palgrave Macmillan.

Doyal L and Pennell I. 1979. *The Political Economy of Health*. New Brunswick, NJ: Rutgers University Press.

Easterly W. 2007. *How the Millennium Development Goals are Unfair to Africa. Global Economy and Development Working Paper 14.* Washington, DC: The Brookings Institution.

Farmer P. 2006. Challenging orthodoxies in health and human rights. Paper presented at the American Public Health Association 134th Annual Meeting and Exposition, Boston. November 5, 2006.

Fogel RW. 2004. *The Escape from Hunger and Premature Death, 1700–2100: Europe, America, and the Third World.* Cambridge: Cambridge University Press.

Forman L. 2007. Trade rules, intellectual property and the right to health. *Ethics and International Affairs* 21(3):337–357.

Fort M, Mercer MA, and Gish O, Editors. 2004. *Sickness and Wealth: The Corporate Assault on Health.* Cambridge, MA: South End Press.

Franco M, Orduñez P, Caballero B, Tapia Granados JA, Lazo M, Bernal JL, Guallar E, and Cooper RS. 2007. Impact of energy intake, physical activity, and population-wide weight loss on cardiovascular disease and diabetes mortality in Cuba, 1980–2005. *American Journal of Epidemiology* 166(12):1374–1380.

Franco S. 1999. *El Quinto: No Matar. Contextos Explicativos de la Violencia en Colombia.* Bogotá: Tercer Mundo.

Fuhrer H. 1996. *A History of the Development Assistance Committee and the Development Co-operation Directorate in Dates, Names, and Figures.* Paris: OECD.

Fukuda-Parr S. 2002. Operationalizing Amartya Sen's ideas on capabilities, development, freedom and human rights—The shifting policy focus on the human development approach. http://hdr.undp.org/docs/training/oxford/readings/fukuda-parr_HDA.pdf. Accessed April 18, 2007.

Glendon MA. 2001. *A World Made New: Eleanor Roosevelt and the Universal Declaration of Human Rights.* New York: Random House.

Global Health Watch. 2005. *Global Health Watch 2005–2006: An Alternative World Health Report.* London: Zed Books.

Gloyd S. 1987. Child survival and resource scarcity. Paper presented at the International Congress of the World Federation of Public Health Associations, Mexico City. March 1987.

Goldfrank WJ. 2000. Paradigm regained? The rules of Wallerstein's world-system method. *Journal of World-Systems Research* XI(2):150–195.

Government of Canada, Department of Foreign Affairs and International Trade. 1995. Canada in the World: Canadian Foreign Policy Review. http://www.dfait-maeci.gc.ca/foreign_policy/cnd-world/menu-en.asp. Accessed May 2, 2007.

———. 2005. Canada's international policy statement: A role of pride and influence in the world. http://geo.international.gc.ca/cip-pic/current_discussions/ips-archive-en.aspx. Accessed May 2, 2007.

Government of the United States of America. 2002. *The National Security Strategy of the United States of America.* Washington, DC: The White House.

Graham C. 2005. Insights on development from the economics of happiness. *World Bank Research Observer* 20(2):201–231.

Gruskin S and Tarantola D. 2005. Health and human rights. In Gruskin S, Grodin MA, Annas GJ, and Marks SP, Editors. *Perspectives on Health and Human Rights.* New York: Routledge Press.

Guevara E. 1960. Discurso a los estudiantes de medicina y trabajadores de la salud. In Ariet Garcia MdC and Deutschmann D, Editors. *Che Guevara Presente.* Melbourne: Ocean Press.

Gunder Frank A. 1972. The development of underdevelopment. In Cockroft J, Frank AG, and Johnson D, Editors. *Dependence and Underdevelopment: Latin America's Political Economy.* Garden City, NY: Anchor Books.

Gwatkin D. 2002. *Who Would Gain Most from Efforts to Reach the Millennium Development Goals for Health? An Inquiry into the Possibility of Progress that Fails to Reach the Poor.* Washington, DC: World Bank.

Halstead SB, Walsh JA, and Warren KS, Editors. 1985. *Good Health at Low Cost: Rockefeller Foundation Conference Report.* New York: Rockefeller Foundation.

Handelman H. 1996. *The Challenge of Third World Development.* Upper Saddle River, NJ: Prentice Hall.

Hazen A and Ehiri JE. 2006. Road traffic injuries: Hidden epidemic in less developed countries. *Journal of the National Medical Association* 98(1):73–82.

Henwood D. 2006. A critique of Jeffrey D. Sachs's *The End of Poverty. International Journal of Health Services* 36(1):197–203.

Hogerzeil HV, Samson M, Casanovas JV, and Rahmani-Ocora L. 2006. Is access to essential medicines as part of the fulfilment of the right to health enforceable through the courts? *Lancet* 368:305–311.

Hsiao WC and Liu Y. 1996. Economic reform and health—lessons from China. *New England Journal of Medicine* 335(6):430–432.

Hunt P. 2006. The human right to the highest attainable standard of health: New opportunities and challenges. *Transactions of the Royal Society of Tropical Medicine and Hygiene* 100(7):603–607.

Independent Commission on International Development Issues. 1983. *Common Crisis North-South: Co-Operation for World Recovery. The Brandt Commission.* Cambridge, MA: MIT Press.

Interagency Task Force on Gender and Water. 2004. A gender perspective on water resources and sanitation. Background Paper submitted to the Commission on Sustainable Development. New York: UNDESA.

International Energy Agency. 2004. Analysis of the impact of high oil prices on the global economy. http://www.iea.org/Textbase/Papers/2004/High_Oil_Prices.pdf. Accessed October 11, 2007.

Jaggar AM. 2002. Vulnerable women and neo-liberal globalization: Debt burdens undermine women's health in the global South. *Theoretical Medicine and Bioethics* 23(6):425–440.

Kapur D, Lewis JP, and Webb R. 1997. *The World Bank: Its First Half Century.* Vol. 1. Washington, DC: The Brookings Institution.

Karl TL. 1997. *The Paradox of Plenty: Oil Booms and Petro States.* Berkeley, CA: University of California Press.

Kassalow J. 2001. *Why Health is Important to US Foreign Policy.* New York, NY: Council on Foreign Relations and Milbank Memorial Fund.

Katz A. 2002. AIDS, individual behaviour and the unexplained remaining variation. *African Journal of AIDS Research* 1(2):125–142.

Kawachi I and Kennedy BP. 2002. *The Health of Nations: Why Inequality is Harmful to your Health.* New York: New Press.

King L, Stuckler D, and Hamm P. 2006. Mass privatization and the postcommunist mortality crisis. Working Paper Series No. 118. Amherst, MA: Political Economy Research Institute, University of Massachussetts Amherst.

Kinney E and Clark BA. 2004. Provisions for health and health-care in the constitutions of the countries of the world. *Cornell International Law Journal* 37(2):285–355.

Lane C and Glassman A. 2007. Bigger and better? Scaling up and innovation in health aid. *Health Affairs* 26(4):935–948.

Laurell AC. 1989. Social analysis of collective health in Latin America. *Social Science and Medicine* 28(11):1183–1191.

————. 1995. *La Reforma de los Sistemas de Salud y de Seguridad Social. Concepciones y propuestas de los distintos actores sociales.* México, DF: Fundación Friedrich Ebert.

————, Editor. 1992. *Estado y políticas sociales en el neoliberalismo.* México, DF: Fundación Friedrich Ebert/UAM-Xochimilco.

Leaning J. 1998. Obituary: Jonathan Mann. *British Medical Journal* 317:754–755.

Lehohla P. 2005. Country indices like the HDI must be read with caution. http://www. statssa.gov.za/news_archive/20October2005_1.asp. Accessed November 4, 2007.

Lopez AD, Mathers CD, Ezzati M, Jamison DT, and Murray CJL. 2006. *Global Burden of Disease and Risk Factor Study.* New York: Oxford University Press and the World Bank.

Malloch Brown M. 2005. Third Forum on Human Development: Cultural identity, democracy and global justice. Statement read at the Third Forum on Human Development, Paris. January 17, 2005. http://content.undp.org/go/newsroom/2005/january/mmb-third-forum-on-human-development.en?categoryID–593045&lang=en. Accessed June 2, 2007.

Mann J. 1997. Medicine and public health, ethics and human rights. *The Hastings Center Report* 27(3):6–13.

Mann J and Tarantola D. 1995. The global AIDS pandemic: Toward a new vision of health. *Infectious Disease Clinics of North America* 9(2):275–285.

Marshall GC. 1947. Remarks of Secretary of State George C. Marshall. http://usinfo.state.gov/products/pubs/marshallplan/marshall.htm. Accessed May 18, 2007.

McKee M. 2007. A UK global health strategy: The next steps. *British Medical Journal* 335(7611):110.

McKeown T, Record R, and Turner R. 1975. An interpretation of the decline of mortality in England and Wales during the twentieth century. *Population Studies* 29(3):391–422.

Men T, Brennan P, Boffetta P, and Zaridze D. 2003. Russian mortality trends for 1991–2001: Analysis by cause and region. *British Medical Journal* 327(7421):964–966.

Merhy EE. 2000. *Saúde: a cartografia do trabalho vivo.* Rio de Janeiro: Editora Hucitec.

Minkler M. 1999. Personal responsibility for health? A review of the arguments and the evidence at century's end. *Health Education & Behavior* 26(1):121–140.

Murphy M, Bobak M, Nicholson A, Rose R, and Marmot M. 2006. The widening gap in mortality by educational level in the Russian Federation, 1980–2001. *American Journal of Public Health* 96(7):1293–1299.

Nasser A. 2003. The tendency to privatize. *Monthly Review* 54(10):22–37.

Natsios A. 2006. Five debates on international development: The US perspective. *Development Policy Review* 24(2):131–139.

Navarro V. 1981. The underdevelopment of health or the health of underdevelopment? An analysis of the distribution of human health resources in Latin America. In Navarro V, Editor. *Imperialism, Health and Medicine.* Amityville, NY: Baywood Publishing Company.

————. 1984. A critique of the ideological and political position of the Brandt report and the Alma-Ata declaration. *International Journal of Health Services* 14(2):159–72.

————. 2002. Neoliberalism, "globalization," unemployment, inequalities, and the welfare state. In Navarro V, Editor. *The Political Economy of Social Inequalities: Consequences for Health and Quality of Life.* Amityville, NY: Baywood Publishing Company.

Navarro V. 2004. Development and quality of life: A critique of Amartya Sen's *Development as Freedom*. In Navarro V and Muntaner C, Editors. *The Political and Economic Determinants of Population Health and Well-being*. Amityville, NY: Baywood Publishing Company.

———. 2007a. Neoliberalism as a cause of class ideology: Or, the political causes of the growth of inequalities. *International Journal of Health Services* 37(1):47–62.

———. 2007b. A Note for the IAHP's History. http://www.healthp.org/node/255. Accessed September 22, 2007.

Navarro V and Muntaner C, Editors. 2004. *The Political and Economic Determinants of Population Health and Well-being*. Amityville, NY: Baywood Publishing Company.

Navarro V, Muntaner C, Borrell C, Benach J, Quiroga A, Rodriguez-Sanz M, Verges N, and Isabel Pasarin MI. 2006. Politics and health outcomes. *Lancet* 368(9540):1033–1037.

OECD. 2003. *External Debt Statistics, 1998–2002*. Paris: OECD.

———. 2005. DAC members' net ODA 1990–2005 and DAC secretariat simulation of net ODA in 2006 and 2010. http://siteresources.worldbank.org/DEVCOMMINT/Documentation/20898324/DCS2006-0006-OECD-DAC.pdf. Accessed March 1, 2007

Ollila E. 2005. Global health priorities—priorities of the wealthy? *Globalization and Health* 1(6).

Packard R. 1989. *White Plague, Black Labor: Tuberculosis and the Political Economy of Health and Disease in South Africa*. Berkeley: University of California Press.

Palmer N, Mueller DH, Gilson L, Mills A, and Haines A. 2004. Health financing to promote access in low income settings—how much do we know? *Lancet* 364(9442):1365–1370.

Paxson C and Schady N. 2007. Does money matter? The effects of cash transfers on child health and development in Rural Ecuador. World Bank Policy Research Working Paper 4226. Impact Evaluation Series No. 15. Washington, DC: World Bank.

Pogge T. 2002. *World Poverty and Human Rights: Cosmopolitan Responsibilities and Reforms*. Cambridge: Polity Press.

———. 2005. Recognized and violated by international law: The human rights of the global poor. *Leiden Journal of International Law* 18:717–745.

———. 2007. Poverty and human rights. http://www2.ohchr.org/english/issues/poverty/expert/docs/Thomas_Pogge_Summary.pdf. Accessed November 10, 2007.

Powles J. 2001. Healthier progress: Historical perspectives on the social and economic determinants of health. In Eckersly R, Dixon J, and Douglas B, Editors. *The Social Origins of Health and Well-being*. Cambridge: Cambridge University Press.

Preston SH. 1980. Causes and consequences of mortality decline in less developed countries during the twentieth century. In Easterlin R, Editor. *Population and Economic Change in Developing Countries*. Chicago: University of Chicago Press.

Reddy SG. 2008. Death in China: Market reforms and health. *International Journal of Health Services* 38(1):125–141.

Reddy SG and Pogge T. 2005. How not to count the poor. http://ssrn.com/abstract=893159. Accessed May 13, 2007.

Reich M. 1994. The political economy of health transitions in the third world. In Chen LC, Kleinman A, and Ware NC, Editors. *Health and Social Change in International Perspective*. Boston, MA: Harvard University Press.

Riley JC. 2001. *Rising Life Expectancy: A Global History*. New York: Cambridge University Press.

Rostow WW. 1960. *The Stages of Economic Growth: A Non-Communist Manifesto*. Cambridge: Cambridge University Press.

Sachs J. 2001. *Macroeconomics and Health: Investing in Health for Economic Development*. Geneva: WHO.

Sagar AD and Najam A. 1998. The human development index: A critical review. *Ecological Economics* 25(3):249–264.

Schofield R, Reher D, and Bideau A, Editors. 1991. *The Decline of Mortality in Europe*. Oxford: Clarendon Press.

Schultz TP. 1993. Mortality decline in the low-income world: Causes and consequences. *American Economic Review* 83(2):337–342.

Schumacher EF. 1973. *Small is Beautiful: A Study of Economics as if People Mattered*. London: Blond & Briggs.

Sen A. 1999. *Development as Freedom*. New York: Oxford University Press.

———. 2004. Interdependence and global justice. New York: UN.

Shah A. 2007. A primer on neoliberalism. http://www.globalissues.org/TradeRelated/FreeTrade/Neoliberalism.asp. Accessed May 25, 2007.

Shakow A and Irwin A. 2000. Terms reconsidered: Decoding development discourse. In Kim JY, Irwin A, Millen JV, and Gershman J, Editors. *Dying for Growth: Global Inequality and the Health of the Poor*. Monroe, ME: Common Courage Press.

Shaw JE, Zimmet PZ, McCarty D, and de Courten M. 2000. Type 2 diabetes worldwide according to the new classification and criteria. *Diabetes Care* 23(Suppl 2):B5–B10.

Stanton E. 2007. The Human Development Index: A history. Working Paper Series No. 127. Amherst, MA: The Political Economy Research Institute, University of Massachusetts Amherst.

Steckel R and Floud R, Editors. 1997. *Health and Welfare during Industrialization*. Chicago: University of Chicago Press.

Steger MB. 2002. *Globalism: The New Market Ideology*. Lanham, MD: Rowan and Littlefield.

Stillwaggon E. 2006. *AIDS and the Ecology of Poverty*. New York: Oxford University Press.

Szreter ST. 1988. The importance of social intervention in Britain's mortality decline c. 1850–1914: A reinterpretation of the role of public health. *Social History of Medicine* 1(1):1–37.

Tapia Granados JA. 2005. Response: On economic growth, business fluctuations, and health progress. *International Journal of Epidemiology* 34(6):1226–1233.

Tarantola D and Gruskin S. 1999. Children confronting HIV/AIDS: Charting the confluence of rights and health. *Health and Human Rights* 3(1):60–86.

Tarantola D, Gruskin S, Brown TM, and Fee E. 2006. Jonathan Mann: Founder of the health and human rights movement. *American Journal of Public Health* 96(11):1942–1943.

Tedeschi S, Brown T, and Fee E. 2003. Salvador Allende: Physician, socialist, populist, and president. *American Journal of Public Health* 93(12):2014–2015.

Tesh SN. 1988. *Hidden Arguments: Political Ideology and Disease Prevention Policy*. New Brunswick, NJ: Rutgers University Press.

Theberge A. 1999. The Latin American debt crisis of the 1980s and its historical precursors. http://columbia.edu/~ad245/theberge.pdf. Accessed June 17, 2007.

Thomas KJA. 2002. Development projects and involuntary population displacement: The World Bank's attempt to correct past failures. *Population Research and Policy Review* 21(4):339–349.

Timmer CP. 1988. The agricultural transformation. In Chenery H and Srinivasan TN, Editors. *Handbook of Development Economics*. Amsterdam: North-Holland.

Truman H. 1949. *Inaugural Address.* http://www.trumanlibrary.org/publicpapers/index.php?
pid=1030&st=development&st1=. Accessed November 22, 2006.

UN. 1948. *Universal Declaration of Human Rights.* New York: United Nations Department
of Public Information.

———. 1986. *Determinants of Mortality Change and Differentials in Developing
Countries—The Five-Country Case Study Project.* New York: UN.

———. 2000. *United Nations Millennium Declaration.* New York: UN

———. 2005. *The Millennium Development Goals Report 2005.* New York: UN.

———. 2006. *World Population Prospects: The 2006 Revision.* http://esa.un.org/unpp.
Accessed June 20, 2007.

UN Committee on Economic Social and Cultural Rights. 2000. General comment No. 14.
The right to the highest attainable standard of health. http://www.unhchr.ch/tbs/doc.nsf/
(symbol)/E.C.12.2000.4.En. Accessed May 14, 2007.

UN Human Rights Council. 2008. *Promotion and protection of all human rights, civil,
political, economic, social and cultural rights: Report of the special rapporteur on
the right of everyone to the enjoyment of the highest attainable standard of physical and mental health, Paul Hunt.* January 31, 2008. http://www.unhcr.org/refworld/
docid/47ce6ddd2.html. Accessed February 9, 2008.

UN Millennium Project. 2007. *Goals, targets and indicators.* http://www.
unmillenniumproject.org/goals/gti.htm#goal1. Accessed March 23, 2007.

UNDP. 1996. *Human Development Report 1996: Economic Growth and Human
Development.* New York: Oxford University Press.

———. 2006. *Human Development Report 2006. Beyond Scarcity: Power, Poverty and
the Global Water Crisis.* New York, NY: Palgrave Macmillan for the United Nations
Development Programme.

UNICEF. 2006. 0.7% Background. http://www.unicef.ca/portal/Secure/Community/502/
WCM/HELP/take_action/G8/Point7_EN.pdf#search=%22Cana. Accessed April 17,
2007.

U.S. Institute of Medicine. 1997. *America's Vital Interest in Global Health: Protecting
our People, Enhancing our Economy, and Advancing our International Interests.*
Washington, DC: National Academy Press.

Virchow R. 1848a. The aims of the journal "Medical Reform." In Rather L, Translator and
Editor. *Collected Essays on Public Health and Epidemiology (1985).* Canton, MA:
Science History Publications.

———. 1848b. The charity physician. In Rather L, Translator and Editor. *Collected
Essays on Public Health and Epidemiology (1985).* Canton, MA: Science History
Publications.

———. 1848c. Report on the typhus epidemic in Upper Silesia. In Rather L, Translator
and Editor. *Collected Essays on Public Health and Epidemiology (1985).* Canton, MA:
Science History Publications.

Vitek C and Wharton M. 1998. Diphtheria in the former Soviet Union: Reemergence of a
pandemic disease. *Emerging Infectious Diseases* 4(4):539–550.

Waitzkin HB. 1983. *The Second Sickness: Contradictions of Capitalist Health Care.*
New York: Free Press.

———. 2001. *At the Front Lines of Medicine: How the Health Care System Alienates
Doctors and Mistreats Patients... and What We Can Do about It.* Lanham, MD:
Rowman and Littlefield Publishers, Inc.

———. 2006. One and a half centuries of forgetting and rediscovering: Virchow's lasting
contributions to social medicine. *Social Medicine* 1(1):5–10.

Wallerstein I. 1974. *The Modern World-System.* New York: Academic Press.

Wellings K, Collumbien M, Slaymaker E, Singh S, Hodges Z, Patel D, and Bajos N. 2006. Sexual behaviour in context: A global perspective. *Lancet* 368(9458):1706–1728.

Wellons PA. 1987. *Passing the Buck: Banks, Government and Third World Debt*. Boston, MA: Harvard Business School Press.

WHO. 2002. *25 Questions on Health and Human Rights*. Geneva: WHO.

———. 2006a. *Obesity and Overweight*. Fact sheet No. 311. Geneva: WHO.

———. 2006b. Water-related diseases: Diarrhoea. http://www.who.int/water_sanitation_ health/diseases/diarrhoea/en/. Accessed March 20, 2007.

———. 2007. Health and Human Rights 2007. http://www.who.int/hhr/en/. Accessed April 13, 2007.

WHO EURO. 2007. *European Health for All Database*. Copenhagen, Denmark: WHO Regional Office for Europe.

Worboys, M. 1976. The emergence of tropical medicine: A study in the establishment of a scientific specialty. In Lemaine G, MacLeod R, Mulkay M, and Weingart P. *Perspectives on the Emergence of Scientific Disciplines*. The Hague: Mouton & Co.

World Bank. 1991. *World Debt Tables 1990-91: External Debt of Developing Countries. Supplement*. Washington, DC: World Bank.

———. 1993. *World Development Report 1993: Investing in Health*. Washington, DC: World Bank.

———. 2003. *Global Development Finance: Striving for Stability in Development Finance*. Washington, DC: World Bank.

———. 2005a. *Dying Too Young: Addressing Premature Mortality and Ill Health due to Non-Communicable Diseases and Injuries in the Russian Federation*. Washington, DC: World Bank.

———. 2005b. *Global Economic Prospects 2005: Trade, Regionalism and Development*. Washington, DC: World Bank.

———. 2006. *World Development Report 2006: Equity and Development*. Washington, DC: World Bank.

———. 2007a. *Global Economic Prospects 2007: Managing the Next Wave of Globalization*. Washington, DC: World Bank.

———. 2007b. *World Development Indicators 2007*. Washington, DC: World Bank.

Yamin AE. 2005. The right to health under international law and its relevance to the United States. *American Journal of Public Health* 95(7):1156–1161.

5

What Do We Know, What Do We Need to Know, and Why it Matters—Data on Health

INTRODUCTION TO HEALTH DATA

The political economy approach to international health provides a theoretical understanding of the distribution of health and sickness in a given country or population, which necessarily rests on the existence of health data. Health-related information, and knowing how to obtain it, is essential to taking action to improve health. Although the policies that affect health—both inside and outside the health services sector—are ultimately determined in the political arena, health data play a vital role in helping to identify needs and shape solutions. Notwithstanding the importance of health information, many countries have limited data collection capacity at national and/or subnational levels, leaving policy makers to rely on extrapolations of older data or data from other countries. Such extrapolated data may be of limited relevance and may even jeopardize population health by indicating erroneous needs and priorities. Additionally, health professionals and other decision makers may overlook the crucial subject of health-related information due to time constraints and/or a lack of training in how to collect, interpret, and disseminate health data. Yet accurate information is the lifeblood of decision making, and the current proliferation of health programs means the demand for reliable data is greater than ever. This chapter will analyze the nature, strengths, and limitations of data collection and analysis at a local and global scale, and examine and critique the various types of health data that are currently used.

Challenges of Health Data

The statistical health and mortality data we come across in books, articles, and the media—such as estimates of average life expectancy and infant mortality rates—appear impressively precise and objective. Global life expectancy in 2006 was estimated at 67 years with average life expectancy at birth ranging from 40 years in Sierra Leone to 83 in Japan. These data are tabulated at national and international levels and are believed to be the unequivocal baseline for public health decision making (WHO 2007b). But not all deaths are equally recorded: most of the approximately 50 million deaths that take place worldwide each year lack medical certification. Moreover, summary statistics do not reflect variations within countries by social class, geographic location, occupation, and other important factors. For example, in Egypt the under-5 mortality rate in 2005 was 74.6/1,000 live births amongst the poorest 20% of the population, and 25.1/1,000 live births amongst the wealthiest 20%, as compared to the national average of 33/1,000 (WHOSIS 2007). In the United States in 2004 the average life expectancy was 81.3 years in Montgomery County, Maryland and just 72.5 years in bordering Washington, DC (Murray et al. 2006) as compared to the national average of 77.9 (Miniño, Heron, and Smith 2004).

Understanding the patterns of health and mortality in a population, and being able to act on this information, also requires knowledge of the social distribution of these patterns and of the constellation of factors that affect the health of populations and individuals. Despite increasing recognition of the influence of social, political, and economic factors on both illness and death, in most settings these variables are insufficiently captured by routine health statistics collection. As well, many variables that directly influence health—such as rainfall, pollution, living conditions, and transportation—do not typically qualify as health statistics, although they may be vital in uncovering and addressing the multiple underlying causes of ill health. For these reasons, a strict reliance on narrowly defined health data may not accurately portray valuable areas of policy development and evaluation.

Agencies and governments often rely on simple numerical indicators to summarize the health status of individuals and populations in order to track patterns over time, compare populations, and evaluate the effects of interventions. Nonetheless, much of the data available might be considered estimations or in some cases "guesstimations." When the basic starting point in decision making and priority setting in public health is derived from flawed or weak data, there are obvious challenges in interpreting the findings and making decisions based on those data. One of the first priorities in public health research, then, must be to secure reliable health statistics collection. But data cost money, and the higher the quality, the greater the cost. In the most underdeveloped countries, where the need for health and social services is acute and resources are perpetually inadequate, the funds allocated for collection and analysis of data fall short of requirements. In general, where disease occurrence is highest, the numbers are the least trustworthy (Hill et al. 2006).

Assumptions Related to Health Data

Along with the expectation that governments can and should collect vital statistics on the population, the use of health statistics rests on two assumptions: first, that disease and death are medicalized processes that are—or should be—certified by trained medical practitioners and publicly recorded, tabulated, and gauged over time; second, that there is an agreed-upon nosology—a disease classification process universally applied by doctors through common diagnostic procedures. Although the *International Classification of Diseases* (ICD) has been revised and agreed upon at periodic international conferences since its development in the 1890s, cultural and economic factors sometimes limit its adoption. These factors include the cost of implementing changes to the ICD in terms of administration and training as well as differing local understandings of disease categories. In many countries, traditional healers practice in parallel to health workers trained in modern allopathic medicine, but with competing ideologies. Healers may adhere to spiritual or supernatural understandings of disease that do not coincide with allopathic nosology. Even where allopathy is widely practiced, political and economic circumstances often limit the distribution and affordability of health services, in turn impeding the collection of health and mortality data.

USES AND LIMITATIONS OF HEALTH DATA

Key Questions:

- For what purposes are health data collected?
- What are the limitations of health data?

Health data are commonly used for a variety of purposes including health services planning, detecting outbreaks, and monitoring and complying with international health regulations (see Table 5–1). Health statistics, including the infant mortality rate, cases of notifiable illnesses, numbers and (if possible) causes of deaths, and certain health services, such as immunization coverage, together with a few socioeconomic, geographic, and other measures, typically make up the raw material for various health policy decisions. Some countries, such as Cuba and Sweden, interpret health policy through a more comprehensive array of data, including the influence of economic, educational, occupational, and housing conditions on health. Health-related data are not only used by government agencies, but also by NGOs, charitable organizations, and academic researchers. Many industries and schools employ health data to make projections about needed services, rates of absenteeism, and other aspects of management. These varied uses make the collection of health statistics—and their limitations—all the more important.

Table 5–1 Some Uses and Limitations of Statistical Health Data

Uses for Statistical Health Data

1. Identify emerging problems	Recognize health issues and identify the demographic groups and geographic areas in which they occur
2. Anticipate future needs	Track changes in population health in relation to changes in the economy, the environment, and demographics; collect data appropriate for public health planning efforts
3. Help determine priorities	Identify the types and distribution of health problems and their impact
4. Estimate budgets	Determine the number of people who must be reached, their characteristics and location, and the severity of problems
5. For use by government in the public sphere	Produce statistics for education campaigns and for presentation to voters, experts, officials, and legislators who control finances
6. Help direct progress toward goals	Follow trends, evaluate programs, and reconfigure programs if necessary
7. For international sharing and comparison purposes	Surveillance of public health emergencies; monitor and report health statistics to global health agencies
8. Monitor progress/setbacks by social groups	Identify health needs of particular social groups

Limitations of Statistical Health Data/What Health Data Cannot Do

9. Make decisions on polices that affect health	Once data are collected and analyzed, they enter into the political and institutional decision-making process as one of a variety of factors to be considered
10. Give causal explanations	Mortality and morbidity data alone do not provide causal pathways, nor do they explain how and why health and disease rates follow particular patterns
11. Determine which variables to include in data collection and analysis	Data collection and analysis are simultaneously technical, ideological, political, and cultural activities; thus the selection of variables is not a neutral process

Source: Points 1–6 adapted from Woolsey (1979).

Health Services Planning and Legislation

Persons responsible for health services use information about the classification, quantity, and distribution of illness to help guide planning and evaluation functions. Statistical data about health are also needed by branches of government at municipal, regional, and national levels. In most countries, health-related legislation originates from a perception of need based on available health statistics. Legal requirements for detecting, reporting, and combating diseases, laws dealing with occupational and environmental hazards, as well as regulations pertaining to hospitals and the training and licensing of professional personnel, all depend on relevant health data.

Gauging Trends and Needs

A primary reason for the collection of health data is to track trends in population health status at the level of countries, geographic regions, and subpopulations (such as particular age groups or marginalized populations). Local, regional, and national governments, nongovernmental sponsors of health and welfare programs, as well as insurance companies and other businesses, employ health data to gauge the success and limitations of particular medical or health promotion interventions, or social and economic policies writ large. Health data are also employed to monitor and compare populations within and between countries and to evaluate the effects of particular programs and policies, ideally in an effort to use successful experiences as examples to be followed. Health improvements (e.g., in infant mortality) can serve to legitimize political decisions, while a deterioration in health status (such as in life expectancy) can demonstrate the failures of particular economic or public health efforts.

Of course, as discussed in Chapter 7, the determinants of health are complex, and comparisons of health status between populations may not always lead to obvious conclusions regarding what should be done (e.g., food security and housing stability may have a much greater impact on child mortality than do hospital beds). Moreover, health data can indicate gross disparities between populations without resulting in political action to address these inequalities.

The need to assess the health implications of a range of policy decisions and programs has led to the recent development of the health impact assessment (HIA). HIA explicitly considers the health impact of both public and private sector policies in diverse arenas including zoning, transportation, labor, energy, and education. The HIA approach also calls for action and accountability on the part of decision-makers for the promotion of health and reduction of health disparities (Krieger et al. 2003).

Monitoring Diseases and Complying with International Health Regulations

To address both domestic and international concerns, every country needs to monitor real and potential threats to the health of its citizens. The health problems likely to be encountered by migrants and visitors also require international collation and dissemination of data. Smallpox was declared eradicated by the World Health Organization (WHO) in 1980 (though it has reemerged as a possible bioterrorist threat), and the problem of widespread plague has been greatly reduced. However, cholera, malaria, AIDS, avian influenza, and other diseases still pose a hazard to many countries. Accurate figures on cases of diseases near eradication, such as polio, are also crucial for monitoring progress.

Under the WHO's Constitution, member countries are obligated to provide certain information in the form of regular reports. They must also report annually on the actions taken and progress achieved in improving the health of their people. Member states must keep the WHO informed of important laws, regulations, official reports, and statistics pertaining to health, and provide statistical and epidemiological reports as determined by the World Health Assemblies. In addition, the *International Health Regulations* (IHR) require that national governments notify the WHO of cases or outbreaks of certain diseases, and of measures taken to prevent their spread.

The IHR's precursor, the *International Sanitary Regulations*, were adopted by the WHO in 1951 as a legal instrument to protect against the international spread of diseases. Originally, diseases subject to international reporting included cholera, plague, yellow fever, smallpox, relapsing fever, and louse-borne typhus. When the IHR were created in 1969, the latter two diseases were dropped, and a new group of diseases "under surveillance" was subsequently added, including malaria and poliomyelitis. In 1981, after it was declared eradicated, smallpox was removed, only to be re-added 25 years later.

Starting in the 1980s the (re)appearance of old and new ailments, including plague in India, cholera in the Americas, SARS in Asia and Canada, and Ebola hemorrhagic fever in Africa motivated the World Health Assembly to review and adapt the scope of the IHR. These emerging diseases, plus emergencies provoked by noninfectious diseases, made apparent the need for improvements in international surveillance of, and coordinated responses to, public health emergencies. In 2005, WHO member states agreed on a revision of the IHR to ensure a broader scope and consistent application. The critical change of the new IHR, which came into effect in 2007, is the requirement that member states notify the WHO of all events that constitute a public health emergency, well beyond the diseases included in the IHR's 1969 surveillance scope.

According to the common understanding developed under the new IHR—the world's first legally binding agreement on disease notification—a public health emergency is considered to be of international concern if it (a) constitutes a public health risk to other states through the international spread of disease; and (b) potentially requires a coordinated international response. The IHR stipulate that the WHO be notified within 24 hours of the first official case of a listed disease. National IHR focal points and individuals at country and regional levels are to provide timely, accurate information flow between member states and the WHO on a 24 hours a day/7 days a week basis. The IHR's legal framework also requires WHO member states (except those that have rejected them or submitted reservations) to respond to public health emergencies and ensure a mechanism for seeking technical assistance from the WHO. For its part, the WHO assesses country reports and information, recommends concrete action, and provides assistance as needed. Once the WHO has determined that a particular event constitutes a public health emergency of international concern, the IHR require the WHO to make "a 'real-time' response to the emergency" through immediate action (WHO 2007a).

Early Detection of Health Problems and Outbreaks

Routine and continuous monitoring of health data is essential, as health statistics derived therein can serve an early warning function—prompt detection of outbreaks can lead to knowledge of their cause, and important steps can be taken to minimize hazards. New conditions can be discovered before larger population groups are exposed. For example, in the 1960s, a syndrome of eye, ear, and heart damage was described in children whose mothers contracted rubella during pregnancy. In the late 1950s and early 1960s, reports of limb malformations in newborns led to the discovery that these were related to maternal use of thalidomide. Both cases resulted in worldwide awareness and control efforts. Similarly, the first cases of what became known as AIDS were detected in the early 1980s through physician reports and CDC epidemiological investigations of an unusual number of cases of Kaposi's sarcoma and *Pneumocystis* pneumonia in a population of young homosexual men in Los Angeles, New York, and San Francisco. Many other similar instances could be cited, including the ongoing surveillance efforts for avian influenza.

Limitations of Health Data

Many politicians, analysts, and advocates are interested in international compilations of statistics to use as a yardstick in comparing their country with others in areas such as life expectancy, the ratio of population to physicians, child mortality, and accessibility of health services. Such data, which may also include information related to socioeconomic development, are highly sensitive and laden with political overtones. One should always be cautious in interpreting health-related data, as it is difficult to define the metrics, hard to get the numbers right, and there may be pressure on local and regional officials and ministries of health to distort figures. Administrators may be tempted, for example, to overestimate the number of inoculations given or to minimize reported rates of sickness or death. Concern with international trade or tourism may prompt cases of cholera to be reported as gastroenteritis, and forthcoming elections may entice a politician into uncharacteristic exaggeration. Such distortions, arising from varied incentives and influences, need not be overemphasized but should be kept in mind when reading and interpreting all health-related data.

At the same time, health data may enter into overtly charged political environments. Epidemiological findings associating cigarette smoking with lung cancer, firearms with accidental shootings, and alcohol with road accidents, for example, have been cited as arguments in favor of restrictive legislation. Proponents and opponents of tobacco, guns, or alcohol have sought, identified, and interpreted data to support their positions. The same is true of partisans on either side of issues such as the construction of nuclear power plants or fetal stem cell research. Health statistics are sometimes provided to officials and to the public by the advocates of a particular cause, who may release biased or selective information in an attempt to attract money and public attention to their cause. At the same time, diseases or conditions with committed advocates may receive disproportionate funding while others languish for lack of organized proponents. Indeed, the global resurgence of tuberculosis in the late 1980s occurred when it was no longer a political priority. This does not mean that health data should be disregarded. Still, it is important to be vigilant about how data are collected, interpreted, and communicated and to be mindful of the underlying assumptions of particular data collection efforts.

TYPES OF HEALTH DATA

Key Questions:

- What are the major kinds of health-related data?
- What are the challenges involved in collecting health data?

The basic categories of health-related data are:

- *Population data*: The number of people in a population and their attributes, such as age, sex, ethnicity, religion, urbanization, geographic distribution, and similar fundamental characteristics.
- *Vital statistics*: Live births; deaths (including fetal deaths) by sex, age, and cause; and marriages. In some countries, migration (internal and external), adoptions, and similar categories are also recorded by vital statistics agencies.
- *Health statistics*: Morbidity by type, severity, and outcome (of illness or accident); data on notifiable diseases, blindness, impairment, incapacity; cancer registries; and so forth. This category is not as clearly defined as the previous two and varies from one jurisdiction to another.
- *Health services statistics*: Numbers and types of facilities and services available; distribution, qualifications, and functions of personnel; nature of the services and their utilization rates; hospital and health center operations; organization of government and private health care systems; costs, payment mechanisms, and related information.
- *Data on social inequalities in health*: Social factors that lead to inequalities in health—rates of absolute and relative poverty, levels of education, and occupational conditions, among others; population groups categorized by social class, race and ethnicity, religion, and sex/gender in order to identify how equally or unequally health (and health care services) are distributed in a population.

Table 5–2 Some Questions About Health Data

---

1. By whom and at what level(s) in the health system will these health data be used? (e.g., village health worker, regional planning officer, provincial or central Ministry of Health, prime minister, medical college, research institute, international organization)

2. For what specific purpose will the data be used? (e.g., prioritization, planning, advocacy, surveillance, monitoring, evaluation, research, multiple uses)

3. If used for monitoring or evaluation, do the health programs have stated objectives, targets, or outcomes relevant to these indicators?

4. Have these or similar indicators been found useful in other programs, districts, or countries in similar circumstances?

5. Are these standard international indicators used or suggested by international or regional organizations to facilitate comparisons?

6. Is the indicator statistically valid? (i.e., does it measure what it is intended to measure?)

7. Is the indicator reliable and consistent? Is it sufficiently sensitive and specific?

8. Is the indicator a direct or a proxy measure? (i.e., does it measure health status directly, or does it measure a determinant of health?)

9. What other information is needed to generate or interpret the indicator?

10. Are conditions in place to process and utilize the indicator? (e.g., staff training and expertise, computer hardware and software, coding systems)

11. Are funds available to collect and manage the data?

Source: Adapted from Graham (1986).

Societal variables—including those that measure social welfare and social security, distribution of power and resources—are increasingly considered vital to health-related decision making, although they are not collected to the same extent as other, more discrete indicators. These will be discussed at length in Chapter 7.

The compilation, analysis, interpretation, and issuance of these health data on a continuing basis entails a great deal of effort and expense for governments (see Table 5–2). This is made even more complex by the need for comparability among countries and over time. A high degree of international cooperation is required to assure that definitions, terminology, diagnostic techniques, certification practices, data-handling methods, and reporting schemes are sufficiently standardized for comparative purposes but flexible enough to take into account diverse national circumstances throughout the world.

Population Data

The demographic characteristics of a population underlie most health data because they provide the base numbers for calculating relevant rates and ratios (see Table 5–3). Population data are usually obtained in two ways: enumeration and registration. Enumeration is done by means of a census of the population, ideally every 10 years. Registration involves collecting vital statistics such as births,

Table 5–3 Commonly Used Health Indicators

Annual crude live birth rate (= birth rate)

$$\frac{\text{Number of births occurring in a defined population during a year}}{\text{Number in that population at midyear of the same year}} \times 1,000$$

Annual crude death rate (= mortality rate, death rate)

$$\frac{\text{Number of deaths occurring in a defined population during a year}}{\text{Number in that population at midyear of the same year}} \times 1,000$$

Annual specific death rate (by age, sex, cause or a combination)

$$\frac{\text{Number of deaths of a specified age, sex, or cause occurring in a defined population during a year}}{\text{Number of the specified age group in that population at midyear of the same year}} \times 1,000$$

Annual infant mortality rate (= infant mortality rate or IMR)

$$\frac{\text{Number of deaths under 1 year of age in a defined population during a year}}{\text{Number of live births occurring in that population during the same year}} \times 1,000$$

Annual neonatal mortality rate

$$\frac{\text{Number of deaths under 28 days of age in a defined population during a year}}{\text{Number of live births occurring in that population during the same year}} \times 1,000$$

Annual post-neonatal mortality rate

$$\frac{\text{Number of deaths between 28 days and 1 year of age in a defined population during a year}}{\text{Number of live births occurring in that population during the same year}} \times 1,000$$

Annual fetal death rate (stillbirth rate)

$$\frac{\text{Number of deaths at 20}^{a}\text{ or more weeks gestational age in a defined population during a year}}{\text{Number of live births occurring in that population during the same year}} \times 1,000$$

Annual maternal mortality rate

$$\frac{\text{Number of deaths from maternal causes}^{b}\text{ in a defined population during a year}}{\text{Number of women of childbearing age in that population during the same year}} \times 100,000$$

Annual maternal mortality ratio

$$\frac{\text{Number of deaths from maternal causes in a defined population during a year}}{\text{Number of live births in that population during the same year}} \times 100,000$$

Proportionate mortality

$$\frac{\text{Number of deaths in a specific category in a defined population during a year}}{\text{Total number of deaths occurring in that population during the same year}} \times 100$$

Annual incidence rate for occurrence of a specified condition

$$\frac{\text{Number of new cases of the condition occuring in a defined population in a year}}{\text{Number of people in that population at midyear in the same year}} \times 10^{n, c}$$

(Point) prevalence of a specified condition

$$\frac{\text{Number of cases of the specified condition existing in a defined population at a particular point in time}}{\text{Number of people in that population at the same point in time}} \times 10^{n}$$

Morbidity rate (crude or specific by age, sex, occupation, etc.)

$$\frac{\text{Number of cases of a specified condition occuring in a specified population during a specific time period}}{\text{Average population in that category during the year}} \times 10^{n}$$

[a] Varies somewhat in different jurisdictions.
[b] As listed in the latest ICD revision or defined nationally.
[c] Multiplier^{n} varies depending on frequency of the condition.

Source: Adapted from Basch (1999), Table 4.3.

marriages, and deaths. Neither enumeration nor registration is done primarily for the purpose of compiling health and vital statistics. Census data have been used for millennia for purposes of taxation and conscription. As early as CE 2 in China, a census was ordered and data were recorded on more than 12 million households, including the heads of families and the name, age, and birthplace of more than 59.5 million people (Hookham 1972). Although internationally sponsored health surveys and programs collect key health data, there is no substitute for permanent, ongoing vital statistics and census data collection—government institutionalization of these systems is the only way to guarantee routine and comprehensive collection.

Census Procedures and Cost

During a census, information is collected on a variety of topics (see Table 5–4). The information obtained from census data permit a population to be characterized by

Table 5–4 Some Topics Recommended by the UN World Population and Housing Census Programme and Various National Census Agencies for Inclusion in a National Population Census

Priority Items	Other Useful Items
Place of usual residence	Religion
Place at time of the census	Language
Place/country of birth	National/ethnic origin
Duration of current residence	Indigenous identity
Place of previous residence	Live births in preceding 12 months
Place of residence at [year]	Infants born and died within last 12 months
Total population	Maternal orphanhood (loss of mother)
Locality	Age of mother at birth of first child
Relationship to household head or other reference member	Household deaths in the past 12 months
Sex	Sector of employment
Age	Years worked
Marital status	Income
Citizenship	Housing conditions
Number of children born alive	Food security status
Number of children living	Access to health care services
Duration of marriage	Disability status
Educational attainment	Educational qualifications
Literacy	Year of arrival (for migrants)
School attendance	
Economic activity status	
Occupation	
Industry	
Status in employment/occupation	

Source: Adapted from UN Department of Economic and Social Affairs (2007).

a variety of classifiers, of which age and sex are most often used, as well as education, literacy status, occupation, and ethnic group, among other features. In an effort to better measure social inequalities in health and their consequences for health status, the WHO's Commission on Social Determinants of Health recommends that additional information be included in routine data collection (see Box 5–1).

Box 5–1 Additional Information to be Included in Routine Data Collection to Enable Measurement of Social Inequalities in Health and Societal Determinants of Health

Social Inequalities in Health

Include information on:
Health outcomes (all cause, age-specific and cause-specific mortality; mental health; early childhood development; morbidity and disability; self-assessed health) stratified by:
  • at least two socioeconomic stratifiers (education, income/wealth, occupational class);
  • sex;
  • ethnic group/race/indigeneity;
  • other contextually relevant social stratifiers;
  • place of residence (rural/urban and province or other relevant geographical unit);
The distribution of the population across these sub-groups.

Consequences of Ill Health

Economic consequences;
Social and psychological consequences.

Determinants of Health

Daily living conditions and social policies
Physical and social environment:
  • water and sanitation;
  • housing conditions;
  • infrastructure, transport, and urban design;
  • air and soil quality;
  • quality and accessibility of nutritious food;
  • social support and networks;
  • neighborhood characteristics, such as community institutions, parks, safety
Working conditions:
  • material working hazards;
  • stress and job control
Personal health characteristics:
  • smoking and alcohol consumption;
  • physical activity;
  • diet and nutrition
Health care:
  • coverage;
  • health care system infrastructure
Social protection:
  • coverage;
  • generosity

(continued)

Box 5–1 Continued

Structural forces underlying social inequalities in health
Gender:
  · norms and values;
  · economic participation;
  · sexual and reproductive health
Race, religion, immigrant status:
  · level of tolerance/discrimination;
  · norms and values
Social inequalities:
  · social exclusion;
  · income and wealth distribution;
  · land tenancy and property;
  · education
Sociopolitical context:
  · participation in community, regional, national, global decision making;
  · distribution of political power;
  · civil rights;
  · level of violence;
  · employment conditions;
  · governance and public spending priorities;
  · macroeconomic conditions.

Source: Adapted (with permission) from Box 16.3 of WHO Commission on Social Determinants of Health (2008, p. 182).

The essential features of a national population census are as follows:

- *Sponsorship*: A legal basis must be established, with administrative machinery to ensure compliance and confidentiality.
- *Defined territory*: The boundaries of national and subnational territorial divisions must be clear.
- *Universality*: Every person physically present and/or residing in the territory should be included.
- *Individual enumeration*: Information should be collected from individuals and households.
- *Simultaneity and specified time*: The collected date should refer insofar as possible to a single point in time.
- *Periodicity*: Censuses should be conducted at regular intervals.
- *Compilation and publication*: Raw data must be put into a useful form and published as soon as possible for maximum utility.

The figures derived from the census serve as denominators for the age- and sex-specific mortality and morbidity rates defined in Table 5–3. Census data of adequate quality make possible more meaningful comparisons of the measures than can be obtained from crude (whole population) figures. As an illustration, the age and sex distributions of the population of five different countries are compared in Figure 5–1. These are known as age pyramids. The shape of each pyramid is affected by birth rates at particular periods in time and death rates for each age group (by sex). The age pyramids portray the childhood and old-age dependency ratios within each population: persons under 14 years of age and over 65 are generally considered to be dependent on the population segment aged 15 to 65. High mortality rates can drastically alter the age pyramid, as seen in the projected effect of HIV/AIDS in South Africa (Fig. 5–2).

The effort and expense involved in completing a census is considerable. The 2000 U.S. census is estimated to have cost US$4.5 billion, or $16 per person. The decennial expenditure just for counting each person in the United States exceeds the total per capita annual health budget of many of the world's least developed countries (UNFPA 2003).

Global Census-Taking

Since 1950, the proportion of the estimate of the world's population that derives from total census enumeration has risen substantially. Almost all developing countries have had some experience in census-taking over the past several decades (UNFPA 2003). In 1995, the UN Statistical Commission, ECOSOC, recommended that all UN member states carry out a population census during the 1995–2004 period, known as the 2000 Round of Census.

A census is a highly complex undertaking in any setting. In India, with the second largest population in the world, each decennial census requires the recruitment and training of 2 million enumerators to survey 150 million households within 25 days in an extensive and highly organized operation. During this exercise, information on the inhabitants of each dwelling is collected and the quality of housing assessed, allowing for measurement of changing living conditions (Jha 2005). Nigeria's 12th census, completed in 2006, needed 6 years of preparation and seven days to carry out. As the most populous country in Africa, with an estimated population ranging between 120 and 150 million people and over 300 different ethnic groups, Nigeria faced an enormous organizational challenge. To ensure the most credible data collection, government authorities imposed a weeklong national stay-at-home order, and for the first time, digital processing of forms and satellite positioning were used to identify census areas. More than 1 million census workers were trained and went door to door across the country.

The high and growing cost of census counts has been compounded by shrinking public sector budgets. Cutbacks in funding for international development assistance, which in the past has been an important source of funding for censuses, has further exacerbated the situation. In the 2000 census round, numerous countries did not do a census at all due to insufficient resources or civil unrest, and many

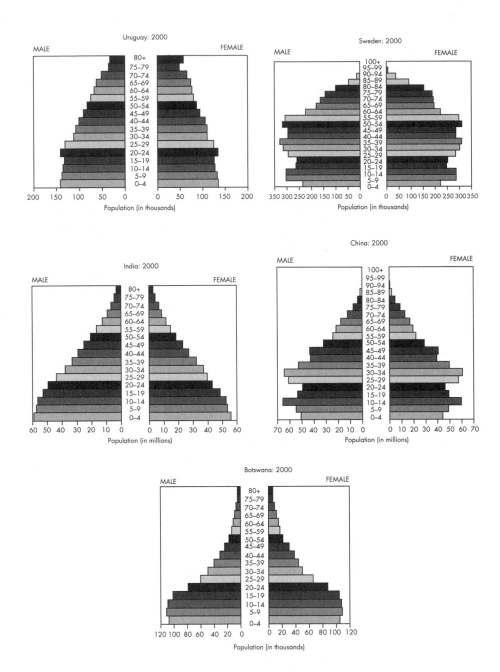

Figure 5–1 Age pyramids for populations of five countries.
Source: U.S. Census Bureau (2006).

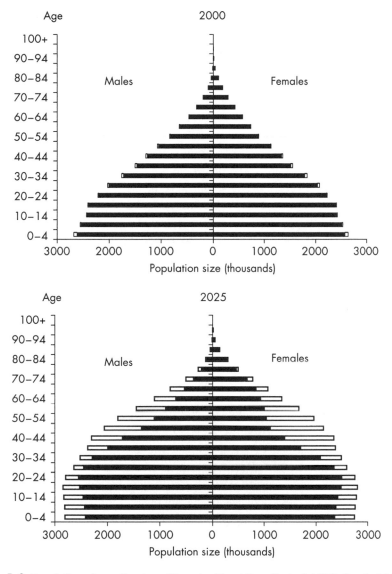

Figure 5–2 Population size estimates with and without the effect of AIDS, South Africa, 2000 and 2025. Outer blocks estimate population size without the effect of AIDS. *Source*: Personal communication based on data from United Nations Population Division, *World Population Prospects: The 2006 Revision*. CD-ROM (United Nations Publication, Sales No. E.0.7.XIII.7). Courtesy of the United Nations Population Division.

others did not achieve the expected or desirable standards of census-taking (UNFPA 2003). Various countries, especially in sub-Saharan Africa, postponed their census, increasing the time interval since the previous one to more than 10 years.

Limitations of Census Data

It may seem that after a national census is budgeted for and planned, enumerators trained, and data processing materials prepared, the rest is a simple matter. In actuality, appraising the completeness and accuracy of census data calls for careful checks and sophisticated techniques. Errors and inaccuracies can tarnish the raw data, particularly when questions are asked of people with low literacy and low education levels who may be unaware of the significance of the census and suspicious of its intent. Coverage of large populations is never perfect, even under the best of circumstances. Each U.S. census, for example, receives thousands of official complaints from communities alleging undercounts which would result in lowered government subsidies, payments for education, and other services based on population size.

The process and standards of a census count vary from country to country depending on a variety of factors and conditions. A country's prior experience with census-taking, available financial and human resources, and existing infrastructure greatly affect census counts. The diversity within a country—including languages spoken, levels of literacy, and existence of nomadic populations—is another factor that makes a population census count a formidable task. Additionally, in countries with civil conflict or in postwar reconstruction, there are unique challenges in census-taking. Countries that lack financial resources may not be able to afford basic computer equipment or software, and limited human resource capacity may compound the difficulties (UNFPA 2003). Regardless of available financial and human resources, complete enumeration of a whole population is nearly impossible. Even in countries with adequate resources to undertake a census, millions of refugees, migrants, and homeless persons are likely to be missed by census counts. The extent to which these deficiencies are addressed through special surveys and adjustments is variable and highly politicized.

Certain categories—such as age and sex—are used similarly by most censuses around the world. Others—such as ethnicity and marital status—vary by local laws and customs, and as such do not lend themselves to universally applicable statistical definitions. Yet even universal categories may lead to ambiguity.

The question of age may be taken as an example of the uncertainty inherent in census-taking. When asked about the number of people in their household, respondents may overlook their children, particularly babies. Many people do not know their age and some may deliberately misstate it. Asking a person for their year of birth rather than their age is considered more accurate, because the former figure remains constant (and is more likely to be recalled correctly) as opposed to the latter, which changes every year. Local customs in reckoning age also vary; in some cultures a child may not be counted until reaching 1 year of age.

Defining the scope of information to be collected on racial and ethnic categories can be problematic. While typologies of humans relating to climatic and geographic features have ancient roots, the contemporary system of classifying people according to such groupings originated with political authorities in the 19th century. They held (erroneously) that humans were composed of distinct, biologically determined races that needed to be distinguished for administrative and political purposes, such as allocation and delivery of social services, natality policies, and workforce projections. These ideological classifications were used to determine domestic economic and industrial policies and to justify imperial expansion and domination (Krieger 2005). As such, the use of racial and ethnic classification on census counts may be both divisive and purposive, in that the way people are classified predetermines the types of conclusions that can be drawn and the way they are addressed.

The most notable recent example of the deliberately racist ends of such categorizations comes from the Apartheid government in South Africa (1948–1994). The Apartheid bureaucracy collected census and vital information according to the following categories: Black (of African descent), White (European), Asian (Indian and Pakistani), and Coloured ("mixed race"). Every public agency in the country used these data to enforce differential treatment under the law, unequal distribution of education and welfare funds, and so on, further reifying these constructed racial categories. Even though the Apartheid system was dismantled in the early 1990s, the South African Department of Health decided to retain these same racial categories in health statistics and census counts, in part to gauge the effect of post Apartheid policies on closing the equity gap between the races.

In the United States, census data are also collected by race and ethnicity, reflecting the country's legacy of slavery, segregation, and discrimination. With the 2000 census, the U.S. government adopted a larger array of racial and ethnic classifications and allowed respondents to self-identify in more than one category, recognizing the growing diversity of the population. While the continued use of racial categories helps to measure the relative standing of these different groups over time, this heavy emphasis on one sociodemographic variable detracts attention from other extremely important population characteristics, such as social class, which may have an even greater bearing on health and well-being.

Indeed, how people are classified, and the classification system as a whole, shape to a great extent the types of policies undertaken to tackle health and other social problems. The disproportionate focus on race and ethnicity in the United States (and its frequent conflation with biological and cultural characteristics) has greatly diverted attention from societal factors that could be modified (e.g., wealth distribution; social protection), implying that health disparities are based on individual characteristics. By contrast, countries that collect health statistics by social class (e.g., the United Kingdom) allow for broader societal approaches to health. As such, the way different countries frame the collection of population data heavily influences the interpretation of the results and the subsequent actions taken.

Vital Statistics

Vital statistics are the data that are normally collected through registration of major life events such as birth, marriage, and death. Registration of vital events is usually done at a legally designated place near the occurrence of the event. Depending on local laws and practice, this may be a police post, courthouse, municipal or district office, special civil registry office, school, or other locale. Compilation of records by administrative divisions (municipalities/provinces/states) and by regions or geographic areas, provides a comprehensive picture of vital events that is essential for the planning and allocation of government services. Together with census data, vital records are essential for estimating future resources and needs for services including public health and medical care. Vital records have many personal and administrative uses, as shown in Table 5–5. Because of these crucial human welfare entitlements, UNICEF's Innocenti Research Centre has declared that "a fully functional civil registration system should be compulsory, universal, permanent and continuous, and should ensure the confidentiality of personal data" (Hawke 2002, p. 2).

Registration systems vary considerably from one country to another. Where an effective registration system exists, the availability of good quality data is often taken for granted, but it is an unfortunate fact that civil registration is still lacking or deficient in numerous settings. Health and demographic surveys have been used in many countries to bridge the gap between the need for accurate data on health and deficient vital statistics coverage. In fact, most available health data do not come from vital statistics systems but from surveys.

Since 1984, the U.S. Agency for International Development (USAID) has supported the demographic and health survey (DHS) program in 75 developing countries. The program funds and provides technical assistance to collect, and make available, data on fertility, family planning, and maternal and child health, as well as infant mortality, HIV/AIDS, and nutrition. The data collected through the DHS are considered accurate and nationally representative and are used not only to underpin national health policy and public health programming but also to compare data

Table 5–5 Some Personal and Administrative Uses of Vital Records

Personal	Administrative
Birth Certificate	
1. Establish date of birth and identity: enter school or government service; obtain work permit, marriage license, driver's license, passport; qualify for voting, retirement, pension	1. Provide basis for child health and immunization, education planning, etc.
2. Establish place of birth: qualify for passport, voting, civil office, social services; determine citizenship at birth, residency	2. Evaluate family planning programs, prenatal clinics, etc.

(continued)

Table 5–5 Continued

Personal	Administrative
3. Establish family relationship: trace descent, prove parentage, birth order; prove legal dependency; qualify for insurance and inheritance benefits	3. Contribute to inter-censal estimate of population size
4. Protect against child labor and military inscription, child trafficking, and violence	4. Aid in family reunification efforts and in delivery of humanitarian assistance during times of war, conflict or disaster

Marriage and Civil Union Certificates[a]

Personal	Administrative
1. Qualify for housing allocation, inheritance, pension, insurance, tax deduction	1. Prove establishment of household for benefit programs
2. Prove legal responsibility of spouse, legitimacy of offspring, and citizenship by marriage	2. Predict population trends
3. Child custody	3. Use as a basis for construction and allocation of housing
4. Medical decision making for spouse/partner	

Divorce Certificate

Personal	Administrative
1. Establish right to alimony or other benefits	1. Determine right to remarry
2. Prove right to remarry	

Death Certificate

Personal	Administrative
1. Establish fact of death: claim pension, insurance, inheritance	1. Provide basis for cause-of-death analysis and specific prevention or control programs, particularly for infant and maternal mortality
2. Establish cause of death: determine indemnity payment	2. Clear files (e.g., electoral rolls, tax or social security registers, disease-case registers)
	3. Contribute to inter-censal estimate of population size

Identity Cards

Personal	Administrative
1. Many countries and jurisdictions require identity cards to be carried at all times, for access to virtually any public service	1. Historically, identity cards have also been used for oppressive purposes (e.g., in South Africa and Nazi-occupied countries), a potential problem which must be considered into the present
2. In some settings, identity cards for minority, indigenous, and Afro-descendant populations certifying lineage are critical for eligibility to land claims, reparations, and other indigenous treaty rights based on indigenous identity	

[a]In countries and jurisdictions where marriage between same sex couples is not legally recognized, marriage certificates and the accompanying eligibility for services are limited to heterosexual marriages. To date, Belgium, Canada, the Netherlands, Norway, South Africa, and Spain legally recognize same sex marriages. Many other jurisdictions recognize same sex civil unions or domestic partnerships, but entitlements are often more limited.

Sources: Based in part on Swaroop (1960); UN Department of Economic and Social Affairs (1973).

across countries. However, the DHS and other survey data are far less effective at estimating youth and adult mortality, and in some countries they impede the development of full-fledged vital statistics systems.

History of Birth, Marriage, and Death Records

The system of registry of births, marriages, and deaths began unevenly in the towns and city-states of early modern Europe, building on the earlier *catastos* (fiscal registries) which were used as a basis for taxation and for compiling urban bills (records) of mortality. Early demographic records were collected and maintained by local parishes, which combined religious and civic-administrative functions. As such, baptisms, burials, and marriages were recorded rather than births and deaths. The first national registry system was founded in England and Wales in 1538, initially as a means of ensuring property rights; other European countries, such as Sweden, soon followed suit. Circa 1600, England established its Poor Law system, which provided locally funded short-term "relief of the poor" in the case of unemployment or destitution. The Poor Laws relied in part on the parish record system, thus ensuring high levels of compliance even among uneducated and marginal populations. This system remained in place for centuries.

In the 19th century, state-run birth and death registries began to be established across Europe, the Americas, and in many colonial settings, often along with census enumerations, for explicit economic and political planning purposes. In an era of rapid industrial growth and inter-imperial rivalries, population size, migration and death patterns, and marriage and birth rates all had considerable bearing on economic output and expansion, military strength, and settlement policies. To the present day, vital statistics records are not only important to demographers, epidemiologists, and health planners but remain central to social and economic policy making writ large. These data contribute to decisions around public transport and economic development, how many schools are needed, and which regions should receive priority, among countless others. The lack of civic registration systems is one of the most important development problems facing the world's poorest countries.

Birth Registration

The right to be registered at birth is recognized under the *International Covenant on Civil and Political Rights*, the 1989 *Convention on the Rights of the Child*, and other human rights charters. UNICEF refers to birth registration as "the first right, the right to an official identity" (Dow 1998), one that is key to fulfillment of other fundamental rights. Birth registration is an essential aspect of vital statistics, particularly because much needed health data rely on accurate birth numbers. Infant mortality rates are considered a strong measure of health status and are used for comparison within and between countries. Without accurate birth records, these figures are extremely difficult to calculate.

Almost 40% of all births in the world are not registered (WHO 2007c), leaving vast numbers of people without the entitlements listed in Table 5–5 during childhood and throughout the life course. A 2004 survey by UNICEF found that within sub-Saharan Africa and South Asia, only one-third to one-half of births were registered. Within the countries categorized as "least developed" 71% of births are not registered (UNICEF 2005). Most such countries are marked by armed conflict and/or conditions of extreme poverty and indebtedness. In total, 48 million of the approximately 136 million births each year go unrecorded (Hawke 2002). As noted by Carol Bellamy, the former director of UNICEF, these children "are in essence nonexistent in the eyes of states.... Not having a birth certificate is the functional equivalent of not having been born" (Crossette 1998).

Mortality

In the middle of the 17th century, during the final years of the Black Death, a London cloth merchant, John Graunt, began a study of the bills of mortality. Using parish registers of births and deaths, he showed that human life conforms to certain predictable statistical patterns. The need for international comparability of cause-of-death data was a prime subject of discussion at the International Statistical Congresses in the 1850s. At the 1855 congress, William Farr of England and Marc d'Espine of Switzerland proposed tabulations that were later merged into a single list of 139 causes applicable to all countries. That list, officially adopted by the congress, formed the basis for subsequent classifications and underwent several revisions during the 19th century.

At the 1893 meeting of the International Statistical Institute, Frenchman Jacques Bertillon proposed a classification system now known as the International Statistical Classification of Diseases and Related Health Problems (ICD). In 1900, the First International Conference for the Revision of the ICD was convened in Paris, and since then, revisions to it have appeared at approximately 10-year intervals. The ICD was greatly modified at the sixth revision in 1948, with the addition of coding rubrics for morbidity as well as for causes of death.

The transition from one ICD revision to another always involves changes in the coding of certain categories. At each revision, some diagnoses are reassigned, resulting in sudden increases or decreases in the reported occurrences of affected categories and breaks in the comparability of statistics. Nevertheless, changes in the ICD are needed from time to time. Identification of new ailments and advances in medical knowledge and diagnostic and therapeutic technology contribute to better ways of defining and distinguishing among the many known diseases and possible causes of death. The latest version, ICD-10, was adopted by WHO member states in 1994, and has more than 2,036 categories, 12,159 subcategories, and 12,420 codes (see Table 5–6). The extensive changes in the ICD-10 required regional and national training programs throughout the world, and gave governments an

Table 5–6 Major Subdivisions of the International Classification of Diseases,
Tenth Revision

Chapter	Subjects	Range of Codes
I	Certain infectious and parasitic diseases	A00–B99
II	Neoplasms	C00–D48
III	Disease of the blood and blood-forming organs and certain disorders involving the immune mechanism	D50–D98
IV	Endocrine, nutritional, and metabolic diseases	E00–E99
V	Mental and behavioral disorders	F00–F99
VI	Diseases of the nervous system	G00–G99
VII	Diseases of the eye and adnexa	H00–H59
VIII	Diseases of the ear and mastoid process	H60–H95
IX	Diseases of the circulatory system	I00–I99
X	Diseases of the respiratory system	J00–J99
XI	Diseases of the digestive system	K00–K93
XII	Diseases of the skin and subcutaneous tissue	L00–L99
XIII	Diseases of the musculoskeletal system and connective tissue	M00–M99
XIV	Diseases of the genitourinary system	N00–N99
XV	Pregnancy, childbirth, and the puerperium	O00–O99
XVI	Certain conditions originating in the perinatal period	P00–P96
XVII	Congenital malformations and chromosomal abnormalities	Q00–Q99
XVIII	Symptoms, signs, and abnormal clinical and laboratory findings not elsewhere classified	R00–R99
XIX	Injury, poisoning, and certain other consequences of external causes	S00–T98
XX	External causes of morbidity and mortality	V01–Y98
XXI	Factors influencing health status and contact with health services	Z00–Z99
XXII	Codes for special purposes	U00–U99

Source: WHO (1992) and updated version for 2007. Note: The ICD-10 has been updated every year since 1996.

opportunity to review and improve the entire flow of health statistics, reformulate data processing systems, and even redesign death certificates.

When a death occurs, a certifier should complete a death certificate (see Fig. 5–3). Medical certification of cause of death is typically the responsibility of the attending physician, when there is one. In cases of sudden, violent, or suspicious death, a coroner or other medico-legal officer could be the certifier. In many countries the certifier may be a midwife, nurse, policeman, village chief, teacher, or lay person, although uniform training seeks to ensure that causes of death are properly classified and can be appropriately analyzed. Many countries include social and economic information on death certificates; however, according to the ICD, only immediate physical and biological factors are considered causes of death. We will discuss the implications of this narrow focus in Chapter 7.

Cause of death		Approximate interval between onset and death
I Disease or condition directly leading to death*	(a)...	....
	due to (or as a consequence of)	
Antecedent causes Morbid conditions, if any, giving rise to the above cause, stating the underlying condition last	(b)...	....
	due to (or as a consequence of)	
	(c)...	....
	due to (or as a consequence of)	
	(d)...	....
II Other significant conditions contributing to the death, but not related to the disease or condition causing it	....	....
*This does not mean the mode of dying, e.g. heart failure, respiratory failure. It means the disease, injury, or complication that caused death.		

Figure 5–3 International form of medical certificate of cause of death.
Source: WHO (1993).

The flow of information following completion of the death certificate varies among countries, but in general a centralized national statistical office eventually receives the individual records and collates the data for administrative purposes, sending summaries to the WHO for compilation. At one point in the system the ICD coding is applied to the data by a coder or nosologist specifically trained for this purpose. In some countries, multiple and/or contributory causes of death are tabulated but usually only the underlying cause of death is coded. It is under this rubric that the data finally appear in the *World Health Statistics* annual and other publications. The U.S. National Center for Health Statistics has developed a computerized program for automated selection of the underlying cause of death.

Mortality statistics are in the first rank of measurements for international health due to their general unambiguity. The advantage of mortality statistics over other statistics relating to health is that they exist on a much more widespread scale. They help to define health problems, monitor the efficacy of health programs, and identify emerging public health concerns. Two categories of mortality rates are of particular significance for international health: the infant mortality rate (IMR) and maternal mortality.

INFANT MORTALITY RATE   The IMR—defined as deaths that occur in the interval between birth and 1 year—differs from all other annual age-specific death rates in several important respects. First, both numerator and denominator are derived directly from registration data, whereas the denominator for other age-specific mortality rates generally comes from census-based estimates. More importantly, the denominator of the IMR is not the number of persons in that age group at midyear but the number of live births occurring in a defined population during the year (see Table 5–3). Unlike other age-specific mortality rates, infant deaths are not uniformly distributed throughout the year, but are highest in the first week and month of life. Another feature of the IMR that distinguishes it from other age-specific death rates is that there appears to be an irreducible lower limit. This minimum mortality rate, consisting primarily of infants congenitally malformed or with other severe birth defects who die shortly after birth, is determined in part by relatively unpreventable genetic, chromosomal, developmental, or physiological complications during development, and in part by controllable environmental factors such as maternal infection and nutrition, behavior, living conditions, and prenatal care.

Although the global IMR has steadily declined over the past several decades, since 1990 child mortality rose in 12 countries (11 of which are in Africa). Recent estimates show that annually between 10 and 11 million infants and children die, mostly from preventable causes, and almost all in poor countries. Six countries account for 50% of worldwide deaths in children under 5, and 42 countries for 90% (see Table 5–7). About 49% of child deaths occur in sub-Saharan Africa and another 32% in South Asia (WHO 2003, 2007b; Black, Morris, and Bryce 2003), but there is considerable variation within countries by region and social class (see Tables 5–8 and 5–9).

The question of statistical artifacts—that is, whether reported rates are correct—always arises when considering infant deaths. Where births are seldom registered and medical attention is lacking, many infant deaths are never recorded and are permanently lost to the statistical system. In Jamaica, a 1996 study found that only 13% of infant deaths were registered, seriously affecting calculation of the IMR (McCaw-Binns et al. 1996). Such discrepancies can be found in many countries with limited vital statistics systems. There is often little parental or community incentive for reporting infant deaths, particularly in areas of economic deprivation where one may expect the toll to be higher than elsewhere. Culture and tradition may render the subject of deceased infants and children unsuitable for discussion, especially with strangers. Statistical coverage is typically better in urban than in rural areas, distorting infant mortality and other vital rates in sometimes unpredictable ways. Underreporting of infant mortality may result in insufficient attention to the factors and conditions that cause infant death.

Fetal deaths, stillbirths, and induced abortions are not always reported, although these are helpful in understanding infant mortality determinants. Such information is important, for example, in ascertaining the harmful prenatal effects of toxic chemicals or other environmental hazards. In the absence of required reporting of miscarriages or spontaneous abortions, these data can be difficult to obtain.

Table 5–7 Countries with Highest and Lowest Infant Mortality Rates (IMR), 2006

Country	IMR	Country	IMR
Afghanistan	165	Iceland	2
Sierra Leone	159	Andorra	3
Liberia	157	Cyprus	3
Angola	154	Czech Republic	3
Niger	148	Denmark	3
Democratic Republic of the Congo	129	Finland	3
Chad	124	Italy	3
Equatorial Guinea	124	Japan	3
Burkina Faso	122	Luxembourg	3
Guinea-Bissau	119	Monaco	3
Mali	119	Norway	3
Central African Republic	114	Portugal	3
Swaziland	112	San Marino	3
Burundi	109	Singapore	3
Lesotho	102	Slovenia	3
Zambia	102	Sweden	3
Nigeria	99	Austria	4
Guinea	98	Belgium	4
Rwanda	97	France	4
Mozambique	96	Germany	4
Botswana	90	Greece	4
Cote d'Ivoire	90	Ireland	4
Somalia	90	Israel	4
Benin	88	Netherlands	4
Cameroon	87	Spain	4
Djibouti	86	Switzerland	4
Gambia	84	Australia	5
Congo	79	Canada	5
Kenya	79	Croatia	5
Mauritania	78	Cuba	5
Pakistan	78	Estonia	5
Uganda	78	Malta	5
Ethiopia	77	New Zealand	5
Ghana	76	Republic of Korea	5
Malawi	76	United Kingdom	5
Yemen	75	Belarus	6
Myanmar	74	Hungary	6

(continued)

Table 5–7 Continued

Country	IMR	Country	IMR
United Republic of Tanzania	74	Poland	6
Azerbaijan	73	Lithuania	7
Madagascar	72	Serbia	7
Togo	69	Slovakia	7
Cambodia	65	Thailand	7
Bhutan	63	USA	7

Source: WHOSIS (2007).

Table 5–8 Infant Mortality in India by State, 2001

State	Infant Mortality per 1,000 Live Births
Andhra Pradesh	66
Arunachal Pradesh	39
Assam	74
Bihar	62
Chhattisgarh	77
Goa	19
Gujarat	60
Haryana	66
Himachal Pradesh	54
Jammu & Kashmir	48
Jharkhand	62
Karnataka	58
Kerala	11 (lowest)
Madhya Pradesh	86
Maharashtra	45
Manipur	20
Meghalaya	56
Mizoram	19
Orissa	91 (highest)
Punjab	52
Rajasthan	80
Sikkim	42
Tamil Nadu	49
Tripura	39
Uttar Pradesh	83
Uttaranchal	48
West Bengal	51

Source: Government of India (2004).

Table 5–9 Infant Mortality Rate by Region, Brazil, 2004

Brazil (National Rate)	22.5 deaths/1,000 live births
North	25.6/1,000
Northeast	33.9/1,000
Southeast	14.9/1,000
South	15/1,000
Central-West	18.7/1,000

Source: Ministério da Saúde (2007).

In addition, criteria for reporting are poorly understood by the medical profession, and countries have differing criteria for registration and publication of perinatal deaths. A further difficulty in deriving fetal death rates is in deciding what to use for the denominator, as it is unreasonable to maintain a registration system for pregnancies.

MATERNAL MORTALITY   A maternal death is defined in the ICD-10 as "the death of a woman while pregnant or within 42 days of termination of pregnancy, irrespective of the duration and the site of the pregnancy, from any cause related to or aggravated by the pregnancy or its management but not from accidental or incidental causes" (WHO 1992). A late maternal death is the death of a woman from direct or indirect obstetric causes more than 42 days but less than 1 year after termination of pregnancy. Maternal deaths are subdivided into two groups:

1. *Direct obstetric deaths*: Deaths resulting from obstetric complications of the pregnant state (pregnancy, labor, and puerperium), from interventions, omissions, incorrect treatment, or from a chain of events resulting from any of the above.
2. *Indirect obstetric deaths*: Deaths resulting from previous existing disease that developed during pregnancy and which was not due to direct causes, but which was aggravated by the physiologic effects of pregnancy.

The Maternal Mortality Ratio (MMR) and the maternal mortality rate (MMRate) should also be distinguished. The MMRate refers to the number of deaths from maternal causes per 100,000 women of reproductive age range (see Table 5–3). The MMR refers to the number of deaths from maternal causes per 100,000 live births, and thus measures the obstetric risk per pregnancy. Sierra Leone and Afghanistan have two of the highest maternal mortality ratios in the world at 2,000 deaths per 100,000 live births and 1,900 deaths per 100,000 live births respectively. The total world MMR is 400 maternal deaths per 100,000 births. Regional differences in the MMR are striking—in developed regions it is 20 per 100,000, while in underdeveloped regions it is 440 per 100,000.

Lifetime risk of maternal death is a more dramatic assessment that takes into account both the probability of becoming pregnant and the probability of dying as a result of that pregnancy cumulated across a woman's reproductive years. Lifetime risk of maternal death is highest in sub-Saharan Africa, with as many as 1 woman in 16 facing the risk of maternal death in the course of her lifetime, compared with 1 in 2,800 in developed regions (WHO 2004a).

LIMITATIONS OF MORTALITY DATA   In many regions of the world most deaths are not medically certified, and those that are recorded are not representative of mortality for the entire region. Only one-third of the estimated 57 million deaths annually are registered (WHO 2007c). A 2005 study on global data and death registration concluded that very few countries have good quality data on mortality, with death registration varying from close to 100% in the WHO European region to less than 10% in Africa (see Fig. 5–4). The study found that globally, only 23 countries have data registration that is more than 90% complete and where ICD-9 or ICD-10 codes are used (Mathers et al. 2005). Of the 193 WHO member states, only 31 provide reliable cause-of-death statistics (WHO 2007c).

Box 5–2 Age-Adjustment

The age structure of different populations is quite varied. The average African population, for instance, has more than twice the proportion of people under 15 and roughly one-fourth as many people over 65 as does the average European population. It would be inappropriate and misleading to compare crude or cause-specific mortality rates between two such groups because their overall mortality experience can be expected to differ on the basis of age structure alone. In order to increase the validity of international comparisons, the crude death rate of one population is apportioned into a set of age-specific death rates, which are then applied to the proportionate age distribution of a second population. This process provides a picture of the mortality experience that one population (population A) would have if it had the same age structure as another population (population B). It also describes the mortality pattern if population B had the same age-specific death rates of population A. In actual practice when many populations are compared, all are adjusted against a standard population, which may be real or a computer model generated for the purpose of the analysis. When a number of populations are being compared, the standard population may be a composite of all of them. Various rates may be made more comparable among populations by adjusting for features other than age, such as educational attainment or economic status.

The underlying cause of death is considered to be the disease or injury initiating the train of events leading directly to death, or the circumstances of the accident or violence producing fatal injury. It is often difficult to ascertain the underlying cause of death even in developed countries where most deaths are attended or certified by a physician. The capability of the certifying physician and the presence of technical facilities (diagnostic laboratory support, pathology reports, and autopsy facilities) vary greatly and affect the reliability of certified cause of death. Globally, fewer than 35% of deaths are registered with a medically certified cause (WHO 2004a). Although death registration data are available for 107 WHO member states,

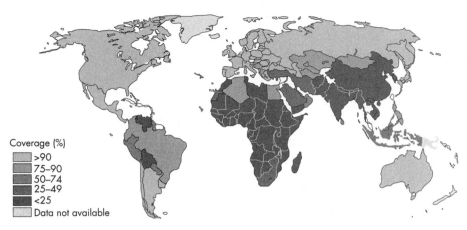

Figure 5–4 Coverage of vital registration of deaths, World, 1995–2003.
Source: WHO (2005).

even these data are limited by coding problems—particularly due to the category of ill-defined causes. The proportion of ill-defined deaths ranges from 4% in New Zealand to more than 40% in Thailand and Sri Lanka (Lopez et al. 2006a).

As people become older and accumulate more chronic illnesses, the specific underlying cause of death (if there is one) becomes murky or undeterminable. An elderly person may die *with* heart failure (and six other serious conditions), but that does not necessarily mean that the person died *of* heart failure. Errors can also occur when coding and transcribing the cause of death, particularly if it relates to a stigmatized condition. Many AIDS-related deaths, for example, may be coded as tuberculosis. Little or no training on this subject is given in most medical schools. Coronary artery disease is often the default diagnosis written on the death certificate.

Many studies have been carried out in different parts of the world to determine the accuracy of the underlying cause of death reported on death certificates. The obvious way to do this is to examine the body shortly after death, but autopsies may not be feasible for this purpose. The rare confirmatory studies that have been done have found major discrepancies between stated causes of death and those determined by careful postmortem analyses. In 1987, 1,023 deaths in the city of Goerlitz in the former East Germany (96.5% of the total) were subjected to a thorough autopsy (Modelmog, Rahlenbeck, and Trichopoulos 1994). For each, an underlying cause of death was assigned by a pathology team, which concluded that 47% of the diagnoses on death certificates differed from those based on autopsy. In 30% of the misclassified deaths, the difference crossed a major disease category—for example, the death certificate said heart failure and the pathologists found that the real cause of death was cancer, or vice versa. As expected, the extent of disagreement was higher for those who died at an older age.

Problems of international comparability of mortality data also include variations in language, terminology, definition of disease, and local differences in medical practice and rules for coding causes of death. In an effort to foster uniformity of diagnosis and terminology, the WHO has published a series of books with accompanying color transparencies of microscopic tissue sections as part of an international histological classification of tumors. Similar publications are issued on standardized classification of atherosclerotic lesions, hypertension, and chronic ischemic heart disease. In underdeveloped countries the application of such criteria is rare, although with increasing rates of chronic diseases there is greater pressure to use international disease codes.

What constitutes death is also a controversial topic in mortality measurements. Recent advances in medical techniques—such as organ transplants—have enabled physicians to keep alive individuals with advanced illnesses or massive injuries who under other circumstances would undoubtedly have died. UN definitions of birth, death, fetal death, and abortion are given in Box 5–3, but may be in need of revision due to current debates surrounding mortality measurement.

Box 5–3 Some Vital Events as Defined by the UN

- *Live birth*: The complete expulsion or extraction from its mother of a product of conception, irrespective of the duration of pregnancy, which after such separation breathes or shows any other evidence of life such as beating of the heart, pulsation of the umbilical cord, or definite movement of voluntary muscles, whether or not the umbilical cord has been cut or the placenta is attached. Each product of such a birth is considered live-born regardless of gestational age.
- *Death*: The permanent disappearance of all evidence of life at any time after live birth has taken place (postnatal cessation of vital functions without capability of resuscitation). This definition therefore excludes fetal deaths.
- *Fetal death*: Death prior to the complete expulsion or extraction from its mother of a product of conception, irrespective of the duration of pregnancy. The death is indicated by the fact that after such separation the fetus does not breathe or show any other evidence of life, such as beating of the heart, pulsation of the umbilical cord, or definite movement of voluntary muscles. Late fetal deaths are those of 28 or more completed weeks of gestation. These are synonymous with the events reported under the pre-1950 term "stillbirth."
- *Abortion**: Any interruption of pregnancy before 28 weeks of gestation with a dead fetus. There are two major categories of abortion: spontaneous and induced. Induced abortions are those initiated by deliberate action undertaken with the intention of terminating pregnancy; all other abortions are considered spontaneous.

*1970 definition.
Sources: (UN 2001, WHO 1970).

In an attempt to ensure more accurate cause-of-death data, some investigators in underdeveloped countries have started to use verbal autopsy (VA) mortality surveillance. In this technique, relatives or others who knew the deceased are interviewed using a structured questionnaire. Specific signs and symptoms of the deceased person, elicited from the respondents, are compared with carefully constructed precoded algorithms based on well-defined diagnostic criteria. Though useful, the VA approach raises vexing ethical issues. The sensitive nature of the questions asked may take an emotional toll on the family of the deceased, and ensuring informed consent may be complicated. As a new method, VA does not yet have fully developed guidelines and mechanisms to regulate and monitor ethical standards (Chandramohan 2005).

Box 5–4 Registrar General of India (RGI) Million Death Study in India

An example of the use of household survey data to gauge mortality patterns is the RGI Million Death Study in India—the world's largest prospective study on the causes of death—carried out in a context of inexistent or weak vital statistics (Jha et al. 2006). More than three-fourths of deaths in India occur at home, and over half of these lack a certified cause. Only one-third of deaths are registered; most do not have a recorded cause or include only a broad category of death. The RGI study is tracking a sample of 14 million people across India for the 1998–2014 period to identify causes of and underlying factors in child and adult deaths (including physical, behavioral, environmental, and, potentially, genetic determinants). Cause of death is documented through VA, with ongoing household monitoring for occurrence of vital events. It is hoped that this model for estimating cause-specific mortality in the absence of routine, comprehensive, sustainable, and reliable measurement of vital statistics may be replicable in other settings.

Problems with Vital Statistics

Sixty percent of all countries, where over 75% of the world population lives—including India, Indonesia, most of sub-Saharan Africa, and China—lack operational vital registry systems. Under the best circumstances, vital statistics provide approximately 95% coverage, with gaps due to nonregistration of temporary or undocumented workers, technical errors, and poor coverage of marginalized populations. For example, in the province of Ontario, Canada—a country known for its strong vital statistics system—more than 3% of live births were found to be underreported due to birth certificate payment requirements. This problem led the province to eliminate these fees in 2006 (Cheney 2006). Where births are underregistered, so are infant deaths. Household surveys, able to provide information on infant mortality levels and trends, remain the primary source for infant mortality data in dozens of countries. However, these methods are far less accurate for determining adult mortality rates. Under the worst circumstances, such as in 55 member states of the UN (42 of which are in Africa), where there are no routine mortality data at all for adults (Lopez et al. 2006b), there is only 15% population coverage of vital statistics information. Overall, there has been little progress in vital statistics expansion in the countries with the lowest GNI per capita (Boerma and Stansfield 2007).

There are many reasons for this unfortunate situation. The Expert Committee on Health Statistics of the WHO has issued numerous technical reports on various aspects of the problems involved. Vital statistics collection requires a sustained and steady budget allocation but is too frequently undervalued and underfunded, and government services are often very thinly dispersed. The absence of a clear administrative mandate is an impediment in some countries since responsibility for parts of this work may be divided among several government departments or ministries: health, finance, planning, census, social security, central statistics, or others. Moreover, trained, competent persons for this complex work are not always available.

Difficulties in obtaining data in developing countries include the isolation of rural populations or inaccessibility of registry offices, a lack of education and knowledge about the system, and suspicion by the public that records may not be kept confidential or that they may be used by the government for taxation, enforced military service, or other purposes considered contrary to their interests. Squatters, undocumented or nonstatus migrants, persons without identity cards, nomads without a fixed residence, persons engaged in illegal activities, and others may have strong disincentives toward registration. Fees or bribes may be demanded by officials for the initial registration or for copies of certificates. A legal requirement for a death certificate before authorization of burial may be a hardship in remote areas and may be overlooked by a bereaved family. Births, marriages, and deaths are accompanied by an infinite variety of cultural and religious customs and rituals, which may be incompatible with the local government's needs for vital statistics data.

Finally, the collection, dissemination, and use of vital statistics are far from neutral activities. A population group or national government may, for various reasons, wish its size to be either overstated or understated or, for reasons of stigma and insurance purposes, may not wish to identify particular causes of death. As well, budgetary and political pressures may result in biased data for ends unrelated to health data per se. The path from data to policy making may be impeded by contradictions between different data sources, insufficient analysis of data, and competition between national and international program needs. As well, health officers in charge of data collection and monitoring may be simultaneously responsible for running programs which themselves are expected to reach particular health goals, generating serious conflicts of interest (AbouZahr, Adjei, and Kanchanachitra 2007).

Health Statistics

Health and illness statistics—commonly referred to as morbidity statistics—are in many ways more useful to health analysts than are data on deaths. Morbidity statistics are numerical representations of the recognized occurrence of ill health in a population. Ideally, they should describe ill health by diagnosis, severity, duration, distribution in place and time, as well as characteristics of the persons affected, such as their age, sex, occupation, and marital status. There are two general categories of sources for morbidity data: records routinely compiled and accumulated by various agencies, and special surveys that obtain information on particular issues. Reliable figures are not always available, even from national and international agencies.

Many institutions and organizations collect illness and disability records. These include: general clinics, health centers, hospitals; public health departments; special clinics (e.g., sexually transmitted infection clinics and maternal and child health clinics); school clinics and factory dispensaries; NGOs; visiting nurses, midwives, physicians and dentists in private practice; military services and veterans, hospitals; workers' compensation programs; census bureaus; police and traffic safety organizations; health insurance and life insurance companies; businesses; and disease-specific registries. Morbidity statistics may be used for the following purposes:

- control of communicable diseases;
- planning for the development of preventive services;
- studies of social factors and health;
- planning for provision of treatment services;
- estimation of economic importance of sickness;
- research into etiology and pathogenesis;
- research on efficacy of preventive and therapeutic measures; and
- national and international studies of distribution of diseases and impairments.

Persons legally responsible for morbidity notification may be physicians and other health workers, school authorities, directors of laboratories in which positive diagnoses are made, or heads of families. There is a great variety of legislation governing notifiable diseases. Some countries require immediate reporting of suspected cases, and others only after laboratory confirmation. Others require notification of certain diseases only by schools, institutions, or resorts. In still others, special regulations require reporting of cases or outbreaks of specified diseases in particular locations, such as on dairy farms or in hospitals, and require that otherwise healthy carriers be reported and registered. Reporting is rarely complete, however. Busy health professionals frequently neglect to notify authorities despite the legal requirement to do so.

With the implementation of the IHR (2005), most countries are now legally bound to report international public health emergencies to the WHO. Still, reporting of disease occurrence in any country is limited to certain notifiable ailments—those for which it is mandatory that cases be brought to the attention of health authorities. The 20th century has seen essentially all countries adopt some form of compulsory notification of certain illnesses within their borders. In most cases these laws refer to highly communicable diseases that pose an immediate threat to the community, but often specific cases of other types must be reported. Botulism, frequently caused by improperly processed canned foods, is such a disease—prompt notification may result in recalls of affected production lots and thus avert additional cases. As conditions change, additional diseases may be added to the list. Rubella became reportable after its association with birth defects was established. Epilepsy may be a notifiable disease when a driver's license is involved. AIDS is reportable everywhere in the world, but due to the stigmatized nature of the disease, the complexity of diagnosis, and a tangle of other factors, case reporting is incomplete. Occupational diseases and work-related injuries are legally notifiable in many countries, in part to gather data for control purposes, and in part for validation of workmen's compensation claims.

Morbidity Data Sources and Measurement

In studying the distribution of particular diseases, a strict case definition is needed. For example, a case of measles can be defined as: a generalized rash of three or more days duration, a fever of 101°F (38.3°C) or more, and a cough, coryza, or conjunctivitis (Orenstein, Bernier, and Hinman 1984). This clinical case definition should distinguish measles from other similar illnesses, but it is not always easy to identify a case. When a good case definition of disease exists, it must be applied to each individual to see if they meet the case criteria. Sometimes that is a relatively simple task, but at times it is very difficult. Applying the clinical case definition of measles, for example, involves observation, the use of a thermometer, and inquiring about duration of illness. For other case definitions, such as tuberculosis, laboratory studies are needed. These can be costly and are often impractical to undertake in the field. The level of diagnostic services needed depends on the purpose and design of the investigation. A relatively straightforward and inexpensive ("quick-and-dirty") clinical survey, with some laboratory backup, may be sufficient to make a policy decision. Such procedures are termed rapid epidemiologic assessments.

In recent years, population-based surveys have been commonly employed to determine the prevalence of particular diseases. To date, these have depended on relatively harmless and inexpensive diagnostic tests. Parasitological surveys for ascariasis or hookworm disease, for example, use stool examination to identify the characteristic worm ova, and population surveys for malaria and filariasis use microscopic examination of blood films. Prevalence estimates of trachoma, sexually transmitted infections such as HIV, childhood diarrhea, hypertension, and nutritional deficiencies also rest on large survey methods.

Screening programs for genetic disorders (e.g., Down's syndrome and sickle cell anemia) and for HIV and cancer, have also been undertaken in varied settings. The objectives of screening programs differ greatly from those of surveys. Surveys attempt to measure prevalence of a disease and do not necessarily lead to treatment, while screening is aimed at secondary prevention of illness. Unless they are universally applied, however, screening programs have a limited impact. Some of the methods of biotechnology, such as DNA hybridization, which can test for the presence and levels of bacteria such as *Shigella* and *Leishmania*, and monoclonal antibody methods may find future application in screening efforts if costs can be greatly reduced.

National registries have been formed in order to monitor the distribution and prevalence of some diseases. The most common of these are cancer registries, but there are also special registries for blindness, childhood disabilities, congenital defects, and diseases of specific local importance. The existence of registries can influence the public health research agenda. For example, because of Canada's comprehensive cancer registry, cancer studies are prominent in population health research efforts.

In addition to counts of disease occurrence, many people have looked for ways to describe the significance of ill health for individuals, communities, and nations. Commonly used indicators include: years of potential life lost (YPLL), quality adjusted life years (QALY), physical quality of life index (PQLI), and healthy years equivalent (HYE). The WHO developed the measure WHOQOL, which produces a profile based on 24 quality of life facets across six broad domains.

Rather than simple yes/no answers (e.g., cancer yes, blindness no), these measures entail some assessment of quality of life. With the YPLL, for example, causes of death that typically strike young people, such as malaria and diarrhea or respiratory diseases, are weighted differently from the chronic diseases characteristic of the elderly. The rationale is that a person who dies in infancy or early childhood loses almost all of his or her life expectancy, while an elderly person who dies loses a few years or, if old enough, none at all. For this metric, the age at death must be known, as well as the expected age at which that person would otherwise have died (not always simple to determine). The potential life lost in a population can be a powerful incentive for policy changes by governments but also de-emphasizes certain chronic diseases among adults. Diabetes, the 12th leading cause of death in 2004 (see Table 5–10), rarely appears on YPLL "top ten" lists.

Howard Barnum of the World Bank refined the concept of days of life lost with the introduction of the "age-productivity profile." As he described it, "the timing of health effects over the life span has implications for the economic contribution of the individual as productive days are lost from acute illness, disability and

Table 5–10 The 12 Leading Causes of Death in the World, 2002 (and rank-order of importance in 2004)

No.	Cause	Estimated Number of Deaths (in Millions)	Percent of all Deaths
1	Ischemic heart disease (1)	7.2	12.6
2	Cerebrovascular disease (2)	5.5	9.7
3	Lower respiratory infections (3)	3.9	6.8
4	HIV/AIDS (6)	2.8	4.9
5	Chronic obstructive pulmonary disease (4)	2.7	4.8
6	Perinatal conditions (10)*	2.5	4.3
7	Diarrheal diseases (5)	1.8	3.2
8	Tuberculosis (7)	1.6	2.7
9	Malaria (14)	1.3	2.2
10	Trachea, bronchus, lung cancers (8)	1.2	2.2
11	Road traffic accidents (9)	1.2	2.1
12	Diabetes mellitus (12)	1	1.7

Source: WHO (2004b, 2008).

*Regrouped for 2004 update into 3 separate categories: prematurity and low birth weight; birth asphyxia and birth trauma; and neonatal infections and other conditions.

premature death" (Barnum 1987, p. 835). Barnum also introduced the idea of health discounting—that is, that we should adjust for the fact that a day of healthy life in the present has a greater intrinsic value to an individual than does a day in the future. By discounting at different rates (adjusting for projected future earnings), the present value of productive life days lost to particular causes changes dramatically. For example, in the unweighted data from a World Bank study in Ghana in 1981, malaria ranked first and cardiovascular disease ranked 22nd in days lost. When both age-productivity weightings and discounting at an extreme 20% rate were applied, malaria ranked fourteenth and cardiovascular disease first in present value of income lost from future productivity (Ghana Health Assessment Team 1981). It is clear that data can be manipulated in a number of ways. Yet age-productivity profiles and discounting are, largely, tools of economists and little understood by most health workers, although they stimulate great controversy.

GLOBAL BURDEN OF DISEASE   The first attempt to quantify the total weight of disease throughout the world was the global burden of disease (GBD) project, commissioned in the early 1990s by the World Bank, and carried out jointly by the WHO and Harvard School of Public Health researchers. Diseases were grouped into three major classifications: Group I includes communicable diseases as well as perinatal conditions and nutritional deficiencies; Group II includes noncommunicable diseases; and Group III includes all injuries. These groups were further subdivided into categories, and then into 107 separate causes of death according to the Ninth Revision of the ICD. The ongoing GBD studies use the disability adjusted life year (DALY) as the measure of comparison (see below for a discussion of the DALY).

In the first GBD study, noncommunicable diseases, including neurological and psychiatric ailments, were estimated at 41% of the global burden of disease in 1990, with 44% due to communicable, maternal, perinatal and nutritional conditions combined, and 15% due to injuries (Murray and Lopez 1996). Fifty-five percent of all deaths worldwide were found to be due to noncommunicable diseases; 35% to communicable diseases; and 10% to injuries. An updated GBD study found that in 2001 58.5% of all deaths and 52.6% of the global burden of disease worldwide were due to noncommunicable diseases; 32.3% of all deaths and 36.5% of the global burden of disease were due to communicable diseases, perinatal conditions, and nutritional deficiencies; and injuries accounted for 9.2% of all deaths and 10.9% of the global burden of disease (Lopez et al. 2006a). As in 1990, approximately one-third of deaths were in Group I (virtually all in low- and middle-income countries); however HIV/AIDS went from 2% of Group I deaths in 1990 to 14% in 2001. Altogether, the three leading causes of death in 2001 were ischemic heart disease, cerebrovascular disease, and lower respiratory infections. These diseases together accounted for almost 20% of all deaths in low- and middle-income countries (see Table 5–11 for 2002 data), demonstrating that there is a simultaneous burden of infectious and

Table 5–11 The 10 Leading Causes of Death by Country Income Level, 2002*

Low- and Middle-Income Countries			High-Income Countries		
Cause	Deaths (Millions)	% of Total Deaths	Cause	Deaths (Millions)	% of total Deaths
Ischemic heart disease	5.70	11.8	Ischemic heart disease	1.36	17.3
Cerebrovascular disease	4.61	9.5	Cerebrovascular disease	0.78	9.9
Lower respiratory infections	3.41	7.0	Trachea, bronchus, and lung cancers	0.46	5.8
HIV/AIDS	2.55	5.3	Lower respiratory infections	0.34	4.4
Perinatal conditions	2.49	5.1	COPD[a]	0.30	3.8
COPD[a]	2.36	4.9	Colon and rectal cancers	0.26	3.3
Diarrheal diseases	1.78	3.7	Alzheimer's and other dementias	0.21	2.6
Tuberculosis	1.59	3.3	Diabetes mellitus	0.20	2.6
Malaria	1.21	2.5	Breast cancer	0.16	2.0
Road traffic accidents	1.07	2.2	Stomach cancer	0.15	1.9

[a]COPD, chronic obstructive pulmonary disease.

Source: WHO (2004b).

* In the latest GBD report (2004 data), the 10 leading causes of death remained the same in high-income countries, but in low- and middle-income countries HIV/AIDS went from the 4th to 6th leading cause due to re-estimates by UNAIDS. As well, there was a marked increase in deaths from diarrheal diseases (from 6th to 5th leading cause of death) and a disaggregation of perinatal conditions. Malaria no longer figured in the top 10 causes. WHO (2008).

noncommunicable diseases (Lopez 2006a). The 2004 update of the GBD showed that the three leading causes of death had increased to comprise 29% of all deaths in low- and middle-income countries (WHO 2008).

The GBD studies have also sought to estimate the burden of disease due to a series of "risk factors" (see Chapter 6 for a critique of this concept). The 2001 study found that undernutrition was the single leading global cause of premature death and disability, followed by high blood pressure, unsafe sex, tobacco, and alcohol use. At the same time, the GBD attributed to unsafe water, sanitation, and hygiene had declined since 1990, mainly due to a worldwide decline in mortality from diarrheal disease (which has since reversed). The disease burden as a result of unprotected sex disproportionately affected women in all regions, and tobacco and alcohol affected men in developed regions the most, though this problem was also growing elsewhere. The study ascribed the steep increase in the burden of noncommunicable diseases worldwide to population aging and increased tobacco use in underdeveloped regions (Lopez et al. 2006a). As discussed in Chapter 4, such a narrow focus on risk factors excludes the role of political and social factors in shaping patterns of disease, and prioritizes biomedico-behavioral solutions.

DISABILITY ADJUSTED LIFE YEAR   In the *World Development Report 1993: Investing in Health*, the World Bank proposed a new composite measure called the disability adjusted life year or DALY (rhymes with rally) as a generic indicator to help set health policy priorities, facilitate comparisons between countries, and standardize health sector decision making. Its major contribution is the incorporation of both mortality and morbidity (in terms of disability) into a single summary statistic. The DALY is defined as "the present value of the future years of disability-free life that are lost as the result of the premature deaths or cases of disability occurring in a particular year" (World Bank 1993, p. x). It combines four elements: (1) levels of mortality by age; (2) levels of morbidity by age; (3) the value of a healthy year of life at specific ages; and (4) a discount rate of 3%. The underlying assumption is that priority should be given to those health problems that cause a large disease

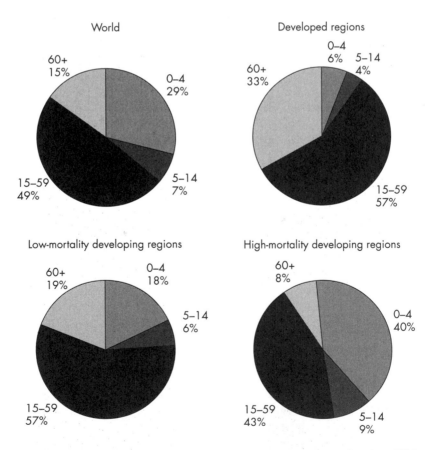

Figure 5–5 Distribution of disease burden (in DALYs) by age group and region, 2002. *Source*: WHO (2003).

Table 5-12 Leading Causes of Disease Burden (in DALYs) for Males and Females Aged 15 Years and Older, Worldwide, 2002*

Males	% of DALYs	Females	% of DALYs
HIV/AIDS	7.4	Unipolar depressive disorders	8.4
Ischemic heart disease	6.8	HIV/AIDS	7.2
Cerebrovascular disease	5.0	Ischemic heart disease	5.3
Unipolar depressive disorders	4.8	Cerebrovascular disease	5.2
Road traffic injuries	4.3	Cataracts	3.1
Tuberculosis	4.2	Hearing loss, adult onset	2.8
Alcohol use disorders	3.4	Chronic obstructive pulmonary disease	2.7
Violence	3.3	Tuberculosis	2.6
COPD	3.1	Osteoarthritis	2.0
Hearing loss, adult onset	2.7	Diabetes mellitus	1.9

Source: WHO (2003).

* In the latest GBD report (2004 data), HIV/AIDS dropped to the 4th leading cause of disease burden for adult men, and road traffic injuries rose to the 2nd cause. HIV/AIDS is currently the 3rd leading cause of disability in adult women, and diabetes has risen to 7th place. While cataracts still represent a significant cause of disability among women, refractive errors (visual impairments) have dropped to 6th place. WHO (2008).

burden and for which generally accepted cost-effective interventions are available (Lopez et al. 2006a).

The accumulated DALYs are used to represent the global burden of disease, as shown in Figure 5–5 and Table 5–12. In 2001, the average global burden of disease across all regions was 250 DALYs per 1,000 people, two-thirds of which were due to premature death. Average numbers often hide regional and population disparities. For example, sub-Saharan Africa had the highest disease burden with over 500 DALYs per 1,000 people (double the global average), and high-income countries had the lowest disease burden with approximately 200 DALYs per 1,000 people (20% less than the global average). The 2004 GBD data show that regional disparties in burden of disease are increasing: Africa's disease burden is 510 DALYs per 1,000 people, compared with 124 DALYs per 1,000 for high-income countries and 237 DALYs per 1,000 people globally WHO (2008). An analysis of regional-, population-, and disease-specific DALYs is useful to demonstrate how marked regional health discrepancies are: sub-Saharan African countries experience a much higher burden of disease than do wealthier nations and those with more redistributive policies. Upon more detailed analysis (e.g., comparing young women in rural Zimbabwe with their counterparts in urban Denmark), DALYs demonstrate an even greater divide.

CRITIQUE OF DALYS   Soon after their appearance, DALYs came under fire on both technical and political/social grounds. The main lines of criticism are (Anand and Hanson 2004; Bobadilla 1996):

- DALYs reflect the social values of a small group of researchers and international professionals. The discount rate, age weights, and disability scores are arbitrary, and were developed with little involvement of health care workers or the public. They do not necessarily reflect the thinking or values of those affected by the analysis.
- Valuing people's lives solely in terms of their current and future productivity is difficult to defend ethically and contradicts the notion of health as a human right. Moreover, valuing future years of life at levels less than present years of life could be used to justify many activities that result in environmental degradation, benefiting the present generation at the expense of future generations.
- DALYs' disability weights devalue the lives of persons who are disabled, and they fail to take account of variations in how disabilities are experienced. Societies differ in their views of specific impairments such as psychosis, AIDS, and infertility, and in the degree to which they stigmatize or aid impaired individuals. A more appropriate measure for disability would account for existing support systems and services that facilitate participation in the workforce and enhance the quality of the daily activities of individuals with impairments.
- DALYs discriminate against the elderly because death at a young age has a higher DALY value than death at an older age. The DALY is also insensitive to variations in the experiences of each life-year lost. The value of 30 years lost by one individual's premature death is equated to 1 year lost by 30 different individuals.
- DALYs are biased in favor of societies that use life-prolonging technologies and overestimate the years of life lost in high mortality countries. Basing calculations on a life expectancy of 80 is clearly unrealistic in countries with a life expectancy of, for example, 60 years.
- DALYs favor narrow, disease-specific interventions that can be used in a cost-effectiveness analysis and do not account for non-health sector interventions that affect health, such as improved social security measures and food subsidies.
- DALYs do not account for differences in socioeconomic status, income, and poverty rates within and across populations.
- Calculating DALYs is expensive as they require large quantities of data that are not readily available.
- Maximizing the number of DALYs gained might not be the goal of the health sector.
- Cost-effectiveness might not be the most desirable criterion to guide health policy making.

Despite these charges, the DALY and corresponding GBD indicators are achieving ever more widespread application.

Challenges of Gathering and Measuring Health Statistics

Deciding which variables to use when collecting health data is a complex and often ideologically driven endeavor. Essential information regarding underlying determinants of health may be overlooked or willfully ignored. As a result, causation may be drawn between specific variables in lieu of searching for missing data. For example, the dearth of data collected on social class in the United States and the abundance of race-related variables, has led many to draw conclusions related to race only, without a deeper analysis of racism, class structure, or other determinants of health. Moreover, a focus on individual and behavioral variables when measuring health status and determinants may lead to data interpretations that "blame the victim" and fail to see beyond so-called lifestyle factors.

The same difficulties inherent in the collection, interpretation, and comparison of vital statistics are evident to a far greater degree when data on health status are being considered. While at least some of the elements underlying all vital statistics are mandated by law, no such compulsion exists for most of the information related to measures of health status. One difficulty, of course, pertains to what to document or measure—that is, how to define health and ill health. Problems of definition and assessment are far more complex in health and sickness data than in mortality statistics. The uniform measurement and reporting of such information is complicated by the varying definitions and interpretations of illnesses and their causes among different social groups—what is considered illness in one group may not be so elsewhere. For example, the Rockefeller Foundation found that hookworm-induced anemia was not considered a disease by poor, rural populations in the southern United States and Mexico in the early 20th century; instead hookworm's key symptom—fatigue— was an expected feature of subsistence agriculture and marginal living conditions.

Many diseases exhibit a wide spectrum of clinical severity ranging from unapparent to extreme. It is likely that most infections go undetected by those harboring them since they may experience only generalized, nonspecific symptoms. As a result, the overwhelming majority of infections never come to medical attention. Serological surveys to determine the prevalence of antibodies to many viruses, for instance, do not necessarily correlate with the apparent distribution of illnesses caused by them in the same population. Furthermore, people have many episodes of sickness during their lifetimes, and very few persons can document their own complete health history.

Researchers often magnify the importance of the diseases they study, as they may not take into account a clear, overall vision of the field and therefore believe their issue to be most important or deserving of funds. However, even if some prevalence estimates are grossly mistaken, certain illnesses are ubiquitous in marginalized populations, such as diarrhea related to malnutrition, lack of sanitation and education, and similar factors associated with poverty.

The quality and completeness of morbidity records vary greatly, as does their accessibility. In many cases information is considered confidential or privileged, particularly when individual patients are identified and where the information forms the basis of legal claims for insurance, inheritance, or compensation. There is a growing trend in some countries to increase privacy protection laws. Personal data of all kinds, particularly those concerned with diagnoses of mental and emotional illnesses, may be specifically sealed off from epidemiological use. Conducting epidemiological analyses can be difficult, if not impossible, if they involve records concerned with stigmatized diagnoses. However, compared with larger issues of data deficiency, these problems seem minor (Helgason 1992).

Finally, a high degree of coordination between regional reporting agencies is seldom achieved, even in the most developed countries, because information is collected differently, for different purposes, and at different intervals. The problems of international comparability of such data are obvious, as are the frustrations that may beset researchers who wish to use those data for the purposes of analysis.

Health Services Statistics

Most countries view information about the internal working of their own health services as an indispensable part of health data. Health services statistics refer not only to resources (facilities, personnel, financing) but also to activities and utilization patterns. This type of information is useful to government agencies, insurance companies, health organizations, and large hospitals, which need to keep track of the numbers and costs of all categories of medical procedures.

The main reasons for collecting health services statistics are to (WHO 2000):

- support the administration, management, and coordination of local, regional, and national health services;
- create short-term and long-term plans/policies;
- assess whether health services are accomplishing their objectives (effectiveness and responsiveness) and whether they are doing so in the best possible way (efficiency and equality/equity);
- keep track of costs and determine when programs should be commenced/ terminated; and
- provide data required by government departments and legislatures, international agencies, health services researchers, and members of the public.

More specifically, health services planners need data regarding the following:

- characteristics of health facilities and personnel;
- acquisition and use of supplies and equipment;
- services provided and their utilization by the community; and
- the costs involved and flow of resources through the system.

Ideally, these data are compiled at a national level and forwarded to the WHO. They then become accessible through the WHO Statistical Information System (WHOSIS) (WHO 2007b). WHOSIS provides a set of core health system and health status indicators. It also has a section dedicated to national health accounts (NHA), which includes information on health spending, system coverage, and epidemiological and demographic indicators. NHA are particularly useful for planning purposes and comparative analyses.

In the past there was little international standardization of preventive and curative activities. In 1978, in conjunction with the release of the ICD-9, the WHO issued a coding manual for medical procedures, now called the *International Classification of Health Interventions* (ICHI). Its utility varied from one country to another. A coded list was not developed for ICD-10, primarily because medical technology developments would require frequent revisions. Currently, a short version of the ICHI is under field trial in various countries that do not have their own intervention classification systems. One proposal for the future ICD-11 is the creation of three volumes—one for primary care practitioners, a second for specialists, and a third for researchers (WHO 2007d).

International standardization of procedures is very complex. Immunizations by conventional methods using fixed doses of a standard vaccine of uniform potency may come close to the ideal of a universally comparable procedure, but what is to be said of a physical examination? How are users and nonusers of services to be identified and characterized, and how are outcomes of treatment to be assessed? In some way, each country must face these kinds of questions if it wants to evaluate the effectiveness of its health services. When efficiency (i.e., value for investment) is considered, these questions become even more pressing. As in the case of mortality and morbidity statistics, many countries also have insufficient health services statistics because of a lack of routine data collection, inadequate information systems, and limited support for health services research (WHO 2000).

Large-scale programs, international in origin and scope, typically standardize their methodologies, activities, and outcomes, and keep appropriate records in an attempt to gauge their effectiveness and impact. A good example is the worldwide malaria eradication program, long defunct, in which field, laboratory, and clinical work as well as assessment procedures were carefully spelled out in universal protocols (see Chapter 13). More recently, the WHO adopted directly observed therapy (DOTS) as a standardized tuberculosis treatment and control measure. However, the five recommendations for standardized funding, screening, treatment, pharmaceutical management, and evaluation have not been followed uniformly, making it difficult to draw conclusions or comparisons (see Chapter 6). Programs of this type represent only a small part of the activities of most countries' health services. They are often organized and administered separately from the other activities of health departments or ministries, impeding the routine and uniform collection of health services data.

The comparison of data on health services in different countries is generally more difficult than similar studies of population, mortality, and morbidity statistics. Whereas human physiology and pathogens are essentially the same everywhere, the organizational patterns of governments and societies are very diverse. In countries where most aspects of life are regulated by a central authority, health facilities and personnel can be identified with relative clarity. Elsewhere, a mosaic of formal and nonformal health services exist, which often differ from place to place. This has been recognized as a challenge at an international level, and current initiatives aim to overcome these difficulties.

Data on Social Inequalities in Health

Key Questions:

- Can health data address larger determinants of health?
- How can health data collection systems monitor social inequalities in health?

A complex array of social, political, economic, and biological factors influence health and longevity. Differences in the health of individuals and populations reflect intrinsic features of the societies in which they live (Marmot 2004). Social inequalities in health (or health inequities, as they are sometimes called) are defined as "avoidable disparities in health or its key determinants that are systematically observed between groups of people with different levels of underlying social privilege, i.e. wealth, power, or advantage" (Braveman and Tarmino 2002, p. 1624).

The importance of documenting social inequalities in health has been recognized for almost two hundred years. One of the earliest studies of the social patterns of disease and death was by Frenchman Louis-René Villermé, an army doctor turned sociomedical researcher, who investigated mortality patterns in different neighborhoods of Paris in the 1820s. He discovered that, in contrast to prevailing beliefs that disease was divinely ordained or influenced by geographic and environmental features, mortality rates in the city's dozen *arrondissements* (neighborhoods) were almost exactly correlated with poverty levels: where there was a higher proportion of poor people, death rates were higher and vice versa. Many other 19th-century reformers including Engels and Chadwick (discussed in Chapter 2) also examined the connections between untoward social conditions and ill health.

More recent interest in the social determinants of health was sparked by the publication of the Black Report—*Inequalities in Health: Report of a Research Working Group*—in Britain in 1980. The report demonstrated persistent (and even growing) inequalities in health by social class—at every stage of the life-cycle—more than three decades after the creation of the country's National Health Service. The authors stressed the importance of material conditions—class-related differences in socioeconomic conditions—in explaining inequalities in health (Black and Research Working Group 1980). In 2008 the WHO's Commission on Social Determinants of Health (launched in 2005) issued its final report, calling for the incorporation of social determinants of health into planning, policy, and technical work at the WHO and in member countries (see Box 5–1). As well, it is advocating for political action to address the structural forces underlying social inequalities in health, including inequitable distribution of wealth, resources, and power (WHO Commission on Social Determinants of Health 2008) (see Chapter 7 for details).

Failure to include socioeconomic indicators in the collection and analysis of health data severely impedes efforts to understand, routinely monitor, and address social disparities in health (Krieger, Chen, and Waterman 2005). It is important to understand how data collection and interpretation affect the measurement of health inequities within and among populations. Much of the data routinely collected and analyzed measuring average levels of health and disease do not reflect disparities in access to services within a population nor do they expose how health is distributed according to different population characteristics (including socioeconomic status, ethnicity, gender, urban or rural residence, and age). Understanding this distribution has important implications for health and other public policies. For example, in the United States there is a 20-year gap in life expectancy between the most and least advantaged populations (Marmot 2005). Uncovering these significant social inequities based on regional, ethnic, and class differences is critical to understanding and addressing their health consequences.

Collection of Data on Social Inequalities in Health

There are many approaches that can be taken to identify and measure social inequalities in health. For example, population groups and their health status can be categorized and studied in terms of economic status, geographic location (e.g., rural–urban or developed–underdeveloped country), occupation, gender, ethnicity, and citizenship status (e.g., immigrant, refugee, migrant worker) (Gwatkin 2000). Poverty and income inequalities are also used as measures of inequalities in health. Absolute and/or relative poverty levels, for example, determine a community's or family's ability to obtain adequate food, shelter, and health care, which in turn affects health status.

In practice, the majority of attention regarding measuring social inequalities in health and disease is given to socioeconomic status (SES) (Braveman et al. 2005). SES follows in the tradition of Max Weber and incorporates measures of income or economic resources, education, and/or prestige. SES, however, stands in sharp contrast to Karl Marx's concept of social class which measures relationship to economic production, property and asset ownership, and overall power differences. As we shall see in Chapter 7, the difference between these two concepts—SES and social class—are not semantic but have enormous implications for the types of policies employed to address inequalities in health.

The importance of implicit assumptions and values regarding health data are perhaps most evidenced in the emphasis on collection of data by race in the United States. As social epidemiologist Nancy Krieger notes:

> Science is at once objective and partisan.... the allegedly neutral stance of leaving out class and focusing on race...is as thoroughly political as overt efforts to augment public health data bases with variables pertaining to social class and the everyday realities of both racism and sexism. The seemingly "apolitical" stance is also fundamentally

invalid, for by failing to address the full range of variation in population patterns of disease, it blocks our scientific efforts and professional duties to understand and improve the public's health (Krieger 1992, p. 422).

CONCLUSION

Learning Points:

- Mortality and morbidity data collection and analysis underpin health policy.
- Reliable health data are essential for national and international health policies and decision making.
- Health data collection and analysis are simultaneously technical, political, and ideological activities.
- The availability of health data in and of itself will not improve health status.

As the old saying goes, "If you don't ask, you don't know, and if you don't know, you can't act" (Krieger 1992, p. 412). Without knowledge of local, national, and international health and illness patterns, action to improve health is highly limited. Though far less palpable than ill health and preventable death, the routine collection of population data, health and vital statistics, health services statistics, and data on social inequalities in health is essential to understanding local and global patterns of disease and illness and to formulating effective actions for health improvement.

To date, international health actors and donors have paid insufficient attention to the problem of health data and vital statistics registration, due to the high cost of establishing and maintaining such systems and the perception that they are less important than disease-control efforts. Yet as global attention to the health of marginalized populations and the problem of social inequalities in health has grown—and as donors demand ever greater monitoring and evaluation of programs—the need for health data is even more pressing (Bchir et al. 2006; Boerma and Stansfield 2007). In order to respond adequately to these major challenges, far more accurate and comprehensive health data and analysis are necessary. Indeed, compiling and assessing health data in an ongoing and permanent fashion—especially in the 60% of countries lacking operational vital statistics registries—should be a global and national health priority.

REFERENCES

AbouZahr C, Adjei S, and Kanchanachitra C. 2007. From data to policy: Good practices and cautionary tales. *Lancet* 369(9566):1039–1046.

Anand S and Hanson K. 2004. Disability-adjusted life years: A critical review. In Anand S, Peter F, and Sen A, Editors. *Public Health, Ethics, and Equity.* Oxford: Oxford University Press.

Barnum H. 1987. Evaluating healthy days of life gained from health projects. *Social Science and Medicine* 24(10):833–841.

Bchir A, Bhutta Z, Binka F, Black R, Bradshaw D, Garnett G, et al. 2006. Better health statistics are possible. *Lancet* 367(9506):190–193.

Black RE, Morris SS, and Bryce J. 2003. Where and why are 10 million children dying every year? *Lancet* 361(9376):2226–2234.

Black SD, Morris J, Smith C, and Townsend P. 1980. *Inequalities in Health: Report of a Research Working Group.* London: Department of Health and Social Security.

Bobadilla JL. 1996. Priority setting and cost effectiveness. In Janovsky K, Editor. *Health Policy and Systems Development: An Agenda for Research.* Geneva: WHO.

Boerma JT and Stansfield S. 2007. Health statistics now: Are we making the right investments? *Lancet* 369(9563):779–786.

Braveman PA, Cubbin C, Egerter S, Chideya S, Marchi KS, Metzler M, and Posner S. 2005. Socioeconomic status in health research: One size does not fit all. *JAMA* 294(22):2879–2888.

Braveman P and Tarimo E. 2002. Social inequalities in health within countries: Not only an issue for affluent nations. *Social Science and Medicine* 54(11):1621–1635.

Chandramohan D, Soleman N, Shibuya K, and Porter J. 2005. Editorial: Ethical issues in the application of verbal autopsies in mortality surveillance systems. *Tropical Medicine and International Health* 10(11):1087–1089.

Cheney, P. 2006. *Ontario to eliminate fees for registering births.* Globe and Mail, July 24.

Crossette B. 1998. Third of births aren't registered, UNICEF says. *New York Times,* July 8.

Dow, U. 1998. Birth registration: The "First" right. In *The Progress of Nations 1998.* New York: UNICEF.

Ghana Health Assessment Team. 1981. A quantitative method of assessing the health impact of different diseases in less developed countries. *International Journal of Epidemiology* 10(1):73–80.

Government of India. 2004. *Ministry of Statistics and Programme Implementation. Statistical Abstract: India 2003.* New Delhi, India.

Graham WJ. 1986. *Health Status Indicators in Developing Countries. A Selective Review.* London: The Commonwealth Secretariat.

Gwatkin DR. 2000. Health inequalities and the health of the poor: What do we know? What can we do? *Bulletin of the World Health Organization* 78(1):3–18.

Hawke A, Editor. 2002. *Birth Registration: Right from the Start.* Florence, Italy: UNICEF Innocenti Research Centre.

Helgason T. 1992. Epidemiological research needs access to data. *Scandinavian Journal of Social Medicine* 20(3):129–133.

Hill K, Croft T, Jones G, Loaiza E, Hancioglu A, Walker N, et al. 2006. Tracking progress towards the Millennium Development Goals: Reaching consensus on child mortality levels and trends. *Bulletin of the World Health Organization* 84(3):225–232.

Hookham H. 1972. *A Short History of China.* New York: New American Library (Mentor Books).

Jha P. 2005. *Prospective Study of One Million Deaths in India: Rationale, Design and Validation Results.* Toronto, ON: Centre for Global Health Research, Public Health Sciences, University of Toronto.

Jha P, Gajalakshmi V, Gupta PC, Kumar R, Mony P, Dhingra N, Petro R, and RGI-CGHR Prospective Study Collaborators. 2006. Prospective study of one million deaths in India: Rationale, design and validation results. *PLoS Medicine* 3(2):e18.

Krieger N. 1992. The making of public health data: Paradigms, politics, and policy. *Journal of Public Health Policy* 13(4):412–427.

Krieger N. 2005. Stormy weather: *Race*, gene expression, and the science of health disparities. *American Journal of Public Health* 95(12):2155–2160.

Krieger N, Chen JT, and Waterman PD. 2005. Painting a truer picture of U.S. socioeconomic and racial/ethnic health inequalities: The public health disparities geocoding project. *American Journal of Public Health* 95(2):312–323.

Krieger N, Northridge M, Gruskin S, Quinn M, Kriebel D, Davey Smith G, Bassett M, Rehkopf DH, and Miller C. 2003. Assessing health impact assessment: Multidisciplinary and international perspectives. *Journal of Epidemiology and Community Health* 57(9):659–662.

Lopez AD, Mathers CD, Ezzati M, Jamison DT, and Murray CJL, Editors. 2006a. *Global Burden of Disease and Risk Factors*. Washington, DC: Oxford University Press and The World Bank.

Lopez AD, Mathers CD, Ezzati M, Jamison DT, and Murray CJL. 2006b. Global and regional burden of disease and risk factors, 2001: Systemic analysis of population health data. *The Lancet* 367(9524):1747–1757.

Marmot M. 2004. Social causes of social inequalities in health. In Anand S, Peter F, and Sen A, Editors. *Public Health, Ethics and Equity*. Oxford: Oxford University Press.

———. 2005. Social determinants of health inequalities. *Lancet* 365(9464):1099–1104.

Mathers CD, Fat DM, Inoue M, Rao C, and Lopez AD. 2005. Counting the dead and what they died from: An assessment of the global status of cause of death data. *Bulletin of the World Health Organization* 83(3):171–177.

McCaw-Binns AM, Fox K, Foster-Williams KE, Ashley DE, and Irons B. 1996. Registration of births, stillbirths and infant deaths in Jamaica. *International Journal of Epidemiology* 25(4):807–813.

Miniño AM, Heron M, and Smith BL. 2006. Deaths: Preliminary data for 2004. *National Vital Statistics Reports* 54(19):1–49.

Ministerio da Saúde, Brasil. 2007. Evoluçao da mortalidade infantil no Brasil. http://portal. saude.gov.br/saude/visualizar_texto.cfm?idtxt=24437. Accessed October 30, 2007.

Modelmog D, Rahlenbeck S, and Trichopoulos D. 1992. Accuracy of death certificates: A population-based complete-coverage one-year autopsy study in East Germany. *Cancer Causes and Control* 3(6):541–546.

Murray CJL, Kulkarni SC, Michaud C, Tomijima N, Bulzacchelli MT, Iandiorio TJ, and Ezzati M. 2006. Eight Americas: Investigating mortality disparities across races, countries, and race-counties in the United States. *PLoS Medicine* 3(9):e260–e271.

Murray CJL and Lopez AD, Editors. 1996. *The Global Burden of Disease: A Comprehensive Assessment of Mortality and Disability from Diseases, Injuries and Risk Factors in 1990 and Projected to 2020*. Cambridge, MA: Harvard School of Public Health/Harvard University Press on behalf of the World Health Organization and the World Bank.

Orenstein WA, Bernier RH, and Hinman AR. 1984. Assessing vaccine efficacy in the field: Further observations. *Epidemiological Reviews* 10:212–241.

Swaroop S. 1960. *Introduction to Health Statistics for the Use of Health Officers, Students, Public Health and Social Workers*. Edinburgh: Livingstone.

UN Department of Economic and Social Affairs. 1973. *The Determinants and Consequences of Population Trends: New Summary of Findings of Interaction of Demographic, Economic and Social Factors*. New York: UN Department of Economic and Social Affairs.

———. 2001. *Principles and Recommendations for Vital Statistics Systems, Revision 2*. New York: United Nations.

———. 2007. *Principles and Recommendations for Population and Housing Censuses, Revision 2.* New York: United Nations.

UNFPA. 2003. Counting the people: Constraining census costs and assessing alternative approaches. In *Population and Development Strategies Number 7.* New York: UNFPA.

UNICEF. 2005. *The 'Rights' Start to Life: A Statistical Analysis of Birth Registration.* New York: UNICEF.

U.S. Census Bureau. 2006. International Data Base Population Pyramids—2000. U.S. Census Bureau—International Database. http://www.census.gov/ipc/www/idb/pyramids. html. Accessed December 18, 2006. Web site updated June 2008.

WHO. 1970. *Spontaneous and Induced Abortion: Report of a WHO Scientific Group.* WHO Technical Report Series No. 461. Geneva: WHO.

———. 1992. *ICD-10: International Statistical Classification of Diseases and Related Health Problems, Tenth Revision and updated version for 2007.* Geneva: WHO.

———. 1993. *International Statistical Classification of Diseases and Related Health Problems, Tenth Revision.* Vol. 2. Geneva: WHO.

———. 2000. *World Health Report 2000. Health Systems: Improving Performance.* Geneva: WHO.

———. 2003. *World Health Report 2003: Shaping the Future.* Geneva: WHO.

———. 2004a. *Maternal Mortality in 2000: Estimates Developed by WHO, UNICEF, and UNFPA.* Geneva: WHO. Updated 2005.

———. 2004b. *World Health Report 2004: Changing History.* Geneva: WHO.

———. 2005. Health System Statistics. Coverage of vital registration of deaths, 1995–2003. In *World Health Statistics 2005.* Geneva: WHO.

———. 2007a. Frequently asked questions about the International Health Regulations (2005). http://www.who.int/csr/ihr/howtheywork/faq/en/index.html#whatis. Accessed June 16, 2007.

———. 2007b. WHO Statistical Information System (WHOSIS). http://www.who.int/whosis/en/index.html. Accessed June 26, 2007.

———. 2007c. New drive to encourage civil registration. http://www.who.int/mediacentre/news/releases/2007/pr57/en/index.html. Accessed November 5, 2007.

———. 2007d. The WHO family of international classifications. http://www.who.int/classifications/en/. Accessed June 26, 2007.

———. 2008. *The Global Burden of Disease: 2004 Update.* Geneva: WHO.

WHO Commission on Social Determinants of Health. 2008. Closing the gap in a generation: Health equity through action on the social determinants of health. Final report of the Commission on Social Determinants of Health. Geneva: WHO.

WHOSIS. 2007. *World Health Statistics 2007.* Geneva: WHO.

Woolsey TD. 1979. Needed development research for measuring the health of populations in the less developed countries. *International Health Planning Methods Series, Volume 10.* Washington, DC: Agency for International Development.

World Bank. 1993. *World Development Report 1993: Investing in Health.* New York: Oxford University Press for the World Bank.

6

Epidemiologic Profiles of Global Health and Disease

Now that we have seen the importance of, and the limits to, data collection, we turn to global, national, and local patterns of health and disease. While all causes of mortality and morbidity have natural histories and pathogenic processes, these causes are often neither natural nor inevitable, but shaped by larger political, economic, and demographic influences.

This chapter examines global health and disease patterns from several perspectives, beginning with an analysis by country, age group, and broad disease categories. We continue with a detailed exploration of specific ailments using a political economy framework, examining communicable and noncommunicable diseases in developing and developed countries. We also analyze some of the broader societal determinants of health and disease patterns.

There are difficulties and drawbacks in the collection of global health data, particularly considering that an estimated two-thirds of deaths are not medically certified. Yet reliable cause-specific disease and death statistics are essential to national and international health policies and planning. For the purposes of this book, we have cited the most accurate data available, whether from routine vital statistics, surveillance systems, disease registries, commissioned surveys, or estimates and projections. Many countries do not have the capacity to keep routine surveillance systems in operation, so they must rely on periodic surveys which are time consuming and expensive. The best solution is to have comprehensive national health information systems for the production of health data and statistics for monitoring purposes, evaluation, and decision making (Boerma and Stansfield 2007).

Before beginning, the reader should review some basic epidemiologic terms that are essential to understanding public health epidemiology (Table 6–1).

Table 6-1 Public Health Epidemiologic Terms

Adjustment	A summarizing procedure for a statistical measure in which the effects of differences in composition of the populations being compared have been minimized by statistical methods. Often performed on rates or relative risks because of differing age distributions in populations that are being compared.
Analytic study	A study designed to examine associations, either putative or hypothesized causal relationships. Usually concerned with identifying or measuring the effects of risk factors or with the health effects of specific exposures.
Association	Statistical dependence between two or more events, characteristics, or other variables. It is present if the probability of occurrence of an event or characteristic, or the quantity of a variable, depends upon the occurrence of one or more other events, the presence of one or more other characteristics, or the quantity of one or more other variables.
Birth rate (crude)	A summary rate based on the number of live births in a population over a given period, usually 1 year. Defined as: $$\frac{\text{Number of live births to residents in an area in a calendar year}}{\text{Average or midyear population in the area in that year}} \times 1{,}000$$
Case fatality rate	The proportion of cases of a specified condition that are fatal within a specified time. Defined as: $$\frac{\text{Number of deaths from a disease (in a given period)}}{\text{Number of diagnosed cases of that disease (in the same period)}} \times 100$$
Census	An enumeration of a population, originally intended for purposes of taxation and military service. See Chapter 5 for further details.
Communicable disease	An illness due to a specific infectious agent or its toxic products; arises through transmission of that agent or its products from an infected person, animal, or reservoir to a susceptible host, either directly or indirectly.
Death rate (crude)	An estimate of the portion of a population that dies during a specified period. The numerator is the number of persons dying during the period; the denominator is the number in the population, usually estimated as the midyear population. Defined as: $$\frac{\text{Number of deaths during a specific period}}{\text{Number of persons at risk of dying during the period}} \times 1{,}000$$
Disability-adjusted life year (DALY)	A measure of the burden of disease on a defined population and the effectiveness of interventions. DALYs are based on adjustment of life expectancy to allow for long-term disability as estimated from official statistics. See Chapter 5.
Endemic disease	The occurrence in a community or region of cases of an illness, specific health-related behavior, or other health-related events clearly in excess of normal expectancy.
Exposure	Proximity or contact with a source of a disease agent in such a manner that effective transmission of the agent or harmful effects of the agent may occur.
Fertility rate	Refined rate measuring production of live offspring; the denominator is restricted to the number of women of childbearing age (i.e., 15–44 or 15–49). Defined as: $$\frac{\text{Number of live births in an area during a year}}{\text{Midyear female population age 15–44 in same area in same year}} \times 1{,}000$$

(*continued*)

Table 6–1 Continued

Incidence	The number of instances of illness commencing, or of persons falling ill, during a given period in a specified population. Compare this to incidence rate: the rate at which new events occur in a population.
	Defined as:
	$$\frac{\text{Number of new events in specified period}}{\text{Number of persons exposed to risk during this period}} \times 10^n$$
Infant mortality rate (IMR)	A measure of the yearly rate of deaths in children less than 1 year old. The denominator is the number of live births in the same year. This is often used as an indicator of the level of health in a community.
	Defined as:
	$$\frac{\text{Number of deaths in a year of children less than 1 year of age}}{\text{Number of live births in the same year}} \times 1,000$$
Life expectancy	The average number of years an individual of a given age is expected to live if current mortality rates continue to apply; i.e., one can have an expectation of life at birth, expectation of life at 50, etc.
Maternal death	Death of a woman while pregnant or within 42 days of termination of a pregnancy, irrespective of the duration and site of pregnancy (i.e., ectopic or not), from any cause related to or aggravated by the pregnancy or its management but not from accidental causes.
MSM	Men who have sex with men (who may or may not self-identify as homosexual).
Notifiable disease	A disease that, by statutory requirements, must be reported to the public health authority in the pertinent jurisdiction when the diagnosis is made; a disease must be deemed of sufficient importance to the public's health to require that it be reported to health authorities.
Observational study	Epidemiologic study that does not involve any intervention, experimental or otherwise. Such a study may be one in which nature is allowed to take its course.
Pandemic	An epidemic occurring worldwide, or over a very wide area, crossing international boundaries, and affecting a large number of people.
Prevalence (rate)	The total number of individuals who have an attribute or disease at a particular time (or during a particular period) divided by the population at risk of having the attribute or disease at this point in time or midway through the period. Problems often arise in defining the time period for the denominator.
Population pyramid	A graphic representation of the age and sex composition of the population, and constructed by computing the percentage distribution of a population, simultaneously cross-classified by age and sex.
Standardization	A set of techniques used to attempt to remove the effects of differences in age or other confounding variables when comparing two ore more populations. The most common method uses weighted averaging of rates specific for age and sex.
Stratification	The process or result of separating a group into several subgroups according to specified criteria, such as age or socioeconomic status. Stratification is used not only to control for confounding effects but also as a way of detecting modifying effects.
Trend	A long-term movement in an ordered series, such as time. An essential feature is that the movement, while possibly irregular in the short term, shows movement consistently in the same direction over the long term.

Source: Last (2001) by permission of Oxford University Press, Inc.

Note: Other health indicators (such as MMR) may be found in Table 5–3. ^{n} Multiplier varies depending on frequency of the condition.

LEADING CAUSES OF MORBIDITY AND MORTALITY

Key Questions:

- Who gets sick and who dies? From what? Where? What are the patterns of mortality across countries? How are they similar or different?
- What are the structural factors causing these patterns of disease?
- What factors make children more susceptible to acute diseases?
- What are some of the underlying causes of high infant mortality in developing countries?

Patterns of disease vary remarkably throughout the world and depend on political, economic, and social contexts as much as on biological susceptibility or climatic conditions. We have chosen three countries to demonstrate the range in causes of death. The countries are grouped according to the income/capita level and redistribution[1] typology developed in Figure 4–6.

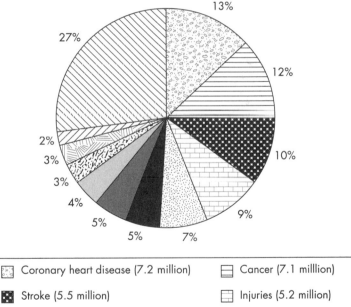

Figure 6–1 Leading causes of death in the world, 2002 (WHOSIS 2007a).

1. High-income/highly redistributive: Denmark
2. Middle-income/partially redistributive: Egypt (formerly marginally redistributive)
3. Low-income/marginally redistributive: Nigeria

Figure 6–1 shows the leading causes of death in the world (without any stratification) reported by the WHO. Even including developing nations, the three leading causes of death are noncommunicable (chronic) conditions: coronary heart disease (CHD), cancer, and stroke (35% combined).

Denmark is a high-income/highly redistributive economy that typifies northern Europe. Denmark has a high degree of economic development, as well as social benefits distributed relatively evenly across all social classes. As a result, life expectancy in Denmark is high (78 years) and the infant and child mortality rates are both below 5 deaths/1,000 live births (among the lowest in the world). Maternal mortality is also low, at 7 deaths/100,000 live births. However, Denmark has a very

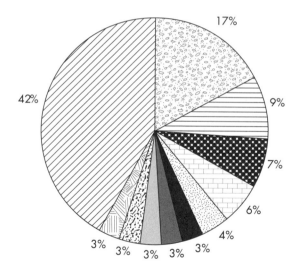

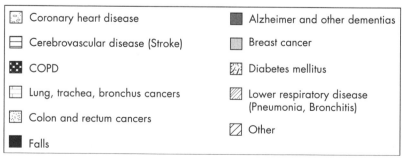

Figure 6–2 Leading causes of death in Denmark, 2002 (WHOSIS 2007a).

high mortality rate from cancer compared to low- and middle-income countries. Figure 6–2 shows a pie chart with the leading causes of death in the country: heart disease, stroke, chronic obstructive pulmonary disease, and cancer.

Egypt is categorized as a middle-income and partially redistributive country. Life expectancy in Egypt is lower than in European countries, at an average of 68 years. The infant and child mortality rates are 25 to 35 deaths/1,000 live births, average for middle-income standards, but still six times higher than Denmark. Maternal mortality is also 10 times higher than in Denmark, at 84 deaths/100,000 live births. Figure 6–3 shows a similar pie chart with the leading causes of death in Egypt: heart disease, stroke, and hypertension. Closely behind are pneumonia (mainly in children), nephritis (from schistosomiasis infection), perinatal conditions, and cirrhosis from chronic hepatitis B infection.

Nigeria is a low-income, marginally redistributive country with very poor health indices. Life expectancy in Nigeria is only 46 years. The infant mortality rate (IMR)

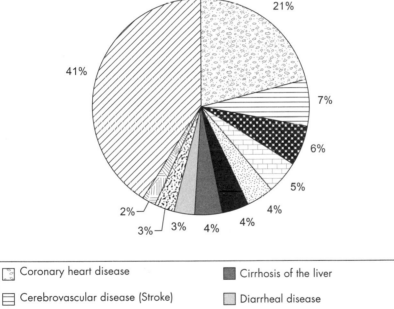

Figure 6–3 Leading causes of death in Egypt, 2002 (WHOSIS 2007a).

is 100 deaths/1,000 live births, and the child mortality rate is 197 deaths/1,000 live births (nearly one child in five dies before his or her fifth birthday). Maternal mortality is extremely high, at 800 deaths/100,000 live births. Figure 6–4 shows the leading killers in Nigeria as all infectious, with HIV/AIDS, malaria, measles, and tuberculosis (TB) combined causing 37% of all deaths. Lower respiratory tract infections and diarrheal diseases contribute another 18%. Over 50% of all causes of death are communicable diseases. Noncommunicable diseases only account for 7% of all deaths.

CHD is present in all countries shown in Figures 6–2 to 6–4. Thus, CHD is not solely a "disease of modernization" or a "disease of rich countries" since it is found in all types of settings.

Mortality inequalities between rich and poor countries exist for both communicable and noncommunicable diseases (see Fig. 6–5) (Gwatkin, Guillot, and Heuveline 1999). In 1990, communicable diseases caused 59% of death and disability among

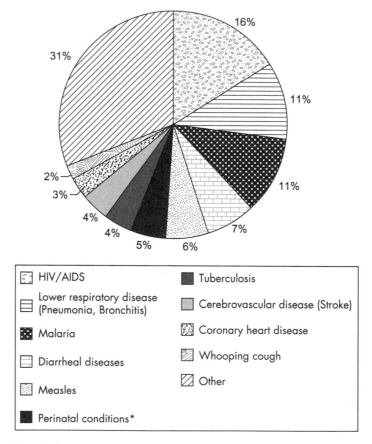

Figure 6–4 Leading causes of death in Nigeria, 2002 (WHOSIS 2007a).

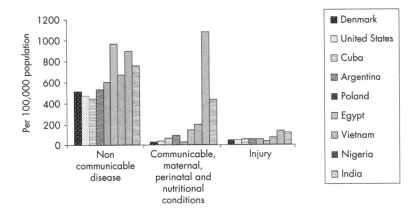

Figure 6–5 Age-standardized mortality rate between selected countries, 2002 (WHOSIS 2007a).

the world's poorest 20%. Among the world's richest, however, noncommunicable diseases caused 85% of death and disability.

The Coming Plagues: Noncommunicable Diseases

In low-income countries, communicable diseases presently result in the highest disability-adjusted life year (DALY) rates over and above noncommunicable diseases and injuries (see Chapter 5 for details). However, noncommunicable diseases are projected to exceed communicable diseases in all income groups by 2015 (Strong et al. 2005).

The consequences of noncommunicable diseases for low-income populations are not well recognized by the international health community. Noncommunicable diseases are often seen as "diseases of the affluent," acquired through poor personal health choices such as smoking, unhealthy diets, and physical inactivity. In reality, noncommunicable diseases are as large a problem in low-income countries, especially among those with fewer resources for pursuing healthy choices.

What will it take to address the growing dominance of noncommunicable disease as a cause of death? Sustained interventions based on primary and secondary prevention have achieved dramatic decreases in heart disease and stroke in countries such as the United States, Japan, and England. It is estimated that in the United States alone, 14 million deaths due to heart disease were averted; more than 30% of the morbidity and 50% of the deaths from noncommunicable diseases are believed attributable to a small number of modifiable "risk factors" (Ezzati et al. 2004). Changing personal risk factors are of course important, such as maintaining a healthy diet, getting regular exercise, and avoiding tobacco. As we shall see in Chapter 7, however, these are not enough. Other larger-scale interventions must be implemented, such as reducing salt in processed food; taxing tobacco products (which simultaneously brings in revenue for local governments);

and increasing the use of disease screening and disease-control measures, as well as medications (many of which are off-patent and very cost-effective) (Epping-Jordan et al. 2005).

Approach to Prevention and Control

The practice of medicine occasionally recognizes the structural determinants of health and illness, but it mainly focuses on biomedical and behavioral prevention and control methods (see Chapter 4). Diet and physical activity are urged to reduce noncommunicable diseases and their precursors (such as obesity), and hand-washing, infant feeding practices, and condom use are recommended to prevent communicable diseases. Biomedical approaches promote medications, immunizations, and other medical interventions, focusing on individuals and specific diseases rather than on the factors affecting multiple diseases simultaneously. International public health, while typically influenced by biomedical and behavioral approaches, also offers the chance to use broad prevention strategies to improve health on a population level.

Prevention activities are often classified as primary, secondary, and tertiary. Primary prevention is undertaken to prevent infection or exposure, avoid the development of disease, and promote overall good health. Some primary prevention measures include immunization, seatbelt use, smoking cessation, condom use, and diet and exercise. Other examples are less intuitive, such as Papanicolaou smear testing (to detect cervical dysplasia or cancer) and fasting lipid panel testing (to measure cholesterol levels). Secondary prevention activities are aimed at early detection of disease to prevent its development. Checking for disease progression through blood pressure monitoring, blood tests, x-rays, or physical examinations is accompanied by treatment or behavioral change measures to stop further development of the disease. Tertiary prevention is similar to disease management and attempts to mitigate the negative effects of, any complications or disability arising from, an illness once a person is diagnosed.

While there is clearly a role for such forms of prevention, they neglect the importance of systematic and structural changes that could prevent illnesses, such as regulating the production and marketing of cigarettes, fast food, or soft drinks; ensuring access to potable water and sanitation systems; enforcing safe work practices and fair remuneration; and providing strong welfare state protections. We discuss how social and political systems affect health in greater depth in Chapters 4, 7, and 13.

Health of Infants and Children

One of the greatest success stories in international health over the past half century has been the dramatic reduction of overall infant and child mortality around the globe. In 1960 there were 20 million deaths of children under the age of 5; by 2006 this had been reduced to 9.7 million (4.8 million in sub-Saharan Africa alone) through improved sanitation, maternal and infant nutrition, vaccination, and primary health care interventions (UNICEF 2008). Despite this progress, the numbers remain appallingly high—equivalent to 26,000 children dying every day, nearly all from preventable causes (see Table 6–2). More than one-third die within the first month of life, usually at home, and without any access to health care. Currently, most deaths in children under the age of 5 occur in only 60 countries and mainly result from treatable or preventable causes such as pneumonia, malaria, measles, diarrhea, and HIV/AIDS.

Between 1960 and 2003, the global childhood mortality rate decreased from 198 deaths/1,000 live births to 72/1,000 (UNICEF 2008). Although rates continue to drop around the world, the gains are not equitably distributed. Advances have been made in many high- and middle-income countries but in low-income countries, especially in sub-Saharan Africa, there has been stagnation and even declines in infant and child mortality relative to the rest of the world (Victora et al. 2003) (see Fig. 6–6). Within many countries, a child from the poorest population group is two to three times more likely to die before his or her fifth birthday than a child from the wealthiest population group; moreover, this gap is widening (WHOSIS 2007b).

Table 6–2 Global Distribution of Cause-Specific Mortality Among Children Under the Age of 5 (2006)

Cause	Deaths	
	Percent	Number in Millions
Lower respiratory tract infections	19	1.8
Diarrheal diseases	17	1.6
Neonatal infections	13	1.3
Preterm birth	10	1.0
Malaria	8	0.8
Birth asphyxia	8	0.8
Measles	4	0.4
Congenital abnormalities	3	0.3
HIV/AIDS	3	0.3
Injuries	3	0.3
Tetanus	2	0.2
Other	10	1.0
Total	100	9.7

Note: Undernutrition is implicated in up to 50% of all deaths in children under 5.

Source: By permission of UNICEF (2008, p. 8).

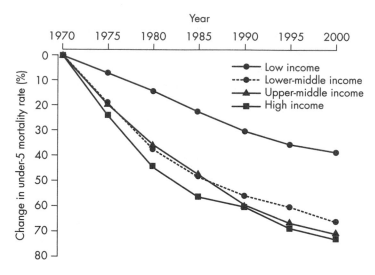

Figure 6–6 Rates of change in under-5 mortality rate by income. *Source*: Reprinted from Victora et al. (2003) with permission from Elsevier.

The IMR is often cited as the most sensitive indicator of a general level of "development" and the state of health of a population. IMRs span a wide range, from 2 deaths/1,000 live births (Iceland) to 165 deaths/1,000 live births (Afghanistan) (see Table 5–7) (WHOSIS 2008). High IMRs reflect underlying inadequacies in socioeconomic and sanitary conditions. Many of the leading causes of infant and child mortality are preventable through structural and redistributive policy approaches.

Malnutrition can increase susceptibility to infectious disease, and is an underlying cause of the majority of child deaths (Black, Morris, and Bryce 2003) (see Fig. 6–7). Chronic undernutrition leads to failure to grow, delayed maturation, impaired learning, and, ultimately, lower productivity in the workforce (see Table 6–3).

A number of childhood illnesses are notable for their short- and long-term effects on child health. Hepatitis B virus (HBV)—which affects 2 billion people globally—is primarily transmitted in utero and during birth (WHO 2008c). Although adults may also become infected with HBV, the earlier a child is exposed to the virus, the higher the likelihood of developing chronic liver conditions later in life. Early exposure to environmental contaminants, such as air pollution, is also associated with early and lifelong health problems. While only 10% of the world's population is under the age of five, this population experiences 40% of the global burden of environmentally related disease (WHO 2007c), leading to at least 3 million child deaths. Chronic obstructive pulmonary disease, asthma, cancers, and fertility problems are some examples of the long-term implications of such exposures.

As with every cause of death, there are multiple levels of causality for child illness and mortality. The immediate cause of death, such as dehydration, may

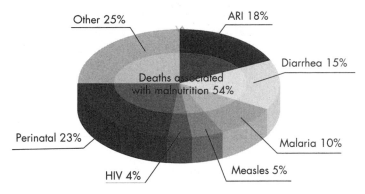

Figure 6–7 Major causes of childhood deaths in developing countries, 2002.
Source: Black, Morris, and Bryce (2003); Adapted from USAID.

Table 6–3 Some Functional Consequences of Deficiency of Selected Micronutrients

Problem	Functional Consequences	Economic Implications
Iodine deficiency in pregnancy and early childhood	Mental retardation	Low educability and diminished productivity
	Growth failure	
	Delayed maturation	
Vitamin A deficiency in early childhood	Blindness	Loss of productivity
	Increased severity of infections	Increased health care costs
	Child mortality	
Iron deficiency anemia in children and adults	Impaired learning	Low educability
	Low work capacity	Loss of productivity
	Low birth weight	Increased health care costs and loss of productivity
	Increased maternal mortality	

appear on a death certificate. Of course, dehydration is determined in large part by living conditions that shape children's health, such as food quality and distribution (including breast milk), exposure to pathogens, water supply, housing stock and neighborhood conditions, and parental educational level. These, in turn, are influenced by the social and political determinants of health (Millard 1994).

According to the conventional public health model, 75% of neonatal and 60% of child deaths could be readily prevented with a set of 20 proven interventions (Bryce, Boschi-Pinto et al. 2005). Examples include providing a skilled attendant at delivery, immunization and antibiotic treatment for pregnant women and newborns, hygienic practices during delivery, and exclusive breast feeding for the first 6 months of life. These interventions focus on the immediate determinants of child and maternal health but fail to address the underlying factors (Lawn et al. 2005). A 2007 review of neonatal intervention packages found that, in most settings, neonatal care was underfunded, lacked a coherent national policy framework, failed to target women before pregnancy, and lacked the comprehensive approach touted as effective for reducing infant mortality (Haws et al. 2007).

In food-insecure areas (such as much of sub-Saharan Africa), breast feeding provides crucial energy, protein, and micronutrients to infants and young children. Early weaning increases malnutrition, morbidity, and death if families cannot afford nutritionally adequate foods for their children. Yet exclusive breast feeding is often impeded by maternal–infant separation for work reasons, maternal illness, or weaning and mixed feeding practices promoted by infant formula companies (see Chapter 9 for details).

Toddlers (aged 12–36 months) are subject to a variety of illnesses, to death related to immature immunological systems, and to dangers in the environment (e.g., indoor pollution). This can create a cycle of disadvantage due to educational and occupational challenges and difficulties in social and physical functioning (Jolly 2007). Interventions to improve child survival include providing potable water, improving sanitation and cooking facilities, and oral rehydration therapy for diarrhea. Of the 60 countries with the highest rates of child mortality, only seven are on track to meet the 2015 targets set by the Millennium Development Goals (Bryce et al. 2003).

Box 6–1 The Health of Children over Five and Young Adults: Unique Realities and Issues

Nearly half the people in the world are under the age of 25, representing the largest youth generation in history (UNFPA 2003). Yet many young persons have few educational and economic opportunities and have limited decision-making capacity. Almost a quarter of the world's youth live in extreme poverty, surviving on less than US$1 a day.

Early education has great consequences on the health and quality of life of young people. For young girls and women, there are particularly important benefits in early education that permit expanded life options beyond child bearing and marriage. Although there is a global increase in access to education for girls at all levels (UNFPA 2003), in many developing countries, less than half of all children continue as far as secondary school, and there is evidence of a sharp decline in female attendance after primary school.

Employment also has an important and direct impact on the quality of life of young people. Worldwide, an estimated 352 million children aged 5 to 17 were working in 2000, most illegally, and nearly 171 million in hazardous conditions (UNFPA 2003). In many developing countries, gender discrimination in education and employment results in higher unemployment among young women.

Many adolescents and youth do not have the ability or social support to delay the age of sexual debut, negotiate safer sex, or protect themselves against unintended pregnancy and sexually transmitted infections. Many countries have inadequate or nonexistent sexual health education programs for youth, limited sexual and reproductive health services, and laws that prohibit providing contraceptive methods to young people or to unmarried women. Globally, half of all HIV infections occur in people aged 15 to 24. Each day an estimated 6,000 youth become infected with HIV/AIDS, the majority of them young women (UNFPA 2003).

Health of Adults

The health of adults (defined by WHO as persons aged 25–60) is distinct from that of children and the elderly because adults typically have greater immunity and recover more readily from acute communicable illnesses. Conversely, adults face more chronic health problems. Rates of many noncommunicable (and some communicable) diseases are much higher in adults than among children (e.g., cancers, cardiovascular disease, and tuberculosis).

Adults form the economic backbone of all countries, but their health typically elicits little attention from policymakers and planners. Few health ministries focus on the main causes of adult deaths; indeed, a landmark book on the subject identified an adult health policy vacuum (Feachem et al. 1990). Yet, as noted in the previous chapter, the decline in life expectancy in some parts of sub-Saharan Africa and Eastern Europe is largely a result of increasing adult illness and death (from HIV and TB, respectively).

Adult deaths, illnesses, injuries, and disabilities reduce productivity and family income. In addition, many adult illnesses are chronic (long-term) and place heavy social and financial burdens on health services and caregivers. As the proportion of adults increases in populations worldwide, greater attention must be given to the prevention and control of adult health problems.

Box 6–2 Disability

WHO estimates that 10% of the global population lives with a disability. Because definitions of disability are shaped by cultural and societal factors, the term impairment is also used, defined as the point at which a person faces "problems in body function or structure," which may be physical, mental, and/or intellectual in nature. In contrast to disability, which may be a result of a confluence of factors—medical, physical, and environmental, primarily determined by discrimination, stigma, and exclusion on a societal level—impairment is more measurable and discrete (WHO 2007j). For example, while a person may be impaired by the loss of a limb or through congenital blindness, these impairments only become disabilities if she or he cannot fully participate in society. Technologies and medical interventions may alleviate impairments, but disabilities are only countered through social change (Durham 2002).

Poverty is both a cause and consequence of disability; 80% of the population with disabilities live in low-income countries, and it is estimated that 20% of the world's poorest people live with disabilities (Thomas 2005). Throughout the world, persons living with disabilities face social exclusion and disadvantages in accessing health and rehabilitation services, and are more likely to be unemployed (WHO 2006e).

People living with disabilities are often in need of specialized rehabilitation programs and therapy. While such interventions can help alleviate some economic and social difficulties, many developing countries do not have the resources to provide such care. For example, in low- and middle-income countries, only 5% to 15% of persons in need of assistive devices (e.g., wheelchairs, hearing aids, prosthetics) have access to them. Furthermore, the devices that are available are frequently of poor quality and prohibitively expensive (WHO 2007b).

International health and development reports rarely explicitly mention disability. Human rights groups are attempting to change this by advocating for greater recognition of disability in international health.

Aging

A "demographic transition" is underway as populations live longer and often healthier lives. In 2000, 600 million people were aged 60 or older, and by 2050, this number will likely grow to 2 billion, with over 80% residing in developing countries. Figure 6–8 shows the predicted growth of the population pyramid between 2002 and 2025, with much of the proportional growth in the groups over age 50. Aging populations are a result of factors such as improvements in health and its determinants throughout the life course, and decreased fertility rates (WHO 2007p).

Aging populations have particular health needs. Many elderly persons have long-term care problems, such as cardiovascular disease or physical impairments, which necessitate continual management as well as measures to prevent further illness (i.e., tertiary prevention). The major health conditions of older people include (WHO 2002a):

- cardiovascular (coronary heart/cerebrovascular) disease;
- hypertension;
- diabetes;
- cancer;
- chronic obstructive pulmonary disease;
- musculoskeletal conditions (arthritis and osteoporosis);
- mental health conditions (dementia and depression); and
- blindness and visual impairment.

Older persons have higher rates of morbidity owing in large part to accumulated life factors that determine illness, such as exposure to environmental toxins or

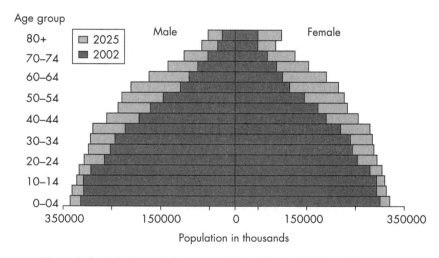

Figure 6–8 Global population pyramid in 2002 and 2025 (WHO 2002a).

poor nutrition. Physical and social environments not supportive of aging contribute to increased health problems, such as falls and depression. Physical and mental impairments—new and exacerbated—are more common among aging populations.

The extent to which adults are able to age with health and dignity largely depends on the same societal and cultural factors that determine lifelong health trajectories and influence the level of care and social support elderly people receive. These include family structure, retirement age and benefits, accessibility of transit systems and infrastructure, and opportunities to engage in mentally and physically stimulating activities.

Sexually Transmitted Infections

Sexually transmitted infections (STIs), also referred to as sexually transmitted diseases (STDs), include viral, bacterial, and parasitic infections transmitted through sex and primarily, although not exclusively, affecting the genitalia and reproductive organs. Some of the most common STIs are:

- syphilis;
- gonorrhea;
- chlamydia;
- herpes simplex virus (HSV);
- human papilloma virus (HPV);
- HIV; and
- pubic lice.

Each year, over 340 million people aged 19 to 44 are infected with one of the first four STIs listed above, with the highest rates in urban areas (WHO 2001a). STIs are the main preventable cause of infertility among women due to chronic, undiagnosed infection, and can lead to adverse perinatal conditions, such as congenital disability and blindness, as well as to increased maternal mortality (WHO 2006c). STIs also increase exposure to HIV through open sores or abrasions.

STIs are largely preventable through barrier methods of protection (e.g., condoms) during sexual activity. However, these methods are not always available or appropriate. The spread of STIs is largely determined by factors beyond choice of contraception, such as commercial sex, forced sex, migrant labor, gender disparities, and an overall lack of access to health services.

Most bacterial STIs are curable through short-course antibiotic therapy, and many viral STIs can be managed through medication and improvements in immunologic status. Factors such as stigma, cost, and availability of services often inhibit people from seeking diagnosis and/or treatment.

Box 6-3 Injecting Drug Use

Substance use and abuse can have acute and long-term detrimental effects on health, such as reduced memory and cognitive function, organ damage, and increased acute injury rates as a result of impaired perceptive capabilities and reflexes. There are an estimated 13 million injecting drug users globally (United Nations Office on Drugs and Crime 2004). Many viral infections are spread through injecting drug use (IDU). Outside of sub-Saharan Africa, 30% of new HIV infections are attributed to IDU (Csete and Wolfe 2007) and in some regions, 80% of HIV infections are due to needle sharing (United Nations Office on Drugs and Crime 2004). Currently, 180 million people (3% of the world's population) are estimated to be infected with hepatitis C virus (HCV), an incurable viral infection transmitted largely through IDU and nonsterile medical injections that can lead to liver cirrhosis and cancer (WHO 2007o). Some HCV transmission may also occur through sex, from mother-to-child in utero, and from blood transfusions. Hepatitis B virus (HBV) is another liver infection that is commonly spread via unsterilized, reused needles and syringes, either in the health care setting or during "recreational" drug use. Although generally transmitted congenitally (and not related to IDU), growing rates of hepatitis B among injection drug users pose a concern in many countries (WHO 2008c).

Addressing IDU and related health effects is complex because the behavior is often illegal and highly stigmatized. Some countries (Britain and Holland) and local municipalities (Vancouver, Canada) have responded by providing injecting drug users with safe injection locations, clean needles and disposal facilities, drug replacement therapy, and nursing and addiction counseling staff. These practices—known as harm reduction strategies—have reduced the spread of disease via shared needles as well as many adverse health effects of IDU. However, many people oppose these practices. The United States is the only government in the world to ban federal funding of needle exchange programs (Csete and Wolfe 2007). Still, some needle exchange programs do exist in the United States, most often funded through private or nonprofit foundations.

Box 6-4 Dental Health

Dental diseases are a major public health concern in most of the world's underdeveloped countries (Dickson 2006). Common problems include dental caries, periodontal (gum) disease (such as gingivitis), tooth loss, oral mucosal lesions and oropharyngeal cancers, HIV-related diseases, and trauma to the teeth as a result of violence, road accidents, unsafe sports, and falls. In industrialized countries, most adults, and 60% to 90% of school-aged children, are affected by dental caries (Petersen et al. 2005). Globally, up to one in five middle-aged adults suffers from severe periodontal (gum) disease. Almost half (40% to 50%) of people living with HIV/AIDS suffer from oral fungal, bacterial, or viral infections (WHO 2007n).

Throughout the world, problems with oral health remain common among underprivileged groups (Petersen et al. 2005; Dickson 2006). Increased consumption of prepackaged commercial foods containing refined sugars, insufficient exposure to fluorides, the prohibitive cost of tooth brushes and dental visits, and poor access to preventive dental care all contribute to this rise.

Despite an increasing need for dental care in low-income countries, the density of dentists is abysmal, with an average of 0.08 dentists/1,000 people in Southeast Asia and 0.03 in Africa, compared with 0.6 dentists/1,000 people in Europe (WHOSIS 2008). In developed countries, dentists remain financially inaccessible to many. In the United States, for instance, poor and near-poor children, regardless of race or ethnic group, have half the chance of receiving preventive dental visits compared to those in middle- or high-income brackets (Watson, Manski, and Macek 2001; Centers for Disease Control and Prevention 2002).

Various health issues are related to a person's sex and/or gender. As discussed in Chapter 7, gender is a social category relating to the roles assigned to men and women, whereas sex is a biological category, distinguished by physical and genetic characteristics. Here we explore the health determinants and status of men and women, which are expressions of both sex and gender differences.

Women's Health

Women in many societies have limited economic and social power, attain lower levels of education than men, and lack legal autonomy. These factors combine to maintain women's disadvantaged social position and result in gender-specific health problems. Violations of health and human rights resulting from unequal power relations include early and coerced onset of sexual activity, early marriage, domestic violence, bride-burning and dowry deaths, high rates of STIs, including HIV/AIDS, sexual trafficking, sexual violence and coercion, and female genital cutting (Willis and Levy 2003; UNFPA 2003). Women also experience higher rates of certain occupational diseases and deaths due to gendered work patterns and unequal power in the workplace.

Although women generally have greater life expectancy than men, they tend to have more illnesses and physical disabilities, as discussed in Chapter 7. For reproductive-age women in developing countries, almost one-fifth of illnesses and deaths are pregnancy related, and more than one woman dies every minute (529,000/year) due to maternal causes (primarily hemorrhage, infection, eclampsia [seizures], obstructed labor, complications from abortion, and ectopic pregnancy) (WHO 2005c).

Of all the health statistics monitored by the WHO, maternal mortality shows the largest discrepancy between developed and developing countries (see Fig. 6–9). Lack of proper infrastructure for prenatal care, poor resource allocation, and a low priority given to women's health result in enormous deficiencies in maternal health care and low presence of skilled birth attendants for delivery and postpartum care in low-income countries (see Fig. 6–10). In Africa, women have a lifetime risk of 1 in 20 of dying from pregnancy-related causes, while in Asia (excluding Japan) it is 1 in 94. By contrast, in developed countries the risk is 1 in 2,000 (WHO 2004c). India alone has more maternal deaths each week than all of Europe has in a year (WHO 2005c).

Barriers to obtaining prenatal and obstetric services include distance from health services, cost (direct fees for medical services as well as the cost of transportation, drugs, and supplies), and women's lack of decision-making power within the family. Three main types of care are essential for pregnant women:

- *Antenatal care*: the percentage of women who seek care during their pregnancies at least once is 63% in Africa, 65% in Asia, and 73% in Latin America and the Caribbean (WHO 2005c).
- *Perinatal care* (during childbirth): almost half of all births in developing countries take place without the assistance of a skilled birth attendant, such as a doctor

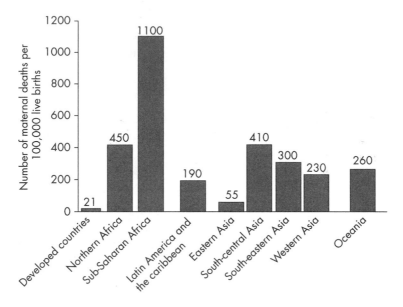

Figure 6–9 Estimates of maternal mortality ratios (UN Secretary General 2001).

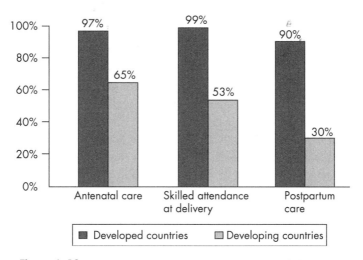

Figure 6–10 Coverage of maternal health services (WHO 1997).

or midwife. A skilled birth attendant is the major factor in reducing maternal mortality (WHO 2005c).

• *Postpartum care*: care after delivery can prevent life-threatening infections and provide support on issues such as breast feeding and birth spacing. The majority of women in developing countries receive no postpartum care.

Poorly performed abortions are an important cause of maternal mortality. Approximately 50 million unwanted pregnancies are ended annually (WHO 2005c). Many abortions are performed in an unsafe manner, largely because women have no access to safe procedures or appropriate treatment for complications. Unsafe abortions cause up to 50% of maternal deaths in some areas (99% of which occur in developing countries) primarily sub-Saharan Africa and Asia (Family Care International 2003). Abortion is legal without restriction in most countries in North America and Europe, and in Cambodia, Cape Verde, China, Guyana, Puerto Rico, Singapore, South Africa, Cuba, the Democratic People's Republic of Korea, Mongolia, Nepal, and Vietnam, as well as in some cities, such as Mexico City (Center for Reproductive Rights 2007).

Another leading cause of maternal death is preventable infections resulting from poor hygiene, primarily in the health care delivery setting, and contamination during childbirth. Although sanitary delivery measures have been practiced for over 150 years in many parts of the world (and have led to a dramatic decrease in maternal mortality), many women still die from these complications.

Women's health is not only linked to reproductive issues, but also to efforts to improve the health, nutritional status, and general well-being of girls and women from infancy through childhood and into the adult years. The health of families is also strongly related to the mother's level of educational attainment and her level of income (UNDP: Gender Unit 2005). Initiatives such as micro credit loans have given some women the means to support their families, but universal education and social security measures have proven much more successful. Child health, and gender and health, will be discussed further in Chapters 7 and 13.

Box 6–5 Mental Health of Adults

Mental health is an immense yet neglected aspect of international health, partly due to the stigma surrounding it, the concentration of mental illnesses in marginalized populations, and difficulties in measurement. One in four people experience a mental health problem at some point during their lifetime (WHO 2001b); 154 million people are estimated to suffer from depression, 106 million from drug and alcohol use disorders, and 25 million from schizophrenia. Mental illness is disproportionately borne by the poor and marginalized, largely due to accumulated lifelong stressors such as precarious living conditions, economic insecurity, social isolation, experiences of oppression and exploitation, as well as lack of health care and social support.

Appropriate mental health services are unavailable in over 30% of countries (WHO 2001b). Not only are mental health care resources scarce, they are inequitably distributed (Saxena et al. 2007). Despite high levels of mental illness in low-income countries, little is spent on care and available services are often institutionally based.

Mental health problems—especially suicide—often accompany other illnesses, particularly noncommunicable diseases. Over 877,000 people commit suicide each year (WHO 2007m). Even though women attempt suicide more often than men, the completed suicide rate is 3.5 times higher among men (WHO 2002b). Mental health disorders affect many aspects of life, including the ability to work productively, engage in community and family events, and enjoy leisure activities. For the family and caregivers of a person suffering from a mental health disorder, care is often complicated by stigma and inadequate social support.

Men's Health

The principal health problems of men have been well studied, perhaps mainly because most prominent health researchers and policy makers are men. They experience higher rates of mortality than women and are overrepresented in many illness categories such as cardiovascular disease, HIV/AIDS (except in Africa), and physical injury.

While some illnesses can be attributed to (biological) sex (e.g., only men can have prostate cancer), many of these differences are a result of gender roles. Men's roles as primary breadwinners in numerous societies may lead them to travel and work in dangerous and/or stressful settings, and result in illness and/or injury. Men smoke, drink alcohol, and engage in armed conflict more than women (accounting for reported injury rates being three times higher in men than in women) (WHO 2002c) and experience more violent deaths and deaths related to smoking and alcohol consumption. In 2000, of the 4.2 million preventable deaths related to tobacco use, 3.4 million occurred in men (WHO 2003).

Lesbian, Gay, Bisexual, and Transgender Health Issues

Lesbian, gay, bisexual, and transgendered (LGBT) populations have particular health concerns that deserve attention. In many societies, these communities fear being identified as homosexual because this may lead to stigma, violence, abuse, or death. Until 1990, homosexuality was listed as a mental disorder by the WHO. At least 40 countries criminalize same-sex behavior in both men and women, and an additional 35 criminalize it solely for men. In many Muslim societies, both civil law and shari'a law criminalize homosexual activity. Police abuse of LGBT people is common in many countries.

For LGBT populations, health concerns go well beyond specific needs, such as reproductive health or surgical services. Societal homophobia (discrimination and prejudice toward persons based on their sexual orientation) and heterosexism (the favoring of heterosexual persons and behaviors) combine to jeopardize LGBT health through discrimination in housing and employment (which in turn affects the ability to purchase food, shelter, and health care); lack of social security benefits (limiting financial security and the ability to obtain health insurance and other social services); harassment and stress (which may provoke mental health and/or substance abuse problems); isolation (which may lead to depression); physical abuse and violence; and imprisonment.

Health of Indigenous Populations

Over 300 million people (approximately 5% of the world's population) identify themselves as indigenous; those who, according to J. Martinez Cobo, have a "historical continuity with preinvasion and precolonial societies that developed on their territories, consider themselves distinct from other sectors of the societies now prevailing in those territories, or parts of them" (UNESCO 2006, p. 10).

Across the world, indigenous groups consistently experience higher mortality rates and worse health than nonindigenous populations (see Table 6–4). In Canada, First Nations communities have higher prevalence rates of heart disease (1.5 times greater), diabetes (3–5 times greater), and TB (8–10 times greater) than the general

Table 6–4 Selected Indigenous Populations and Related Health Indicators

Area of the World/ Indigenous Group (year of statistics)	Estimated Numbers of Indigenous People[a]	As % of Total Population	Selected Health Disparities
China (2007)	100 million[b]	7.6	Under-5 mortality rate National average: 39.7/1,000 Xuar: 65.4/1,000
India (2001)	84.3 million	8.2	IMR National average: 65/1,000 Kuttiya Kandhs: 200/1,000
Mexico (2001)	12–13 million	12–13	Life expectancy National average: 74 Indigenous population: 69
Guatemala (2004)	7.2 million	66	IMR National average: 40/1,000 Indigenous population (Alta Verapaz): 192/1,000
Bolivia (2004)	5.7 million	71	IMR Nonindigenous population: 54/1,000 Quechua: 81/1,000
United States (2005)	2.9 million	1	IMR National average: 6.8/1,000 American Indians & Alaska Natives: 8.5/1,000
Canada (2001)	1.1 million	4.1	Life expectancy (males) National average: 77.1 First Nations: 70.4
Brazil (2000)	332,000	0.2	IMR National average: 31/1,000 Xavante: 106/1,000
New Zealand (2001)	590,000	15.4	IMR National average: 4/1,000 Maori: 8.6/1,000
Australia (2005)	501,236	2.4	Life expectancy (females) National average: 77 Indigenous: 59

(continued)

Table 6–4 Continued

Area of the World/ Indigenous Group	Estimated Numbers of Indigenous People[a]	As % of Total Population	Selected Health Disparities
Cambodia (1998)	101,000[b]	0.9	N/A
			N/A
Pygmy/Batwa	400,000, mostly in Central Africa		N/A
Democratic Republic of Congo (2000)	270,000	0.5	N/A
Burundi (2000)	40,000	0.6	N/A
Cameroon (2000)	34,000	0.2	N/A
Rwanda (2000)	28,000	0.2	N/A
Central African Republic (2000)	20,000	0.5	IMR
			National average: 9.8%
			Aka: 20% to 22%
Congo-Brazzaville (2000)	20,000	0.7	N/A
Uganda (2000)	4,000	0.02	IMR
			National average: 9.7%
			Twa: 20% to 21%
Inuit	167,000, worldwide		
United States (1998)	57,000	0.02	
Canada (1998)	50,000	0.17	Life expectancy (females)
			National average: 82.2
			Inuit: 70.2
			Life expectancy (males)
Greenland (1998)	50,000	90	Greenland: 66
Denmark (1998)	8,000	0.15	Denmark: 76
Russia (1998)	1,700	0.1	Unknown

[a]Counts of indigenous populations may be inaccurate due to censuses that do not distinguish among ethnic groups and differences in identification of indigenous populations. For example, while some populations are classified as indigenous based on language, others rely on self-identification. As well, various ethnic groups fall under the term indigenous within a country. In Canada, the term "Aboriginal peoples" encompasses Inuit, First Nations, and Métis (people of mixed European and indigenous ancestry), while in Ecuador, indigenous groups are distinguished from the mestizo population (who are descendants of mixed European and indigenous heritage).

[b]Historically, these national governments have denied the presence of indigenous groups.

Sources: African Commission on Human and Peoples' Rights and International Work Group on Indigenous Affairs (2005); Anderson et al. (2006); Bjerregaard et al. (2004); Castro, Erviti, and Leyva (2007); Central Intelligence Agency (2007); Government of Cambodia (1998); Government of Canada (2001, 2005); Government of India (2001); Human Rights in China and Minority Rights Group International (2007); Indian Health Service (2006); Montenegro and Stephens (2006); Ohenjo et al. (2006); Statistics New Zealand (2001); Stephens et al. (2006); Trewin and Madden (2005); UNICEF (2007); United Nations (2000); United States Census Bureau (2005); WHO (2007g).

population (Health Canada 2000; 2006). In the United States, mortality rates for indigenous peoples are 533% greater for TB and 249% greater for diabetes than in the general population (PAHO 2002). Most telling is the enormous life expectancy differential: Canadian indigenous peoples have a life expectancy 7 years shorter than the nonindigenous population, while in Australia there is a 20-year gap (Government of Canada 2005; Trewin and Madden 2005).

Social inequalities in health between indigenous peoples and dominant groups are related to historic colonization processes and to the ongoing practices of social, economic, political, and cultural oppression. While other groups (e.g., the working class, women, LGBT groups) share certain aspects of this oppression, among indigenous populations and slave descendants, the effects are compounded over time owing to the loss of historic majority and the profound effects of colonization on their spiritual and material ways of life.

Between one-third and one-half of indigenous inhabitants of the Americas were killed in the colonial invasions of the 16th and 17th centuries by warfare, forced labor, and infectious disease epidemics. While these extremely high death rates have been attributed to the fact that previously unexposed, "virgin," indigenous populations were exposed to new diseases, this mortality was also the result of the military, economic, and social aspects of the colonial conquest (McCaa 1995; Cook 1998; Alchon 2003), including loss of means of subsistence, cultural practices, and social systems. In some places, indigenous populations such as the Taino of Cuba and the Beothuk of Newfoundland, Canada, were entirely wiped out.

Descendants of African slaves in North America, Brazil, the Caribbean, and elsewhere have also experienced unspeakable loss of freedom, social disruption, death and sickness, and physical and psychological abuse (Jones 1999). Nonetheless, the legacy is not uniform across regions: slave descendants comprise the majority population in some countries and have realized important sociopolitical gains (e.g., in Barbados), whereas in other settings (e.g., the United States), there is reified racial discrimination and persistent "embodied" oppression, as among indigenous populations (see Chapter 7). Mainstream public health authorities and researchers typically seek biomedical and behavioral explanations for the health inequalities between indigenous and nonindigenous groups, citing genetic and dietary differences, different rates of mental health disorders, and supposed differences in proclivity to violence. Recently, increasing attention has focused on socioeconomic factors, including poor living conditions, substandard schools, chronic unemployment, and persistent discrimination.

DISEASE TYPOLOGIES

Key Questions:

- How can we move beyond traditional categories used in population health?
- What are the underlying causes of diarrheal diseases worldwide?

- What measures must be taken to reduce malaria and other marginalization diseases in low-income countries?
- What is leading to soaring rates of Type II diabetes?
- What are the primary determinants of the spread of drug-resistant TB around the world?
- Are the factors leading to the transmission of HIV more biologic, social, or economic?

While dichotomies of developed/developing and communicable/noncommunicable disease offer a useful snapshot of different disease patterns across the world, these fail to fully explain the complexity of the factors influencing and underpinning the health–disease process in a global context.

The epidemiological transition (see Chapter 2) assumes a one-way path of industrialization and "progress." However, as evidenced in settings as varied as the former Soviet Union (where deindustrialization has led to a resurgence of preventable infectious diseases such as diphtheria) and the U.S. state of Mississippi (where, despite the United States being classified as "developed," infant mortality rates have climbed in recent years), patterns of health and disease and their determinants may follow complex pathways. The emergence of various infectious diseases (e.g., SARS) and the increased predominance of some health concerns (e.g., road deaths) also demonstrate the fallacy of assuming a one-way trajectory of improvement of health patterns. This chapter uses the following typology to describe patterns of health and illness, one that differs from the standard communicable/noncommunicable disease dichotomy:

- diseases (ailments) of marginalization and deprivation;
- diseases of modernization and work; and
- diseases of marginalization and modernization.

Because the quality of much international morbidity data is poor, this chapter focuses more on mortality patterns, while recognizing the importance of morbidity to population health.

Diseases of Marginalization and Deprivation

Many diseases occur primarily as a result of marginalization and deprivation—that is, extreme poverty, substandard living conditions, geographic isolation, and political oppression. Many, if not all, of these ailments have been nearly eliminated in developed countries and among the elite. For example, it is rare for a rich person to fall ill from cholera, Chagas disease, or even TB, whether in Mali or Luxembourg. Yet a broad swath of people face a range of diseases that are largely, if not wholly, preventable and controlled in societies with universal social welfare provisions, including some developing countries. These ailments often result from exposure to pathogens and toxins in contaminated water, air, food, and physical environments. Populations living in chronic poverty—who lack social benefits and healthy environments—not only face greater exposure to pathogens and toxins, but are also more susceptible and less resistant to illness due to compromised immune systems from conditions such as malnutrition. They are therefore more likely to become ill or disabled, to remain sick longer, and to die earlier.

Diarrhea

Diarrhea can result from infection, or from the effects of a pathogen's toxin on the body. There are approximately 4 billion cases of diarrhea throughout the world every year, causing 2.2 million deaths (4% of all deaths). Globally it is the leading cause of death among children. Although deaths from diarrhea have fallen dramatically over the past 40 years, the number of cases has remained constant (and high), at over three episodes per year for children living in developing countries (Kosek, Bern, and Guerrant 2003).

Box 6–6 Cholera

Cholera occurs in pandemic waves, often related to conflict, displacement, and weather and climate changes, all of which alter living patterns and access to potable water and sanitation. The current (eighth) pandemic of cholera began in Southeast Asia in the early 1990s and spread to Latin America through the discharged ballast of a ship, killing tens of thousands of people (see Fig. 6–11). In Peru alone, there have been over 1 million identified cases and over 10,000 deaths. In 2005, there were 131,943 cases of cholera and 2,272 deaths reported globally, 58% occurring in West Africa. However, these numbers are likely underestimates, given the difficulty in accurately diagnosing each episode of diarrhea and the fear of trade- and travel-related sanctions (WHO 2006a).

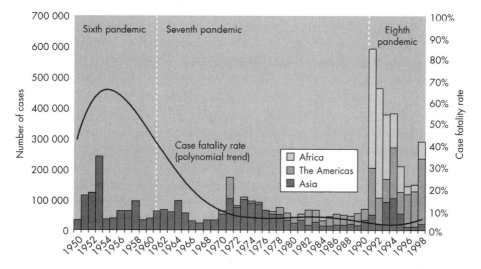

Figure 6–11 Reported number of cholera cases and case fatality rates, 1950–1998 (WHO 2000, p. 41).

Mass diarrheal infection often results from large-scale contamination of a common water source, such as a river. The lack of adequate facilities to dispose of and treat human waste increases the likelihood of widespread infection, as does using contaminated water to prepare food and consuming raw foods that have not been peeled. Bottle-feeding with powdered milk or formula mixed with bacteria-laden water may lead to the death of infants very quickly. Leading diarrhea-causing agents are listed in Table 6–5.

The main determinants of diarrhea are structural factors such as water quality and level of sanitation, as well as overall health-promoting and immune-boosting determinants, such as sufficient food of good quality and overall health status since birth (Werner and Sanders 1997). Thus, persons with suppressed or weakened immune systems, particularly those infected with HIV, are more susceptible to frequent diarrhea.

Because the agents of diarrhea are generally found in food and drink, it is theoretically possible to prevent many diarrheal diseases. Preventive measures can be undertaken at the individual level by changing biology (immunization) or behavior

Table 6–5 Some Enteric Agents that Can Cause Acute or Chronic Diarrhea

Viruses
  Rotaviruses
  Norwalk-like agents
Bacteria
  Campylobacter jejuni
  Clostridium difficile
  Escherichia coli: enterotoxigenic, enteropathogenic, enterohemorrhagic, or enteroinvasive
  Salmonella species
  Shigella species
  Vibrio species, including *V. cholerae* and *V. parahemolyticus*
  Yersinia enterocolitica
Protozoa
  Entamoeba histolytica
  Cryptosporidium parvum
  Cyclospora species
  Giardia lamblia
  Balantinium coli
Helminthes (worms)
  Ascaris lumbricoides (roundworm)
  Strongyloides stercoralis
  Taenia solium (pork tapeworm)
  Trichuris trichiuria (whipworm)

(education and training); at the community level (collective organization); or at the environmental level (water supply). Improved access to clean water and to sanitary disposal of waste are the cornerstones of diarrheal disease control by environmental means. An important intervention against diarrheal illness, and many other child-hood diseases, is the promotion of exclusive breast feeding.

Oral rehydration therapy (ORT) has proven an effective treatment that has saved the lives of many, perhaps millions, of children in developing countries since WHO approved its use in 1969. ORT replaces lost fluids orally rather than intravenously. It is cheap, relatively simple, requires only basic training, can be done at home by parents or even older siblings, and involves no time delay. But, this method requires clean water, something often not available in areas with high diarrhea rates.

Measures such as ORT, education regarding sanitary practices and, for a few pathogens such as rotaviruses and cholera, newly developed vaccines, may contribute to the control of diarrheal diseases. In the long run, serious reductions in illness and death are likely to occur only after there have been substantial improvements in social and economic conditions and basic betterment of the living standards of the world's disadvantaged populations. An example of effective reduction of diarrheal disease mortality is found in Cuba, where concerted public health programs have improved sanitation and nutrition, promoted breast feeding, provided medical care, and educated the public since 1963. As a result, reported rates of acute diarrheal disease mortality in infants fell from 12.9 deaths/1,000 live births in 1962 to 0.3/1,000 in 1993, while in the same period reported diarrheal mortality rates among 1- to 4-year-olds went from 6.4 to 0.1 deaths/10,000 (Riverón Corteguera 1995; Werner and Sanders 1997).

Neglected Tropical Diseases

Some diseases no longer attract world headlines, and have largely been ignored, although they still pose an enormous burden on people living in poverty, mainly in tropical and subtropical areas of the world (Ehrenberg and Ault 2005). Due to strong lobbying by Médecins Sans Frontières (MSF), among others, many diseases are now referred to as "neglected tropical diseases," or NTDs. The term "neglected" is used because most countries are not required to report the prevalence of these diseases; they occur below the threshold of surveillance and detection, usually not developing into immediate health crises. Yet at least 1 billion people suffer from at least one NTD (see Table 6–6). Usually the populations most afflicted are also the poorest and most vulnerable—minority populations, indigenous groups, infants, the elderly, migrant workers, and slum dwellers—leading some to argue that it is people, rather than diseases that are neglected. NTDs are among the most common infections in the estimated 2.7 billion people who live on less than US$2/day.

The main determinants of NTDs are nonpotable water, poor sanitation and hygienic practices, and lack of access to health care services. In aggregate, NTDs cause approximately 534,000 deaths annually, a relatively low toll, yet their impact

Table 6–6 Descriptions of "Neglected Tropical Diseases"

Neglected Tropical Disease	Global Prevalence (Millions)/Population at Risk (Millions)	Description
Buruli ulcer	ND/ND	• Caused by bacterial infection • Most frequent near waterways • Leads to destruction of skin and soft tissue and long-term aesthetic and functional disability
Chagas disease	8–9/25	• Caused by infection via Triatominae insects, transfusion of infected blood, or mother-to-child transmission • Causes 13,000 deaths/year • Leads to lymphatic and organ infection, including fatal heart and digestive tract infection
Dengue/dengue hemorrhagic fever	ND/ND	• Viral infection transmitted through mosquito bites • Leads to flu-like symptoms, hemorrhage, convulsions • Causes 21,000 deaths/year
Dracunculiasis (guinea worm)	0.01/ND	• Parasitic infection by ingesting water containing guinea worm larvae • 11,000 cases reported in 2005, all in sub-Saharan Africa • Leads to intestinal and skin infection, rarely fatal
Endemic treponematoses (yaws, pinta, endemic syphilis)	ND/ND	• Transmitted through bacterial infection by contact with the skin of an infected person • Cause lesions and eventual deformities of the skin, cartilage, and bones • Rarely fatal, but can lead to permanent disfiguration
African trypanosomiasis (sleeping sickness)	0.3/60	• Parasitic protozoa infection via bite of a tsetse fly • Found only in sub-Saharan Africa • Leads to fatigue, damage to lymphatic system, spleen, neurological, and endocrine system • Causes 50,000 deaths/year, due to coma
Human leishmaniasis	12/350	• Parasitic infection through sandfly bites • Approximately 2 million new cases/year • Causes 59,000 deaths/year • Leads to skin lesions, soft tissue deterioration, and organ inflammation

(continued)

Table 6–6 Continued

Neglected Tropical Disease	Global Prevalence (Millions)/Population at Risk (Millions)	Description
Leprosy	0.4/ND	• Transmitted through human-to-human contact • 410,000 new cases/year; 4,000 deaths/year • Causes infection of skin, nerves, and mucous membranes, lesions on skin and nerves leading to loss of sensitivity, atrophy, and severe disfiguration
Lymphatic filariasis	120/1,300	• Parasitic infection transmitted through bites from infected mosquitoes • Causes damage to the lymphatic system and kidneys; elephantiasis
Onchocerciasis	37/90	• Parasitic worm transmitted through blackfly bites • Second leading cause of blindness globally • 99% of infected live in sub-Saharan Africa • Leads to lesions, visual impairment, and elephantiasis
Schistosomiasis	207/779	• Infection via contact with freshwater parasites • More than 80% of infected people live in sub-Saharan Africa • Causes 15,000 deaths/year • Causes bladder cancer, damage to the intestines, spleen, and kidneys
Soil-transmitted helminthiasis	576/3,200	• General term for worms (e.g., roundworm, hookworm, whipworm, tapeworm) which cause gastrointestinal and occasionally liver infections • Transmitted by ingesting food contaminated with helminth eggs, or by direct infection through contact with contaminated soil • Together with schistosomiasis, cause 1 billion infections worldwide—300 of which are severe

Sources: Centers for Disease Control and Prevention (2007); WHO (2002d, 2006d, 2007e).
Note: ND = No Data.

on health care services and economic development can be quite large. Some diseases have lifelong consequences and may lead to consistent morbidity (particularly diarrhea and long-term malnutrition and anemia due to poor nutrient absorption capacity), physical disability, and/or disfigurement. Other NTDs are not chronic, but rather cause severe and acute infections; these may lead to death or to social stigma and abuse. The cumulative effects of chronic illness with NTDs often undermine education and work productivity, and may worsen pregnancy outcomes and negatively influence fetal and child development, leading to lifelong and inter-generational effects (Hotez et al. 2007). Millions of agricultural laborers work in areas with endemic NTDs, which have high prevalence in fertile regions.

Effective drugs are available for prevention and control of some NTDs, but they are infrequently used because major pharmaceutical companies see no profit in their distribution, since the affected populations are unable to purchase them. For example, antibiotic treatment has helped nearly eliminate leprosy and trachoma. For the control of many NTDs such as filariasis, onchocerciasis, schistosomiasis, and soil-transmitted nematode infections, large-scale, regular treatment plays a central role. Regular chemotherapy against intestinal worms reduces mortality and morbidity in preschool children, improves the nutritional status and academic performance of schoolchildren, and improves the health and well-being of pregnant women and their babies. Ultimately, the control of many NTDs cannot be effectively carried out at the individual level, since most infectious agents are in the wider environment and affect communities as a whole, requiring improvements in water, housing, sanitation, and the environment, and access to health care.

Although NTDs are for the most part, as per the designation, neglected, there have been some important recent successes in their control. Since 1985, multidrug therapy has cured 14.5 million patients of leprosy; fewer than 1 million people are currently affected by the disease. Since the late 1980s Merck has donated hundreds of millions of Mectizan treatments against onchocerciasis and, more recently, lymphastic filariasis. The Guinea-Worm Eradication Program, supported by the Carter Center in Atlanta, has reduced global prevalence from 3.5 million to 10,000, with complete eradication possible in our lifetime (WHO 2007e).

Malaria

Malaria is the most important vector-transmitted disease in the world. It is transmitted to humans by female *Anopheles* mosquitoes, found worldwide throughout the tropics. *P. falciparum* causes the majority of deaths, but *P. ovale* and *P. vivax* can produce a dormant form of infection that can persist from a few months to 3 to 4 years, causing relapses of illness. Resistance to the primary malaria drug, chloroquine, is common around the world. Malaria's biological features interact with social and economic conditions, creating intractable health problems.

As far back as records extend, malaria has been endemic in much of Asia, Africa, and Latin America—but also in temperate climates such as Russia, North America, and Europe—causing millions of deaths annually. Malaria's role as an obstacle first to colonial conquest, then to the productivity of colonized peoples, and more recently to economic development, has kept the disease on the international health agenda for well over a century. Emboldened by successful control in the United States and Europe during World War II, international health authorities turned to malaria control through DDT spraying to demonstrate the possibilities of disease control for development and as a tool of anticommunist efforts amidst the Cold War. In 1955, the eighth World Health Assembly held in Mexico City approved the Global Malaria Eradication Campaign and urged member states to adopt malaria eradication as a national policy, despite some delegates' misgivings. Incredibly, African countries were left out of these plans from the beginning. Because African malaria was regarded as intractable, the WHO and its major funders did not want to set themselves up for failure.

Although some malaria control efforts led to decreased infection rates in Asia and Latin America, today more people are dying of malaria worldwide than in the 1950s. An estimated 500 million malaria cases occur in the world each year, primarily among pregnant women, young children, and nonimmune adults. Figure 6–12 depicts the malaria problem across the globe, with inflated state/territory size indicating areas with higher disease burden. Sub-Saharan Africa is disproportionately afflicted by malaria, with other regions suffering to a far less degree. It is estimated that more than 1 million children a year, mainly under 5 years of age, die of malaria in sub-Saharan Africa alone, equivalent to one child dying every 30 seconds (WHO 2007k).

In addition to its mortality burden, malaria's high morbidity results in significant economic effects. These include direct costs for treatment and prevention, as well as indirect costs from lost work productivity, time spent seeking treatment, and diversion of household resources. These costs are estimated to be over US$1 billion/year.

The demise of the Global Malaria Eradication Campaign in the late 1960s, and the subsequent rise in cases of malaria, was complex and many-faceted (see Chapters 3 and 13). Currently malaria control centers on mosquito control, interruption of transmission, and treatment. Yet the *Anopheles* mosquito has proven resilient to control. Home spraying with insecticide and use of insecticidal bed nets can take place in conjunction with environmental measures, such as destruction of mosquito breeding sites (i.e., areas of stagnant water). Until World War II, malaria control efforts were based on killing *Anopheles* mosquito larvae in their natural aquatic habitats. This was done by draining swamps and spraying stagnant water with larvicidal oils. Although quinine had been used for malaria treatment and prevention for centuries, the development of synthetic antimalarials in the 1930s made treatment more practical.

DDT, developed in the mid-1940s to protect Allied troops from malaria in the Pacific area, made it possible to spray houses and kill mosquitoes. As a result, many countries reported great reductions in malaria morbidity and mortality. Malaria was eliminated from North America and much of Europe in the first decade after World War II, coinciding with economic recovery from the Depression and large-scale economic developments such as swamp drainage, sanitary housing, plumbing, and road building.

One type of malaria control that was common in early 20th century Europe and North America was the use of screens, bed nets, clothing, repellents, mosquito coils, and the like, which can be quite effective in reducing transmission. Today,

A

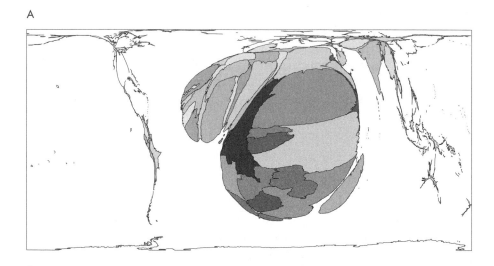

B

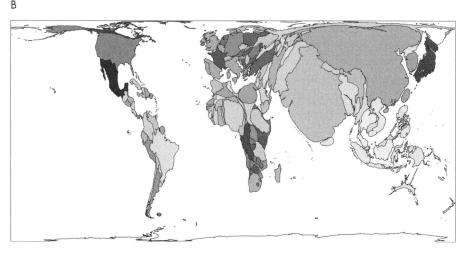

Figure 6–12 Number of estimated cases of malaria in proportion to population of each country. *Source*: http://www.worldmapper.org/display.php?selected=229. (A) Bulging or shrunken depictions of the countries indicate the proportion of the world's population with malaria who live in that territory. (B) Country depictions show the proportion of the world's population with malaria if the rate of malaria infection were identical in each territory. © Copyright 2006 SASI Group (University of Sheffield) and Mark Newman (University of Michigan).

the use of modern insecticide-treated bed nets in a home not only reduces transmission in that household, but also benefits persons living in adjacent houses (Hawley et al. 2003). Because of the encouraging results from bed net use, there is international momentum to include them as part of basic child intervention packages that provide free prenatal care and childhood vaccines (Bryce, Black et al. 2005).

Yet some advocates of "social marketing" campaigns oppose such a move, arguing that items distributed for free are not valued. Various social marketing campaigns for bed nets have not given credence to this position. Halfway through a campaign which sold nets in Malawi in 2000, only 5% of rural children were reported to be sleeping under a bed net on any given night (Holtz et al. 2002). The nets often cost the equivalent of a full week's wages for the family.

The other major strategy for malaria prevention and treatment is the use of drugs. However, there are problems of cost, possible side effects, and parasite resistance. Drug resistance is increasing much faster than the ability of the pharmaceutical chemists to produce and test new compounds. The reduced effectiveness of chloroquine in treating malignant *falciparum* malaria was reported independently in Colombia and in Thailand in 1960 and has since become widespread throughout almost all endemic areas. Resistance to the other drug largely used in Africa, sulfadoxine-pyrimethamine (SP), is now also common across the continent. As in the case of mosquitoes resistant to multiple insecticides, strains of *Plasmodium* are now known to be resistant to virtually every drug, including quinine, further compounding the therapeutic dilemma. At the end of the 1990s, a new antimalarial was introduced: the artemisinin group of compounds, derived from a plant native to China. Because they are cleared from the blood in a short time, the artemisinins must be given in combination with other drugs to remain effective in killing all stages of the parasite. One major impediment to use of artemisinins is cost; at their cheapest, they cost at least 10 times as much as chloroquine.

Respiratory Infections

Acute respiratory tract infections (ARIs) are a broad mix of various illnesses, all affecting the lungs and respiratory tract through viral or bacterial infection. Measles can cause subsequent pneumonia in young children, and can be included in this category. Although virtually everyone experiences mild upper respiratory tract (throat) infections, ARI death rates from lower respiratory tract infections overwhelmingly affect marginalized populations.

Box 6-7 Measles

Despite the existence of a vaccine, measles causes 30 to 40 million cases annually, with around 600,000 deaths, 98% of which occur in developing countries (WHO 2007l). Measles most severely affects children in the poorest communities of the countries with the least financial and human resources. However, rates of measles vaccination vary widely within countries. For example, in Bangladesh, the vaccine is given to 60% of children from the poorest quintile, but to 90% from the wealthiest quintile (WHOSIS 2007b). The WHO estimates that measles alone is responsible for more child deaths than any other cause, due to the ensuing complications of pneumonia, diarrhea, and malnutrition. Measles is also the main cause of preventable blindness throughout the world (Hoekstra et al. 2006; WHO 2007l).

(continued)

Box 6–7 Continued

There is only one effective vaccine for lifelong protection from measles infection. Global efforts to expand the use of this vaccine since 2000 have resulted in a remarkable reduction in under-5 mortality from measles, with annual deaths reduced by 48% from 871,000 in 1999 to 454,000 in 2004. While most children in developed countries receive the vaccine, this is not the case in many parts of the world, including Nigeria, where measles is the fifth leading cause of death. Currently, aerosolized vaccines are being tested to replace the traditional syringe method. Of course, as with other health interventions, improved nutrition could both prevent the development of disease and aid in speeding up recovery time.

There are also an estimated 150 million episodes of childhood pneumonia in the developing world each year. Pneumonia kills more children than any other illness— more than AIDS, malaria, and measles combined. Respiratory infections claim the lives of nearly 2 million children under the age of 5 annually, accounting for almost one in five deaths in these children. The majority of these deaths are in sub-Saharan Africa, Southeast Asia, and the Eastern Mediterranean, where vaccination rates remain low (see Fig. 6–13).

The consequences of respiratory tract infections are wide-ranging. In people with strong immune systems, viral infections usually clear up on their own or with minimal medical intervention. Bacterial infections are much more serious, and generally

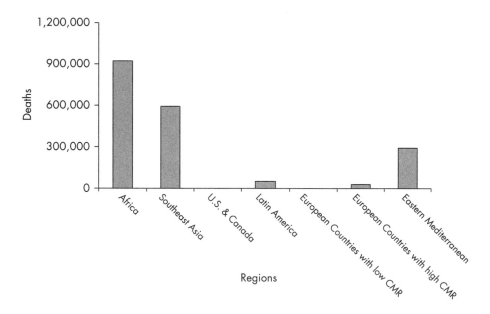

Figure 6–13 Estimated deaths caused by acute respiratory infection worldwide (WHO 2005c).
Note: CMR refers to case mortality rate (from acute respiratory infection).

require antibiotic treatment. For the many children in developing countries who lack access to proper housing, medical care, food, and water, these infections are often fatal. Moreover, respiratory tract infections are a leading cause of missed work and wage losses.

Pediatric pneumonia can be prevented through immunization (with the *Haemophilus influenzae* type b, measles, and pneumococcal vaccines), adequate nutrition (e.g., through exclusive breast feeding and zinc intake), and reduction of indoor air pollution (Wardlaw et al. 2006). Prompt antibiotic treatment is lifesaving for children and adults because most severe cases are bacterial. Practices of self-medication and indiscriminate use of antibiotics have led the WHO to warn of increasing antibiotic resistance (to penicillin and other commonly used antibiotics) around the world.

Diseases of Modernization and Work

As most societies shift from rural, agriculturally based economies to urban, industrially based economies, their populations face ailments related to work, transport, stress, toxic exposures, and consumption patterns. Yet largely agrarian societies are not shielded from such problems: use of toxic chemicals, and dangerous machinery and work methods have multiplied in recent years as countries have been pressured to reduce health and safety measures in order to compete on the global market. As such, not only acute infectious diseases, but also noncommunicable diseases and injuries are on the rise.

Cardiovascular disease

Cardiovascular disease (CVD) refers to both CHD and cerebrovascular disease (stroke). Although CVD caused fewer than 10% of all deaths in the early 20th century, since 1990 it has been the leading cause of death globally. And while death rates have declined in many developed countries, they are increasing in developing countries. The WHO estimates that 7.2 million people (3.8 million men and 3.4 million women) die of CHD each year; 80% of these deaths occur in developing countries. Even in countries with a high prevalence of HIV and other infectious diseases, CHD is often the second leading cause of mortality (Gaziano 2005; WHO 2005c, 2007i).

A stroke occurs when there is a lack of oxygen to parts of the brain, causing damage to brain tissue. Major strokes have much more severe consequences, including paralysis, disability, and death. Each year, 5.5 million people die from stroke (3 million men and 2.5 million women). China, Russia, and India report the most deaths from stroke, and in most developed countries, stroke is the third leading cause of death. Death rates and cases of stroke are highest in developed countries, but many developing countries, such as Libya, have rapidly increasing stroke rates, particularly in younger populations (Mackay and Mensah 2004).

The main biological determinants of CVD are high blood pressure and uncontrolled high cholesterol levels, which lead to blockage of coronary arteries and reduced levels of oxygen flowing to the heart and brain. CVD is mostly seen in older populations, possibly owing to the cumulative effects of lifetime exposures, but the disease can manifest even before age 50. The existence of other ailments, such as diabetes, also increases the likelihood of stroke. High cholesterol levels and blood pressure are often attributed to low levels of physical activity, tobacco use, and consumption of foods high in saturated fats. These biological and behavioral determinants are, in turn, influenced by societal factors which can determine patterns of consumption and production, the affordability and availability of nutritious food, employment patterns (including job security and levels of occupational stress), and overall stress levels related to employment and income. Because of these factors, lower-income groups experience disproportionately higher rates of CVD fatality.

Caring for a patient after a stroke can be expensive, time consuming, and difficult, particularly when there is a lack of social support. Rehabilitation is often time consuming and costly, with support centers typically located in urban centers. Without rehabilitative services, caregivers often become responsible for dressing, bathing, and feeding the patient, as well as communicating for him/her and taking over his/her responsibilities. In developing countries, younger family members are the most likely to be involved in providing home care of sick parents or elders, effectively diminishing their income-earning capacity.

Many CVD interventions emphasize ceasing tobacco use, increasing physical activity, reducing fatty food intake, and increasing consumption of fruits and vegetables. Medications to reduce blood pressure and cholesterol levels are commonly prescribed, and surgical interventions may be performed to clear arterial blockage and keep damaged arteries open. These dominant approaches focus on individual behavior and medical interventions without adequately addressing issues of affordability of nutritious food, time and safe spaces for exercise, sedentary occupations, high levels of workplace stress, racial discrimination, political disempowerment, and sexual harassment, among others.

Cancer

Cancer is the overarching term used for over 100 different conditions characterized by an abnormal division of cells. In 2007, cancer caused 13% of all deaths (7.9 million); 72% of cancer deaths occur in low- and middle-income countries. Overall, five cancers account for the majority of cancer deaths (WHO 2008a):

- lung (1.4 million deaths/year);
- stomach (866,000 deaths/year);
- liver (653,000 deaths/year);
- colon (677,000 deaths/year); and
- breast (548,000 deaths/year).

The causes of cancer range from workplace exposure to chemicals and other substances, to environmental toxins encountered in the home or community, to inherited genes that are activated by viral infections, to infectious diseases. Unlocking the key to cancer causation and treatment is one of the most challenging problems of modern epidemiology and medicine. Tobacco use is believed to be the single largest cause of cancer, and is related not only to lung cancer, but to cancers of the mouth, esophagus, stomach, kidney, bladder, and cervix. In the United States, tobacco has been linked to 30% of all cancers, and nearly one in five deaths from heart disease and stroke, with mortality rates higher in lower-income groups.

Other environmental toxins linked to cancer include radiation, chemical and material pathogens (such as asbestos and vinyl chloride), and even contaminated food (causing liver and stomach cancers). Infectious disease links to cancer include hepatitis B and C virus and liver cancer, HPV and cervical cancer, *H. pylori* bacteria and stomach cancer, schistosomiasis and bladder cancer, and HIV and Kaposi's sarcoma and lymphomas. Over 20% of cancers are thought to be due to chronic infections, which occur more commonly among working and marginalized classes. Developed countries have large disparities in cervical cancer incidence and mortality rates by socioeconomic status and race, with the most disadvantaged groups having the highest rates. Poor women die from cervical cancer largely due to lack of medical services; in many cases regular Papanicolaou testing (Pap smears) would detect early signs of cancer and enable treatment (Garner 2003).

Just as there are many different forms of cancer, so too are there differing methods of prevention and treatment and rates of survival. The Disease Control Priorities project categorizes cancers into three groups, depending on the degree to which they can be prevented and effectively treated. The first group of cancers—liver, esophageal, lung, and pancreatic—are extremely difficult to treat and cure and have high case fatality rates. Interventions often focus on primary prevention, such as environmental measures, smoking cessation, and reduction in infectious agents. The second group includes cancers for which screening and secondary prevention measures are available. In particular, there are proven methods of early detection and treatment for breast, bowel, and cervical cancers. Screening for cervical cancer is done via pelvic exam, which may include examination of the cervix, DNA testing for HPV, and/or the Pap smear. One screening for cervical cancer can lower a woman's likelihood of developing cervical cancer by 25% to 35%. The third group includes cancers for which treatment is much more difficult and costly, such as leukemia and lymphoma. Detection and treatment of these cancers rely on high-cost and highly technological interventions, necessitating trained medical staff and infrastructure, often over a long period of time (Brown et al. 2006).

The WHO estimates that over 40% of cancers are preventable, and many curable if detected early. Methods of cancer prevention involve minimizing exposure to damaging environmental pathogens such as asbestos, air pollution, and tobacco smoke. Cancers caused by infectious agents can often be prevented by immunization and the regulation of food preparation. Many prevention messages focus on individuals and their behaviors, and emphasize smoking cessation, physical activity, and diets higher in fruit and vegetable consumption.

The first cancer prevention vaccine was introduced by the Merck pharmaceutical company in 2006 and has been adopted by the United States and several other high-income countries. This vaccine (Gardasil), administered to young women, prevents some strains of HPV infection and lowers the subsequent risk for cervical cancer but remains controversial. Some groups feel that it will promote sexual activity, others are concerned that it has been insufficiently tested for safety, and still others believe it generates a false sense of security against STDs. The manufacturer (Merck) is heavily promoting the high-priced vaccine. At US$120/dose (three are needed), it is far too expensive for most developing countries.

Road Traffic Injury and Death

Road traffic crashes cause considerable injury and death and are the leading cause of death in persons aged 10 to 24. Throughout the world, men and people of low socio-economic status are disproportionately killed and injured in road incidents. Over the past three decades, traffic fatality and injury rates have dramatically declined in developed countries, primarily owing to regulations regarding seatbelt use and speeding, and the implementation of punitive measures for alcohol use before or while driving, rest periods for long haul drivers, vehicle safety laws, and road design improvements. Improved public transit has also helped reduce vehicle fatalities. At the same time, road injuries and deaths have increased in developing countries; these regions now have fatality and morbidity rates six times higher than developed countries (Nantulya and Reich 2003), with limited adoption of safety regulations.

In addition to immediate injuries and deaths from vehicle trauma, long-term ailments and impairments are also associated with traffic-related injuries, particularly loss of limbs, mobility, mental stress, and chronic pain. Consequences often include job and income loss, and depression.

Diseases of Marginalization and Modernization

Although the ailments of marginalization and deprivation are typically associated with the most underdeveloped countries, they are also present in marginalized populations within developed societies whose social welfare systems are patchy or have been undermined by underfunding and deregulation. Similarly, given rapid industrialization and urbanization across the developing world, diseases of modernization have proliferated.

As such, in most of the world, modernization and marginalization and their corresponding ailments coexist to varying degrees. Marginalized populations not only experience TB and malaria, but also have increasing rates of CVD, cancer, and diabetes. The pie charts at the beginning of the chapter showing causes of death for Egypt and Nigeria illustrate the point that diseases associated with marginalization and with modernization can overlap in the same place. For example, China is nowhere near eliminating diseases of marginalization, but is already experiencing high rates of cancer and respiratory diseases related to industrialization. Indeed, environmental toxins and air pollution disproportionately affect marginalized populations throughout the world.

In this section we discuss a set of globally prevalent diseases that are present in settings where modernization and marginalization coexist.

Diabetes Mellitus

Diabetes is a noncommunicable chronic disease characterized by disturbances in blood sugar regulation and metabolism. Type I diabetes occurs when the pancreas produces little/no insulin (typically has childhood onset). Type II is diagnosed when a person cannot effectively use the insulin that the pancreas produces; 90% of diabetics have Type II diabetes. In developed nations such as the United States, diabetes is one of the top 10 causes of death, but its rank is likely higher, since it often goes unrecorded on death certificates. The rate of diabetes in developing nations is skyrocketing (it is already the leading cause of death in Mexico), although much diabetes in the developing world remains undiagnosed. Over 180 million people (projected to increase to 366 million by 2030) have Type II diabetes globally (WHO 2006b). Diabetes is estimated to be related to as many as 3 million deaths/year (1 million in developed countries and 2 million in developing countries, equal to 5.2% of all deaths) (Roglic et al. 2005).

The main biological and behavioral determinants of diabetes are low physical activity levels and diets high in processed sugars and fats (or processed food in general), as well as advanced age. As developing countries modernize, it becomes increasingly difficult for their populations to maintain physical activity and the healthy eating traditions of the past, due to increased production and marketing of food high in sugar and saturated fat and the shift from agricultural to sedentary factory work. This trend will likely worsen, as corporations selling low-cost mass-produced food further expand into developing countries. Rates of diabetes are significantly higher in certain ethnic and indigenous populations whose ways of living have undergone rapid change (such as in Samoa and among Canadian aboriginals); overall, rates of Type II diabetes are highest among the lowest socioeconomic groups (Colagiuri et al. 2006). Low birth weight, followed by rapid weight gain in childhood, especially common in developing countries and in marginalized populations throughout the world, is also a determining factor of future diabetes (Phipps et al. 1993, Phillips et al. 1994).

Diabetes affects blood vessels, nerves, and major body organs, commonly resulting in visual impairment and blindness, kidney failure, CHD, and stroke (the cause of 50% of diabetes-related deaths). Diabetes can also cause severe end-nerve damage, leading to pain, numbness, and weakness in the outer limbs. As a result, foot ulcers and amputations are common in diabetic patients. Psychological health problems are also common among people with diabetes, including depression, anxiety, and low levels of self-reported health and well-being.

Type II diabetes is largely preventable and many of its consequences can be delayed, if not avoided altogether. Diabetes interventions can be categorized into four broad approaches: medical, surgical, educational, and social policy-related (Colagiuri et al. 2006). Medical approaches include modification of diet and exercise, and pharmacologic management. Surgical interventions focus on secondary prevention of further end-nerve and arterial damage to extremities. Educational efforts include counseling, tests, and health promotion. While these behavioral and medical approaches may help manage diabetes, they must be complemented by efforts that address the structural factors associated with the rise of diabetes, including food production and marketing patterns, safe, convenient, and affordable spaces for physical activity; the high cost of healthy food (and the difficulty in obtaining it in many settings); work schedules that do not provide time for exercise and food preparation; and poverty.

Colagiuri et al. found that broader changes in the social environment were essential for sustainable prevention and management of Type II diabetes. As such, social policy approaches, such as collaboration among different sectors to promote healthy societies (e.g., creating a unified policy in agriculture, transportation, health, education, public planning, and labor) are essential.

Chronic Obstructive Pulmonary Disease

Chronic obstructive pulmonary disease (COPD) is an umbrella term for a number of diseases (e.g., chronic bronchitis and emphysema) characterized by decreased airflow in the lungs. Two hundred ten million people worldwide have COPD, and 3 million people died of it in 2005; 90% of these deaths occurred in developing countries. It is the fifth leading cause of death in high-income countries, accounting for 3.8% of total deaths, and in low-income countries it is the sixth leading cause of death, accounting for 4.9% of deaths (Mannino and Buist 2007).

The global data suggest a 9% to 10% prevalence of COPD in adults older than 40; estimates are lacking from many underdeveloped countries (Wouters 2007). Prevalence is higher in men, older adults, undereducated persons, and those with high exposure to smoking. As the global population ages and smoking rates rise in developing countries (as tobacco companies market aggressively), COPD rates will likely increase. China's rapid development without adequate controls on industrial pollution has already led to soaring COPD rates (WHO 2007d, 2008b).

In developed countries, most COPD mortality is related to tobacco smoke (although outdoor air pollution may also be important), whereas in low- and middle-income countries, indoor air pollution from indoor stoves (which kills an estimated 1 million women and children a year—see Chapter 10) plus outdoor air contamination are more important than tobacco smoke. Other factors that increase or exacerbate COPD include crowding, poor nutrition, inadequate access to health care, early-age respiratory infections, and occupationally related dust and vapors (Mannino and Buist 2007).

Most importantly, COPD is a preventable disease, and primary, secondary, and tertiary prevention measures exist. These interventions include smoking reduction measures, early detection and treatment of disease, and occupational and environmental health measures. Although tobacco regulations are most heavily emphasized, occupational and safety standards can also decrease exposure, or level of vulnerability, to COPD-provoking agents through protective gear and changes in work practices. Similarly, outdoor air pollution measures such as emissions limits on industries and automobiles, could significantly reduce COPD. Because the most marginalized populations live and work in the most dangerous environments, they benefit least from COPD-reducing efforts.

Tuberculosis

Tuberculosis (TB) is an airborne disease that commonly affects one or both lungs, causing pneumonia and slow destruction of lung cells. TB can also cause disease in nearly every part of the body. Infection with TB occurs through inhalation of airborne particles containing *M. tuberculosis*, its causative agent. These particles are transmitted when a person who has TB disease coughs, sneezes, talks, or spits. A healthy and strong immune system can prevent an infected person from becoming sick for many years. Conversely, those with weakened or compromised immune systems fall ill sooner. General symptoms of pulmonary tuberculosis include prolonged, constant coughing and chest pain, fevers with night sweats, weight loss, and fatigue. Without treatment, TB is fatal in most patients, though a diseased person may live for many years before dying. In the pre-antibiotics era, a small proportion of patients survived without pharmacologic treatment—some through improved nutrition, others through fresh air cures. At times, more drastic measures were taken to effect cure.

TB is estimated to have killed more people in the history of the world (≈2 billion) than any other infectious disease (Ryan 1992). The discovery in ancient skeletons of deformities consistent with tuberculosis suggests that the disease was common in Egypt at least 4,000 years ago (Nerlich et al. 1997). Tuberculosis prevalence in Europe increased during the 17th century, as the population moved into rapidly growing cities, under crowded living conditions. By the early 19th century, TB was responsible for one quarter of all European deaths, as a result of industrialization and concentrated urban misery. As housing and sanitation improved toward the end of the 19th century, tuberculosis rates began to decline. However, European colonialism to Africa and Asia was accompanied by TB. In India and China, TB rates reached epidemic levels at the turn of the 20th century, and European immigration to sub-Saharan Africa, Indonesia, and Southeast Asia also spread TB, even as low population density in Africa limited its impact at the time (Stead et al. 1995).

TB's decline in the developed world starting in the 19th century was aided by improvements in labor and housing conditions, and subsequent advances in public health such as the introduction of the Bacille Calmette-Guérin (BCG) vaccine, followed by antibiotics in the late 1940s. This was followed by a steady decline in TB rates in North America and Europe until the 1980s. By the early 1990s rising racial and socioeconomic inequalities, along with poverty, increased homelessness, and crowded housing, all contributed to an increase in TB rates. Extremely costly and intrusive TB control efforts enabled a marked decline in rates in the United States and Europe. But other parts of the world did not attract this level of attention at the time, and TB rates were soaring by the early 1990s.

At the turn of the 21st century, TB remains a major health threat. Worldwide there were an estimated 8.8 million new cases of TB in 2005. The incidence and mortality rates vary widely by region (Fig. 6–14). Developing countries bear the brunt of the epidemic—in precisely the places with the fewest resources for combating the problem—with 95% of the world's cases and 98% of the TB deaths. On one hand, in part due to international control programs, the WHO estimated in 2007 that global incidence rates and death rates of TB had been falling for several years. On the other hand, the WHO also estimated that the global incidence (absolute number of new cases per year) of TB is growing at roughly 1%/year, owing to the growing caseload in sub-Saharan Africa and countries of the former Soviet Union (Eastern Europe and Central Asia), as well as to population growth (WHO 2007h).

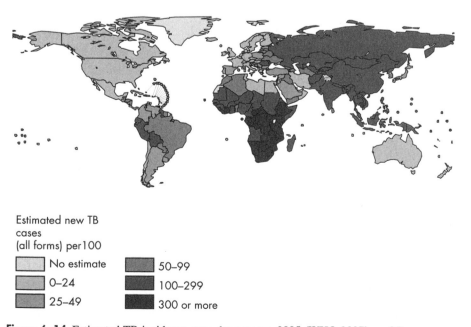

Estimated new TB
cases
(all forms) per 100

	No estimate		50–99
	0–24		100–299
	25–49		300 or more

Figure 6–14 Estimated TB incidence rates, by country, 2005 (WHO 2007h, p. 25).

Despite the availability of antibiotics, TB resists effective control in many regions, chiefly owing to the inadequacy of public health services, the spread of HIV, and the emergence of drug-resistant TB. TB is not only a matter of infection, it is also a reflection of resource distribution within and between countries. It is the preeminent disease of poverty. Rates of TB today are telling indicators of a country's level of wealth and inequality (Kim et al. 2005). The emerging worldwide epidemic of drug-resistant tuberculosis is entirely a human-made problem—indeed, an entirely treatable problem became untreatable due to inaction, apathy, and political disempowerment of the billions of people living in poverty. The natural selection of drug-resistant strains occurs when treatment is inconsistent or interrupted, when the wrong drugs are prescribed for the wrong amount of time, when drugs of inferior quality are given, or when the drug supply is unreliable.

Strains are identified as "MDR TB" (multidrug-resistant TB) if resistant to at least isoniazid and rifampin, the two most important drugs used to treat TB (Espinal 2003). When susceptibility to these two core drugs is lost, more toxic and more expensive drugs (known as "second-line") must be used. A case of MDR TB can take up to 2 years to treat and costs a TB program over 100 times more than a drug-susceptible case. Tuberculosis patients in Eastern Europe and Central Asia are 10 times more likely to have MDR TB than patients in the rest of the world (WHO 2004b). Globally, approximately 5.3% (490,000) of all new TB cases are MDR TB.

Extensively drug-resistant tuberculosis (XDR TB) was described in 2005 (Centers for Disease Control and Prevention 2006a) as MDR TB that is also resistant to any fluoroquinolone and to one of the three second-line injectable drugs (Centers for Disease Control and Prevention 2006b). The most recent reports have noted XDR TB in 45 countries on six continents, but most commonly in Asia and Eastern Europe. Even the most successful treatment efforts are estimated to cure only 30% to 40% of XDR TB (Holtz et al. 2005). In 2006, South African investigators reported the occurrence of XDR TB in HIV-infected persons enrolled in antiretroviral treatment programs, whose case fatality was alarmingly high (98%) despite adequate response to drugs (Gandhi et al. 2006). A large proportion of patients had never had TB before, and several were health care workers, raising questions about transmission in health care facilities and infection control practices in that region. The specter of virtually untreatable strains of TB being propagated throughout sub-Saharan Africa threatens to undo years of TB control work in the region.

One of the primary causes of the resurgence in TB is the increase in HIV infection, including in rural areas. HIV suppresses the body's immune system, which promotes progression to active tuberculosis in people with tuberculosis infection. Between 1990 and 1999, the incidence of TB in sub-Saharan Africa increased by over 250% (WHO 2005b), with an estimated one-third of all new TB cases among HIV-infected people. In areas of high tuberculosis prevalence, therefore, TB is one of the most common opportunistic infections associated with AIDS and is thought to be the primary cause of death in 40% of deaths among people with HIV (de Jong et al. 2004).

In the face of rising TB rates, the WHO declared TB a "global emergency" in 1994 and launched a five-component program called directly observed therapy, short-course (DOTS). The Global Strategy was updated in 2006 to include addressing TB/HIV and drug-resistant TB; contributing to health system strengthening; engaging all public and private providers in TB control; empowering people with TB and their communities; and promoting research into new drugs, new vaccines, and new diagnostic methods (the standard sputum smear method is over 120 years old) (Stop TB Partnership 2006). Critics maintain that DOTS has prioritized public health over individual rights, excluded "low priority patients," understressed the need for new diagnostics and new drug development, and ignored those who return for retreatment of TB. The structure of the DOTS framework has also been criticized as being too rigid to be universally applied to every social context (Lienhardt and Ogden 2004; Hakokongas 2005). Nevertheless, the DOTS strategy remains one of the most cost-effective public health measures in the developing world.

In 2000, the WHO formulated a strategy that provides for the treatment of patients with MDR TB using second-line medications. Given their expense, the STOP TB Partnership set up a "Green Light Committee" to allow access to reduced price second-line medications through a bulk-purchasing mechanism for those programs demonstrating an effective DOTS strategy. Prices of the drugs fell drastically owing to this pressure (Kim et al. 2005). Even in resource-poor areas with high rates of MDR TB, community-based treatment programs can deliver medical treatment that was once called "not cost-effective" (Mitnick et al. 2003). Treatment success rates are now approaching 65% to 70% in these programs (Leimane et al. 2005).

HIV/AIDS

The human immunodeficiency virus (HIV) is a retrovirus (i.e., it can use a host's DNA to self-replicate) and is the infectious agent that causes acquired immunodeficiency syndrome (AIDS). HIV attacks the body's infection-fighting CD4 cells, and slowly disables a person's immune system, which normally fights off common infections. AIDS is the term given to a collection of illnesses and symptoms found in persons with advanced HIV (and similar viruses). There is often a long time lapse—as much as 5 to 10 years—between initial HIV infection and progression to AIDS.

AIDS was first labeled as a distinct clinical entity in 1981, although in retrospect a few cases, puzzling to physicians, had probably been seen in the late 1960s and may have existed in humans as early as 1959. Infection and disease did not become epidemic until the late 1970s. The virus has since spread throughout the world.

The WHO estimated that the global number of deaths due to AIDS in 2007 was 2.1 million (that is, between 1.9 and 2.4 million), with a cumulative total of 25 million deaths since the epidemic was recognized. In 2007, there were approximately 2.5 million new infections, or 6,800 new infections every day (10% in children, with approximately 600,000 infants infected with HIV annually) (UNAIDS 2008). Overall, an estimated 33.2 million people (30.6–36.1 million) are living with HIV/AIDS (UNAIDS 2007).

While HIV/AIDS has been a pandemic for many years, 10 years passed before deaths from HIV in developing countries elicited a global response. The initial phase of HIV/AIDS in the early 1980s was one of severe discrimination and human rights violations against people infected with the disease, or perceived to be at risk for infection, primarily gay men. HIV/AIDS stigma and discrimination have been so great that Jonathan Mann, the founding director of the WHO's Global Program on AIDS, stated they are as central to the global AIDS challenge as the disease itself (Mann 1987). Public health prevention and control measures adopted during the 1980s often further exacerbated the discriminatory associations with the disease, including proposals for mandatory HIV testing, isolation of people with AIDS, and exclusion of people with AIDS from schools and workplaces (Mann 1999). In the United States, over 100 HIV-infected Haitian political refugees were quarantined at the U.S. Naval base in Guantánamo Bay, Cuba, rather than permitted asylum in the United States.

Today sub-Saharan Africa bears the brunt of the global epidemic, as seen in Figure 6–15 (latest data from 2007). Only 10% of the world's population resides there, but it is home to almost 68% of the global HIV-infected population. In 2007 it was estimated that 20.9 to 24.3 million people were living with HIV/AIDS in the subcontinent, with 1.4 to 2.4 million people newly infected and 1.5 to 2.0 million people dying from AIDS that year. Nine in every ten children and three out of every four people living with HIV in the world reside in sub-Saharan Africa (UNAIDS 2007). HIV seroprevalence rates vary across the continent, ranging from less than 1% in Mauritania to nearly 30% in Botswana and Swaziland. Southern Africa, with less than 2% of the world's population, accounted for 32% of all new HIV infections and AIDS deaths in 2007. The impact on mortality in sub-Saharan Africa has been immense. In seven African countries, life expectancy is 13 years lower than it was 10 years ago. In Zambia, Zimbabwe, and Swaziland, among the hardest-hit countries, life expectancy may drop below age 35 by 2010 (UNAIDS 2004).

Collecting HIV prevalence data and estimating its global burden is challenging. Estimates of HIV infection in developing countries are not based on a comprehensive national surveillance system (often these do not exist), but rather on data from antenatal clinics where HIV prevalence in pregnant women is periodically monitored (Boerma and Stansfield 2007). The Joint UN Program on HIV/AIDS and the WHO have used a six-step method to estimate HIV-infection prevalence in adults. Since 2000, however, national demographic and health surveys (DHS) and other surveys have been employed to generate population-based estimates of HIV infection. By 2007, HIV trends were better understood through these population-based surveys, and adjustments were made in existing mathematical models. As a result, the estimate of HIV worldwide for 2007 was 16% lower than the estimate for 2006

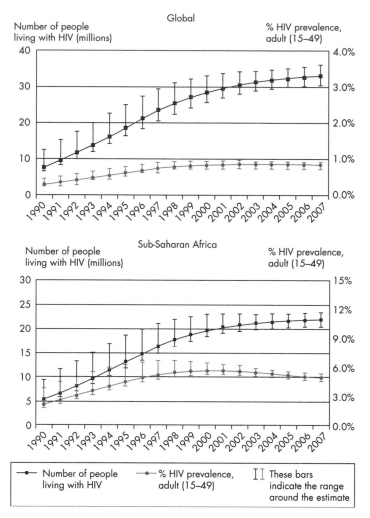

Figure 6–15 Estimated number of people living with HIV and adult HIV prevalence. Global HIV epidemic, 1990–2007; and HIV epidemic in sub-Saharan Africa, 1990–2007 UNAIDS (2008, p. 35). *Source:* www.unaids.org. Reproduced by kind permission of UNAIDS.

(39.5 million [34.7–47.1 million]). Of note, an intensive exercise to assess India's HIV epidemic showed that it has surpassed South Africa as the country with the largest number of people living with HIV/AIDS (over 5 million).

Notwithstanding the global response to the pandemic in the last decade, there is significant potential for an increase in HIV infection or AIDS in the near future. In India and China, the two most populous countries in the world, HIV/AIDS has been fueled by a lack of political commitment to early prevention efforts, compounded by poverty, illiteracy, population mobility, and gender inequality.

Epidemiologic explanations of HIV/AIDS typically focus on individual "risk behaviors" (e.g., unprotected sex and drug use) without considering the societal-level root causes that determine and limit individuals' choices and options. The underlying assumption of this approach is that individuals make decisions in isolation of their contexts. However, HIV/AIDS is a disease of marginalization; poverty and vulnerability are both cause and consequence of the disease. At a global level, the distribution of infection reflects regional economic and political inequities; the majority of people infected live in the developing world, in some of the poorest regions. At a societal level, the most marginalized groups continue to be the most affected by the disease. In 2001, the UN General Assembly Special Session on HIV/AIDS recognized that "poverty, underdevelopment, and illiteracy are among the principal contributing factors to the spread of HIV/AIDS" (UN 2001).

Biologically, HIV is spread in the following ways:

- Sexual activity with no barrier protection (i.e., condoms), with improper use of protection, or with ineffective protection, leading to a transfer or exchange of bodily fluids.
- Blood inoculation by transfusion of blood products, shared intravenous needles by drug users, contaminated dental tools, or accidental needlestick (in laboratory personnel, doctors, nurses).
- Medical injection with a contaminated needle or syringe.
- Injection of prepared blood fractions and products such as clotting factors used by hemophiliacs.
- Organ or tissue transplantation.
- Semen donation for artificial insemination.
- Mother-to-child transmission (MTCT) during childbirth or breast feeding.

The majority of HIV infections in children are a result of MTCT. Without preventive interventions, on average, there is about 5% to 10% transmission in utero, 10% to 20% intrapartum, and 5% to 20% during breast feeding.

Antiretroviral drugs (ARVs) can reduce antenatal and intrapartum transmission rates by 50% or more, and investigators are currently testing prophylaxis strategies during breast feeding. The potential for MTCT continues throughout breast feeding, which has led to a debate about whether or not HIV-infected women should breast-feed their children. Increasing evidence shows that exclusive breast feeding for the first 6 months is more protective against postnatal HIV transmission than early mixed feeding, in large part because exclusively breast-fed babies have fewer diarrheal and respiratory diseases. There is also increasing evidence that early mortality is higher for non-breast-fed HIV-exposed children living in resource-limited settings, erasing any potential benefit from reduced HIV transmission. Most programs now encourage informed choice on infant feeding for HIV-infected mothers. Replacement feeding from birth is only recommended when it can be safely practiced, primarily in areas with potable water and secure supplies of formula feeding.

Box 6–8 Social Cost of HIV/AIDS in Sub-Saharan Africa

The disruption of social and family life owing to AIDS in parts of sub-Saharan Africa is extreme. By 2010, an estimated 20 million children in sub-Saharan Africa will have been orphaned due to HIV/AIDS (UNAIDS 2004). In countries with the highest prevalence rates—Botswana, Lesotho, Swaziland, and Zimbabwe—more than 1 in 5 children will be AIDS orphans. It is not unusual for grandmothers in these countries to care for a dozen or more children orphaned by AIDS. Orphans are usually cared for in female-headed households, increasing the likelihood of living in poverty. Being an orphan decreases chances of survival, owing to the lack of education, malnourishment, and physical and sexual exploitation, and an increased vulnerability to HIV infection. Orphans are also less likely to be educated, and may be forced into lives of crime, violence, and exploitative sex. Orphans must not only cope with the emotional aspects of losing a parent but also with the stigma and discrimination associated with the disease, while at the same time facing an uncertain future. The number of orphans will continue to rise well after the prevalence rates of HIV/AIDS have decreased, and even as larger numbers of people gain access to treatment.

AIDS is also depriving the region of the skills and knowledge base necessary for social and economic development. By 2020, AIDS will have claimed 20% of the agricultural workforce in Africa. It already causes 20% to 53% of deaths in government workers in the health care sector (UNAIDS 2004). Teachers are dying at almost the same rate as they can be trained, undermining an already fragile education system (Harries 2005). The world will be dealing with the dire consequences of the AIDS crisis in subsequent generations long after treatment and prevention have been scaled up.

AIDS presents special problems in its prevention and treatment:

- Efforts must address not only the health and economic aspects of the disease, but also the associated fear and prejudice, the routes of transmission, and the needs of the marginalized groups most vulnerable to the disease.
- The groups most affected by HIV/AIDS are poor and marginalized and may face social, economic, and legal barriers in accessing community resources.
- Some consider the causes of transmission and preventive measures to be offensive and socially unacceptable topics, thereby inhibiting public discussion and education. Issues such as sexuality and homophobia, gender and gender oppression, marriage and extramarital relations, as well as drug use and harm reduction programs, are often controversial.
- Illiteracy and distrust of the state make it difficult for some groups to receive necessary health information if it is not accessible and culturally appropriate.
- Fear of discrimination discourages people from taking measures to learn their status and prevent transmission to others. Many people infected with HIV have no symptoms but may be infectious to others.
- Case detection is very costly and may not be budgeted for in national health ministries. In some settings, national budgets have shrunk, and there is a shortage of appropriate facilities.
- Medical care costs for AIDS patients are very high. In the numerous developing countries that have been pressured to provide cost-effective priorities, AIDS treatment may not be publicly provided. In developed or developing country settings, few people are able to purchase a lifelong supply of medication.

Where there are high rates of poverty and no national health insurance system, appropriate nutrition, and access to health care are also unaffordable.

Condoms serve as an effective barrier against possible infection through sexual intercourse. Condom promotion, the cornerstone of prevention, faces multiple obstacles including public resistance due to cultural and religious mores. In some settings, the linking of condoms to HIV/AIDS prevention has led to their becoming synonymous with infidelity and/or HIV infection.

Trials in the 1990s showed a large reduction in mother-to-child transmission when nevirapine is given at delivery. As a result, the PMTCT Initiative (prevention of mother-to-child transmission) was launched in 2002. It was later renamed PMTCT-Plus to include long-term medications for the mother. Despite the operation of PMTCT-Plus initiatives in many countries, coverage is not universal. Only 1 in 10 women in low- and middle-income countries are offered PMTCT-Plus services, and in sub-Saharan Africa only 5% of eligible women receive them.

In 1988, the World Health Assembly affirmed that preventing discrimination against people with HIV infection and AIDS is a critical part of national and global AIDS strategies (Mann 1999). For the first time, efforts to prevent such discrimination became an integral element in the global strategy for infection and disease control. In developed countries, where the disease disproportionately affected the gay community early on, activists used the human rights approach to call for increased attention, funding for treatment, and research on HIV/AIDS. In other countries, such as Brazil, the recognition of health as a human right helped mobilize the government and nongovernmental organizations to take up the responsibility of ensuring the right to health care of persons living with HIV/AIDS.

For those infected with HIV, treatment with ARVs can dramatically slow the progression of HIV to AIDS and reduce transmission to others by maintaining the viral load in the bloodstream. In the early 1990s, researchers found highly active

---

Box 6–9 Brazilian National AIDS Program

The Brazilian National AIDS Program is widely recognized as the leading example of an integrated HIV/AIDS prevention, care, and treatment program (Berkman et al. 2005). In the early 1990s, the World Bank estimated that 1.2 million Brazilians would have HIV/AIDS by 2000. Due to aggressive HIV prevention efforts and universal access to free HIV treatment, Brazil cut that number nearly in half (UNAIDS 2005). Brazil's epidemic initially affected mainly men who have sex with men, as well as injecting drug users. As the epidemic matured, the infection has spread, with women increasingly affected. In 1996 the government of Brazil began offering universal and free access to ARVs, reaching 160,000 persons in 2005.

Brazil has achieved its success through widespread distribution of condoms, needle exchange and harm reduction programs, and HIV testing campaigns. Prevention programs have addressed sexuality, focusing on condom use while also combating stigma and discrimination and supporting sexual diversity. The government has supported community-based prevention programs that work with men who have sex with men, sex workers, and youth (Berkman et al. 2005).

(continued)

Box 6–9 Continued

An engaged civil society, activist NGOs, and organizations led by people living with AIDS (PLWAs) have helped reduce stigma, educate the public, and provide care and support for other PLWAs.

In 1992, during negotiations with the World Bank for the first loan to support Brazil's national HIV/AIDS program, Brazil successfully resisted World Bank demands that it drop its free distribution of AZT (which it had begun several years earlier) as a condition to the loan agreement (Berkman et al. 2005). Brazil has also successfully resisted U.S. threats challenging its generic manufacture of some ARVs. In 2005, the Brazilian government refused the remaining US$40 million in a 5-year grant from USAID to protest restrictions on funding that required all recipient organizations to agree to a declaration condemning prostitution.

---

antiretroviral therapy (HAART) to be the most effective and important intervention for reducing morbidity and mortality in HIV/AIDS patients. HAART is a combination of several ARVs (typically three or four). While it has been widely employed for publicly insured patients in most developed countries, less than one quarter of the eligible population in developing countries has access to HAART. Where treatment has become available, many more people have sought to be tested.

Two nonprofit organizations made early efforts to deliver HAART to poor populations: the Nobel Peace Prize–winning Médecins Sans Frontières (MSF) (Doctors without Borders), and Boston-based Partners In Health (PIH). Ignoring critics who charged that ARVs were too complicated and expensive to be delivered in Africa, MSF launched initiatives in South Africa and Malawi on a small scale. PIH also set up community-based treatment programs in Haiti, Rwanda, and low-income areas of the United States, demonstrating that delivering complex health interventions in low-income settings is possible (Mukherjee et al. 2006). MSF continues to advocate for improved access to existing medical tools, and to stimulate the development of better ones (vaccines, diagnostics, medicines), through the Campaign for Access to Essential Medicines

Recently, the goal of "universal treatment" has obtained greater support. WHO has been successful in driving down the price of ARVs from US$2,500/year to US$300/year, with more progress to follow (WHO 2004a). It also provides drugs free of charge to those who are unable to pay. The largest funders for ARVs worldwide are the Global Fund to Fight AIDS, Tuberculosis and Malaria, and the U.S. President's Emergency Plan for AIDS Relief (PEPFAR) (see Chapter 3 for details).

As of the end of 2007, it was estimated that nearly 3 million people in low-and middle-income countries persons were receiving ARVs, a ten-fold increase from 2001 (see Fig. 6–16). It is also estimated, however, that over 6 million people in developing countries still need access to ARVs (see Fig. 6–17). The unmet needs are greatest in sub-Saharan Africa and Asia, where 94% of the untreated reside (WHO, UNAIDS, and UNICEF 2007). In total, by 2007 it was estimated that only 31% of the 9.6 million people in need of treatment had received it. However, the number of new HIV infections continues to outstrip the increase in the number of people on ARVs each year. For every two people who start taking ARVs, another five become newly infected (UNAIDS 2008).

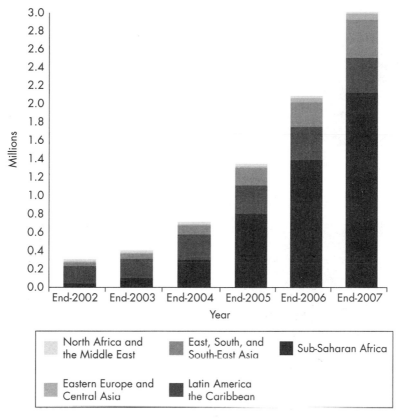

Figure 6–16 Number of people receiving ARV therapy in low- and middle-income countries by region, 2002–2007. *Note*: Even though HIV prevalence stabilized in sub-Saharan Africa, the actual number of people infected continues to grow because of ongoing new infection and increasing access to antiretroviral therapy. *Source*: UNAIDS (2008, p. 131), www.unaids.org. Reproduced by kind permission of UNAIDS.

DISEASES OF EMERGING GLOBAL SOCIAL AND ECONOMIC PATTERNS

Key Questions:

- What biologic and structural factors allow some emerging diseases to spread rapidly, while others take years to spread?
- What methods can we use to both prevent and detect emerging infectious diseases?

Over the past few decades, new infectious diseases have emerged along with factors common to rapid modernization and globalization. Also, increased surveillance for new diseases has improved our ability to detect them. Industrialization

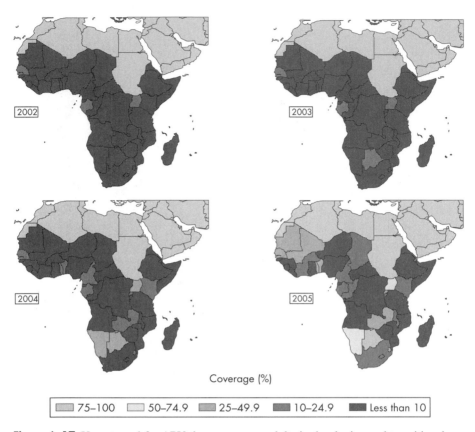

Coverage (%)

| 75–100 | 50–74.9 | 25–49.9 | 10–24.9 | Less than 10 |

Figure 6–17 Unmet need for ARV therapy among adults in developing and transitional countries in sub-Saharan Africa, 2002–2005 (UNAIDS 2006, p. 153).
Source: www.unaids.org. Reproduced by kind permission of UNAIDS.

and urbanization have dramatically shifted many living and production patterns from rural to urban areas, yet disease transmission occurs in both directions. For example, there is evidence in a number of countries of men who work in urban areas, become infected with TB or HIV, and then bring the infection back to their home villages. Highly dense urban centers are often high-stress contexts for workers, with low levels of worker protection and crowded housing, providing easy pathogen transmission to an increased pool of individuals. At the same time, increasing wages for workers have outpaced the prevention activities needed to stem these diseases and their determinants. In some cases, protective bodies and regulatory frameworks have been undermined by neoliberal policies and the collapse of the welfare state. In the wake of these changes, new disease entities have emerged, often defying public health efforts to control them.

In a rash of misplaced optimism in the 1960s, a number of scientists suggested that infectious diseases had become a thing of the past. Nobel Laureate Sir Frank MacFarlane Burnet wrote, "one can think of the middle of the 20th century as the end of one of the most important social revolutions in history—the virtual elimination of the infectious disease as a significant factor in social life" (Burnet and White 1962, p. iii). Similarly, U.S. Surgeon General (1964–1969) William Stewart opined, "the time has come to close the book on infectious diseases" (Stewart 1967, p. 1). Despite these convictions, the threat of infectious diseases is perhaps higher now than ever. Some have argued that many common infectious diseases, such as pertussis, TB, or cholera, never really disappeared; instead, authorities in industrialized countries lost interest in these ailments and only perceived them to be "reemerging" when they began to threaten high-income settings (Farmer 1996).

The term emerging infectious diseases (EIDs) has become part of the official lexicon and the basis of a thriving academic field. Many multisectoral agencies have been involved. These include the WHO, through management of the Global Outbreak Alert and Response Network (GOARN), and the U.S. Centers for Disease Control and Prevention, through publication of the *Emerging Infectious Diseases Journal* (www.cdc.gov/eid/), the *Strategic Plan for Addressing Emerging Infections in the United States* (1994 and 1998), and the Global Disease Detection Network, as well as through training and fellowship programs.

In general, emerging infectious diseases are those that have newly appeared in a population or that previously existed but are rapidly increasing in incidence or geographic range (Morse 1995). Table 6–7 lists a number of commonly cited EIDs. They can be viewed as falling into one of three groups:

1. Truly new diseases, such as severe acute respiratory syndrome (SARS) in 2002, avian influenza, and HIV/AIDS in the late 1970s and early 1980s.

Table 6–7 Some Emerging Infections and Probable Factors in Their Emergence

Disease (or Agent Causing Disease)	Factors Contributing to Emergence
Bovine spongiform encephalopathy (cattle)	Agricultural practices (changes in rendering processes; human cases of variant Creutzfeldt-Jakob disease (vCJD) thought to be linked to consuming infected cattle products)
Viral Syndromes/Diseases	
Argentine, Bolivian hemorrhagic fever	Changes in agricultural practices favoring rodent hosts
Chikungunya fever	Probably introduction of virus into areas with suitable indigenous mosquito vectors; increased international travel; breakdown of public health measures
Dengue hemorrhagic fever	Transportation, travel, migration, urbanization, sanitation deficiencies (i.e., stagnant water)
Ebola, Marburg	Initial cases through contact with infected natural host (probably a bat); subsequent cases through contaminated injection equipment in clinics or close contact with patient, bodily fluids by caregivers
Hantavirus	Ecological or environmental changes increasing contact with rodent hosts

(continued)

Table 6–7 Continued

Disease (or Agent Causing Disease)	Factors Contributing to Emergence
Hepatitis B, C	Transfusions, organ transplants, contaminated hypodermic apparatus/needles, sexual transmission, transmission from mother to child
Human immunodeficiency virus (HIV) infection	Probably originally introduced through handling nonhuman primates used as food animals, so-called "bushmeat." Marginalization, discrimination, migration, travel, sexual transmission, transmission from mother to child, transfusions, organ transplants, contaminated hypodermic apparatus/needles
Influenza, Avian (H5N1)	Food animal agriculture (infected poultry or products)
Influenza (pandemic)	Pig–duck–chicken agriculture, contact with humans facilitating reassortment of avian and mammalian viruses
Lassa fever	Human settlement patterns (e.g., near diamond mines), favoring rodent exposure in homes
Rift Valley fever	Dam building, agriculture, irrigation
SARS (Severe Acute Respiratory Syndrome)	Food animal agricultural practices (from handling infected food animals that acquired virus from other species in live animal markets); contact with infected bodily fluids, especially in health care settings; international travel
West Nile fever	Introduction of virus into area with suitable indigenous mosquito vectors
Yellow fever	Conditions favoring mosquito vectors
Bacterial Syndromes/Diseases	
Brazilian purpuric fever	Mutation of new strain
Cholera	International shipping, travel, poor sanitation, contaminated beverages, raw seafood consumption; facilitated by water chlorination
Helicobacter pylori	Likely to be common, newly recognized. Infection risk possibly associated with domestic cats
Hemolytic uremic syndrome	Mass food processing technology allowing *E. coli* 0157:H7 contamination of meat, or contamination of other products with infected cattle manure
Legionella (Legionnaire's disease)	Cooling and plumbing systems
Lyme borreliosis (*Borrelia burgdorferi*)	Reforestation around homes and other conditions favoring tick vector with deer (a secondary reservoir host)
Streptococcus, group A (invasive, necrotizing, "flesh-eating")	Unknown
Toxic shock syndrome (*Staphylococcus aureus*)	Ultra-absorbent tampons
Parasitic Diseases/Agents	
Cryptosporidium, Cyclospora, other waterborne pathogens	Transnational trade in food and produce, contaminated surface water, faulty water purification
Malaria	Travel, migration, global climate change
Schistosomiasis	Dam building

Source: Adapted from Morse (1995).

Table 6–8 Some Factors in the Emergence of Infectious Diseases

Category	Factors	Examples of Disease
Ecological changes	Agriculture, dams, changes in water ecosystems, deforestation and reforestation, flood and drought, famine, climate changes	Schistosomiasis, Rift Valley fever, Argentine hemorrhagic fever, Hantavirus pulmonary syndrome, hemorrhagic fever with renal syndrome, malaria
Human demographics, behavior	Societal events, population growth and migration, urbanization, war and civil conflict, urban decay, sexual behavior changes, injection drug use	Introduction of HIV, spread of dengue fever, spread of HIV and other sexually transmitted infections
International travel and commerce	Worldwide movement of goods and people, transcontinental air travel	SARS, introduction of cholera to South America, dissemination of *V. cholerae* 0139
Technology and industry	Globalization of food supplies, changes in food processing and packaging, organ and tissue transplantation, drugs causing immune suppression, widespread use of antibiotics	Hemolytic uremic syndrome (*E. coli* contamination of meat), bovine spongiform encephalopathy, transfusion-associated hepatitis B and C, opportunistic infections in immunosuppressed patients, Creutzfeldt-Jakob disease from contaminated batches of human growth hormone
Microbial adaptation and change	Response to human-related selection factors, microbial evolution	Antibiotic-resistant bacteria (multidrug-resistant and extensively drug-resistant TB), "antigenic drift" in influenza virus
Breakdown in public health measures	Curtailment or reduction in prevention programs, inadequate sanitation and vector control measures, lack of infection control measures	Resurgence of TB and multidrug-resistant TB in Eastern Europe and Africa, cholera in Africa, resurgence of diphtheria in the former Soviet Union

Source: Adapted from Morse (1995).

2. Newly recognized entities, such as amebic infection of the sinuses and brain, which have always occurred but were not recognized until recently.
3. Diseases that are increasing greatly in areas where they were previously absent or infrequent, such as cholera in Africa and Latin America, or extensively drug-resistant TB (XDR TB) in sub-Saharan Africa and Eastern Europe.

Most emerging infections are caused by organisms already present in the environment, which become prominent through some change in conditions, such as those shown in Table 6–8.

SARS

A disease that demonstrated the potential of rapid spread of infectious disease is SARS (Severe Acute Respiratory Syndrome). Although it likely started in late 2002, the first signs of SARS were only reported in February 2003 from Guangdong Province, China, where over 100 persons died from a mysterious atypical pneumonia. A physician who had treated some of the patients became infected and subsequently traveled to Hong Kong, where he infected at least 13 other guests and visitors in his hotel. These infected individuals then traveled and inadvertently seeded large outbreaks in Vietnam, Singapore, and Toronto. The virus spread quickly to six other countries in Asia and major urban centers of Canada. Thousands of people were quarantined for weeks in order to stop the spread of SARS. By the time the outbreak was declared contained in July 2003, there had been 8,098 cases of probable or confirmed SARS—over 5,000 in China alone—with 774 deaths reported in 29 countries.

The causative agent was a new pathogen, the SARS-coronavirus (SARS-CoV), almost identical to a virus found in civet cats, raccoon dogs, and bats in animal markets in southern China. Close crowding of animal species sold for consumption in Chinese markets proved a fertile ground for transmission to humans. The rapid spread to so many corners of the globe was facilitated by air transit of many patients, and respiratory droplet spread of the virus.

On the global level, health care workers accounted for 21% of all SARS cases. Early in the outbreak, health care facilities were recognized as an extremely conducive environment for SARS transmission after a patient hospitalized in Guangdong for just 18 hours infected more than 18 hospital staff. Health care workers were particularly vulnerable because: (a) SARS patients were most infectious during their second week of illness, when they were seeking care; (b) health care workers often had close contact with SARS patients to administer care; and (c) aerosol-generating procedures (such as intubation) used during patient management exposed health workers to the virus (Stockman and Parashar 2004).

SARS cases were similar to other episodes of atypical pneumonia: fever, cough, shortness of breath, and/or difficulty breathing. The overall case fatality rate was 9.6%. Advanced age and coexisting illnesses such as diabetes were found to be associated with poor outcomes. In persons over 60, case fatality rates reached 50%.

SARS was contained through the traditional approach to an easily transmissible disease, using available technology. The pathogen was identified and the laboratory diagnostics were developed extremely rapidly. Without drugs or a vaccine, it was vital to institute appropriate infection control measures, identify and manage contacts, and quarantine those potentially exposed. SARS has clearly shown that inadequate surveillance and response capacity in one country has global implications (Heymann 2004). The outbreak tested WHO's international response capability, and generated a coordinated international response based on information and evidence obtained in real time, through the medium of electronic communication.

Influenza

There are approximately 1 billion cases of influenza (the flu) each year, with about 3 to 5 million severe cases and 300,000 to 500,000 deaths annually. Throughout history there have been a number of influenza epidemics. Many fatalities have occurred in young, healthy populations not previously exposed to the virus and thus susceptible to infection (WHO 2005a). On a yearly basis, health authorities plan for the most likely strain of influenza and create vaccines accordingly. Often targeted to people with lowered immune systems and those who work with them, these vaccines may prevent specific, but not all, strains of the flu. As dominant strains change over time, influenza vaccines must also change.

New strains of influenza A viruses can be transmitted to humans from other species, most often poultry and swine. An influenza pandemic occurs when one of these novel strains of influenza is introduced and adapts to become easily transmissible from human to human. While seasonal influenza kills 30,000 to 40,000 people in the United States annually, a "medium" pandemic could kill up to 200,000 since no one would have immunity to the novel strain (WHO 2007a).

There were three influenza pandemics in the 20th century: the Spanish flu (1918), the Asian flu (1957), and the Hong Kong flu (1968). While the Asian and Hong Kong flus were relatively mild pandemics with the highest mortality rates seen in the elderly and small children (similar to seasonal flu trends), the Spanish flu killed young, healthy adults at an extremely high mortality rate. Seasonal flu mortality is normally less than 0.1%, but the Spanish flu killed 2% to 20% of those infected— some 40 to 100 million people over 10 months (Patterson and Pyle 1991).

Another potentially serious public health problem is avian influenza. The strain of concern (known as H5N1) was first documented in 1996. This new strain of bird influenza initially posed only a mild threat to humans. The threat rose when the virus spread rapidly through bird flocks in numerous countries (hundreds of millions of birds became infected and more than 100 million chickens were culled to slow the spread of the disease). It then became a larger human health concern when the virus crossed the species barrier and infected persons living and working with birds in Southeast Asia. In 2004, the first documented case of probable human-to-human transmission occurred in Thailand (WHO 2007f). Countries in Eastern Europe and Central Asia began detecting avian influenza in local flocks starting in 2005. As of late 2008, cases of avian influenza in humans were confirmed by the WHO in more than a dozen countries, with most deaths concentrated in: Cambodia, China, Egypt, Indonesia, Thailand, and Vietnam.

Case fatality rates are around 60%. A potential consequence of the H5N1 virus is a large-scale human influenza epidemic. The WHO has stated that the virus has all of the necessary characteristics for an epidemic, but lacks the means of efficient and sustainable human-to-human transmission. As the virus continues to mutate, human-to-human transmission could increase.

Anticipating a possible pandemic of influenza H5N1, researchers are working to develop a vaccine. Since influenza strains mutate over time, developing a vaccine in response to the first signs of a pandemic would take 6 months. In the meantime, a version of an H5N1 vaccine has been created and is being used in clinical trials throughout Asia (as a "pre-pandemic" vaccine). However, some countries refuse to share viral samples collected from infected patients, fearing (with apparently good reason, in the case of Indonesia) that viral strains will be passed on to pharmaceutical companies, which could produce a vaccine for profit rather than for public health (and without sharing the benefits). In response, the WHO has provided grants to Brazil, India, Indonesia, Mexico, Thailand, and Vietnam to upgrade local vaccine development facilities and to allow local officials to respond to an outbreak of disease and keep it localized.

CONCLUSION

Learning Points:

- Communicable and noncommunicable diseases affect all nations, with patterns of disease are shaped by social, political, and economic factors as well as biology.
- Global disease patterns can be categorized according to macro-structural causes as: (a) diseases of marginalization and deprivation; (b) diseases of modernization and work; and (c) diseases of marginalization and modernization.
- Treatment and preventive measures are available for many of the world's leading causes of morbidity and mortality, but there are myriad structural barriers to implementation.

This chapter began with an examination of communicable and noncommunicable disease patterns from selected countries. On the surface, some of these mortality profiles reflect different stages in the "epidemiological transition," as discussed in Chapter 2. Yet the reality is far more complex. Populations in all countries experience morbidity and mortality due to communicable diseases as well as from CHD, diabetes, and cancer. The relative weight of these causes is linked to the economic structure and sociopolitical features of different societies (e.g., level of urbanization, class relations, and age structure) as well as to biological factors.

For most childhood diseases, there are simple and effective interventions. There have been great strides in international child health in the past 50 years, with millions of lives saved. Yet up to 10 million children continue to die each year, mostly from preventable causes. There are large inequalities in infant and child morbidity and mortality and maternal mortality between developed and developing countries as well as within these settings. Our inability to prevent child deaths and maternal mortality is as much a failure of politics as it is of public health.

Malaria, measles, and diarrhea continue to plague developing countries. The immediate determinants, such as nonpotable water, poor sanitation and hygiene, and lack of access to health care services, are influenced by larger structural factors. The challenge of reaching those in need of seemingly simple interventions should not obscure the need for larger societal change. Most tellingly, although the ailments of marginalization and deprivation are typically associated with the most underdeveloped countries, they are also present among the marginalized populations of developed societies, where inequalities have worsened and social welfare systems have been undermined by defunding and deregulation.

Modernization has brought great benefits, but has also exacerbated chronic noncommunicable diseases. Again, biological factors are intertwined with societal patterns of consumption and production, the affordability and availability of nutritious food, employment patterns (including job security and levels of occupational stress), and overall stress levels, which relate to the politics and distribution of power and wealth. At the confluence of marginalization and modernization, we also see increased rates of diabetes, lung disease, TB, and HIV/AIDS. Claiming the lives of millions, these diseases fall along the fault lines of poverty and discrimination, with social and economic dynamics fueling the AIDS pandemic more than any inherent characteristics of the virus.

The next chapter will explore the societal determinants of health at global, national, community, and household levels and how social inequalities within societies shape patterns of ill health and premature death.

NOTE

1. The extent to which wealth is evenly spread through a population via taxation and social policies (see Chapter 4 for details).

REFERENCES

African Commission on Human and Peoples' Rights, and International Work Group on Indigenous Affairs. 2005. Report of the African Commission's Working Group of Experts on Indigenous Populations/Communities. Copenhagen, Denmark: IWGIA.

Alchon SA. 2003. *A Pest in the Land: New World Epidemics in a Global Perspective.* Albuquerque, NM: University of New Mexico Press.

Anderson I, Crengle S, Leialoha Kamaka M, Chen T, Palafox N, and Jackson-Pulver L. 2006. Indigenous health in Australia, New Zealand and the Pacific. *Lancet* 367(9524):1775–1785.

Berkman A, Garcia J, Muñoz-Laboy M, Paiva V, and Parker R. 2005. A critical analysis of the Brazilian response to HIV/AIDS: Lessons learned for controlling and mitigating the epidemic in developing countries. *American Journal of Public Health* 95(7):1162–1172.

Bjerregaard P, Young K, Dewailly E, and Ebbesson SOE. 2004. Indigenous health in the Arctic: An overview of the circumpolar Inuit population. *Scandinavian Journal of Public Health* 32(5):390–395.

Black RE, Morris SS, and Bryce J. 2003. Where and why are 10 million children dying every year? *Lancet* 361(9376):2226–2234.

Boerma JT and Stansfield SK. 2007. Health statistics now: Are we making the right investments? *Lancet* 369(9563):779–786.

Brown ML, Goldie SJ, Draisma G, Harford J, and Lipscomb J. 2006. Health service interventions for cancer control in developing countries. In Jamison DT, Breman JG, Measham AR, Alleyne G, Claeson M, Evans DB, Jha P, Mills A, and Musgrove P, Editors. *Disease Control Priorities in Developing Countries.* New York: Oxford University Press.

Bryce JB, Black RE, Walker N, Bhutta ZA, Lawn JE, and Steketee RW. 2005. Can the world afford to save the lives of 6 million children each year? *Lancet* 365(9478):2193–2200.

Bryce JB, Boschi-Pinto C, Shibuya K, Black RE, and WHO Child Health Epidemiology Reference Group. 2005. WHO estimates of the causes of death in children. *Lancet* 365(9465):1147–1152.

Bryce JB, El Arifeen S, Pariyo G, Lanata CF, Gwatkin D, Habicht J-P, and The Multi-Country Evaluation of IMCI study group. 2003. Reducing child mortality: Can public health deliver? *Lancet* 362(9378):159–164.

Burnet FM and White DO. 1962. *Natural History of Infectious Disease, Third Edition.* Cambridge: Cambridge University Press.

Castro R, Erviti J, and Leyva R. 2007. Globalización y enfermedades infecciosas en las poblaciones indígenas de México. *Cadernos de Saúde Pública* 23(Supp 1):S41–S50.

Center for Reproductive Rights. 2007. *The World's Abortion Laws. Fact Sheet.* New York: Center for Reproductive Rights.

Centers for Disease Control and Prevention. 2002. Section 17: Social and economic impact of oral disease. Oral Health, U.S. 2002 Annual Report. http://drc.hhs.gov/report/17_1. htm. Accessed February 10, 2008.

———. 2006a. Emergence of Mycobacterium tuberculosis with extensive resistance to second-line drugs—worldwide, 2000–2004. *Morbidity and Mortality Weekly Report* 55(11):301–305.

———. 2006b. Notice to readers: Revised definition of XDR-TB. *Morbidity and Mortality Weekly Report* 55(43):1176.

———. 2007. Fact Sheet—Leishmania infection. http://www.cdc.gov/ncidod/dpd/parasites/leishmania/factsht_leishmania.htm. Updated September 17, 2007. Accessed September 20, 2007.

Central Intelligence Agency. 2007. Greenland. https://www.cia.gov/library/publications/the-world-factbook/geos/gl.html. Accessed June 26, 2007.

Colagiuri R, Colagiuri S, Yach D, and Pramming S. 2006. The answer to diabetes prevention: Science, surgery, service delivery or social policy? *American Journal of Public Health* 96(9):1562–1569.

Cook ND. 1998. *Born to Die: Disease and New World Conquest.* Cambridge: Cambridge University Press.

Csete J and Wolfe D. 2007. *Closed to Reason: The International Narcotics Board and HIV/AIDS.* Toronto/New York: Canadian HIV/AIDS Legal Network and the International Harm Reduction Development Program of the Open Society Institute.

de Jong BC, Israelski DM, Corbett EL, and Small PM. 2004. Clinical management of tuberculosis in the context of HIV infection. *Annual Review of Medicine* 55(1):283–301.

Dickson M. 2006. *Where There Is No Dentist.* Berkeley, CA: The Hesperian Foundation.

Durham M. 2002. *Poverty, Disability and Impairment in the Developing World.* London: DFID and KAR.

Ehrenberg JP and Ault SK. 2005. Neglected diseases of neglected populations: Thinking to reshape the determinants of health in Latin America and the Caribbean. *BioMed Central Public Health* 5(1):119–131.

Epping-Jordan JE, Galea G, Tukuitonga C, and Beaglehole R. 2005. Preventing chronic disease: Taking stepwise action. *Lancet* 366(9497):1667–1671.

Espinal MA. 2003. The global situation of MDR-TB. *Tuberculosis* 83(1–3):44–51.

Ezzati M, vander Hoorn S, Rodgers A, Lopez AD, Mathers CD, and Murray CJL. 2004. Potential health gains from reducing mutiple risk factors. In Ezzati M, Lopez AD, Rodgers A, and Murray CLJ, Editors. *Comparative Quantification of Health Risks: Global and Regional Burden of Disease Attributable to Selected Major Risk Factors.* Geneva: WHO.

Family Care International. 2003. *Saving Women's Lives: The Health Impact of Unsafe Abortion.* The Partnership for Safe Motherhood and Newborn Health. New York: Family Care International.

Farmer PE. 1996. Social inequalities and emerging infectious diseases. *Emerging Infectious Diseases* 2(4):259–269.

Feachem R, Kjellstrom T, Murray CJL, Over M, and Phillips MA. 1990. *The Health of Adults in the Developing World.* Washington, DC: Oxford University Press for the World Bank.

Gandhi NR, Moll A, Sturm AW, Pawinski R, Govender T, Lalloo U, et al. 2006. Extensively drug-resistant tuberculosis as a cause of death in patients co-infected with tuberculosis and HIV in a rural area of South Africa. *Lancet* 368(9547):1575–1580.

Garner EIO. 2003. Cervical cancer: Disparities in screening, treatment and survival. *Cancer Epidemiology Biomarkers & Prevention* 12(Suppl):242S–247S.

Gaziano T. 2005. Cardiovascular disease in the developing world and its cost-effective management. *Circulation* 112(23):3547–3553.

Government of Cambodia. 1998. *Country Census.* Phnom Penh.

Government of Canada. 2001. *Country Census.* Ottawa.

———. 2005. Aboriginal peoples. http://www.tbs-sct.gc.ca/report/govrev/05/ann304_e.asp. Accessed June 26, 2007.

Government of India. 2001. *Scheduled Tribes.* New Delhi: Government of India.

Gwatkin DR, Guillot M, and Heuveline P. 1999. The burden of disease among the global poor. *Lancet* 354(9178):586–589.

Hakokongas L. 2005. *Running Out of Breath? TB Care in the 21st Century.* Geneva: Médecins Sans Frontières.

Harries A. 2005. HIV/AIDS: The epidemic, its impact and turning the tide. *International Journal of Tuberculosis and Lung Disease* 9(5):471–474.

Hawley WA, Phillips-Howard PA, ter Kuile FO, Terlouw DJ, Vulule JM, Ombok M, et al. 2003. Community-wide effects of permethrin treated bed nets on child mortality and malaria morbidity in western Kenya. *American Journal of Tropical Medicine and Hygiene* 68(4 Suppl):121–127.

Haws RA, Thomas AL, Bhutta ZA, and Darmstadt GL. 2007. Impact of packaged inter-ventions on neonatal health: A review of the evidence. *Health Policy and Planning* 22(4):193–215.

Health Canada. 2000. *Diabetes among Aboriginal (First Nations, Inuit and Métis) people in Canada: The Evidence.* Ottawa, ON: Aboriginal Diabetes Initiative.

———. 2006. First Nations and Inuit Health: Diseases and other conditions. http://www.hc-sc.gc.ca/fnih-spni/diseases-maladies/index_e.html. Accessed June 26, 2007.

Heymann DL. 2004. The international response to the outbreak of SARS in 2003. *Philosophical Transactions of the Royal Society of London Series B: Biological Sciences* 359(1447):1127–1129.

Hoekstra EJ, McFarland JW, Shaw C, and Salama P. 2006. Reducing measles mortality, reducing child mortality. *Lancet* 368(9541):1050–1052.

Holtz TH, Marum L, Mkandala C, Chizani N, Roberts JR, Macheso A, et al. 2002. Insecticide-treated bed net use, anaemia, and malaria parasitemia in Blantyre District, Malawi. *Tropical Medicine and International Health* 7(3):220–230.

Holtz TH, Riekstina V, Zarovska E, Laserson KF, Wells CD, and Leimane V. 2005. XDR-TB: Extreme drug-resistance and treatment outcome under DOTS-Plus, Latvia, 2000–2002. *International Journal of Tuberculosis and Lung Disease* 9(Suppl 1):S258.

Hotez PJ, Molyneux DH, Fenwick A, Kumaresan J, Sachs SE, Sachs JD, and Savioli L. 2007. Control of neglected tropical diseases. *New England Journal of Medicine* 357(10):1018–1027.

Human Rights in China and Minority Rights Group International. 2007. *China: Minority Exclusion, Marginalization and Rising Tensions*. New York: Human Rights in China.

Indian Health Service. 2006. Facts on Indian health disparities. http://info.ihs.gov/Files/DisparitiesFacts-Jan2006.pdf. Accessed June 26, 2007.

Jolly R. 2007. Early childhood development: The global challenge. *Lancet* 369(9555):8–9.

Jones C. 1999. *Maori-Pakeha Health Disparities: Can Treaty Settlements Reverse the Impacts of Racism?* Wellington, New Zealand: Ian Axford Fellowships.

Kim JY, Shakow A, Mate K, Vanderwarker C, Gupta R, and Farmer P. 2005. Limited good and limited vision: Multidrug resistant tuberculosis and global health policy. *Social Science and Medicine* 61(4):847–859.

Kosek M, Bern C, and Guerrant RL. 2003. The global burden of diarrhoeal disease, as estimated from studies published between 1992 and 2000. *Bulletin of the World Health Organization* 81(3):197–204.

Last JM. 2001. *A Dictionary of Epidemiology, Fourth Edition.* New York: Oxford University Press.

Lawn J, Cousens S, Darmstadt GL, Martines J, Paul VK, Bhutta ZA, et al. 2005. The Executive Summary of the Lancet Neonatal Survival Series. http://www.who.int/child_adolescent_health/documents/pdfs/lancet_neonatal_survival_exec_sum.pdf. Accessed July 15, 2007.

Leimane V, Riekstina V, Holtz TH, Zarovska E, Skripconoka V, Thorpe LE, et al. 2005. Clinical outcome of individualised treatment of multidrug-resistant tuberculosis in Latvia: A retrospective cohort study. *Lancet* 365(9456):318–326.

Lienhardt C and Ogden JA. 2004. Tuberculosis control in resource-poor countries: Have we reached the limits of the universal paradigm? *Tropical Medicine and International Health* 9(7):833–841.

Mackay J and Mensah G. 2004. Deaths from stroke. In *The Atlas of Heart Disease and Stroke*. Geneva: WHO.

Mann J. 1987. Statement at an informal briefing on AIDS Paper read at 42nd session of the United Nations General Assembly, October 20, New York, cited in R. Parker and P. Aggleton. 2002. HIV and AIDS-Related Stigma and Discrimination: A Conceptual Framework and Implications for Action. Rio de Janeiro: Associação Brasileira Interdisciplinar de AIDS and London: Thomas Coram Research Unit.

————. 1999. The transformative potential of the HIV/AIDS pandemic. *Reproductive Health Matters* 7(14):164–172.

Mannino DM and Buist SA. 2007. Global burden of COPD: Risk factors, prevalence, and future trends. *Lancet* 370(9589):765–773.

McCaa R. 1995. Spanish and Nahuatl views on smallpox and demographic catastrophe in the conquest of Mexico. *Journal of Interdisciplinary History* 25(3):397–431.

Millard AV. 1994. A causal model of high rates of child mortality. *Social Science and Medicine* 38(2):253–268.

Mitnick C, Bayona J, Palacios E, Shin SS, Furin JJ, Alcántara F, et al. 2003. Community-based therapy for multidrug-resistant tuberculosis in Lima, Peru. *New England Journal of Medicine* 348(2):119–128.

Montenegro R and Stephens C. 2006. Indigenous health in Latin America and the Caribbean. *Lancet* 367(9525):1859–1869.

Morse SS. 1995. Factors in the emergence of infectious diseases. *Emerging Infectious Diseases* 1(1):7–15.

Mukherjee JS, Louise I, Fernet L, Paul F, and Heidi B. 2006. Antiretroviral therapy in resource-poor settings: Decreasing barriers to access and promoting adherence. *Journal of Acquired Immune Deficiency Syndrome* 43(Suppl 1):S123–S126.

Nantulya VM and Reich MR. 2003. Equity dimensions of road traffic injuries in low- and middle-income countries. *Injury Control and Safety Promotion* 10(1–2):13–20.

Nerlich AG, Haas CJ, Zink A, Szeimies U, and Hagedorn HG. 1997. Molecular evidence for tuberculosis in an ancient Egyptian mummy. *Lancet* 350(9088):1404.

Ohenjo N, Willis R, Jackson D, Nettleton C, Good K, and Mugarura B. 2006. Health of indigenous people in Africa. *Lancet* 367(9526):1937–1946.

PAHO. 2002. Health of Indigenous people: A challenge for public health. http://www.paho.org/english/DPI/100/100feature32.htm. Accessed June 26, 2007.

Patterson KD and Pyle GF. 1991. The geography and mortality of the 1918 influenza pandemic. *Bulletin of the History of Medicine* 65(1):4–21.

Petersen PE, Bourgeois D, Ogawa H, Estupinan-Day S, and Ndiaye C. 2005. The global burden of oral diseases and risks to oral health. *Bulletin of the World Health Organization* 83(9):661–669.

Phillips DIW, Hirst S, Clark PMS, Hales CN, and Osmond C. 1994. Fetal growth and insulin secretion in adult life. *Diabetologia* 37(6):592–596.

Phipps K, Barker DJ, Hales CN, Fall CH, Osmond C, and Clark PM. 1993. Fetal growth and impaired glucose tolerance in men and women. *Diabetologia* 36(3):225–228.

Riverón Corteguera RL. 1995. Strategies and causes of reduced infant and young child diarrheal disease mortality in Cuba, 1962–1993. *Bulletin of the Pan American Health Organization* 29(1):70–80.

Roglic G, Unwin N, Bennett PH, Mathers C, Tuomilehto J, Nag S, et al. 2005. The burden of mortality attributable to diabetes. *Diabetes Care* 28(9):2130–2135.

Ryan F. 1992. *Tuberculosis: The Greatest Story Never Told.* Worcestershire, UK: Swift Publishers.

Saxena S, Thornicroft G, Knapp M, and Whiteford H. 2007. Resources for mental health: Scarcity, inequity, and inefficiency. *Lancet* 370(9590):878–889.

Statistics New Zealand. 2001. *Census.* Wellington: Statistics New Zealand.

Stead WW, Eisenach KD, Cave MD, Beggs ML, Templeton GL, Theon CO, and Bates JH. 1995. When did Mycobacterium tuberculosis infection first occur in the New World? An important question with public health implications. *American Journal of Respiratory and Critical Care Medicine* 151(4):1267–1268.

Stephens C, Porter J, Nettleton C, and Willis R. 2006. Disappearing, displaced and under-valued: A call to action on Indigenous health worldwide. *Lancet* 367(9527):2019–2028.

Stewart WH. 1967. *A Mandate for State Action.* Washington, DC: Association of State and Territorial Health Officers.

Stockman LJ, and Parashar UD. 2004. Review of the epidemiology of severe acute respiratory disease. *Business Briefing: Clinical Virology and Infectious Disease* 1–6.

Stop TB Partnership. 2006. *The Global Plan to Stop TB, 2006–2015*. Geneva: WHO.

Strong K, Mathers C, Leeder S, and Beaglehole R. 2005. Preventing chronic diseases: How many lives can we save? *Lancet* 366(9496):1578–1582.

Thomas P. 2005. Disability, poverty and the millennium development goals: Relevance, challenges and opportunities for DFID. London, UK: Disability Knowledge and Research.

Trewin D and Madden D. 2005. *The Health and Welfare of Australia's Aboriginal and Torres Strait Islander Peoples*. Canberra: Australian Bureau of Statistics.

UN. 2001. Declaration of commitment to HIV/AIDS. Paper read at United Nations General Assembly, at New York.

UNAIDS. 2004. *2004 Report on the Global AIDS Epidemic*. Geneva: UNAIDS.

———. 2005. Brazil country profile. http://www.unaids.org/en/CountryResponses/ Countries/brazil.asp. Accessed January 20, 2008. and updated http://data.unaids.org/ pub/Report/2008/brazil_2008_country_progress_report_en.pdf

———. 2006. *2006 Report on the Global AIDS Pandemic*. Geneva: UNAIDS.

———. 2007. *AIDS Epidemic Update*. Geneva: UNAIDS and WHO.

———. 2008. *2008 Report on the Global AIDS Pandemic*. Geneva: UNAIDS.

UNDP: Gender Unit. 2005. *En Route to Equality: A Gender Review of National MDG Reports*. New York: UNDP.

UNESCO. 2006. *UNESCO and Indigenous Peoples: Partnership to Promote Cultural Diversity*. New York: UNESCO.

UNFPA. 2003. *Annual Report*. New York: United Nations Population Fund. New York: UNFPA.

UNICEF. 2007. At a glance: Guatemala. http://www.unicef.org/infobycountry/guatemala. html. Accessed June 26, 2007.

———. 2008. *State of the World's Children: Child Survival*. New York: UNICEF.

United Nations. 2000. Latin America: Infant mortality by selected indigenous group. http://www.eclac.org/prensa/noticias/comunicados/3/27523/graficoCP3panosocENG. pdf. Accessed June 26, 2007.

United Nations Office on Drugs and Crime. 2004. World Drug Report. New York: UNODC.

United States Census Bureau. 2005. *Census Statistics*. Washington, DC: Census Bureau.

UN Secretary General. 2001. *Roadmap Towards the Implementation of the United Nations' Millennium Declaration*. Geneva: United Nations.

Victora CG, Wagstaff A, Schellenberg JA, Gwatkin D, Claeson M, and Habicht J-P. 2003. Child Survival IV: Applying an equity lens to child health and mortality: More of the same is not enough. *Lancet* 362(9379):233–241.

Wardlaw T, Salama P, Johansson EW, and Mason E. 2006. Pneumonia: The leading killer of children. *Lancet* 368(9541):1048–1050.

Watson MR, Manski RJ, and Macek D. 2001. The impact of income on children's and adolescents' preventive dental visits. *Journal of the American Dental Association* 132(11):1580–1587.

Werner D and Sanders D. 1997. *Questioning the Solution. The Politics of Primary Health Care and Child Survival*. Palo Alto, CA: HealthWrights.

WHO. 1997. *Coverage of Maternal Care: A Listing of Available Information, Fourth Edition*. Geneva: WHO.

———. 2000. *Report on Global Surveillance of Epidemic-Prone Infectious Diseases*. Geneva: WHO.

————. 2001a. *Global Prevalence and Incidence of Selected Curable Sexually Transmitted Infections: Overview and Estimates.* Geneva: WHO.

————. 2001b. Mental health: New understanding, new hope. In *World Health Report.* Geneva: WHO.

————. 2002a. *Active Ageing: A Policy Framework.* Geneva: WHO.

————. 2002b. *Gender and Mental Health: Department of Gender and Women's Health.* Geneva: WHO.

————. 2002c. *Gender and Road Traffic Injuries: Department of Gender and Women's Health.* Geneva: WHO.

————. 2002d. Reducing risks, promoting healthy life. In *World Health Report.* Geneva: WHO.

————. 2003. *Gender, Health and Tobacco: Department of Gender and Women's Health.* Geneva: WHO.

————. 2004a. *"3x5" Progress Report.* Geneva: WHO.

————. 2004b. *Antituberculosis Drug Resistance in the World: Third Global Report.* Geneva: WHO.

————. 2004c. *Maternal Mortality in 2000: Estimates Developed by WHO, UNICEF, UNFPA.* Geneva: WHO.

————. 2005a. Avian influenza: Assessing the pandemic threat. http://www.who.int/csr/disease/influenza/WHO_CDS_2005_29/en/. Updated January 2005. Accessed July 2007.

————. 2005b. *Global Tuberculosis Control: Surveillance, Planning, Financing.* Geneva: WHO.

————. 2005c. *World Health Report 2005: Make Every Mother and Child Count.* Geneva: WHO.

————. 2006a. Cholera 2005. *Weekly Epidemiological Record* 81(31):297–308.

————. 2006b. Diabetes. Fact Sheet No. 312. http://www.who.int/mediacentre/factsheets/fs312/en/index.html. Updated September 2006. Accessed February 2008.

————. 2006c. *Prevention and Control of Sexually Transmitted Infections: Draft Global Strategy.* Geneva: WHO.

————. 2006d. Schistosomiasis and soil-transmitted helminth infections—preliminary estimates of the number of children treated with albendazole or mebendazole. *Weekly Epidemiological Record* 81(16):145–163.

————. 2006e. World report on disability and rehabilitation. http://www.who.int/disabilities/publications/dar_world_report_concept_note.pdf. Accessed July 15, 2007.

————. 2007a. Acute respiratory infections: Influenza. http://www.who.int/vaccine_research/diseases/ari/en/index.html. Accessed July 16, 2007.

————. 2007b. Assistive devices/technologies. http://www.who.int/disabilities/technology/en/. Accessed July 15, 2007.

————. 2007c. *Children's Environmental Health.* http://www.who.int/ceh/en/. Accessed July 15, 2007.

————. 2007d. Chronic respiratory disease. http://www.who.int/respiratory/en/index.html. Accessed July 16, 2007.

————. 2007e. Control of neglected tropical diseases (NTD). http://www.who.int/neglected_diseases/en/. Updated August 14, 2008. Accessed July 16, 2007.

————. 2007f. Cumulative number of confirmed human cases of Avian influenza A/(H5N1) Reported to WHO. http://www.who.int/csr/disease/avian_influenza/country/cases_table_2007_05_31/en/index.html. Updated 31 May 2007. Accessed July 16, 2007.

————. 2007g. Denmark. http://www.who.int/countries/dnk/en/. Accessed June 26, 2007.

WHO. 2007h. *Global TB Control—Surveillance, Planning, Financing*. Geneva: WHO.

————. 2007i. Health and the Millennium Development Goals. http://www.who.int/mdg/en/. Accessed July 18, 2007.

————. 2007j. International classification of functioning, disability, and health. http://www.who.int/classifications/icf/site/intros/ICF-Eng-Intro.pdf. Accessed July 15, 2007.

————. 2007k. Malaria. Fact Sheet No. 94. http://www.who.int/mediacentre/factsheets/fs094/en/. Updated May 2007. Accessed July 16, 2007.

————. 2007l. Measles. http://www.who.int/vaccine_research/diseases/ari/en/index1.html. Accessed July 16, 2007.

————. 2007m. Mental health. http://www.who.int/mental_health/en/. Accessed July 16, 2007.

————. 2007n. Oral health. Fact Sheet No. 318. http://www.who.int/mediacentre/factsheets/fs318/en/print.html. Accessed February 10, 2008.

————.2007o. Viral cancers: Hepatitis C. http://www.who.int/vaccine_research/diseases/viral_cancers/en/index2.html. Accessed July 16, 2007.

————. 2007p. The world is fast ageing: Have we noticed? http://www.who.int/ageing/en/. Accessed July 15, 2007.

————. 2008a. Cancer. Fact Sheet No. 297. http://www.who.int/mediacentre/factsheets/fs297/en/index.html. Updated July 2008. Accessed September 15, 2008.

————. 2008b. Chronic obstructive pulmonary disease (COPD). http://www.who.int/mediacentre/factsheets/fs315/en/index.html. Updated May 2008. Accessed September 9, 2008.

————. 2008c. Hepatitis B. Fact Sheet No. 204. http://www.who.int/mediacentre/factsheets/fs204/en/. Updated August 2008. Accessed September 9, 2008.

WHO, UNAIDS, and UNICEF. 2007. *Towards Universal Access: Scaling up Priority HIV/AIDS Interventions in the Health Sector*. Geneva: WHO.

WHOSIS. 2007a. Core health indicators. http://www.who.int/whosis/database/core/core_select_process.cfm. Accessed July 15, 2007.

————. 2007b. *Inequities in Health*. http://www.who.int/whosis/en/. Accessed July 16, 2007.

————. 2008. Core health indicators. http://www.who.int/whosis/database/core/core_select.cfm. Accessed September 10, 2008.

Willis BM and Levy BS. 2003. Child prostitution: Global health burden, research needs, and interventions. *Lancet* 359(9315):1417–1422.

Wouters EF 2007. COPD: A chronic and overlooked pulmonary disease. *Lancet* 370(9589):715–716.

7

Societal Determinants of Health and Social Inequalities in Health

In 2004, Costa Ricans lived, on average, to the age of 77, an almost identical life expectancy to that in the United States. Yet the U.S. per capita income was more than four times that of Costa Rica (WHO 2006). Even more striking, in 2000, inhabitants of the southern Indian state of Kerala, earning, on average, less than US$3,000 per year, had a life expectancy of 74.6 (Government of Kerala 2005), while Washington, DC residents, with almost $30,000 per capita annual income, had a life expectancy of 72.6 years (Phillips and Beasley 2005; U.S. Government 2005).

What makes Costa Ricans and Keralites so healthy, and why does U.S. wealth not enable greater longevity? The answer to this question has far less to do with the *nature of the people* living in these settings than with the *structure of their societies*. The political economy of health framework developed in Chapter 4 examined the role of the distribution of power and of social, economic, and political resources in shaping the health of populations, showing that factors such as genetic endowment, health behavior, and medical care explain only a small fraction of health and disease patterns.

In Chapter 6, we examined the range and distribution of health and disease problems across the world. Here we discuss these patterns from the perspective of the societal determinants of health and social inequalities in health.[1] We begin by outlining a range of factors that influence health at personal, household, community, national, and global levels. Next, we turn to the role of social inequalities in explaining persistent differences in health status. We then discuss the gradient in health— whereby at each rung down the "social ladder" people experience a deterioration in health and lower life expectancy—offering a series of explanations for these inequalities in health. We conclude by presenting a set of theories that explain *how* social inequalities affect health and explore their implications for local, national, and global policies.

The Societal Determinants of Health: What Makes the Underlying Determinants of Health Societal as Opposed to Individual?

Most of us experience ill health as individuals. Yet virtually every bout of ill health or injury can be understood in societal terms. For example, picture a construction worker who takes a 10-storey fall from a scaffolding and dies. On one level, he may have been inattentive and insufficiently conscious of safety. But if we look to the societal context in which this worker lives, we learn that he was exhausted due to his long commute to work—he can only afford to reside in a distant slum—and his inability to get a good night's sleep, because the thin walls of his dwelling fail to block out nighttime noise. At an intermediary level, we learn that his low earnings derive from poor enforcement (and inadequate levels) of minimum wages and his precarious status as an undocumented worker. Lack of government oversight and poor regulation also contribute to the meager safety training he received from his employer and the poor quality materials the company purchased to build the scaffolding. At the highest level, we may understand the fall to be linked to a free market economic system where profits come before worker safety and working class efforts to organize and ensure social security and occupational measures are constrained by threats of job loss and repression. In sum, the construction worker's fall may be construed as a personal accident, but when viewed through a lens of societal determinants can be clearly understood as the product of interlocking social, economic, and political factors.

At a population level, patterns of premature death and disability can also be examined in societal terms. Population health is linked to and explained by a range of societal factors and conditions, from neighborhood conditions to the work environment, availability of and access to social services, such as education and health, to the overall class and political structure. Accordingly, though the term *social determinants of health* is widely used, here we employ *societal determinants of health* to refer to the structural forces that affect health. Strictly speaking, the social determinants of health refer to those factors related to interactions among people and communities, whereas societal determinants emphasize a broader array of structural influences.

Box 7–1 Definitions

- *Social determinants of health* are "the social characteristics within which living takes place" (Tarlov cited in WHO Commission on Social Determinants of Health 2007a, p. 4).
- *Societal determinants of health* are the political, economic, social, and cultural structures that shape health and health patterns.
- *Health inequalities* may be understood as (a) individual health differences; (b) differences in health between population groups; or (c) health differences between groups linked to broader social inequalities and unequal societal structures (Graham 2007, p. 4).

(continued)

Box 7–1 Continued

- *Social inequalities (or inequities) in health* refer to "health disparities, within and between countries…that systematically burden populations rendered vulnerable by underlying social structures and political, economic, and legal institutions" (Krieger 2001, p. 698).
- *Equity in health* is the "absence of systematic and potentially remediable differences in one or more aspects of health across socially, demographically, or geographically defined populations or population subgroups" (Starfield 2006, p. 13).
- The term *health disparities* (mostly used in the United States) "implies differences in health status without necessarily implying the presence of injustice" (Thomson et al. 2006, cited in Graham 2007, p. 8).

The societal determinants of health framework illustrates how political economy of health pathways operate—how health and ill health are produced and reproduced at the societal level. As seen in Figure 4–2, these determinants function on multiple levels simultaneously. The most immediate determinants of health shape exposure, susceptibility, and resistance to death and illness at household and community levels. For example, without adequate housing, maintaining healthy levels of sanitation and hygiene are next to impossible. Unhealthy activities, such as smoking and violence, are shaped by neighborhood conditions, cultural and social factors, and the available means to relieve stress and resolve conflict. Similarly, narcotic drug use, while certainly addictive, is heavily mediated by economic insecurity, organized crime, and social breakdown.

At the next level are a range of determinants that manifest themselves largely in terms of social policy and governmental regulation. These include societal poverty levels, education, nature of employment, environmental conditions, and human rights. These determinants may directly or indirectly affect health and disease, for example, through social security protections (guaranteeing unemployment support, "old age" security, health care, maternity leave, etc.); inadequate regulation of pollution emissions (exacerbating respiratory and other ailments); or discriminatory policing (causing excess deaths and higher incarceration rates, as well as stress-related ailments, among particular racial/ethnic groups).

The final level includes the underlying social, political, economic, and historical context. Key determinants include class and social structure, distribution of wealth and power, and international trade regimes. Again, these conditions affect health directly and indirectly. Unaccountable and unrepresentative governments fail to protect their citizens or residents from economic and physical insecurity. Trade agreements often eliminate price protections for small farmers, leading to declines in land tenure, food production for export rather than local consumption, and concomitant income declines and nutritional deficiencies, all affecting health. Of course, other structural factors may yield positive consequences: land redistribution and fair trade policies can improve farmer livelihood; democratization of power may strengthen the welfare state, increase economic redistribution, ensure regulation of the environment and the workplace, and improve housing and sanitary infrastructure.

In other words, the societal determinants of health are the "causes of the causes" of health and disease (Marmot 2005). The following section explores a selection of societal determinants of health from each level of the framework. We begin by examining individual characteristics and experience.

INDIVIDUAL CHARACTERISTICS AND EXPERIENCE

As discussed in Chapter 4, the behavioral and medical models of health largely attribute ill health to personal features and actions, and ascribe its resolution to individual and medical measures. However, other than major genetic conditions passed down through Mendelian inheritance patterns, every occurrence of disease, death, or disability includes varying degrees of societal influence. Moreover, the health outcomes of genetic conditions, too, are socially mediated. Here we review how societal and personal determinants interact and consider the shortcomings of viewing ill health primarily at the individual level.

Many personal features affect health, all of which are linked in some way to societal determinants of health. The importance of agency (decisions and actions taken at the individual or collective level) and the ability of individuals to influence health derive from a mix of personal endowment, family circumstances, social class, and larger political conditions. Illness, injury, and disability affect subsequent health status; at the same time, they are affected by preventive, regulatory, and curative measures as well as various other societal determinants of health. Congenital and perinatal conditions, for example, are affected by prenatal care and maternal well-being, which are in turn influenced by nutrition, household resources, employment, housing, social security measures, and health policies.

Life-course Trajectories

A lifecourse perspective helps explain how disadvantage (or advantage)—produced through societal determinants of health—accumulates over time in an individual (Kuh et al. 2003). For example, child health and childhood social class are a strong determinant of adult health (Irwin, Siddiqi, and Hertzman 2007). Physiological and psychological stresses beginning in childhood and workplace exposures during adulthood also influence health in older age (Middlebrooks and Audage 2008). A life-course perspective addresses past social conditions, the resulting influence on present-day health status, and possible future directions of health, exploring the interaction of these experiences, individual biology, and health (Blane 1999).

Health "Behaviors"

As discussed in Chapter 4, behavioral understandings of health largely ascribe health status to personal practices and habits, including unsafe sexual behavior, smoking, alcohol and drug consumption, poor diet, inadequate hygiene, excessive stress, and insufficient physical activity. This has become known as the "lifestyle approach" to health (Lalonde 1974). While there is no doubt that individual behaviors have a bearing on health outcomes (i.e., reckless driving can lead to automobile fatalities), behaviors are mediated by political, economic, cultural, and other societal determinants of health. For example, notwithstanding the well-known correlation between smoking and lung cancer, lung cancer mortality is considerably higher among working-class smokers than upper-class smokers. As well, smoking cessation and education efforts have been far more successful among privileged populations who are better able to relieve stress or cope with the challenges of quitting smoking.

What is wrong with the individual perspective? Is it not important to live a healthy life? Of course it is, but this approach covers only one small component of multiple levels and influences on health. It assumes that people are perfect decision makers with day-to-day control over work and neighborhood conditions—not to mention production, pollution control, trade, and marketing patterns—in order to improve their health, ignoring the clear evidence that life chances are structurally constrained. Moreover, in placing the blame on the individual for poor health, the individual approach removes responsibility for change from government, private business, and other actors. With this in mind, we turn to the influence of living conditions on health.

THE INFLUENCE OF LIVING CONDITIONS

Living conditions refer to housing and neighborhood characteristics, availability of potable water and adequate sanitation, food quality and security, maternal and child health facilities and policies, income and work/household roles, quality of and access to social services such as public health and transportation, and social stress (and its mitigators, such as support from friends and leisure activities). Many of the cultural and religious aspects of health, which also play out at national and regional levels, intertwine with and affect health at household and community levels. Numerous ailments result from poor living conditions, in particular cardiovascular, respiratory, gastrointestinal, endocrine, nutritional and metabolic diseases, injuries, and violence (Marmot 2006). Each year, 18 million deaths (more than one-third of all deaths worldwide) are directly attributable to the conditions of poverty (Pogge 2005), with women, children, and indigenous populations disproportionately affected. These numbers say nothing of the untold millions of deaths *indirectly* linked to poverty.

Box 7-2 Interactions of the Determinants of Health: Living Conditions

"The concomitants of poverty are often poor nutrition [either insufficient calories, protein, and fresh fruit and vegetables, or excessive energy-dense, nutritionally deficient, but cheap food]; overcrowded, damp, and inadequately heated housing; increased risk of infections; and inability to maintain optimal hygiene practices" (Shaw, Dorling, and Davey Smith 1999, p. 216).

Water and Sanitation

Water is fundamental to life, yet over one-sixth of the world's population lives without an adequate supply of safe water. Approximately one-third of the world's population lives on lands with moderate to severe water stress (McMichael 2001; Dauvergne 2004). Competition for water also precipitates conflict, as evidenced in the Middle East and many other settings over thousands of years (Gleick 2006). Almost half the world's population (2.6 billion people, mostly in rural areas) lacks access (unpaid or paid) to even the most basic sanitation and must resort to using pit latrines, fields, and ditches. This leads to water and soil contamination and increased rates of communicable diseases, especially diarrhea (UNDP 2006). Water and sanitation-related illnesses kill some 3 million people each year and are among the leading causes of preventable mortality and morbidity (WHO and UNICEF 2001). Diarrhea alone causes 2 million annual deaths, mostly among children (UNICEF 2007).

As shown in Figure 7–1, access to an in-house water connection is closely associated with infant mortality—in general, where water access is high, infant mortality is low, and vice versa. This general trend is countered under some circumstances, as indicated by the outliers in Figure 7–1. For example, despite fairly high rates of in-house water connections (73% of the population), Iraq has experienced a 150%

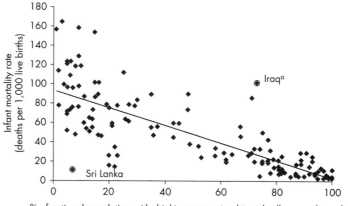

% of national population with drinking water piped into dwelling, yard, or plot[b]

Figure 7–1 Water connection rates and infant mortality rates, 2006.
[a]Iraq's infant mortality rate is contested. Although the current WHOSIS database indicates a rate of 37 deaths/1,000 live births, as recently as 2004, the official rate in WHOSIS was 102/1,000. Save the Children has documented similarly high figures, which we use in this table.
[b]Many with household or community access to a water connection or protected source must pay steep fees in order to use this water. Moreover, piped water is not always potable.
The countries above the line have higher than average infant mortality given the proportion of households with water connections, whereas those below the line have lower than average infant mortality given the water connection rate.
Data Sources: Save the Children (2007); WHO and UNICEF (2008); WHOSIS (2008).

jump in child and infant mortality (the world's highest rate of increase) since the first Gulf War in 1991, which has been exacerbated by the U.S. invasion of Iraq in 2003 (Save the Children 2007). This is because Iraq's relatively high official water connection rate does not reflect interruptions in and contamination of water supplies due to numerous bombings. Water access is of course not the only factor influencing Iraq's elevated infant mortality rate, which has suffered enormously from the health and nutrition effects of sanctions, repression, and violence (see Chapter 8 for further details). Sri Lanka, by contrast, has an infant mortality rate of 11 deaths/1,000 live births, even though less than 10% of the population has an in-house water connection. This is partially explained by extensive community, rather than household, water coverage—82% of the total population has access to "improved water sources" (see Chapter 10). Sri Lanka has also invested heavily in many other social programs that influence infant mortality (see Chapter 13).

Thus, the connection between water/sanitation and health is complex. For instance, the WHO argues that hand-washing can reduce diarrheal diseases by close to 50% (WHO 2004b). However, this is not simply a matter of personal habits, but rests on sufficient access to clean water (and soap). Indeed almost half of the mortality decline in the United States during the first three decades of the 20th century can be attributed to water purification. Paradoxically, poorer populations tend to pay more for water use than richer ones, who typically live closer to utility systems (UNDP 2006). Women, girls, and refugees are particularly affected by poor water supply. They typically bear responsibility for collecting water, often over great distances, subjecting them to injury from heavy loads and assault, and jeopardizing school attendance and other activities.

Nutrition and Food Security

Feeding children is a foremost family and societal responsibility. A healthy diet is essential to child development and growth and to human flourishing. Food security refers to availability of and access to sufficient quantities of nutritious food. Food sovereignty, by contrast, refers to self-determination in the production and consumption of foods in terms socially, economically, and culturally consistent with local practices and conditions (Via Campesina 2002).

Over 50% of child deaths are the result of poor nutrition or undernutrition (Sanchez et al. 2005), and it is estimated that hunger and malnutrition kill more people per year than do AIDS, malaria, and TB combined (WHO 2002a). The mainstream medical community addresses hunger and malnutrition almost exclusively through clinical approaches, leaving the structural factors of food distribution and production unaddressed. This is one of the reasons that a societal determinants of health approach is a necessary counterpart to the biomedical approach.

In the past, both hunger and malnutrition were a matter of insufficient calories, protein, fresh fruits, and vegetables. Today, malnutrition is increasingly associated

with so-called empty calories—chemically processed foods with high sugar and
fat content—that are cheaper (due to agricultural subsidies and mass production),
widely available, and heavily marketed in many societies. Not only does this food
have little nutritional value, its consumption can lead to obesity, cardiovascular disease, certain cancers, dental caries, low birth weight babies, diabetes, and vitamin
deficiencies (WHO EURO 2003). Throughout the world, 2 million people suffer
from nutrient shortages, even when their daily caloric needs are met or exceeded
(Sanchez et al. 2005).

Box 7-3 Food Quality and the Societal Determinants of Health

In mid-19th century Britain, Friedrich Engels found that the health effects of contaminated food
were disproportionately borne by the working class and poor. Because workers typically received
their weekly wages on Saturday evening, they were only able to reach the market:

> "after the best food has been purchased in the morning by the middle classes...But even if
> it were still there, [they] probably could not afford to buy it. The potatoes purchased by the
> workers are generally bad, the vegetables shrivelled, the cheese stale and of poor quality, the
> bacon rancid. The meat is lean, old, tough, and partially tainted. It is the produce either of
> animals which have died a natural death or of sick animals which have been slaughtered. Food
> is generally sold by petty hawkers who buy up bad food and are able to sell it cheaply because
> of its poor quality... The workers are cheated in other ways by the greed of the middle clas-
> ses. Producers and shopkeepers adulterate all food stuffs in a disgraceful manner, with a scan-
> dalous disregard for the health of the ultimate consumer" (Engels 1845, pp. 80–82).

Personal, household, and community food (in)security are determined by a
number of factors. For approximately one-seventh of the world's population, hunger
is a severe problem. Although global food production far exceeds the nutrient and
caloric needs of the world's population, over 850 million people go hungry every day.
Nobel economist Amartya Sen has demonstrated that hunger and famines are caused
more by the economics of maldistribution than by food shortages. In Bengal's 1943
famine (in which 3 million people died), poor people starved because they lacked
purchasing power (due to unemployment and wage declines), while excess food
rotted in the storehouses of wealthy landowners and food retailers or was exported
at high prices (Sen 1981; Ravallion 1987; Sen 1990). Over 60 years later, although
reducing hunger is one of the MDGs (see Chapters 3 and 4), hunger is increasing in
the Middle East, Asia, and sub-Saharan Africa (FAO 2005).

For billions of other people, poor nutrition is the main problem. While some
public health authorities attribute poor diet to bad individual choices and lack of
education, these issues are rooted in the mass production and marketing of food.
For example, marbled (fatty) meat is a result of an industrial meat processing system that overfeeds livestock, uses growth hormones, and limits animals' exercise.
Ubiquitous sales and advertisements of sugar and fat-laden convenience foods—and
the consequences of their mass consumption—have affected almost every society.

Although tradition, culture, and household resources play an important role, dietary patterns are increasingly influenced by the industrialization of food production, which has made processed food cheaper per calorie than fresh produce and basic foodstuffs, despite the multiple ingredients and complex production methods, marketing costs, and distribution chains it entails. In Seattle, United States, for example, "the differential in energy cost between refined sugar and sugar in fresh raspberries [is] approximately 10,000%" (Drewnowski and Barratt-Fornell 2004, p. 164). In many poor neighborhoods, and even in places where fresh produce is abundant, healthy food selection in grocery stores or *bodegas* may be limited and expensive. For households with restricted food storage and cooking facilities, and/ or in which household members work long hours or in noncoinciding shifts, "fast food" is indeed convenient.

The "cornification" of the United States and other societies—thanks to vast agricultural supports given to corn farmers in recent decades—means that corn-based products are present in most foods, either in the form of feed for animals or as high carbohydrate, low nutrition corn syrup, a ubiquitous food additive. Corn subsidies in the United States (which also support production of corn-based ethanol, a problematic gasoline alternative—see Chapter 10) have artificially lowered prices on the global market, forcing hundreds of thousands of small farmers out of business in Mexico and other developing countries. All told, large-scale industrial corn production leaves a trail of pollution where it is grown, of misery where it can no longer be grown, and of health problems where it is (often unknowingly) consumed (Pollan 2006).

Food production and consumption affect health in other ways. Pesticide residues, industrial chemical run-off in soil and waterways (e.g., petroleum in the soil of the Niger Delta; mercury in the North American Great Lakes), and other contaminants in food cause a variety of cancers and infertility. In addition, food-borne illnesses due to contamination in the production and distribution process affect millions of people each year (WHO 2007).

World food production and trade are big business, and power is increasingly concentrated in a few large corporations. One-third of global grocery sales are in the hands of 30 food retailers, and 90% of world grain trade is controlled by just five companies (Eagleton 2005). This affects another determinant of health—local sustainable farming practices—especially since over 50% of the population in developing countries works in agriculture.

Housing and Human Settlements

Along with food and water, shelter is a basic human need that (ideally) provides safety, stability, rest and leisure, and conditions that foster physical and mental health. Moreover, since societies require both economic production (the conversion of labor into goods) and social reproduction (the making—biologically and socially—of more members of society), households or family units take center stage in the continuation of any social group. Poor housing, by contrast, not only inhibits these factors, for example due to unsafe plumbing, cooking, or sleeping facilities, but can also cause or exacerbate a range of health problems. For example, housing that is cold, damp, and/or moldy can lead to upper- and lower-respiratory tract diseases, meningococcal infections, and asthma (Ineichen 1993). Furthermore, housing in which open stoves are used for heating or cooking have high rates of fire accidents and lung disease (Shaw, Dorling, and Davey Smith 1999).

Overcrowding and inadequate ventilation and sanitation facilitate the spread of air-borne, water-borne, and skin ailments, including TB, diarrhea, lice, and scabies. Beds shared by many increase the spread of disease and the possibility of the molestation of minors. Flimsy structures provide little or no protection from storms, fires, and earthquakes, and recycled industrial materials and lead paint can cause fatal poisonings and severe neurological and cognitive problems. All of these aspects of housing also affect psychological well-being.

Of course, a prime role of housing is to provide protection against the elements, animals, and violence. In areas with endemic malaria, dengue, and other vector-borne diseases, door and window screens (usually prohibitively expensive) or bed nets are the main impediment to mosquito bites. If there is no indoor plumbing or regular refuse collection, water storage containers often serve as mosquito breeding sites. In areas where Chagas disease is endemic, low-cost thatched roofs can pose a problem because trypanosomes spend daylight hours hidden in them, only to descend and bite in the night.

The most extreme housing problem is homelessness. Estimates of global homelessness range from 100 million to 1 billion people (Tipple and Speak 2005). In high-income European countries, 2 million people depend on homelessness services. More than 7 million U.S. residents have experienced homelessness at some point in their lives, with over 600,000 people homeless every night. Homelessness estimates in developing nations range from 1.5 million homeless people in South Africa to 18.5 million in India (Kellett and Moore 2003).

The death rate among homeless people is 2 to 10 times higher than the death rate of the nonhomeless (Hwang 2000; Cheung and Hwang 2004). This differential is partially mitigated by social services—for example, the death rate among homeless people in Toronto (where there is universal health care) is 58% lower than in Philadelphia, where health and other services are more limited (Hwang 2000). But even societies with extensive social services for the homeless—including free health care, accessible shelters, food banks, and employment training programs—cannot compensate for the health effects of not having a permanent home. In many locales, homeless people may be jailed or abused by the police. Children who live on the streets in cities across Latin America and other regions are subject to violence by shopkeepers, gangs, or political authorities. The desperate conditions of homelessness can also lead to drug use, sex work, and deterioration of mental health.

While these material dimensions of shelter (or homelessness) are extremely important to population health outcomes, housing is also tied to identity, self-expression, and other socially and psychologically meaningful dimensions (this is why people decorate and adorn their homes). In fact, whether one takes pride in and enjoys being in one's home appears to be significantly tied to measures of self-reported physical and mental health (Dunn 2002).

Neighborhood Conditions

Neighborhood conditions affect the quality of housing, water and sanitation, food availability, and other determinants of health. But neighborhood also transcends these determinants, affecting health via quality and availability of infrastructure and institutions, including schools, health and social services, parks, stores, transport, and recreation and community spaces. Other less tangible neighborhood features, such as unemployment rates, crime, stress levels, community solidarity and organization, social, racial, and cultural tolerance, political empowerment, and civic engagement also affect health (Pickett and Pearl 2001).

Across the world, nearly 1 billion people (32% of the world's urban population, and 43% of the "developing" world's urban population) live in "slums" characterized by open sewers, stagnant water, rotting garbage, toxic dumpsites, an unstable land base, shoddy housing, abandoned lots and buildings, unpaved roads; inadequate electricity, sanitation, schools, clinics, and other infrastructure; poor quality of housing; overcrowding; gang violence; high eviction rates; and few legal protections. Because factories and waste facilities located near slums often evade regulations, air and soil pollution in slums is often extensive. Although not all slum dwellers are poor, they include large numbers of destitute migrants from rural areas (many of whom are socially marginalized), and chronically unemployed and exploited, long-time urban residents (Riley et al. 2007). These conditions generate poor health from infectious diseases such as TB, HIV, and diarrhea, as well as cancer, trauma, and stress-related cardiovascular disease. Other ailments that particularly affect slum dwellers include salmonella, plague, and other diseases that have rodent vectors.

"What good does it do to treat people's illnesses...then send them back to the conditions that made them sick?" (Michael Marmot, at "Tackling Health Inequalities" conference, London, October 2005).

Public Health and Health Care Services

A range of community-level public health activities are important determinants of health. These include food safety inspection and standards; epidemic and chronic disease surveillance, control, and clinics; collection and disposal of refuse; road safety; monitoring of sanitation and water quality; environmental health monitoring; school health services (and school lunches); maternal and child health programs; housing regulations and inspection; workplace safety and inspection, among others. These activities influence other determinants of health and can have a significant role in reducing mortality.

For the approximately 10% of premature deaths preventable through medical care and the many other ailments treated through the health care system, provision of health care services is a key determinant of health (Chapter 12 will discuss health systems in detail). The health system itself can also promote or jeopardize health, depending on how equitably it is financed (i.e., the presence or absence of user fees and national health insurance), its accessibility and quality (especially to rural populations and slum dwellers), and the extent to which it prioritizes preventive services and public health over curative services (Gilson et al. 2007).

The strength of integrating primary health care with other determinants of health in countries such as Cuba and Costa Rica partially explains why health indicators are high even when economic indicators are not. Costa Rica's 1970s health system reform, for example, emphasized primary care for underserved areas together with nutritional and educational improvements. In the 15 years following the reform, infant mortality rates dropped from 60/1,000 to 19/1,000, and life expectancy increased dramatically (Starfield, Shi, and Macinko 2005).

Culture and Religion

Although people often think of culture in terms of literature, music, and art, to anthropologists culture refers to socially transmitted frameworks of meaning—frameworks that form the basis through which people interpret and engage with the world. Just as language is shared by members of the same linguistic group but employed with varying proficiency and originality by each speaker, cultural understandings are broadly shared but by no means identical from one cultural member to another. Cultural meanings are derived from national, ethnic, religious, institutional, or transnational values or symbols, and the social relations, rituals, practices, and traditions in which these symbols are embedded. Culture shapes how people see the world and their place in it and gives meaning to personal and collective experience.

Health reflects cultural priorities and practices (e.g., individualism, materialism, solidarity) in a variety of ways (Eckersley 2005). Cultural beliefs influence the ways in which health and illness are defined and understood. Notwithstanding more than a century of use of the International Classification of Diseases (see Chapter 5), most people view health through cultural filters other than the biomedical lens (which is itself an assemblage of cultural values, symbols, preferences, rituals, practices, and traditions). Learning and understanding what these filters mean is important to any cross-cultural health effort whether carried out locally or internationally. In some cultures, pregnancy is medicalized and treated as though it were a disease; in others, it is understood in spiritual or kinship terms. Among the Maya, a fever may be understood as an ailment rather than a symptom; in wine-loving France, general malaise is often referred to as a "liver crisis"; and in the United States, chronic fatigue syndrome is recognized as a disease that usually afflicts young urban professionals working long hours. The dietary practices of some religions, such as the Jewish prohibition on eating pork, arose from a health concern—the presence of trichinosis in pork meat.

Identifying cultural influences on health is fraught with issues of cultural relativism and misunderstanding. What one cultural group determines is harmful to health is unlikely to be universally viewed as such by all cultures. Sometimes what are believed to be cultural views of health may be subsumed under social conditions. For example, the fatigue-inducing anemia accompanying chronic malnutrition may not be viewed as a disease at all by subsistence farmers, but rather as an inevitable part of their lives.

Culture influences what actions may be taken to prevent or treat illness, and which healing authorities to consult. In developed countries, this can be particularly important in relation to subcultures, and dominant and minority groups. For instance, biomedical care may not be sought by some (im)migrant and minority populations who do not share cultural frames with the dominant group. Anthropologists can be helpful in ascertaining how health programs and policies can be more effective or acceptable in particular contexts (e.g., the importance of integrating local healers and traditional medicinal practices in health campaigns).

However, cultural influences on health can be overemphasized, particularly when the illness and/or treatments are considered "exotic" or are sensationalized. For example, most HIV/AIDS prevention work in sub-Saharan Africa focuses primarily on sexual practices, to the neglect of larger structural issues such as migration, immunological susceptibility due to poor nutrition and housing, and extremely limited access to safe employment and social services. Critical medical anthropology emphasizes how political and economic forces, including the exercise of power, shape health, disease, illness experience, and health care (Castro and Singer 2004).

Certain cultural values—such as cooperativism—can be particularly protective of health. For example, the Bhutan government's emphasis on "gross national happiness" (GNH), is distinct from the dominant global cultural norm emphasizing gross domestic product (GDP). There are four main pillars of GNH: (1) promotion of equitable and sustainable socioeconomic development; (2) preservation and promotion of cultural values; (3) conservation of the natural environment; and (4) establishment of good governance. Although Bhutan's household incomes have remained among the world's lowest, life expectancy increased by 19 years following the implementation of GNH measures (Revkin 2005).

Transport

Transport influences health through a variety of mechanisms: road injuries and fatalities, air quality, places for exercise and human interaction, interpersonal security, cost, and overall quality of urban life (WHO EURO 2003). As well, inadequate or unaffordable transport can affect other determinants, such as school attendance, employment, and preventive health care (e.g., prenatal care visits or control of chronic ailments). Most directly, road traffic accidents are the second leading cause of death for children between 5 and 14 years of age.

Traffic fatality and injury rates vary by class, income, geography, and education levels, with poor and working classes disproportionately affected. There has been a steady decline in traffic fatalities in high-income regions over the past three decades (due to a combination of increased road and automobile safety, legal restrictions and sanctions, and trauma care), but significant increases elsewhere. Much of the difference has to do with safety measures: in high-income countries, most casualties are among drivers and passengers, whereas in low- and middle-income countries, pedestrians, cyclists, and public transport passengers account for 90% of casualties, reflecting poor vehicle and road regulation. In Haiti, the *molue* (local transport) is known as the "moving morgue," and in southern Nigeria, the *danfo* are called "flying coffins" (Nantulya and Reich 2003).

SOCIAL POLICIES AND GOVERNMENT REGULATIONS

A range of social, political, and economic policies and their implementation influence health. These include education, health services, taxation, union organization, freedom of the press, human rights, and environmental protections. In the following sections, we will examine the health consequences of several of these.

Income and Poverty

Extreme poverty is characterized by very low income and lack of access to the basic necessities of life—food, shelter, and water. As discussed in Chapter 4, living on less than US$1/day is the indicator of extreme poverty used by international agencies (UN 2003; World Bank 2008). While income-related poverty is a crucial determinant of the ability to purchase the necessities for health and well-being, many researchers argue that poverty entails more than a lack of income and that measurements of poverty must include questions of empowerment, security, dignity, and social acceptance (Nussbaum and Sen 1991; Marmot 2006). Others have made the case for an index of material deprivation, which would include indicators such as access to clean water, sanitation, shelter, education, information, food, and health (Townsend 2005).

"The test of our progress is not whether we add more to the abundance of those who have much; it is whether we provide enough for those who have too little" (Franklin Delano Roosevelt, 32nd President of the United States).

Regardless, absolute poverty alone does not explain global mortality patterns. Although per capita income and health are roughly correlated up to a level of approximately US$5,000 (see Chapter 11), above this level, the correlation is far hazier (Kawachi, Wilkinson, and Kennedy 1999). This seeming discrepancy is somewhat mitigated by the role of relative income levels (or income inequalities), but other factors are also at play (see ahead).

Education

Education has long been associated with higher health status through two primary means: increased likelihood of better-paid, safer jobs with benefits and room for advancement; and the ability to take, or advocate for, protective health measures (Cutler and Lleras-Muney 2007) understood at the broadest level. People who are more educated are empowered to improve their health through their range of employment possibilities, neighborhood selection, political participation, and understanding of, and ability to avoid or respond to, a variety of impediments to health. Moreover, early childhood development and education can help ameliorate some of the negative effects of social disadvantage, with an impact throughout the life span (Irwin, Siddiqi, and Hertzman 2007, p. 7).

In general, people who are better educated have lower levels of hypertension, emphysema, diabetes, anxiety, and depression, improved physical and mental functioning, and healthier behaviors (e.g., lower rates of smoking, heavy drinking, obesity, and drug use; higher rates of exercise and screening procedures; better management of stress and chronic health conditions) (Carr 2004). For instance, in St. Petersburg, Russia, education level is negatively correlated with all-cause mortality and cardiovascular disease (see Figs. 7–2 and 7–3).

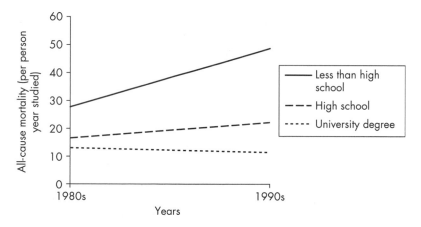

Figure 7–2 All-cause mortality among men 40–59 in St. Petersburg, Russia, by education level. *Data Source*: Plavinski, Plavinskaya, and Klimov (2003).

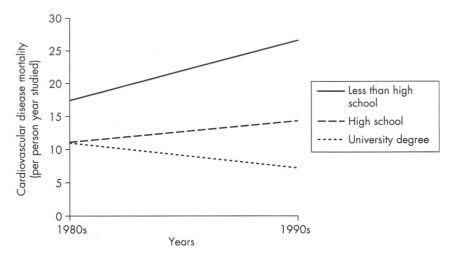

Figure 7–3 Cardiovascular mortality among men 40–59 in St. Petersburg, Russia, by education level.
Data Source: Plavinski, Plavinskaya, and Klimov (2003).

Education barriers can be understood in terms of access and quality. For example, in growing numbers of underdeveloped countries, students must pay user fees (and fees for books, uniforms, and supplies) in order to attend school, excluding millions of children from formal education. Girls' ability to attend school is particularly jeopardized by these fees (and other impediments to access, such as lack of toilets and unsafe conditions) as their families may favor having girls contribute to household work over paying for their school fees, and boys may be perceived as potentially benefiting more from education. As well, in many countries, deregulation and reductions in social sector spending have led to a marked deterioration in the quality of education. In some settings, the ranks of educators have been decimated in recent decades by high rates of migration to developed countries, civil conflict, and HIV/AIDS. Neighborhood conditions (safety, existence of schools, transport) and the household environment (e.g., space, a quiet environment, light to study by, economic and family care-giving responsibilities, and family health) also affect school attendance.

Work Conditions/Employment Status

Work conditions affect health at four levels and may have long-lasting effects:

1. through exposure to dangerous chemical, physical, and biological agents (including repetitive motion strain, unsafe equipment and activities, and toxins), and the degree to which workers are protected against them;
2. via hierarchy and worker control, workplace stress, and the right to organize;

3. according to the extent of fair pay, benefits, and stability of employment; and
4. in terms of sexual, racial, and other forms of harassment.

Globally, there are annually 250 million occupational injuries, 350,000 injury-related deaths (on the job or job-related), and 1.6 million occupationally-related deaths. Typically, those who are employed in many of the most dangerous employment sectors (forestry, fishing, agriculture, construction, and transport) are not covered by workers' compensation for any injury (Driscoll et al. 2005). Only 10% of workers in developing countries are covered by occupational health and safety laws (LaDou 2003) (see Chapter 9 for more details).

The psychosocial bases of stress are exacerbated in work environments where there is low or no worker control and inadequate rewards (WHO EURO 2003). Seasonal employment, including construction and agricultural migrant work, also generates high levels of stress and danger because employment from year to year is not guaranteed, and seasonal workers usually lack benefits, workplace protections, or recourse against abuse, such as lack of payment and physical violence. In addition, location in the production process and degree of decision making at the micro and macro levels are key determinants of stress-related diseases, including heart disease, stroke, and cancer (Theorell et al. 1992; Marmot et al. 1997; Marmot et al. 1999; Johnson and Lipscomb 2006).

Employment and its exposures, workplace stress, and variable compensation can have major negative health effects, but unemployment is even more deleterious. Precarious or no employment increases stress, anxiety, and mental health problems, leading to excess ill health and mortality, particularly following job loss. Developing countries have unemployment rates of approximately 30% compared with developed countries' rates of 4% to 12% (Benach, Muntaner, and Santana 2007), with concomitant health effects. During periods of severe recession or depression, unemployment soars to much higher rates. Health begins to be affected at the time when people anticipate unemployment, but are still working (job insecurity, threat of job loss); health effects increase when there are inadequate or no social benefits to cushion job loss (Bartley, Ferrie, and Montgomery 1999).

Ill health and disability also affect employment. Those who are ill may be more likely to lose a job, be unable to keep a steady job, and become sicker as a result of stress and anxiety, inability to pay for care, and so on. In many societies, persons with disabilities are unable to find steady employment due to discrimination. Although in general being unemployed is worse than being employed (in health terms), not all employment is protective of health: the most hazardous jobs, such as farm work, coal mining, minibus driving in huge cities, commercial sex work, and work involving chemicals can be more detrimental to health than unemployment.

Income from employment is a key determinant of health but employment is also important in providing social protections such as health benefits and pensions (in some societies), and in offering education and training, social networks, labor organizing, and solidarity.

Environment

As we will see in Chapter 10, environmental conditions are one of the key determinants of health. Environmental problems and their health consequences derive from two key processes: depletion and contamination. Depletion of water, forests, the earth's protective ozone layer, soil, and flora and fauna generally affect human health by limiting availability of and access to basic necessities and arable land, and impeding livelihoods. Contamination, which occurs largely through industrial production and consumption processes, leads to human exposure to a variety of chemical, biological, and physical agents, with endocrinological, physiological, genetic, and other effects (Briggs 2003). As well, greenhouse gas emissions have led to global warming, which decreases land productivity, water availability, and biodiversity, and threatens climate disasters among other effects on human health.

Violence and Health

Violence is an important determinant of health due to the deaths and disability it causes but also because it generates fear and destruction and restricts day-to-day activities and dreams for the future. The *World Report on Violence and Health* (WHO 2002b) categorizes violence as: (a) self-directed, including suicide, and self-mutilation; (b) collective, which may be socially, economically, or politically motivated; and (c) interpersonal, including partner or family violence and violence in settings outside the home. Of the 5 million deaths from injuries in 2000, approximately 1.6 million were the result of violence: 49% from suicides; 18% due to war; and 31% from homicides (WHO 2004a).

Currently rates of violent death are two to three times higher in low- or middle-income countries than in high-income countries due to high poverty rates, political and economic inequality, rapid urbanization, competition for resources, military conflict, and repressive political regimes. During the 20th century, almost 200 million people lost their lives directly or indirectly as a result of wars, with civilians constituting over half of those killed (WHO 2002b). Weapon use (e.g., machetes, landmines, guns, and bombs) can cause acute physical trauma, followed by long-term disability (e.g., loss of limbs, reduction in sensory abilities, fistulae). Men, particularly those between the ages of 15 and 29, are disproportionately killed in violent conflict. However, sexual violence—both within families during conflict and as a weapon of war—affects women in particular (see Chapter 8 for further details).

Social Inclusion/Exclusion, Social Support, and Social Capital

Social inclusion/exclusion describes the ability/inability of certain groups (e.g., people who are homeless or poor, racial and ethnic minorities, or immigrants) to fully participate in civic life. Social exclusion may be the result of structural inequalities, lack of access to resources (economic, social, political, and/or cultural), discrimination, and stigma (Galabuzi and Labonte 2002). Social inclusion provides access to resources and social support networks, adequate housing, education, and transportation (Shaw, Dorling, and Davey Smith 1999). Social exclusion has been found to lead to premature death, increased illness, poor physical and mental health, and increased levels of societal violence (WHO EURO 2003).

Being included in various aspects of civil life may be described in terms of "social capital," which gauges the extent to which individuals experience trust, a feeling of social cohesion, and shared norms with other members of society (Putnam, Leonardi, and Nannetti 1993; Putnam 2000; Islam et al. 2006). While advocates of social capital theory claim that these shared experiences and norms lead to improved health outcomes, they overlook the issue of how social capital is generated in the first place.

A broader societal view based on a political economy framework goes beyond recognition that lack of social cohesion leads to social inequalities and ill health to posit that class structure creates social inequalities *and* reduced social capital, *both* of which negatively affect health (Muntaner and Lynch 1999).

Moreover, nesting ideas of social inclusion and reciprocity in a capitalist framework ignores the detrimental societal and health effects of capitalism itself (Navarro 2002). Ignoring the larger structures shaping factors such as social capital may in fact lead to worse health outcomes and unduly place the onus on communities and individuals to fend for themselves (i.e., generate their own social capital) in a system that has prioritized markets over the welfare state (Pearce and Davey Smith 2003). Moreover, social inclusion is both determined by, and determines, levels of civic engagement and participation in political and social processes, and thus is strongly correlated with democratic governance and the welfare state (WHO EURO 2003).

Human Rights and Political Freedoms

A society's articulation and enforcement of human rights is a key determinant of health and is associated with many other determinants relating to civil, political, economic, employment, and other conditions. While human rights is an abstract concept to some, its use as a means of realizing gains in human well-being transforms this concept into concrete—and measurable—features (Yamin 2005).

Health and human rights are linked through multiple pathways. While the right to health is itself a key component of the WHO Constitution, many human rights treaties protect the right to societal determinants of health as well, such as the right to education, food and nutrition, an adequate standard of living, social security, civil participation, the benefits of scientific progress, and protection from all forms of violence and discrimination (see Chapters 4 and 14).

Other National-Level Policies

Industrial policies and subsidies affect health through the determinants of work and environmental conditions, food production, and trade. Redistributive mechanisms, including social security systems, particular social welfare measures (including unemployment insurance, minimum wages, housing protection, pensions, health services, etc.), and tax policy, all have a profound influence on health. These are discussed further in other sections.

SOCIAL, POLITICAL, ECONOMIC, AND HISTORICAL CONTEXT

At the broadest level, the societal determinants of health can be understood in relation to social, political, economic, and historical forces played out in national and global arenas. At the national level, these forces include forms of stratification such as patriarchy, racism, and class structure, the nature of land tenure, immigrant status, and the structure of the political system. At the international level, these forces include trade agreements and international financial instruments. Many other societal forces highlight the interplay between national and global levels. These include militarism, colonialism, and imperialism. In the following section, we detail how these national and global forces affect population health. Importantly, while we identify these forces one by one, they remain highly interrelated (Waitzkin 2007).

Income/Wealth Distribution

Half the world's population controls just 1% of global wealth, living on less than US$730 per person per year. To put it more starkly, there is a 10,000 to 1 difference between the wealthiest 10% of Americans and the poorest 10% of Ethiopians (Birdsall 2005). These inequalities are not new, but they do counter notions that global economic growth automatically brings shared prosperity (see Chapters 4 and 9).

Wealth and income inequalities have been increasing over the last four decades within countries as diverse as Colombia, Indonesia, Zambia, Poland, China, South Africa, India, and the United States (Almas 2004). Four-fifths of the world's population lives in countries that have seen large increases in income inequality. In Brazil, for example, the poorest 10% of the population earns just 0.7% of national income, while the wealthiest 10% amasses 47% (UNDP 2005).

Richard Wilkinson and his colleagues have argued that income inequality affects population health, with greater inequality in income distribution leading to decreased life expectancy and vice versa (Kawachi, Wilkinson, and Kennedy 1999). In the early 1990s, Wilkinson found that OECD countries with the longest life expectancy were those with the smallest proportion of people living in relative poverty, not the ones with highest levels of national income. He argued that this resulted from the psychosocial impact of relative deprivation and low levels of social cohesion, with levels of well-being growing as groups climbed up the rungs of the socioeconomic ladder (Wilkinson 1994).

While Wilkinson did not include developing countries in his work, a recent World Bank study has found similar stepwise differences in health indicators by wealth quintile, as shown in Figures 7–4 and 7–5. For instance, in Peru, child mortality is almost five times higher for children of the lowest wealth quintile than those of the highest

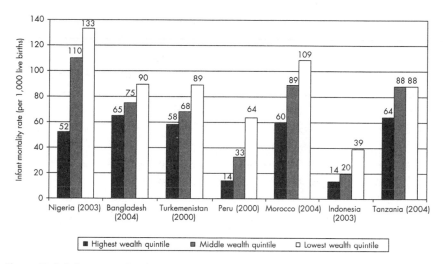

Figure 7–4 Infant mortality by wealth quintile, selected countries.
Data Source: Gwatkin et al. (2007).

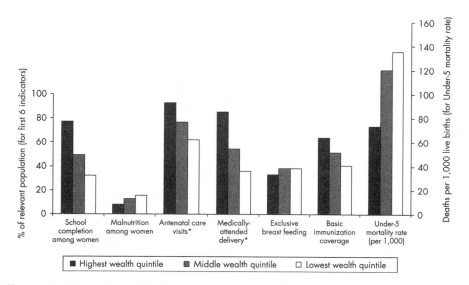

Figure 7–5 Maternal and child health indicators in developing countries, by wealth quintile.
*Includes doctors, nurses, and midwives.
Data Source: Gwatkin et al. (2007).

wealth quintile, whereas Tanzania, which is a less unequal society, has higher infant mortality rates overall but smaller differences by wealth quintile (see Fig. 7–4).

But the relationship between income inequality and health outcomes is more complex than Wilkinson's findings suggest (Lynch et al. 2004). With the exception of the United States, income inequality is not a major determinant of population health differences within or between high-income countries. (Its effect in developing countries with small elites is yet to be determined.) Moreover, seeking to understand socioeconomic status (SES) without addressing class structure does not explain how and why income inequalities are generated and, as such, places undo emphasis on community-level determinants of health. Without addressing the structural roots of inequalities, these analyses may lead to a "community-level version of 'blaming the victim'" (Muntaner and Lynch 1999, p. 525).

Though raising the incomes of the poorest would help to lift people out of absolute poverty and reduce health inequalities, the maldistribution of political influence and power associated with income and far greater wealth inequalities (which take into account property, stock, interest, and other nonincome assets) would likely persist. As such, universal and redistributive social policies are likely to have a far greater impact than income redistribution per se (Starfield and Birn 2007).

Class Stratification

Important as income appears as a direct and indirect determinant of health, it does not tell the whole story. Nor can income inequalities completely explain health and mortality patterns within and across societies. Social class, theorized by Karl Marx to define people's relation to the production process—that is whether one is an owner, a worker, or in an intermediate or contradictory class position (a manager or administrator)—explains health outcomes at a level even beyond income. As we shall see, social class appears to be the largest determinant of social inequalities in health.

Another way of measuring social standing is SES. Deriving from the ideas of sociologist Max Weber, SES refers to individuals' position in society in terms of three variables: income, education, and prestige. This classification uses education and the perception of status to sidestep the limits of income alone. In socially stratified systems, resources may be allocated differentially along SES lines (education, occupation, income, assets, wealth, prestige) (House and Williams 2004), enabling people to achieve health or other desired goals between and across generations. Useful as SES is in elaborating how assets and characteristics intertwine to create social differences within and between societies, SES does not include work and ownership relations—the major feature of power in capitalist societies.

Gender

Gender inequalities and gender discrimination are an important determinant of health. Gender refers to social conceptions and roles rather than biological differences.

In other words, health differences due to sex-based differences in biology are not gendered per se, whereas health differences between women and men (whether heterosexuals, transsexuals, gays, lesbians, bisexuals, or persons of ambiguous sexuality) due to their differing household responsibilities, decision-making power, occupational roles, or legal rights are considered to be gendered differences. Gender-based differences in health status vary over time and place, just as gender roles vary according to era and context. That said, in most societies, women, together with sexual minorities, bear the brunt of gender oppression and prejudice. As such, much work regarding gender equality and health is focused on women (Doyal 2003).

Even health issues that are largely biological may be inextricably linked to gender. For example, although only women experience childbirth, the lifelong effects of nutrition, previous illness, and social support, as well as access to health care, are all influenced by gender roles and in turn affect the health of women during pregnancy and delivery. In most high- and middle-income countries today, women experience lower levels of mortality and longer life expectancy (though higher morbidity) than men do, in large part due to reductions in childbirth-related deaths over the past century. Yet in many developing countries, maternal mortality remains extremely high, shortening women's life expectancy.

Gendered roles by no means consistently favor men. In the former USSR, men have disproportionately higher mortality rates as well as higher rates of smoking, alcohol consumption, and obesity. Men are also more likely to be involved in road traffic accidents (Denton, Prus, and Walters 2004). Globally, violence is a gendered phenomenon, with women experiencing much higher rates of domestic and sexual violence (Ostlin, George, and Sen 2003) and men experiencing higher rates of homicide (WHO 2002b).

The connections between gender and health are complex. Often, there is greater social stress associated with female gender roles, and greater economic stress associated with male gender roles (Denton, Prus, and Walters 2004), but this is changing with women's greater insertion into paid and income-generating positions. The sexual division of labor leads to differential health outcomes, with men more likely to undertake dangerous or high-stress employment outside of the home, while women—especially in developing countries—are exposed to dangerous household activities such as cooking and water collection. Moreover, women are also engaged in significant numbers in some of the most hazardous occupations, including farming and sex work. Although women generally benefit from higher levels of social support through friends and kin, this support can be a demand as well as a resource, potentially increasing stress levels.

Gender interacts with class, race, and other categories of difference and discrimination in determining access to education, employment, health, and social services. Poverty increases morbidity and mortality for both men and women, but women typically have less control over the material and social conditions of life that foster good health. Yet in societies such as Kerala, where there have been investments in education for girls and an emphasis on increasing women's participation in civil and political life, there have been improvements not only in gender equity but also in population health in general (Ostlin, George, and Sen 2003).

Race and Racism

Race, like gender, is a social construction that is used to classify groups into categories based on arbitrary, usually visible, characteristics (e.g., skin color, shape of eyes, etc.). Historically, racial distinctions have been created by dominant societal groups in order to establish or maintain power and privilege at the expense of "the other" group (Krieger 2003). These distinctions vary based on the particular context, as discussed in Chapter 5.[2] Racism—distinguished from race—is the enactment of structural and systematic forms of oppression and discrimination against particular racial groups by individuals and/or institutions, with racial definitions themselves arising from oppressive systems of race relations.

Racism negatively affects health through eight main pathways (Krieger 2003; House and Williams 2004):

1. Economic and social deprivation, which restricts ability to obtain quality education and well-paying, safe, and secure employment;
2. Greater exposure to toxic substances and hazardous conditions, often experienced as a result of segregated living and working conditions;
3. Socially inflicted trauma, such as verbal, sexual, physical, and emotional abuse and the resulting psychological stress, anxiety, and injury;
4. Targeted marketing of substances and activities that are harmful to health;
5. Lower access to appropriate and quality care, leading to inadequate and degrading medical treatment;
6. Exclusion from political power and decision making;
7. Unequal treatment by law and order (police and justice) systems; and
8. State oppression, including inadequate state responses to unfair treatment.

Racial/ethnic health inequities are observed in numerous health outcomes. In the United States, for example, the infant mortality rate among African-Americans is more than twice that of the population of European descent, and the death rate from heart disease, lung, and colorectal cancer is also higher among African-Americans than the population as a whole (Kington and Nickens 2001).

Racial inequalities in health are interpreted in one of three ways. First—as in the Human Genome Project and similar studies—they are theorized to reflect biological differences in susceptibility to disease. This approach disregards the overwhelmingly social rather than biological basis of race, and may in itself reinforce racial discrimination by researchers, doctors, educators, and society-at-large. Moreover, because of the genetic heterogeneity within socially designated "racial/ethnic groups," it is implausible that innate genetics alone can explain patterns and trends in racial/ethnic health inequities. Studies carried out in Brazil, the United States, and the United Kingdom show that phenotype does not correlate to genotype for all sorts of traits (including skin color and genomic African ancestry), precisely because of population "admixture"(Goodman 2000; Feldman, Lewontin, and King 2003; Parra, Kittles, and Shriver 2004).

Second, race is often conceptualized as a proxy for social class. This is based on the reality of many societies in which racial minority groups—including immigrants—are disproportionately poor, and does not address the coexistence of racial and class-based inequalities. The third conceptualization attempts to address racial and class differences as existing independently, but also operating synergistically, and is of central importance in understanding inequalities in health (Kawachi, Daniels, and Robinson 2005).

If, as current research suggests, the basis of racial/ethnic health inequities is not genes, then what? Certainly, the rate of poverty is higher among African-Americans than among most other ethnic/racial groups in the United States. But higher poverty rates do not explain everything: death rates among African-Americans are higher than Euro-Americans in every social class. This is the result of the past legacy of slavery and oppression, and the continued and pervasive effects of institutional and everyday racism. Currently, a small but rapidly growing body of research, conducted in the United States, the United Kingdom, Canada, New Zealand, and other countries, is documenting the impact of racial discrimination on somatic health, mental health, and health behaviors, including self-rated health, blood pressure, preterm delivery, obesity, and tobacco and other substance use (Krieger 1999; Williams, Neighbors, and Jackson 2003; Paradies 2006; Mays, Cochran, and Barnes 2007). As well, the effect of life-course trajectories and intergenerational experience means that adults who were materially and socially deprived as children may continue to experience the effects of deprivation even if their life circumstances improve (Krieger 2005b). In sum, *both* poverty/social class *and* racism, among other societal factors, explain the existence and persistence of racial inequalities in health in the United States.

In South Africa, the legacy of the racist apartheid system of state-sanctioned discrimination continues to manifest itself in unequal health conditions, with a three- to four-fold difference in infant mortality rates between blacks and whites (Burgard and Treiman 2006). In New Zealand, research shows that taking into account experiences of racism and economic deprivation substantially reduces health inequities between Māori- and European-descended populations (Harris et al. 2006). Discrimination has also been shown to be hazardous to the health of aboriginal populations in Canada (Iwasaki, Bartlett, and O'Neil 2004). Global data reveal a consistent pattern: in each society, groups subjected to racial discrimination—tied to racial ideologies involving conquest of indigenous populations, slavery, and subjugation—typically have the worst health status.

Yet, whether in South Africa, New Zealand, Brazil, North America, or Europe, not all people of African (or Asian, or Latin American, or indigenous, or religious minority group, etc.) origin are poor and not all poor people are of these various origins. Most importantly, there is nothing inherent (genetically or culturally) that correlates race with poverty. Rather, it is *racism* and its social application in everyday life that explains the poverty and poor health status of many blacks in South Africa and the United States and of other racialized groups—such as immigrants to Europe from its former colonies in Africa and Asia—around the world. In sum, worse health status among historically oppressed and marginalized groups is a reflection of *both* racism *and* classism and must be analyzed as such.

Box 7–4 Immigrant, Migrant, and Refugee Status

Migration status can be extremely important in shaping health and is often linked to many other societal determinants of health, including social inclusion/exclusion, working and living conditions, political repression, stress, income, and social class. Moving within and across borders permanently or temporarily—whether voluntarily or forced by war, economic, political, cultural, or environmental conditions—may lead to immediate and lifelong health repercussions (Loue and Galea 2007).

Almost 200 million people—3% of the global population—live "outside their place of birth" (International Organization for Migration 2008). This figure does not include undocumented migrants. There may be considerable positive health repercussions for voluntary immigrants—particularly professionals—who choose to leave their homes to seek economic betterment, advanced education, family reunification, or cultural acceptance. These include improved income, better employment conditions and opportunities, and greater social satisfaction. Still, this "healthy immigrant effect" tends to dissipate over time (Wilkins et al. 2008). Moreover, in the new setting, voluntary migrants may also experience racial or cultural discrimination, psychological stress, poor working conditions, loss of family and social support, and may lack political representation or social benefits.

People are obliged to migrate within and outside national borders for many reasons, including political causes, unemployment, and being forced off their land due to famine, ecological disasters, and inability to sustain their livelihood. Those who must move often face immiseration, marginalization, unstable housing situations, loss of family and support networks, and discrimination—and their resultant health consequences—in addition to the problems outlined above. Undocumented migrants, who may have crossed borders unofficially and lack legal status, are particularly subject to employer and police abuse as well as social exclusion due to the continuous threat of deportation and extremely limited legal protections.

Similarly, migrant workers—such as seasonal agricultural workers and temporary laborers in the service and informal sectors—often face the synergistic effects of workplace exploitation, dangerous occupations, violence, and lack of civil and social protection (social security, education, health insurance, unemployment benefits, etc.). Such precarious and exploitative conditions increase susceptibility and exposure to ill health and often preclude the possibility of medical treatment and care, exacerbating premature mortality and disability. Human trafficking—forced sex work by children and women, involuntary servitude in sweatshops, households, factories, and informal work—generates further dire health consequences associated with slavery conditions, including physical injury and disability, sexually transmitted and other infectious diseases, stress disorders, and other mental health conditions (Loue and Galea 2007).

As discussed in Chapter 8, there are tens of millions of refugees and internally displaced persons around the world—forcibly displaced due to armed conflict. These suffer among the worst mix of unhealthy societal determinants and associated health conditions, including political persecution, injuries, trauma, communicable diseases, neonatal problems, malnutrition, and the loss of family members, home, livelihood, and community (Shaw, Dorling, and Davey Smith 1999).

Indigenous Status

Across the world there are marked discrepancies in the health status of indigenous versus nonindigenous populations (see Chapter 6). In virtually every society (Russia, throughout Latin America, China, North America, Iceland, Australasia, and elsewhere), indigenous status is associated with oppression and worse health. These inequalities result from historical subjugation that has denigrated traditional ways of life, kinship structures, and spiritual beliefs—generating near universal patterns of racial and cultural discrimination against indigenous groups (PAHO 2002).

The colonization process and continued discrimination against indigenous peoples—including violence, forcible removal from ancestral lands, denial of heritage, loss of livelihood, government neglect, and absence of social protections—has many consequent health effects. In Australia and Canada, thousands of indigenous children were forced from their families and communities into residential schools for almost a century, where they faced violence, overcrowding, poor nutrition, and forced labor. Almost one-fourth of students in residential schools died of tuberculosis in early 20th-century Canada (Bryce 1907).

The marginalization of indigenous populations is reflected in disproportionate poverty rates, limited access to potable water and quality housing stock, and high levels of exposure to environmental toxins. In Canada, indigenous groups have twice the poverty rate of nonindigenous populations, and in El Salvador, 95% of water sources that are used by indigenous populations are contaminated (PAHO 2002). In Mexico, almost 90% of indigenous communities live in extreme poverty (Castro, Erviti, and Leyva 2007).

The poor health status of many indigenous populations is compounded by lack of access to health care. Throughout the Americas, 40% of indigenous groups do not receive health services for geographical and economic reasons, and often there are large cultural, linguistic, and social barriers to care (Montenegro and Stephans 2006). Indigenous groups have had little voice in public health reporting and policy making, but there is growing recognition of the need for bona fide involvement of indigenous populations in addressing the multiple oppressions they face.

Some countries have achieved better results than others in reducing inequalities in health between indigenous and nonindigenous populations. Currently Canada is the only country with a national-level institute focused on aboriginal health. In New Zealand, the 1840 Treaty of Waitangi officially recognized Māori sovereignty and outlined reparations and agreements. While the treaty was long criticized for not meaningfully engaging indigenous voices, in recent years its implementation has improved. Māori perspectives on health and illness have been incorporated into national and regional health plans, the fruition of longtime Māori involvement in public health activities. The New Zealand government has also prioritized housing and infrastructural needs of the Māori people—providing potable water, affordable housing, and an indigenous justice system on Māori lands. While these policies have not eliminated inequalities in New Zealand, they demonstrate the role of deliberate policy making in improving the health of indigenous populations, especially when contrasted with neighboring Australia's failure to effectively address the entrenched inequalities between indigenous and nonindigenous groups (Ross and Taylor 2002; Anderson et al. 2006).

Land Tenure

While property ownership is a key feature of assets and wealth in most societies, land tenure is particularly salient where there is small-scale agricultural production and subsistence farming because holding and farming the land is often the sole source of livelihood. In settings where sharecropping or tenant farming is practiced, farmers are subject to the control and demand of large landowners and may be compelled to purchase seed, equipment, and other goods from the owner and to sell farm products at depressed prices. In some countries, land redistribution to rural populations has been a key feature of political movements and revolutions and has served as a means of raising the living conditions of millions of small-scale farmers.

As agricultural production has become industrialized over the past two centuries, big business interests and free trade policies have squeezed out small rural landholders through a variety of mechanisms. In 19th-century Britain, collective landholdings were forcibly split after reform of official inheritance laws: smaller and smaller plots were no longer sustainable. At the same time, guaranteed crop prices were abandoned by the state (with repeal of the Corn Laws), driving small farmers off the land and forcing them into factories. More recently, large agri-businesses have used technologies and unfair competitive practices to drive down prices, similarly squeezing out small landholders. In Brazil, for example, recent corporate takeovers by Nestlé and Parmalat have caused 50,000 small dairy farmers to lose their livelihoods. In various countries, governments have nationalized large swaths of land—forcing local farmers or nomadic hunters and pastoralists onto unproductive land—only to resell the property to private interests. Millions of landless farmers in South Asia, Latin America, and elsewhere have been forced to migrate to urban settings and are among the most marginalized of the world's population, even as they have begun to organize politically, as through Brazil's Landless Workers' Movement.

As environmental scientist-activist Vandana Shiva has poignantly demonstrated, the rise of agri-business, free trade agreements, and the marketing of genetically modified (GM) seeds in India has had devastating effects. Unlike local varieties, GM seeds are patented (and expensive) even when seeded naturally through pollination; many farmers lured into GM seed dependence soon become indebted. Millions of small farmers have lost their livelihoods, unable to survive against large competitors, and since 1997 more than 40,000 farmers in India have committed suicide (Editorial 2006; Navdanya 2007) .

International Trade Regimes

The global trade system is one of the ways in which unequal power is created and maintained. In many developing countries, primary materials and labor-intensive goods are extracted and produced at far lower cost than in higher-income countries. The cost of business is minimized through low wages, lax environmental and occupational standards, and few, if any, taxes. Producer countries receive few gains (although corrupt politicians often benefit enormously), as they have little control over commodity pricing. Moreover, in many countries a combination of subsistence living and political repression makes it difficult for workers to unionize and form effective political movements to create more protective measures.

Free trade agreements often undermine worker rights and environmental protection policies, while promoting privatization of public sectors, such as water, health care, and education; reductions in tariffs and taxes lower state income that could have been spent on social services (Gershman, Irwin, and Shakow 2003). Trade agreements also protect businesses from "impediments to competition" (such as subsidies for local industries, price caps for essential goods, occupational protections, social insurance taxes, etc.) at the expense of small-scale farmers and laborers protected by these measures (Labonte 2003) in both developed and developing countries. The role of international trade patterns and agreements are discussed in detail in Chapter 9.

International Financial Instruments and Policies

At the broadest global and structural level, the economic instruments (loans, currency supports) and policies (conditionalities) of international financial agencies, commercial banks, and dominant corporate interests affect health in a variety of ways. These international policies have shaped national policies and environments regarding work, production and economic patterns, and social welfare. The neoliberal economic paradigm that emerged in the 1980s supposes that economic growth through integration into global markets—and deregulation, privatization, and a reduced role for the state—are tools for poverty alleviation and reduction in national and international disparities. However, economic integration has had the opposite effect, with inequality increasing over the past three decades. When economic growth has led to poverty reduction, most notably in China, vulnerability and insecurity have often increased alongside dangerous work and environmental conditions, lack of regulation, and deterioration of health and social infrastructure (Gershman, Irwin, and Shakow 2003; Reddy 2008).

Loan conditionalities—most prominently structural adjustment programs (SAPs) and poverty reduction strategies (PRSPs) (see Chapters 3 and 9)—of

recent decades have affected health in the following ways (SAPRIN 2001;
Guttal 2003):

1. Agriculture and mining sector reforms have undermined the viability of small
   producers, weakened food security, and damaged the natural environment;
2. Privatization and civil and labor sector reforms have led to increased unemployment, precarious employment, and weakened worker protections;
3. Deregulation has led to increased environmental contamination, occupational
   exposures, and hazards in the home and community;
4. Privatization, user fees, and social spending cuts have decreased access to
   essential social services, including education, health care, and housing;
5. Real wages have deteriorated and inequality has increased;
6. The burden of these policies has been borne disproportionately by the poorest
   and most vulnerable populations (children, women, indigenous groups, and
   small-scale farmers), while the benefits have been disproportionately enjoyed
   by local and international elites, large private sector enterprises, and transnational corporations; and
7. Local industries, especially small and medium enterprises, have been devastated and replaced with larger and multinational companies that often flout
   protective legislation (Jubilee USA 2003).

IFI policies are discussed in greater detail in Chapters 3, 4, and 9.

The Political System: Welfare Regime, Distribution of Power, and Accountability

As discussed in Chapter 4, the welfare state, whereby "the state plays a key role
in the protection and promotion of the economic and social well-being of its
citizens...based on the principles of equality of opportunity, equitable distribution
of wealth, and public responsibility for those unable to avail themselves of the
minimal provisions for a good life" (Britannica Online 2008), has been recognized
as a key determinant of population health due to its central functions of ensuring income redistribution, protecting against immiseration, unemployment, and ill
health, providing universal public health care and education, and improving occupational health and safety standards (Chung and Muntaner 2007).

In examining the main types of welfare states within OECD nations, Haejoo
Chung, Carles Muntaner, and Vicente Navarro (among others) have found a high
correlation between the strength of the welfare state and population health outcomes including life expectancy and infant mortality. The most successful welfare states—in terms of desirable health outcomes—are characterized by strong
unionized labor movements and socialist political parties, high corporate taxes, progressive income taxes, high expenditures on social security and health care, high
levels of employment, particularly in the public sector, near universal health and

social services coverage, and low rates of poverty, wage disparities, and income inequalities (Navarro and Shi 2001). The main welfare state policies correlated with health are high rates of female employment, high levels of unemployment compensation, universal access to health care, and adequate subsidies to single mothers and divorced women (Chung and Muntaner 2007).

Ultimately the more egalitarian the country is on political, economic, and social grounds, the fewer inequalities are found in health, pointing to the centrality of reducing differences in social conditions and of redistributing economic and other societal resources through political processes. While there is limited systematic research on these questions outside high-income countries, the experiences of Cuba, Costa Rica, Kerala, and a few other settings where there are substantial social and economic redistribution and good health outcomes (see Chapters 11 and 13) substantiate the evidence based on OECD countries.

Militarism, Colonialism, and Imperialism

The legacies of colonialism, militarism, and imperialism have shaped the historical trajectories of many, if not all, societal determinants of health. Domination and oppression influence health through various channels, including a lack of sovereignty and political self-determination, limited control over resources, social policy, law and order, and so on, whether within or between countries. Although few colonies remain, the current global political structure reflects geopolitical relations that have been in place for centuries. Systems of trade and commodity pricing, debt and global finance regimes, and international organizations for the most part maintain the power imbalances between colonizer (high-income, developed, industrialized) and colonized (low-income, underdeveloped) countries. See Chapters 2, 8, and 9 for further details.

Militarism escalates all forms of violence within and between countries, with extremely damaging consequences to soldiers and civilians alike. Militaristic societies often have excessively harsh judicial systems. For example, the United States has the highest number of people (2.3 million) and proportion of the population (1%) in prison in the world. Those incarcerated are disproportionately poor, young men of color (Aizenman 2008). Military spending also channels resources away from social and infrastructural endeavors—building parks, schools, quality housing, investing in safe employment, and so on. The diamond production and trade business provides one example of the damage that militarism and imperialism can wreak on global health. Recent civil wars in Angola, the Democratic Republic of Congo, and Sierra Leone— where over 5 million people have died—were largely fueled and financed by trade in "conflict diamonds" (Amnesty International 2007). Poor populations of countries with valuable primary resources rarely benefit from them: internal and external competition for control over resources can explode into civil war; extraction causes environmental damage; and profits go into the hands of foreign and domestic elites, with virtually nothing left for social infrastructure and other public needs (Olsson 2007).

As we have seen, the societal determinants of health are both distinguishable from one another *and* interrelated at progressive levels (Starfield 2007; Krieger 2008). Poverty, for example, is both the outcome of local, national, and global policies and activities and is accompanied by material deprivation leading to, among other things, inadequate access to nutritious food, clean water, housing, unsafe neighborhoods, and so on (Marmot 2005). These factors, in turn, increase exposure and susceptibility to, and reduce resistance and recovery from, disease and disability. Ultimately, patterns of political power and resource distribution interact with biological processes, leading to differing gradations of health or ill health in individuals.

The next section explores how these processes take place, that is, how social and political inequalities manifest themselves in unequal health patterns; what brings them about; how and why inequalities in health add up to more than the sum of individual determinants; and how they might be addressed.

SOCIAL INEQUALITIES IN HEALTH

Key Questions:

- How are social inequalities in health produced?
- What is the relationship between societal determinants of health and social inequalities in health?
- What explains why people in certain societies with relatively low income per capita enjoy longer and healthier lives than those in some much wealthier societies?

As Charles Dickens observed of the French Revolution in *A Tale of Two Cities*, "it was the best of times, it was the worst of times." So we could speak of the status of health today. On *average* people across the globe live far longer and healthier lives than did our ancestors: global life expectancy has increased by at least 37 years over the past 200 years, with increases of 45 years in some countries (Riley 2001). Yet the benefits of these gains have not been shared equally. In 1960, China had a life expectancy of 36 years, some 4 years less than the sub-Saharan African average of 40 years. Almost five decades later, Chinese life expectancy is 71 years, while the average life expectancy in sub-Saharan Africa is just 46 years (Jamison et al. 2006). In some regions, such as the former Soviet Union and parts of Africa, life expectancy has even fallen (WHO 2006).

Even more striking than the differences between countries (and regions) are the persistent inequalities in health *within* countries, which are as great or even greater than the more widely cited differences between countries. Marked inequalities in health exist in countries as diverse as China, Chile, and Russia with gaps in life expectancy across segments of society having widened over time. China's rapid industrialization and transition to a capitalist economy over the past three decades has produced urban–rural life expectancy gaps of over 10 years, reflecting not just "a slower rate of increase in health improvement in rural areas, but in many cases an actual net decline in the health of the poor," with infant mortality rates climbing by 25% in the 1980s (Evans et al. 2001, p. 7). China's inequalities are so great that health conditions among some are similar to those seen in Namibia, while the health of other groups are closer to levels in Western Europe (UNDP 2005).

Just as Dickens's novels portrayed the simultaneous glory and brutality of 19th-century industrialization in England (depending on whether you were among the small elite of factory owners who lived to 60 years on average or among the exploited class of factory workers who lived to less than 30 years), today's inequalities show that the best off in society live longer, healthier lives than those worst off. These inequalities manifest themselves in terms of differences in premature death, disability, and life expectancy. In many countries—from Senegal to Vietnam—child mortality rates are twice as high in rural as in urban areas (WHOSIS 2007).

The terms "social inequalities in health," "inequities in health," and "health inequalities" are often used interchangeably, though there are important—if subtle—distinctions between them, as laid out at the beginning of the chapter and in Box 7–5. Here we will principally use the term social inequalities in health (or health inequalities as a shortcut) to refer to the systematic and persistent differences in health between and among different social classes, genders, racial and ethnic groups, occupational groups, and so on, as linked to underlying power and structural differences.

Box 7–5 Differences between Inequalities and Inequities in Health

"The concept of equity is inherently normative—that is, value based, while equality is not necessarily so...However...strictly speaking these terms are not synonymous. The concept of health equity focuses attention on the distribution of resources and other processes that drive a particular kind of health inequality—that is, a systematic inequality in health (or in its social determinants) between more and less advantaged social groups, in other words, a health inequality that is unjust or unfair" (Braveman and Gruskin 2003, p. 255).

A Brief History of Documenting Social Inequalities in Health

Great Britain has a long tradition of collecting national mortality statistics and is one of the most class-conscious societies in the world. Thus, it is no surprise that it was one of the first countries to document persistent inequalities in health. Following path-breaking work on the direct relationship between neighborhood poverty rates and mortality carried out by Louis-René Villermé in 1820s Paris (which he attributed to moral shortcomings rather than climatic, topographic, or divine causes), Edwin Chadwick and Friedrich Engels documented similar patterns in 1840s England (see Chapters 2 and 5). As with Villermé's findings, not only did they identify mortality differences between rich and poor, but they also found shorter life expectancy (higher mortality) at each rung down the social class ladder. In his *Report into the Sanitary Conditions of the Labouring Population of Great Britain* Chadwick argued that crowded, squalid living conditions were linked to illness, in turn leading to immorality, limited work capacity, and the downward cycle of poverty. Drawing from his findings, Chadwick called for drainage and sewage disposal, clean water supplies, and regular refuse collection, all to be overseen by a district medical officer. These recommendations aimed to improve living conditions but did not address the core issue of poverty.

Engels's documentation of mortality differentials by class of neighborhood and housing in Manchester led him to a different explanation: he believed that the root cause of social inequalities in health was the capitalist economic system and the exploitation of the working class. As such, political action was necessary to address poverty (and its health effects). Engels argued that power and resource inequalities had to be addressed in order to achieve permanent improvements in living conditions, an argument that remains as relevant today as it was two centuries ago.

Evidence of Inequalities in Health

Evidence documenting the existence of, and even increases in, social inequalities in health continues to mount in most countries. But how is this gap conceptualized, that is, how can we understand how these inequalities emerge, persist, and even worsen in spite of growing worldwide attention to health? Once the essential human needs of food and shelter are satisfied—along with secondary needs of employment, social services, basic health and sanitation, and relative peace and democracy—the *size* of resources becomes secondary to their *distribution* within society. Because much of the world's population lives in relative poverty (i.e., whereby nobody lacks the basic material necessities of life but lower classes are poor in comparison to higher classes) rather than absolute poverty, it is important to understand and address the health implications of relative poverty.

The Black Report and the Whitehall Studies

Modern attention to health inequalities was spurred by the 1980 "Black Report," which documented class-based health patterns in the United Kingdom from the 1930s through the 1970s. Despite general improvements at the aggregate level, the report found persistent differences in health by socio-occupational class. For example, while the United Kingdom's overall infant mortality rate fell for all social classes between 1930 and the 1970s, infant mortality remained higher among children born to unskilled laborers (Class V) than to partly skilled laborers (Class IV), whose rates were higher than among children born to skilled manual laborers (Class III), and so on up through managerial (Class II) and professional (Class I) classes. At the extremes, infant mortality was almost five times higher in the lowest class than in the highest class (see Fig. 7–6). The report found analogous stepwise class difference for all causes of death and a particularly strong association with respiratory diseases (Black and Research Working Group 1980). Similar stepwise differences in infant mortality and in access to maternal and child health measures by wealth quintile (income class) may be seen in current developing country data (see Figs. 7–4 and 7–5).

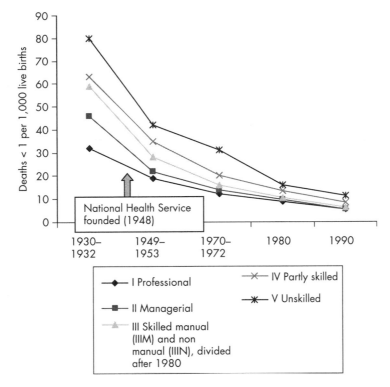

Figure 7–6 Social class and infant mortality in the United Kingdom: The Black Report and beyond. Infant mortality rates show a continued downward trend in more recent data from 1993 to 1995, with persistent and stepwise social class differentials. These data are not included because the lines cannot be distinguished due to the scale of the graph.
Data Sources: Black and Research Working Group (1980); UK Office for National Statistics Series DH3 Nos. 9 and 24; Botting (1997).

Moreover, these health differences between classes, already present in the 1930s, continued long after the establishment in 1948 of Britain's tax-funded, universal National Health Service. The Black Report argued that the persistence of mortality and life expectancy differentials by social class (which continue to the present—see Fig. 7–7) were the result of differences in living and working conditions, *not* differences in health care access and utilization.

The report concluded that class-based mortality differences do not exist naturally but are "socially or economically determined" and therefore amenable to change through social and economic policies. Of course, such changes are subject to political processes; the Black Report was commissioned by a Labour Party government minister (Sir Douglas Black), but it was released (in the most cloaked fashion possible) under a newly elected Conservative government. The report's recommendations for child benefits, preschool education, housing, and workplace improvements, among others, were summarily rejected as unaffordable.

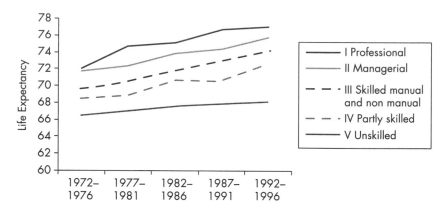

Figure 7–7 Life expectancy by social class for men (England and Wales) since the Black Report. *Data Sources:* Fitzpatrick and Dollamore (1999); Hattersley (1999).

Almost concurrently, another British study uncovered a "social gradient in health" in the absence of poverty or material deprivation. Marmot and colleagues studied 17,350 British civil servants (the initial of several "Whitehall studies") between 1967 and 1969. This first study researched the health of male civil servants, selected because of their large numbers, accessibility, permanent and stable employment, and ease of tracking over time. The study found an inverse relationship between employment class and death from coronary heart disease, with men in the lowest occupational grades bearing the highest death rate from heart disease, and with the rate decreasing progressively from the lowest to the highest class (Rose and Marmot 1981).

This social gradient manifested itself in a clear stepwise fashion, even though none of the study subjects were poor and all had "white collar" office jobs with stable incomes and employment benefits. The social gradient and its effects on health have also been found to continue throughout life with cumulative effects (WHO EURO 2003).

The second Whitehall study (which included women) was begun in the mid-1980s and confirmed that the social gradient found in the first study persisted (see Fig. 7–8). The key explanatory factors for the social gradient relate to position in the work hierarchy and include: extent of control over work processes; variation in tasks; and the pace of work (Job Stress Network 2008).

The next section explores these factors in greater depth.

Understanding and Explaining Social Inequalities in Health

Five main models seek to explain inequalities in health and the distribution of the societal determinants of health:

1. The biology and social selection model, arguing for inherent differences that evolve over time;

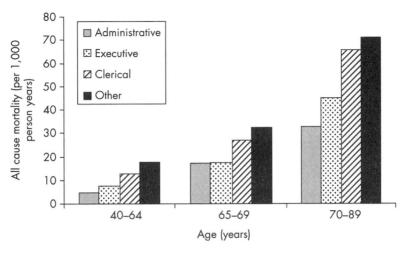

Figure 7–8 Whitehall all-cause mortality over 25 years according to level in occupational hierarchy. *Data Source*: Marmot and Shipley (1996).

2. The lifestyle and behavior model, maintaining that inequalities in health are the product of personal choices over how to live, what to eat, where to work, forms of recreation, exercise, etc.;
3. The psychosocial model, positing that physiological (somatic) manifestations of perceptions of inequality influence health via stress pathways;
4. The political economy of health model, focusing on the structural causes of inequalities (class hierarchies, political and economic processes, unequal access to power and resources) and their material and health manifestations; and
5. The eco-social model, which views illness and health as the biological embodiment of relations of power and other social processes which accumulate over the life-course and intergenerationally.

Biology and Social Selection Model

According to this model, personal health derives from one's genetic heritage and individual constitution (physiology and overall biology). Health, in turn, determines one's ability to thrive, benefit from "opportunities," and, ultimately, attain a favorable socioeconomic position. The biology and selection approach is sometimes associated with personality typologies, characterizing people's ability to withstand stress based on their calm or excitable nature. Because the sick and weak are less able to benefit from social and economic opportunity, according to this model they drift downwards into lower social classes. (This is one of the unsubstantiated theories as to why so many people diagnosed with schizophrenia are found in the lowest social class.) The remedies, according to this model, are found in personal medical and genetic interventions.

However, even though class and heath status interact, social position almost always precedes ill health, as in the case of schizophrenia. Most importantly, the directional weight of causality is not of equal magnitude: though ill health is one of the factors that can lead to poverty, poverty is the primary determinant of ill health. Various researchers have found the effect of social selection on the social gradient to be small; as such, social mobility does little to explain inequalities in health (Blane and Manor cited in WHO Commission on Social Determinants of Health 2007a). Instead, the determinants of health appear to influence both social position and health over the life course.

Lifestyle and Behavior Model

Healers have always proffered advice to the infirm on diet and climate, but it is only in recent decades that individual behavior has taken on scientific pretenses as a primary determinant of health. In 1974, Canada's Minister of National Health and Welfare Marc Lalonde issued a report stating: "good health is the bedrock on which social progress is built. A nation of healthy people can do those things that make life worthwhile, and as the level of health increases so does the potential for happiness...The health care system, however, is only one of many ways of maintaining and improving health" (Lalonde 1974, p. 5). In discounting the primacy of medical care in shaping health, Lalonde's report proposed that:

> [O]minous counter-forces have been at work to undo progress in raising the health status...They include environmental pollution, city living, habits of indolence, the abuse of alcohol, tobacco and drugs, and eating patterns which put the pleasing of the senses above the needs of the human body (Lalonde 1974, p. 5).

This official articulation of the "lifestyle model" brought legitimacy to the notion that health is a *personal* responsibility and that individuals can *choose* to be either healthy or unhealthy. The report also helped ignite the health promotion movement (see Chapter 13), which, though framed broadly in terms of societal influences on health, has been interpreted in an increasingly narrow behavioral fashion by the WHO and many governments (WHO 1999).

Canada's Lalonde Report reverberated across Europe, the Americas, and beyond, with many governments adopting its basic tenets just as neoliberal processes of deregulation and privatization were emerging (see Chapter 4). The lifestyle approach was thus ideologically consistent with (and justified) policies aiming to enhance the role of the private sector and diminish the responsibility of government in providing for social welfare in the United Kingdom, the United States, and many other countries.

The key argument of this model—applied since in countless superficial studies (that simply reiterate presuppositions) and misguided public health policies—is that "human behavior is the single most important determinant of variations in health outcomes" (Satcher and Higginbotham 2008, p. 401). Yet there is abundant evidence that decisions are shaped by far more than individual will, and that lifestyles can-not explain patterns of social inequalities in health. For example, conventional risk factors and behaviors for coronary heart disease (CHD) (smoking, hypertension, cholesterol, diet, physical activity, alcohol consumption) do not account for between 15% and 40% of social inequalities in CHD (Lynch et al. 2006). The first Whitehall study also found that the social class gradient in health persisted even when adjusted for such factors, indicating that there was far more than differential class patterns of "risky behavior" involved in the gradient (Marmot et al. 1978).

Placing the onus on individuals to eat and exercise right, wear seatbelts, avoid alcohol or drug abuse, practice safe sex, and so on, while certainly helpful advice, has deep consequences. First, it deflects attention away from other equally or more important levels and determinants of health, many of which interact with behavioral determinants. Second, it reduces government responsibility for ensuring the health of populations.

Moreover, the lifestyle approach overlooks the reality that people make decisions on how they live their lives within their social context. In environments where there are few outlets for stress relief, more people abuse alcohol, food, and drugs, as these serve as a means of coping with difficult circumstances (Wilkinson 1996). When low quality housing conditions and neighborhood stores, high prices, and difficult work shifts impede nutritious meal preparation (and in milieus where convenience foods are heavily advertised), people tend to have worse diets. Long work hours, expensive childcare, and parks that are in poor shape or unsafe, all inhibit regular exercise (Raphael et al. 2003).

Psychosocial Model

A prominent explanation for the social gradient in health identified by the Whitehall studies has to do with the psychosocial effects of inequalities. According to this model, the psychological effect of one's (unfavorable) location on the social hierarchy translates into a physiological response of stress and resentment, raising blood pressure and depressing the immunological system, and in turn affecting cardiovascular health and a range of other health problems. Here, it is the *perception* of precarious, unfair, or inferior status that counts, not the *reality* of unequal control, limited decision-making latitude, etc. (discussed in the political economy model next).

According to the psychosocial model, "macro- and meso-level social processes lead to perceptions and psychological processes at the individual level...and these psychological changes can influence health through direct psychobiological processes or through modified behaviours and lifestyles" (Martikainen, Bartley, and Lahelma 2002, p. 1092) (see Fig. 7–9).

The psychosocial model draws partly from studies of hierarchy and stress among baboons (Sapolsky 1994) as applied to humans. It is also associated with notions of social capital and social cohesion (discussed earlier), whereby the negative psychosocial effects of living in hierarchical societies are exacerbated and reinforced by

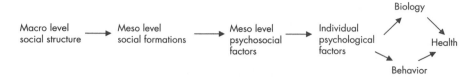

Figure 7–9 Schematic representation of psychosocial pathways.
Source: Adapted from Martikainen, Bartley, and Lehelma (2002, p. 1092).

lower levels of community involvement and interaction (conversely, societies that are more equal enjoy greater communal unity).

Stated differently, societies with greater income disparities are less cohesive and have greater social distance between groups. As distrust and suspicion mount, support for society-wide institutions and infrastructure, such as public education, youth and social programs, public parks, and universal health care decreases. Those at the bottom end of the income distribution may be socially excluded, disrespected, and may themselves lose self-respect, with dire health consequences (Wilkinson 1996). In other words, in "comparing their status, possessions, and other life circumstances with those of others, individuals experience feelings of shame, worthlessness, and envy that have psychobiological effects upon health" (Raphael 2006, p. 658). For example, reactions to stress from inequality, loss of income, housing and food insecurity, among other factors are believed to weaken the immune system and lead to increased insulin resistance and greater incidence of lipid and clotting disorders, all of which are precursors to disease (Stansfeld and Marmot 2002). Moreover, unhealthy behaviors, such as overeating and tobacco and alcohol (ab)use—adopted as coping mechanisms to relieve stress—have further negative effects on health.

According to this theory, even those at the top end of the income scale experience worse health than do people living in more egalitarian societies, because they fear losing their position or assets and may be isolated from other groups. As such, in high-income countries the way that people interpret their position in the social hierarchy strongly influences health inequalities (Kawachi and Kennedy 2002).

One of the main shortcomings of the psychosocial model's understanding of inequalities in health is that it is based on a series of unverified assumptions: that unequal status is largely experienced psychologically; and that psychological perceptions create stress, which is implicated in numerous disease pathways, including unhealthy behavior that jeopardizes health. These assumptions are epitomized in a recent World Bank/USAID study, which narrowly locates health (care) inequalities in individual and psychological characteristics:

> [A]n individual's lack of power and status often translates into a lower likelihood of taking preventive health measures and seeking and using health care. The striking differences in health status among different economic groups reflect inequalities in access to information, to facilities that provide decent standards of care, and to the means to pay for good care (Ashford, Gwatkin, and Yazbeck 2006, p. 3).

Political Economy of Health Model

As we have seen, the psychosocial model reduces the manifestations of the societal determinants of health to individual-level behaviors and "opportunities." However, as discussed throughout the text, the political, social, and economic context into which people are born and live contributes significantly to health status. An alternative to the psychosocial approach, then, is a model that takes the class-based organization of society as the fundamental explanation for social inequalities in health (Keating and Hertzman 1999).

By definition, the capitalist system is one of struggle for power between the capitalist class and the working class. According to the political economy model, the structures, institutions, and relations of the capitalist economic system generate and are reflected in social inequalities. In classical Marxist thought, class location is determined in relation to production—whether one is an owner of the means of production or a worker—and, therefore, the main inequalities are between owners and workers. In more recent decades, neo-Marxist thinkers have elaborated on class structure theory to include the concept of contradictory class location (Wright 1985)—characterizing people who are simultaneously owners and workers (e.g., factory workers with pension plans tied to company profits) or neither owners nor solely workers (e.g., managers, administrators, teachers who both exploit and are exploited)—and other finer class gradations.

Rather than focusing solely on the health effects of differential social status, the political economy of health approach seeks to understand the causes of social-class differentials in health as manifested through various mechanisms. To begin, the material conditions of life, as discussed throughout this chapter, have an enormous bearing on health: these conditions, whether referring to neighborhoods, assets and possessions, or workplace environments, indicate material advantage or disadvantage over the life span (Shaw, Dorling, and Mitchell 2002). Material conditions are associated with physical (infections, malnutrition, chronic disease, and injuries), developmental (delayed or impaired cognitive, personality, and social development), educational (learning disabilities, poor learning, early school leaving), and social (difficulties with socialization and in preparation for work and family life) problems.

Other key mechanisms have to do with structures of power in the polis and in the workplace. Where there are more inequalities in political structures and institutions (to the disadvantage of the working class), there is less redistribution of material resources, social services, economic and social security, and democratic decision making, reflected in inequalities in virtually every other determinant of health. In the workplace, class struggle and class inequality have enormous effects on inequalities in health. The lower one is in a workplace hierarchy, the less decision-making latitude and employment security one has, the more oversight there is, the more repetitive activities one has to do. These all lead to higher stress levels and negative health consequences.

Where workers have less political power (i.e., where unions are constrained or illegal), stress is compounded by precarious work conditions, with higher exposure to workplace hazards, fewer protections against dangers and job loss, and more repression. While social democratic societies with universal and comprehensive social security systems and strong unions, such as Sweden, experience less inequality than less redistributive societies, class-based inequalities remain and redressing them is a prime societal concern (Raphael 2006; Vallgarda 2007).

Eco-Social Model

The emerging multilevel eco-social model, developed by Harvard epidemiologist Nancy Krieger, seeks to integrate political, social, and biological understandings of the determinants of health, with health outcomes as the biologic expression, or "embodiment," of living conditions, social relations, and structures of power over the life course and across generations. This holistic model sees:

> Embodiment [a]s literal. The eco-social premise is that clues to current and changing populations patterns of health, including disparities in health, are to be found chiefly in the dynamic social, material, and ecological contexts into which we are born, develop, interact, and endeavor to live meaningful lives. The contrast is to pervasive aetiological hypotheses concerned mainly with decontextualised and disembodied "behaviors" and "exposures" interacting with equally decontexualised and disembodied "genes." The distinction is more than simply between "determinants" and "mechanisms." Consider, for example, contending and long-standing claims about racism compared with "race" as causes of racial/ethnic disparities in health. An embodied approach promotes testing hypotheses to ascertain if the observed disparities are a biological expression of racial discrimination, past and present; by contrast, a disembodied and decontextualised approach promulgates research focused on detrimental genes and/or lifestyles (Krieger 2005a, p. 350).

Together with embodiment, eco-social theory employs two key concepts: the "cumulative interplay of exposure, susceptibility, and resistance"—whereby past and ongoing biological incorporation of social relations of power are integrated into present health and disease experience—and "accountability and agency, historically and dynamically," which, like the political economy approach, understands the relations of power not simply in the abstract, but through concrete actors, institutions, and actions. Eco-social theory also helps to bridge the false distance between so-called upstream and downstream approaches by showing how unequal power manifests itself at all levels (Starfield 2007; Krieger 2008).

The eco-social approach goes beyond the search for particular determinants of health, instead pursuing the mechanisms through which societal conditions and biological processes interact to produce health or ill health (Krieger 2005a). In contrast to the psychosocial perspective, an eco-social framework examines both how underlying causal factors generate social inequalities in health *and* how these conditions lead to different experiences of and reactions to physical, biological, social, and chemical exposures.

Thus, the eco-social model can be understood as a continuation of the political economy approach to health, one that specifies not just macro-, but also microlevel mechanisms through which social inequalities are manifested in population health.

Policy Implications of Different Understandings of Social Inequalities in Health

Depending on the explanatory model adopted, different policy implications to address social inequalities in health ensue. A biological model may seek medical interventions (including genetic testing) to "treat" the effects of inequality. A life-style understanding focuses on behavioral aspects of disease prevention and health promotion, whereas a psychosocial approach may include environmental and community measures to increase social cohesion as well as individual level interventions to enhance psychological well-being. Chapter 13 will recount how various countries, regions, and cities have responded to inequalities in health and will outline the challenges they have experienced in putting plans into action. Sweden, Sri Lanka, and Costa Rica, for example, have implemented nation-wide policies based on materialist and class-based interventions, and even some new eco-social ideas, whereas numerous "healthy city" approaches focus more on lifestyle and psychosocial approaches.

"The existing gross inequality in the health status of the people particularly between developed and developing countries as well as within countries is politically, socially, and economically unacceptable and is, therefore, of common concern to all countries" Declaration of Alma-Ata (WHO 1978, p. 1).

ADDRESSING INEQUALITIES IN HEALTH

While particular strategies to reduce or eliminate health inequalities are per force context specific, a number of generic and global strategies merit attention. At the microlevel, health care providers should be educated to see beyond a person's presenting problem to consider the conditions in which a patient lives, loves, works, and plays. Public health efforts should emphasize collective protections: political and societal determinants of health should serve as a baseline, with behavioral approaches subsidiary to these. As well, governments need to recognize that "nearly all social determinants of health fall outside the direct control of the health sector" (Chan 2008) and thus demand to be addressed through concerted political struggle and moral leadership. For their part, international agencies should be urged to go beyond a poverty alleviation focus, which typically overlooks the role of social inequalities and the imbalance of power producing them. These approaches do not need to be separated: indeed, addressing social inequalities includes poverty alleviation (Krieger 2007). At the global level, an equitable system of global governance should be developed, allowing for fair terms of trade and democratic distribution of political and economic power that is socially and environmentally sustainable.

The WHO Commission on Social Determinants of Health

Mounting evidence and the mobilization of public health researchers and practitioners has generated international impetus for addressing the societal determinants of health. In March 2005, the WHO established a Commission on Social Determinants of Health (CSDH), at least in part to counter the narrow recommendations of the WHO's 2000–2002 Commission on Macroeconomics and Health, which called for ill health to be addressed through "cost-effective" health care interventions as a means of reducing poverty and helping economies to grow (see Chapter 11 for details).

The CSDH's mandate was to apply the findings of growing national and cross-national research on the social (and what this chapter has referred to as societal) determinants of health and to encourage further research and applications of these studies to enhance policy making, country by country, and internationally. The Commission was chaired by British epidemiologist Sir Michael Marmot (lead researcher of the Whitehall studies) and included 19 other commissioners from developing and developed countries representing the fields of politics, civil society, and academia. It was also supported by the work of hundreds of experts and advocates contributing through "knowledge networks."

The goal of the CSDH has been to strengthen health equity by searching for the "causes of the causes" of social inequalities in health. It has aimed to do so by "catalyzing policy and institutional change to address social determinants of health within countries, among institutions working in global health, and within WHO itself" (Irwin et al. 2006, p. 750). The commission focused on five action areas:

1. Improving living and learning conditions in early childhood;
2. Strengthening social programs to provide fair employment conditions and access to labor markets;
3. Emphasizing policies and interventions to protect people in informal employment;
4. Promoting intersectoral policies to improve living conditions in urban slums; and
5. Implementing programs to address the major determinants of women's health.

Nine autonomous knowledge networks were established to report on specific societal determinants and make recommendations to inform the CSDH's final report: Early Child Development, Employment Conditions, Globalization, Health Systems, Measurement and Evidence, Priority Public Health Conditions, Social Exclusion, Urban Settings, and Women and Gender Equity.

On August 28, 2008, as this textbook was going to press, Sir Marmot officially presented the final CSDH report, *Closing the Gap in a Generation*, to the WHO Director-General, Dr. Margaret Chan. The report begins with a compelling opening statement—"Social justice is a matter of life and death"—and follows with a comprehensive set of well-documented findings and bold recommendations.

> **Box 7–6** The Commission on Social Determinants of Health's Overarching Recommendations and Principles of Action (WHO Commission on Social Determinants of Health 2008)
>
> 1. Improve the conditions of daily life—the circumstances in which people are born, grow, live, work, and age.
> 2. Tackle the inequitable distribution of power, money, and resources—the structural drivers of those conditions of daily life—globally, nationally, and locally.
> 3. Measure the problem, evaluate action, expand the knowledge base, develop a workforce that is trained in the social determinants of health, and raise public awareness about the social determinants of health.

The CSDH report documents the daily living conditions—urban infrastructure and governance, early childhood development and education, employment conditions, social protection measures, and health care—and the reforms in "power, money, and resources" relating to taxation and debt, market conditions, gender equity, global governance, and political empowerment that are necessary to combat the killing fields of social injustice. According to WHO Director-General Chan, the Commission's principal finding is straightforward: "The social conditions in which people are born, live, and work are the single most important determinant of good health or ill health, of a long and productive life, or a short and miserable one... This ends the debate decisively" (Chan 2008). Indeed, the CSDH's final report offers a wholesale indictment of neoliberal economic policy, which has exacerbated social inequalities over the past 30 years.

Though *Closing the Gap in a Generation* has been ignored by much of the mainstream press in the United States, its powerful principles of action have been lauded by progressive scholars (Davey Smith and Krieger 2008) and by advocacy/activist groups, such as the People's Health Movement, at least for its thorough diagnosis (Woodward 2008). While the Commission's recommendations include an explicit call to governments to fulfill their role and meet their obligations of creating the material and social conditions for health, many of these recommendations are buried or remain in the side reports produced by the knowledge networks, and the adoption and implementation plans are unclear. Yet another recommendation states: "Where government lacks capacity or political will, there must be technical and financial support from outside, and a push from popular action" (WHO Commission on Social Determinants of Health 2008, p. 35). The question of how this might be carried out, however, remains to be answered.

The CSDH has also been critiqued for failing to build on previous WHO efforts surrounding the 1978 Alma-Ata conference on primary health care and the "health for all" movements (see Chapters 3 and 12); for not exploring in sufficient depth why primary health care initiatives worked to improve equity in some countries but not in others (i.e., why Cuba's health equity remains consistently good while China's has deteriorated); for not taking on the most powerful political and economic structure—unbridled market capitalism—that drives the societal determinants of health; and for not outlining concrete steps that countries can take toward creating more just societies (Banerji 2006; Navarro 2006; WHO Commission on Social Determinants of Health 2007b). Indeed, given the subversion of the aims of the Declaration of Alma-Ata in the 1980s and the failure to achieve "health for all" by 2000, much attention, activism, and action will be needed to fulfill the goal of "closing the gap in a generation."

Depending on how these inherently political issues are addressed, the CSDH may or may not be able to fundamentally address health inequalities. Moreover, given the five different approaches to understanding health inequalities outlined in this chapter, the CSDH's recommendations could take on remarkably distinct forms.

For instance, targeting the poorest of the poor is easier to implement than a more comprehensive approach (and targeting has certainly been widely employed by the World Bank and other large donors in recent years), is affordable in some contexts, and potentially easy to monitor and evaluate. However, such targeting confuses the "symptom," that is, the poor themselves, with the "disease," the organizing principles that produce and sustain poverty in the first place, and in so doing undermines the cooperation and distributive justice principles necessary for sustainable population-wide support for such efforts. As well, even if the targeted group does better, it will still remain poor in relative terms, and the needs of the "near poor" will remain neglected. Finally, and most importantly, targeting the poor does not address the fundamental inequalities of political power that shape virtually every determinant of health.

On a more hopeful note, *Closing the Gap in a Generation* has taken up socio-economic redistribution as a priority. In particular, it emphasizes the importance of supporting the development and expansion of welfare states that provide comprehensive and universal services and protections to their populations. If the CSDH is able to put its clout behind such recommendations, then it has a bona fide chance of improving human dignity and well-being and of reducing social inequalities in health. Of course, governments need to be willing, ready, supported, and able to adopt such recommendations, and social and political movements (civil society) must help push the local political environment—and compel the international trade and financial context—to become conducive to such reforms.

Box 7–7 Ten Tips for American Public Health Researchers and Workers

1. Recognize that societal determinants of health such as income and its distribution, employment security and working conditions, health and social services, and housing and food security are the primary determinants of population health and the source of health inequalities.
2. Consider that the United States—despite being the second wealthiest nation (behind Luxembourg) in per capita gross domestic product—has one of the worst population health profiles among wealthy—and some not so wealthy—developed nations.

(continued)

Box 7–7 Continued

3. Reflect upon the reality that public policy in the United States is among the least developed, and among the most threatening to the overall population health of its citizens, among wealthy developed nations.
4. Accept the finding that these shortcomings in health-supporting public policy interact with class, race, and gender to create profound inequalities in health among Americans.
5. Explore and integrate developments in population health, public policy in support of health, and the societal determinants of health that are being developed in other nations into U.S. health policy.
6. Demand that governmental authorities support research into the impact of the societal determinants of health and their public policy and political antecedents (Navarro and Shi 2001). Data collection that includes income and social class data as well as indicators of other living conditions is imperative.
7. Recognize that health policy will always be *political* and that human health is produced, quite literally, by political forces that shape the material and social conditions in which people live, work, and play.
8. Stand up to the political forces that consider such intellectual inquiries as being "un-American" and "promoting class warfare."
9. Urge your professional organizations and health and service agencies to support a new, broadened health policy agenda.
10. Communicate the importance of these health policy issues to your fellow Americans.

Source: Adapted with permission from Raphael (2007, p. 108).

CONCLUSION

In this chapter, we have examined patterns of health from the perspective of the societal determinants of health and of the politics of these determinants. After reviewing the factors that influence health at personal, household, community, national, and global levels, we turned to the role of social inequalities in explaining persistent differences in health status. We also covered a set of theories that grapple with how and why social inequalities affect health.

Learning Points:

- The societal determinants of health refer to a broad array of structural influences that take place simultaneously and synergistically at the level of individual experience, living conditions, government social policies, and broad political and economic forces.
- The more redistributive a society in political, economic, and social terms, the fewer social inequalities in health exist.
- Though most international health analyses emphasize the health disparities between developed and developing countries, the persistent inequalities in health *within* countries are as great or even greater.
- Systemic and persistent differences in health among different social classes, genders, racial and ethnic groups, occupational groups, and so on are linked to underlying inequalities in power and resources.

- The explanatory model adopted (e.g., biological, lifestyle, psychosocial, political economy, or eco-social) has significant policy implications in terms of how social inequalities in health are explained, and as a consequence, addressed.

Notwithstanding ample and growing knowledge about social inequalities in health, few countries or international agencies use these findings to develop social and economic policies. Is this because the evidence is not credible to policy makers, or because it questions the fundamentals of capitalist societies, making those in power unwilling to seriously consider the impact of societal distribution of power and resources on health? These are fundamentally *political* issues: whether societies adopt solidarity or individualism as an organizing principle has repercussions for virtually every aspect of life. Social movements that battle for healthy and just social policies and against social inequalities can play a meaningful role in reducing health inequalities. We will explore these matters further in Chapter 13.

NOTES

1. The preponderance of examples in this chapter come from developed countries due to their larger research infrastructure. This is also the result of deficiencies in basic health data collection in many developing countries (see Chapter 5 for details). The lack of studies in and from developing countries does not mean that we universally endorse the implementation of findings from developed to developing countries. See Almeida Filho et al. (2003).

2. Under South Africa's legalized racial categories, the population was stratified into four groups: Black, White, Asian, and Coloured. In the United States, previous census categories of Black, White, Hispanic, Native American, and Asian/Pacific Islander (which in turn replaced a complex of "racial" categories based on national origins) have evolved into further gradations, allowing for multiple forms of self-identification. Yet the older categories prevail in many government activities and societal domains.

REFERENCES

Aizenman NC. 2008. New high in U.S. prison numbers. *Washington Post*, February 29, A01.

Almas H. 2004. Regional income inequality in selected large countries. IZA Discussion Paper No. 1307. http://ssrn.com/abstract=592322. Accessed November 28, 2007.

Almeida Filho N, Kawachi I, Pellegrini Filho A, and Dachs JNW. 2003. Research on health inequalities in Latin America and the Caribbean: Bibliometric analysis (1971–2000) and descriptive content analysis (1971–1995). *American Journal of Public Health* 93(12):2037–2043.

Amnesty International. 2007. Conflict diamonds. http://www.amnestyusa.org/business-and-human-rights/conflict-diamonds/page.do?id=1051176. Accessed May 15, 2007.

Anderson I, Crengle S, Leialoha Kamaka M, Chen T-H, Palafox N, and Jackson-Pulver L. 2006. Indigenous health in Australia, New Zealand and the Pacific. *Lancet* 367(9524):1775–1785.

Ashford LS, Gwatkin DR, and Yazbeck AS. 2006. *Designing Health and Population Programs to Reach the Poor.* Washington, DC: Population Reference Bureau.

Banerji D. 2006. Serious crisis in the practice of international health by the World Health Organization: The Commission on Social Determinants of Health. *International Journal of Health Services* 36(4):637–650.

Bartley M, Ferrie J, and Montgomery S. 1999. Living in a high-unemployment economy: Understanding the health consequences. In Marmot M and Wilkinson R, Editors. *Social Determinants of Health*. New York: Oxford University Press.

Benach J, Muntaner C, and Santana V. 2007. Employment conditions and health inequalities: Final report to the WHO Commission on Social Determinants of Health. Geneva: WHO.

Birdsall N. 2005. Rising inequality in the new global economy. WIDER Annual Lecture. Helsinki: United Nations University World Institute for Development Economics Research. *Wider Angle* 2:1–3.

Black SD and Research Working Group (Morris JN, Smith C, Townsend P). 1980. *Inequalities in Health: Report of a Research Working Group*. London: Department of Health and Social Security.

Blane D. 1999. The life course, the social gradient and health. In Marmot M and Wilkinson R, Editors. *The Social Determinants of Health*. New York: Oxford University Press.

Botting B. 1997. Mortality in childhood. In Drever F and Whitehead M, Editors. *Health Inequalities (Decennial Supplement)*. Series DS No 15. London: Office for National Statistics.

Braveman P and Gruskin S. 2003. Defining equity in health. *Journal of Epidemiology and Community Health* 57(4):254–258.

Briggs D. 2003. Environmental pollution and the global burden of disease. *British Medical Bulletin* 68:1–24.

Britannica Online. 2008. Welfare state. http://info.britannica.com. Accessed January 15, 2008.

Bryce PH. 1907. *Report on the Indian Schools of Manitoba and the North West Territories*. Ottawa: Government Printing Bureau.

Burgard S and Treiman DJ. 2006. Trends and racial differences in infant mortality in South Africa. *Social Science and Medicine* 62(5):1126–1137.

Carr D. 2004. Improving the health of the world's poorest people. *Health Bulletin* 1. Washington, DC: Population Reference Bureau.

Castro A and Singer M, Editors. 2004. Anthropology and health policy: A critical perspective. In *Unhealthy Health Policy: A Critical Anthropological Examination*. Walnut Creek, CA: Altamira Press.

Castro R, Erviti J, and Leyva R. 2007. Globalización y enfermedades infecciosas en las poblaciones indígenas de México. *Cadernos de Saúde Pública* 23(Supp 1):S41–S50.

Chan M. 2008. Launch of the Final Report of the Commission on Social Determinants. Statement to the press. August 28, 2008. http://www.who.int/dg/speeches/2008/20080828/en/index.html. Geneva: WHO.

Cheung A and Hwang S. 2004. Risk of death among homeless women: A cohort study and review of the literature. *Canadian Medical Association Journal* 170(8):1243–1247.

Chung H and Muntaner C. 2007. Welfare state matters: A typological multilevel analysis of wealthy countries. *Health Policy* 80(2):328–339.

Cutler D and Lleras-Muney A. 2007. *Education and Health: Evaluating Theories and Evidence. Policy Brief No. 9*. Ann Arbor, MI: National Poverty Center.

Dauvergne P. 2004. Globalization and the environment. In Ravenhill J, Editor. *Global Political Economy*. Oxford: Oxford University Press.

Davey Smith G and Krieger N. 2008. Tackling health inequities. *British Medical Journal* 337(7669):529–530.

Denton M, Prus S, and Walters V. 2004. Gender differences in health: A Canadian study of the psychosocial, structural and behavioural determinants of health. *Social Science and Medicine* 58(12):2585–2600.

Doyal L. 2003. Sex and gender: The challenges for epidemiologists. *International Journal of Health Services* 33(3):569–579.

Drewnowski A and Barratt-Fornell A. 2004. Do healthier diets cost more? (Policy Update). *Nutrition Today* 39(4):161–168.

Driscoll T, Takala J, Steenland K, Corvalan C, and Fingerhut M. 2005. Review of estimates of the global burden of injury and illness due to occupational exposures. *American Journal of Industrial Medicine* 48(6):491–502.

Dunn JR. 2002. Housing and inequalities in health: A study of socioeconomic dimensions of housing and self reported health from a survey of Vancouver residents. *Journal of Epidemiology and Community Health* 56(9):671–681.

Eagleton D. 2005. *Power Hungry: Six Reasons to Regulate Global Food Corporations.* Johannesburg: ActionAid International.

Eckersley R. 2005. 'Cultural fraud': The role of culture in drug abuse. *Drug and Alcohol Review* 24(2):157–163.

Editorial. 2006. Farmers' suicides nothing but genocide, says Vandana Shiva. *The Hindu,* May 9.

Engels F. 1845. *The Condition of the Working Class in England, 1958 Edition.* Translated by Henderson WO and Chaloner WH. Stanford, CA: Stanford University Press.

Evans T, Whitehead M, Diderichsen F, Bhuiya A, and Wirth M, Editors. 2001. *Challenging Inequities in Health: From Ethics to Action.* New York: Oxford University Press.

FAO. 2005. *The State of Food Insecurity in the World* 2005. Rome: FAO.

Feldman MW, Lewontin RC, and King MC. 2003. Race: A genetic melting-pot. *Nature* 424(6947):374.

Fitzpatrick J and Dollamore G. 1999. Examining adult mortality rates using the National Statistics Socio-Economic Classification. *Health Statistics Quarterly* 2:33-40.

Galabuzi G and Labonte R. 2002. Social inclusion as a determinant of health: Summary of a paper presented at The Social Determinants of Health Across the Life-Span conference, Toronto. http://www.phac-aspc.gc.ca/ph-sp/oi-ar/pdf/03_inclusion_e.pdf. Accessed December 20, 2007.

Gershman J, Irwin A, and Shakow A. 2003. Getting a grip on the global economy: Health outcomes and the decoding of development discourse. In Hofrichter R, Editor. *Health and Social Justice: Politics, Ideology, and Inequity in the Distribution of Disease.* San Francisco, CA: Jossey-Bass.

Gilson L, Doherty J, Loewenson R, and Francis V. 2007. *Challenging Inequity Through Health Systems. Final Report Knowledge Network on Health Systems.* Geneva: WHO Commission on Social Determinants of Health.

Gleick P. 2006. *Water Conflict Chronology.* Oakland, CA: Pacific Institute.

Goodman AH. 2000. Why genes don't count (for racial differences in health). *American Journal of Public Health* 90(11):1699–1702.

Government of Kerala. 2005. *Human Development Report 2005: Kerala.* Thiruvananthapuram, India: Government of Kerala State Planning Board.

Graham H. 2007. *Unequal Lives: Health and Socioeconomic Inequalities.* Maidenhead: Open University Press.

Guttal S. 2003. Missing the mark, or deliberately misleading?: The World Bank's assessments of absolute poverty and hunger. In *Anti Poverty or Anti Poor? The Millennium Development Goals and the Eradication of Extreme Poverty and Hunger.* Bangkok: Focus on the Global South.

Gwatkin DR, Rutstein S, Johnson K, Suliman E, Wagstaff A, and Amouzou A. 2007. *Socio-Economic Differences in Health, Nutrition, and Population within Developing Countries: An Overview.* Washington, DC: World Bank.

Harris R, Tobias M, Jeffreys M, Waldegrave K, Karlsen S, and Nazroo J. 2006. Effects of self-reported racial discrimination and deprivation on Māori health and inequalities in New Zealand: Cross-sectional study. *Lancet* 367(9527):2005–2009.

Hattersley L. 1999. Trends in life expectancy by social class—an update. *Health Statistics Quarterly* 2:16–24.

House JS and Williams DR. 2004. Understanding and reducing socioeconomic and racial/ethnic disparities in health. In Hofrichter R, Editor. *Health and Social Justice: Politics, Ideology and Inequity in the Distribution of Disease.* San Francisco, CA: Jossey-Bass.

Hwang S. 2000. Mortality among men using homeless shelters in Toronto, Ontario. *Journal of the American Medical Association* 283(16):2152–2157.

Ineichen B. 1993. *Homes and Health: How Housing and Health Interact.* London: E & FN Spon.

International Organization for Migration. 2008. About migration. http://www.iom.int/jahia/Jahia/pid/3. Accessed September 23, 2008.

Irwin A, Valentine N, Loewenson R, Solar O, Brown H, Koller T, and Vega J. 2006. The Commission on Social Determinants of Health: Tackling the social roots of health inequalities. *PLoS Med* 3(6):e106 (749–751).

Irwin L, Siddiqi A, and Hertzman C. 2007. Early child development: A powerful equalizer. *Final Report for the World Health Organization's Commission on Social Determinants of Health.* Geneva: WHO.

Islam K, Merlo J, Kawachi I, Lindstrom M, and Gerdtham U. 2006. Social capital and health: Does egalitarianism matter? A literature review. *International Journal for Equity in Health* 5:3, doi: 10.1186/1475-9276-5-3.

Iwasaki Y, Bartlett J, and O'Neil J. 2004. An examination of stress among aboriginal women and men with diabetes in Manitoba, Canada. *Ethnicity & Health* 9(2):189–212.

Jamison D, Breman J, Measham J, Alleyne G, Claeson M, Evans D, Jha P, Mills A, and Musgrove P, Editors. 2006. *Priorities in Health.* Washington, DC: The World Bank.

Job Stress Network. 2008. The Whitehall Study. www.workhealth.org/projects/pwhitew.html. Accessed October 10, 2007.

Johnson JV and Lipscomb J. 2006. Long working hours, occupational health and the changing nature of work organization. *American Journal of Industrial Medicine* 49(11):921–929.

Jubilee USA. 2003. *Structural Adjustment: Making Debt Deadly.* Washington, DC: Jubilee Network USA.

Kawachi I, Daniels N, and Robinson D. 2005. Health disparities by race and class: Why both matter. *Health Affairs* 24(2):343–352.

Kawachi I and Kennedy B. 2002. *The Health of Nations: Why Inequality Is Harmful to Your Health.* New York: New Press.

Kawachi I, Wilkinson R, and Kennedy B. 1999. Introduction. In Kawachi I, Kennedy B, and R Wilkinson, Editors. *The Society and Population Health Reader: Income Inequality and Health.* New York: New Press.

Keating DP and Hertzman C, Editors. 1999. *Developmental Health and the Wealth of Nations.* New York: Guilford Press.

Kellett P and Moore J. 2003. Routes to home: Homelessness and home-making in contrasting societies. *Habitat International* 27(1):123–141.

Kington RS and Nickens HW. 2001. Racial and ethnic differences in health: Recent trends, current patterns, future directions. In Smelser N, Wilson W, and Mitchell F, Editors. *America Becoming: Racial Trends and Their Consequences.* Washington, DC: National Academy Press.

Krieger N. 1999. Embodying inequality: A review of concepts, measures, and methods for studying health consequences of discrimination. *International Journal of Health Services* 29(2):295–352.

———. 2001. A glossary for social epidemiology. *Journal of Epidemiology and Community Health* 55(10):693–700.

———. 2003. Does racism harm health? Did child abuse exist before 1962? On explicit questions, critical science and current controversies: An ecosocial perspective. *American Journal of Public Health* 93(2):194–199.

———. 2005a. Embodiment: A conceptual glossary for epidemiology. *Journal of Epidemiology and Community Health* 59(5):350–355.

———. 2005b. Stormy weather: *Race*, gene expression, and the science of health disparities. *American Journal of Public Health* 95(12):2155–2160.

———. 2007. Why epidemiologists cannot afford to ignore poverty. *Epidemiology* 18(6):658–663.

———. 2008. Proximal, distal, and the politics of causation: What's level got to do with it? *American Journal of Public Health* 98(2):221–230.

Kuh D, Ben-Shlomo Y, Lynch J, Hallqvist J, and Power C. 2003. Life course epidemiology. *Journal Epidemiology of Community Health* 57(10):778–783.

Labonte R. 2003. Globalization, trade and health: Unpacking the links and defining health public policy options. In Hofrichter R, Editor. *Health and Social Justice: Politics, Ideology and Inequity in the Distribution of Disease*. San Francisco, CA: Jossey-Bass.

LaDou J. 2003. International occupational health. *International Journal of Hygiene and Environmental Health* 206:303–313.

Lalonde M. 1974. *A New Perspective on the Health of Canadians: A Working Document*. Ottawa, ON: Government of Canada.

Loue S and Galea S. 2007. Migration. In Galea S, Editor. *Macrosocial Determinants of Population Health*. New York: Springer.

Lynch J, Davey Smith G, Harper S, and Bainbridge K. 2006. Explaining the social gradient in coronary heart disease: Comparing relative and absolute risk approaches. *Journal of Epidemiology and Community Health* 60(5):436–441.

Lynch J, Davey Smith G, Harper S, Hillemeier M, Ross N, Kaplan GA, and Wolfson M. 2004. Is income inequality a determinant of population health? Part 1. A systematic review. *The Milbank Quarterly* 82(1):5–99.

Marmot M. 2005. The social determinants of health inequalities. *Lancet* 365(9464):1099–1104.

———. 2006. Health in an unequal world. *Lancet* 368:2081–2094.

Marmot M and Shipley MJ. 1996. Do socioeconomic differences in mortality persist after retirement? A 25-year follow-up of civil servants from the first Whitehall Study. *British Medical Journal* 313(7066):1177–1180.

Marmot M, Bosma H, Hemingway H, Brunner E, and Stansfeld S. 1997. Contribution of job control and other risk factors to social variations in coronary heart disease. *Lancet* 350(9073):235–239.

Marmot M, Rose G, Shipley M, and Hamilton PJ. 1978. Employment grade and coronary heart disease in British civil servants. *Journal of Epidemiology and Community Health* 32(4):244–249.

Marmot M, Siegrist J, Theorell T, and Feeney A. 1999. Health and the psychosocial environment at work. In Marmot M and Wilkinson R, Editors. *The Social Determinants of Health*. New York: Oxford University Press.

Martikainen P, Bartley M, and Lahelma E. 2002. Psychosocial determinants of health in social epidemiology. *International Journal of Epidemiology* 31(6):1091–1093.

Mays VM, Cochran SD, and Barnes NW. 2007. Race, race-based discrimination, and health outcomes among African Americans. *Annual Review of Psychology* 58:201–225.

McMichael AJ. 2001. *Human Frontiers, Environments and Disease: Past Patterns, Uncertain Futures.* Cambridge: Cambridge University Press.

Middlebrooks JS and Audage NC. 2008. *The Effects of Childhood Stress on Health Across the Lifespan.* Atlanta, GA: Centers for Disease Control and Prevention, National Center for Injury Prevention and Control.

Montenegro R and Stephans C. 2006. Indigenous health in Latin America and the Caribbean. *Lancet* 367(9525):1859–1869.

Muntaner C and Lynch J. 1999. Income inequality, social cohesion and class relations: A critique of Wilkinson's neo-Durkheimian research program. *International Journal of Health Services* 29(1):59–81.

Nantulya VM and Reich MR. 2003. Equity dimensions of road traffic injuries in low- and middle-income countries. *Injury Control and Safety Promotion* 10(1–2):13–20.

Navarro V. 2002. A critique of social capital. *International Journal of Health Services* 32(3):423–432.

———. 2006. What is happening at the World Health Organization? The coming election of the WHO Director-General. http://www.phmovement.org/cms/en/node/279. Accessed November 2006.

Navarro V and Shi L. 2001. The political context of social inequalities and health. *Social Science and Medicine* 52(3):481–491.

Navdanya. 2007. *Corporate Hijack of Land Grab.* New Delhi: Navdanya.

Nussbaum M and Sen A, Editors. 1991. *The Quality of Life.* Oxford: Clarendon Press.

Olsson O. 2007. Conflict diamonds. *Journal of Development Economics* 82(2):267–286.

Ostlin P, George A, and Sen G. 2003. Gender, health and equity: The intersections. In R. Hofrichter, Editor. *Health and Social Justice: Politics, Ideology, and Inequity in the Distribution of Disease.* San Francisco, CA: Jossey-Bass.

PAHO. 2002. Health of indigenous people: A challenge for public health. http://www.paho.org/english/DPI/100/100feature32.htm. Accessed June 26, 2007.

Paradies Y. 2006. A systematic review of empirical research on self-reported racism and health. *International Journal of Epidemiology* 35(4):888–901.

Parra EJ, Kittles RA, and Shriver MD. 2004. Implications of correlations between skin color and genetic ancestry for biomedical research. *Nature Genetics* 36(suppl):S54–S60.

Pearce N and Davey Smith G. 2003. Is social capital the key to inequalities in health? *American Journal of Public Health* 93(1):122–129.

Phillips J and Beasley R. 2005. *Income and Poverty in the District of Columbia: 1990–2004.* Washington, DC: Government of the District of Columbia, DC Office of Planning, State Data Center.

Pickett KE and Pearl M. 2001. Multilevel analyses of neighbourhood socioeconomic context and health outcomes: A critical review. *Journal of Epidemiology and Community Health* 55(2):111–122.

Plavinski SL, Plavinskaya SI, and Klimov AN. 2003. Social factors and increase in mortality in Russia in the 1990s: Prospective cohort study. *British Medical Journal* 326(7401):1240–1242.

Pogge T. 2005. World poverty and human rights. *Ethics and International Affairs* 19(1):1–7.

Pollan M. 2006. *The Omnivore's Dilemma: A Natural History of Four Meals.* New York: Penguin.

Putnam R. 2000. *Bowling Alone: The Collapse and Revival of American Community.* New York: Simon & Schuster.

Putnam R, Leonardi R, and Nannetti R. 1993. *Making Democracy Work: Civic Traditions in Modern Italy.* Princeton, NJ: Princeton University Press.

Raphael D. 2006. Social determinants of health: Present status, unanswered questions, and future directions. *International Journal of Health Services* 36(4): 651–677.

———. 2007. Public policies and the problematic USA population health profile. *Health Policy* 84(1):101–111.

Raphael D, Anstice S, Raine K, McGannon KR, Rizvi SK, and Yu V. 2003. The social determinants of the incidence and management of Type 2 diabetes mellitus: Are we prepared to rethink our questions and redirect our research activities? *Leadership in Health Services* 16(3):10–20.

Ravallion M. 1987. *Markets and Famines.* Oxford: Clarendon Press.

Reddy SG. 2008. Death in China: Market reforms and health. *International Journal of Health Services* 38(1):125–141.

Revkin A. 2005. A new measure of well-being from a happy little kingdom. *New York Times,* October 4.

Riley JC. 2001. *Rising Life Expectancy: A Global History.* Cambridge: Cambridge University Press.

Riley LW, Ko AI, Unger A, and Reis MG. 2007. Slum health: Diseases of neglected populations. *BMC International Health and Human Rights* 7(2), doi:10.1186/1472-698X-7-2.

Rose G and Marmot MG. 1981. Social class and coronary heart disease. *British Heart Journal* 45(1):13–19.

Ross K and Taylor J. 2002. Improving life expectancy and health status: A comparison of indigenous Australians and New Zealand Māori. Joint Special Issue. *Journal of Population Research and NZ Population Review* 219–238.

Sanchez P, Swaminathan MS, Dobie P, and Yuksel N, Editors. 2005. UN Millenium Project Task Force on Hunger. 2005. *Halving Hunger: It Can Be Done.* London: Earthscan.

Sapolsky RM. 1994. *Why Zebras Don't Get Ulcers.* New York: WH Freeman.

SAPRIN. 2001. *The Policy Roots of Economic Crisis and Poverty: A Multi-Country Participatory Assessment of Structural Adjustment.* Washington, DC: Structural Participatory Review International Network.

Satcher D and Higginbotham EJ. 2008. Commentary: The public health approach to eliminating disparities in health. *American Journal of Public Health* 98(3):400–403.

Save the Children. 2007. *State of the World's Mothers 2007: Saving the Lives of Children under 5.* Westport, CT: Save the Children.

Sen A. 1981. *Poverty and Famines: An Essay on Entitlements and Deprivation.* Oxford: Clarendon Press.

———. 1990. Food, economics and entitlement. In Dreze J and Sen A, Editors. *The Political Economy of Hunger, Vol. 1 Entitlement and Well-being.* Oxford and New York: Clarendon Press.

Shaw M, Dorling D, and Mitchell R. 2002. *Health, Place and Society.* Harlow, UK: Prentice Hall.

Shaw M, Dorling D, and Davey Smith G. 1999. Poverty, social exclusion, and minorities. In Marmot M and Wilkinson RG, Editors. *Social Determinants of Health.* New York: Oxford University Press.

Stansfeld SA and Marmot M, Editors. 2002. *Stress and the Heart: Psychosocial Pathways to Coronary Heart Disease.* London: BMJ Books.

Starfield B. 2006. State of the art in research on equity in health. *Journal of Health Politics, Policy and Law* 31(1):11–32.

———. 2007. Pathways of influence on equity in health. *Social Science and Medicine* 64(7):1355–1362.

Starfield B and Birn A-E. 2007. Income redistribution is not enough: Income inequality, social welfare programs, and achieving equity in health. *Journal of Epidemiology and Community Health* 61(12):1038–1041.

Starfield B, Shi L, and Macinko J. 2005. Contribution of primary care to health systems and health. *The Milbank Quarterly* 83(3):457–502.

Theorell T, Karasek R, Johnson J, Hall E, Stewart W, and Alfredsson L. 1992. Medical correlates of poor work content. *International Journal of Psychology* 27(3–4):598.

Tipple G and Speak S. 2005. Definitions of homelessness in developing countries. *Habitat International* 29(2):337–352.

Townsend P. 2005. An end to poverty or more of the same? *Lancet* 365(9468):1379–1380.

UN. 2003. *Indicators for Monitoring the Millennium Development Goals*. New York: United Nations.

UNDP. 2005. *Human Development Report 2005, International Development at a Crossroads: Aid, Trade and Security in an Unequal World*. New York: UNDP.

———. 2006. *Human Development Report 2006. Beyond Scarcity: Power, Poverty and the Global Water Crisis*. New York: UNDP.

UNICEF. 2007. *Facts on Children: Water and Sanitation*. New York: UNICEF.

U.S. Government. 2005. Average life expectancy at birth by state for 2000 and ratio of estimates and projections of deaths: 2001 to 2003. http://www.census.gov/population/projections/MethTab2.xls. Accessed November 10, 2007.

Vallgarda S. 2007. Health inequalities: Political problematizations in Denmark and Sweden. *Critical Public Health* 17(1):45–56.

Via Campesina. 2002. Declaration NGO forum FAO summit Rome +5. http://www.viacampesina.org/main_en/index.php?option=com_content&task=view&id=418&Itemid=38. Accessed October 12, 2007.

Waitzkin H. 2007. Political economic systems and the health of populations: Historical thought and current directions. In Galea S, Editor. *Macrosocial Determinants of Population Health*. New York: Springer.

WHO. 1978. *Declaration of Alma-Ata*. International Conference on Primary Health Care. Alma-Ata, USSR.

———. 1999. *Healthy Living: What is a Healthy Lifestyle?* Copenhagen: WHO Regional Office for Europe.

———. 2002a. *World Health Report 2002: Reducing Risks, Promoting Healthy Life*. Geneva: WHO.

———. 2002b. *World Report on Violence and Health*. Geneva: WHO.

———. 2004a. *Handbook for the Documentation of Interpersonal Violence Prevention Programs*. Geneva: WHO.

———. 2004b. *Water, Sanitation and Hygiene Links to Health: Facts and Figures*. Geneva: WHO.

———. 2006. *World Health Report 2006: Working Together for Health*. Geneva: WHO.

———. 2007. Food safety and foodborne illness. Fact Sheet No. 237. http://www.who.int/mediacentre/factsheets/fs237/en/. Accessed May 11, 2007.

WHO and UNICEF. 2001. *Global Water Supply and Sanitation Assessment 2000 Report*. New York: UNICEF; Geneva: WHO.

———. 2008. *World Health Organization and United Nations Children's Fund Joint Monitoring Programme for Water Supply and Sanitation. Progress on Drinking Water and Sanitation: Special Focus on Sanitation*. New York: UNICEF; and Geneva: WHO.

WHO Commission on Social Determinants of Health. 2007a. *A Conceptual Framework for Action on the Social Determinants of Health*. Geneva: WHO.

WHO Commission on Social Determinants of Health. 2007b. Civil Society Report. October, 2007. http://www.who.int/social_determinants/resources/cso_finalreport_2007.pdf. Accessed January 24, 2008.

———. 2008. *Closing the Gap in a Generation: Health Equity through Action on the Social Determinants of Health*. Final Report of the Commission on Social Determinants of Health. Geneva: WHO.

WHO EURO. 2003. *Social Determinants of Health: The Solid Facts, Second Edition*. Wilkinson R and Marmot M, Editors. Copenhagen: WHO EURO.

WHOSIS. 2007. WHO statistical informaton system: Inequities. http://www.who.int/whosis/en/. Accessed July 16, 2007.

———. 2008. Core health indicators. http://www.who.int/whosis/database/core/core_select. cfm. Accessed September 15, 2008.

Wilkins R, Tjepkema M, Mustard C, and Choinière R. 2008. The Canadian census mortality follow-up study, 1991 through 2001. *Health Reports* 19(3):25–43.

Wilkinson, Richard G. 1994. The epidemiologic transition: From material scarcity to social disadvantage? *Daedalus* 123(4):61–77.

———. 1996. *Unhealthy Societies: The Afflictions of Inequality*. New York: Routledge.

Williams DR, Neighbors HW, and Jackson JS. 2003. Racial/ethnic discrimination and health: Findings from community studies. *American Journal of Public Health* 93(2):200–208.

Woodward D. 2008. Commission on Social Determinants of Health: Good diagnosis— now for the prescription. http://www.phmovement.org/cms/en/node/843. Accessed September 24, 2008.

World Bank. 2008. PovertyNet Overview. http://go.worldbank.org/K7LWQUT9L0. Accessed March 14, 2008.

Wright EO. 1985. *Classes*. London: Verso.

Yamin AE. 2005. The right to health under international law and its relevance to the United States. *American Journal of Public Health* 95(7):1156–1161.

8

Health under Crisis

In December, 1988, a 6.9 magnitude earthquake (and 5.8 aftershock) struck Spitak, Armenia, killing 45,000 people. Two-thirds of the deaths were estimated to be among children attending school. One year later, in Loma Prieta, California, a 6.9 magnitude earthquake struck at peak rush hour, causing only 57 deaths and 3,700 injuries. Why such a marked difference in casualties, for earthquakes of the same intensity? No doubt differences in geology, population density, and timing were all important, but even these factors are insufficient to explain the full extent of differential impact.

As we will explore in this chapter, a crucial set of factors has to do with the social conditions and physical infrastructure in the respective locales. In addition, emergency response to disasters reflects inequalities in preparedness between societies. Most, but not all, high-income countries invest in public health preparedness exercises and emergency care following disasters. Many underdeveloped countries have difficulty preparing for and addressing disasters (Spiegel 2005). Prevention rarely receives adequate attention, nor does the role of international political–economic factors in provoking or exacerbating these crises. While many disasters are termed "natural," the context and consequences of these events are anything but natural.

Indeed, more than 90% of deaths from disasters occur in poor countries. Crises exacerbate the ongoing deprivation already felt by the most disadvantaged communities, as seen with the enormous impact of the 2004 tsunami on Aceh Province, Indonesia and with the 2005 Kashmir earthquake in Pakistan (where 74,000 died and hundreds of thousands were wounded or displaced). The extensive and long-term impairments that accompany crises (and often go unaddressed), contribute to the existing cycles of poverty, disaster, disease, and death.

Nonetheless, the scale of crises can be deceptive. With few exceptions, they may have a large impact locally and may provoke significant morbidity and social disruption, yet they contribute to just a small proportion of global mortality. Even the 227,000 people who lost their lives in the December 2004 Asian tsunami is a small proportion of all those that died a premature death that year. Close to 10 million children die every year from preventable causes, the equivalent of two and a half "9/11" attacks occurring every day of the year. This is not to diminish the importance of such crises, but to put them in perspective.

This chapter begins with an examination of a series of recent ecological disasters and their health implications and the role of the international health community in addressing them. We then explore complex humanitarian emergencies (CHEs), their scope and impact on nutrition, mental health, vulnerable groups, and population displacement. Next, we turn to militarism, war, and public health, the effects of nuclear, chemical, and biologic weapons, and the long-standing effects for refugees and displaced populations. We conclude with a political economy analysis that outlines the factors that instigate and exacerbate CHEs and disasters and how they might be mitigated.

Box 8–1 Definitions and Classifications

Crude mortality rate (CMR)—an estimate of the portion of a population that dies during a specific period of time, calculated by dividing the number of persons that have died during the period by the estimated number of people in the population (usually mid-year). During emergencies this rate is frequently reported as deaths per 10,000 persons per day.

Wasting—nutritional measurement of weight loss. It is defined as weight for height less than –2 Z score (an indicator of malnourishment that is calculated using weight, height, head circumference, and body mass index).

Disaster—a significant disruption, either natural or human-made, that causes ecologic damage, injury, illness, or loss of human life that cannot be managed by routine procedures and quickly overwhelms local capacity, necessitating a request for external assistance (Landesman 2005).

Crisis—a critical incident which involves death, serious injury, or a threat to a significant number of people or animals, or damage to the environment.

Humanitarian emergency—a crisis characterized by large population displacement, food shortages, and social disruption.

Complex humanitarian emergency (CHE)—a situation of civil strife, armed conflict or war, competition for power and resources or political instability (Brennan and Nandy 2001) resulting in social disruption and excess mortality. Although called emergencies, CHEs may be protracted in duration. CHEs and disasters, as defined in this chapter, can differ in terms of the size of the population involved, the magnitude of the health impact, the speed and nature of the response, and the final human cost, especially in marginalized communities.

Refugee—as defined by the 1951 UN Convention Relating to the Status of Refugees, a person who has fled their own country because of well-founded fears of persecution based on race, religion, nationality, membership of a particular social group, or political affiliation (UNHCR 2000).

Internally displaced person (IDP)—a person who has been forced from his/her home for similar reasons as a refugee, but who remains within the internationally recognized borders of his/her country. IDPs are not protected by UN refugee rights.

Ecological disaster—a natural disaster that causes significant ecologic damage or loss of human, animal, or plant life.

"NATURAL DISASTERS" AND THEIR IMPLICATIONS

Key Questions:

- What are the public health implications of hurricanes, tsunamis, heat waves, floods, earthquakes, and related disasters?
- What is the role of international actors and agencies in disaster assessment and response?

Until this point in the book, we have focused on the continuous health consequences of poverty, inequality, and a host of other determinants of health at the household, societal, and global levels. This chapter discusses health under crisis conditions provoked by ecological events or wars that cause a great deal of suffering and mortality, and often elicit considerable response from the public and certain private donors (at least in the short term). So-called "natural disasters" often lay bare inequalities that are otherwise not considered public health priorities. Other events, such as the 800,000 killed in the genocide in Rwanda and war in the Democratic Republic of Congo, garner attention but little or no effective response. War and its effects by continent may garner uneven and delayed attention. Clearly, responding in times of crisis is one of the most visible roles for international health actors. In this section we review three forms of "natural disasters"—water disasters, earthquakes, and famines—and explore the health implications of and forms of response to these events.

Hurricanes, Floods, and Tsunamis

Water disasters are particularly devastating, and can wipe out an entire community's infrastructure, such as housing, schools, roads, and health centers. As illustrated by Hurricane Katrina in the United States and the South Asian tsunami, recent water-related disasters separated by just a few months, the effects of flooding were most devastating to the most vulnerable populations.

Hurricane Katrina in the United States

On August 29, 2005, Hurricane Katrina struck the southern U.S. coastline. The hurricane caused a storm surge of over 20 feet on the Gulf coastline, resulting in massive damage to the states of Louisiana and Mississippi. More than 75% of New Orleans' 500,000 residents became internally displaced within hours. The following day, Lake Pontchartrain's waters breached the levees and flooded most of New Orleans. Although tens of thousands of people fled the city before the storm hit, many more had no means of transportation to leave town, particularly poor and elderly people living alone. While school buses for evacuation lay idle in parking lots, and emergency responders had already left town, residents in flooded neighborhoods were forced into enclosed attics and rooftops awaiting rescue. As the water level rose above many houses, residents were reduced to hacking holes in their roofs in order to escape the rising waters.

Many people drowned in their homes, or died trying to escape through the water. The hurricane killed over 1,200 people and destroyed many local hospitals, clinics, and public health facilities in addition to thousands of homes (Fig. 8–1). Full-scale disaster assistance took several days to arrive, prompting criticism of the U.S. government's Federal Emergency Management Agency (FEMA).

In response to this crisis, FEMA director Michael Brown stated "I don't make judgments about why people chose not to leave, but, you know, there was a mandatory evacuation of New Orleans" (CNN 2005). His comment implies that everyone had the same resources available to follow the hurricane warnings. Few provisions, however, were provided for people without vehicles (or other resources) to evacuate.

Media outlets reached stranded residents more quickly and efficiently than official government rescue efforts, which took several days to arrive in the city. Water shortages in the New Orleans Superdome (a sports stadium used as a shelter after the hurricane) led to skirmishes among stranded residents, and thousands of people went without food for several days. Virtually everyone in the disaster lost many of their personal possessions in the flooding, including records of births, deaths, family memorabilia, pictures, and heirlooms. The poorer sections of New Orleans, however, bore the brunt of the destruction.

Because of the inability to promptly restore utilities to the area (Centers for Disease Control and Prevention 2006a) many people had to rely on gasoline-powered generators to provide power, leading to 27 incidents of carbon monoxide poisoning

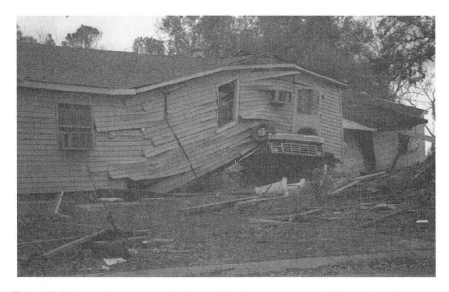

Figure 8–1 New Orleans, post Katrina, 2005. Photo courtesy of Victoria M. Gammino.

and 10 deaths (Centers for Disease Control and Prevention 2006b). Katrina was the deadliest U.S. hurricane since 1928, and became the country's costliest disaster on record (over US$200 billion in losses) (Centers for Disease Control and Prevention 2006d).

Damage from a major hurricane on the U.S. Gulf Coast was a disaster waiting to happen. Over the years, acres of marshland designed to protect against a storm surge were drained and paved by near-sighted city planners. The levee system, built to maintain part of the city below sea level, was only designed to withstand a category 3 storm. One year before, the U.S. Army Corps of Engineers' request for US$100 million in repairs to the New Orleans' levees was only funded at US$40 million. City administrators had done no serious disaster planning, despite repeated warnings from the scientific community, and despite a 2001 U.S. government FEMA report that listed a hurricane-related disaster striking New Orleans as the third most likely disaster to occur (after an earthquake in San Francisco, and a terrorist attack in New York City) (Krugman 2005). Public infrastructure in the United States continues to be more neglected than in virtually every other high-income country (Editorial 2005). (Indeed, 2007 witnessed a steam pipe explosion in New York city, a bridge collapse in Minneapolis, and a mine collapse in Utah.)

While the health effects of geological and weather-related events cannot be entirely prevented, thorough preparedness makes it possible to mitigate the impact of and reduce casualties from "natural disasters." One country with an exceptional record of responding to hurricane damage, despite its low per capita income, is Cuba. Like all Caribbean islands, Cuba is hit by tropical storms of varying severity every year. In 2004's Hurricane Jeanne, over 3,000 Haitians died from flooding and mudslides. However, in neighboring Cuba no one died. Cuba performs several storm preparation exercises every year, encouraging universal community participation. Activities include assuring communication networks among neighbors; preparing drinking water, food, and other supplies; securing roofs, doors, and other loose objects that can break free; cleaning debris from living and working environments; and repairing buildings at risk of collapse. As a result, Cuba's hurricane casualties remain very low. The United Nations (UN) has praised Cuba's Civil Defense System as a model for developing countries preparing for "natural disasters" (Bermejo 2006). As Katrina showed, this model is relevant for industrialized countries as well.

Hurricane Katrina revealed the inequalities present in most countries, whether wealthy or poor. The disaster may have been provoked by a natural event, but social forces—specifically racism and classism—determined who lived and who died (Hartman and Squires 2006). The vast majority of those who could not escape the storm were impoverished and marginalized. The majority were also African-American. Those who stayed and bore the full impact of the hurricane had neither cars nor ready access to organized transport for evacuation. Despite ample evidence of social inequalities in health in the United States, the dramatic and visible

manifestations of the isolation of poor, black populations on television were shocking. As *New York Times* columnist David Brooks, noted, "floods wash away the
surface of society. They expose the underlying power structures, the injustices, the
patterns of corruption, and the unacknowledged inequalities" (Brooks 2005).

What was briefly noted but quickly forgotten in the aftermath of Hurricane
Katrina was that the health of the survivors was a reflection of social relations:
those who were left behind had the least power. For a few brief weeks, the deep
social and economic divisions in the United States were uncovered by the hurricane. Yet the notion of collective responsibility that accompanied the loss after the
storm soon disappeared from the media, the public, and the attention of the U.S.
government relief agencies.

Yet while the New Orleans flooding was disastrous in itself, the ensuing catastrophe is ongoing. Three years after the storm, residents are still struggling to regain
something resembling a normal life. In addition to lost jobs, homes, and disrupted
education and family separation across nearly all 50 U.S. states, long-time community institutions and organizations were wiped out. Returning residents found a city
only half its previous size.

The political economy implications of disasters is evidenced in comparisons
between Hurricane Katrina's effects in New Orleans and the prevention, preparedness, and response to periodic earthquakes and fires in wealthy Californian communities. There, building codes and rescue missions in recent decades have limited
mortality to a handful of cases. Indeed, the ultimate magnitude of human harm due
to hurricanes, tsunamis, and earthquakes depends just as much on human social
organization and the political economy of the prevention and response as it does
on the actual ecologic event.

Tsunami in South Asia

The Indian Ocean tsunami that struck 14 countries in South Asia on December 26,
2004, killing upward of 227,000 people in a single day, is an extreme example of
devastation (Telford and Cosgrave 2006). Hundreds of thousands of people were
completely taken by surprise by the wall of water that hit miles of coastline with
tremendous force. Many were swept away in the flood water, never to be seen again.
Others were miraculously saved by holding onto trees and poles for hours, picked up
later by rescuers. Entire coastal communities were leveled in seconds, unprotected
from the open ocean. The sudden impact of the wave was over in a matter of minutes, but the coastal flooding continued for days in many areas. In Aceh Province,
Indonesia, most injuries occurred from blunt force trauma due to moving debris.

Following the tsunami and flooding, several myths associated with sudden
impact disasters were again raised by the media: that there is a high risk of communicable disease outbreaks following such disasters, that unburied human remains
pose an infectious disease threat, and that the most urgent need is for international
medical teams and equipment such as field hospitals (De Ville de Goyet 2004).

Epidemics of cholera and dysentery have actually been uncommon after large-scale disasters in the past three decades, and no large outbreaks were detected in Aceh, Indonesia. In general, the risk of infection from unburied dead bodies is overstated. Communicable disease transmission among the displaced is of greater concern (Morgan, Tidball-Binz, and Van Alphen 2006). Dysentery and other gastrointestinal diseases occurred in the large displacement centers, due to high-density dwelling with little ventilation.

The first to respond to the disaster in Indonesia were the affected communities themselves, followed by national military and civil groups. In Aceh, it was the Indonesian army and marines already in the province (due to a brutal military occupation that began in the late 1980s in response to an independence movement) that started delivering supplies of food and water, clearing the roads, and repairing bridges in the immediate aftermath of the disaster. The rescue was thus complicated by the fact that the most capable responders were the same military forces who were occupying Aceh, committing widespread human rights abuses, and causing thousands of civilian deaths.

Following the tsunami there was a massive outpouring of international assistance. Agencies to assist the survivors proliferated. At one point there were more than 160 international nongovernmental organizations (INGOs) registered in Aceh Province, many of which were unnecessary or duplicative. A number of agencies arrived with private funding and thus failed to coordinate with UN agencies or other NGOs. Governments of 13 countries sent military contingents to Aceh. Compared to ongoing emergencies elsewhere in the world, the tsunami response was extremely well funded. In total, US$6.2 billion was committed to the relief effort from all parts of the globe (Relief Web 2007). All the same, hundreds of thousands of people are still experiencing grief, loss, and guilt from the 2004 South Asian tsunami (van Griensven et al. 2006).

Earthquakes

Apart from massive floods and hurricanes, earthquakes cause the greatest damage to public health infrastructure. On December 26, 2003, an earthquake struck Bam, Iran killing an estimated 50,000 of the city's 200,000 people and leaving over 100,000 homeless. Over 60% of the city's buildings, many built of mud brick, were destroyed (including the 2,000-year old Citadel). The high death toll was due to lax enforcement of municipal construction regulations.

The world's third-deadliest "natural disaster" of the last 25 years occurred in neighboring northern Pakistan when a massive 7.6 magnitude earthquake struck on October 8, 2005. Due to the remote, widespread, and mountainous nature of the earthquake zone, rescue assistance was delayed. An estimated 74,650 people lost their lives, with 76,000 injured, 2.8 million left homeless, and 2.3 million with insecure access to food and essential goods (Fig. 8–2) (Brennan and Waldman 2006).

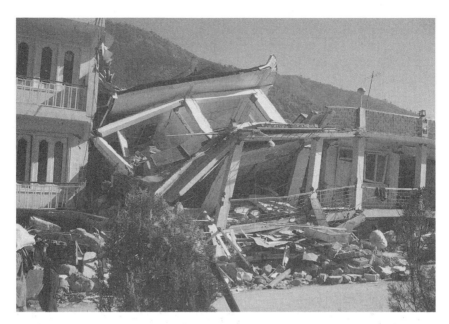

Figure 8–2 Damage from the earthquake in Balakot, Pakistan, 2005. Photo courtesy of Holly Solbergh.

Emergency response crews undertook mass vaccination for measles and established water and sanitation facilities. Since over 50% of the region's health facilities were destroyed, the provision of ongoing health services became the primary focus of the relief. Overcrowding, poor sanitation, and limited access to potable water hampered the effort.

The real public health challenges came as winter set in and millions suddenly faced food deprivation and exposure to the cold. Tents set up for survivors, relief workers, and as health facilities were not suitable for the harsh conditions and collapsed under heavy snow. The efforts were also hampered by "relief fatigue," as the South Asian tsunami 10 months earlier had occupied so much attention on the global stage. For those who survived that winter, the road ahead was difficult. Economic opportunity in this region is scarce, and the possibilities for rebuilding are limited. Though causing an estimated US$5 billion in damages, the World Bank delivered just US$470 million in recovery aid.

A crucial part of the earthquake response was ensuring gender equity. Anecdotal evidence suggested that many injured women could not obtain care from doctors due to a lack of female care providers. Consequently, relief agencies staffed clinics with female doctors and nurses thus raising the proportion of women care providers to more than 50% in some areas (Brennan and Waldman 2006).

The UN first implemented its new "cluster" approach in the Pakistan earthquake. A lead agency was identified within each sector to improve coordination, quality, consistency, and predictability of the relief effort. Ten main cluster groups were established, focusing on health, emergency shelter, water and sanitation, logistics, camp management, protection, food and nutrition, information technology, communication, education, and reconstruction. Lack of coordination has been identified as a contributing cause of death in disasters (Brennan 2007).

Famine and Food Insecurity

As with massive storms and earthquakes, scenes of starvation are often subject to graphic media attention, which neglects the underlying reasons for caloric deprivation. Food insecurity is experienced by millions of people every day. Acute food insecurity can lead to malnutrition and illness, and chronic food shortages can cause stunting in children, marasmus (protein-calorie malnutrition), and increased mortality. As the degree of food security worsens, the CMR and level of wasting in the community rises. Declaring a famine, however, is a highly political act. There are no agreed upon criteria set by the international aid community regarding how to define a famine. Using malnutrition alone is problematic, because it does not take into account the social-political aspects of the problem (Feinstein International Center 2006). One proposed scale to distinguish food insecurity from famine is presented in Table 8–1, which includes descriptors of social and economic conditions and coping strategies that are used to survive (Howe and Devereux 2004).

Lack of food sovereignty, which can lead to food insecurity and famine, entails a broader problem of inappropriate, unsustainable, and inequitable food production and distribution due to a range of agri-business and export-oriented pressures, including monoculture, overcropping, and the use of damaging pesticides, fertilizers, and seeds.

Box 8–2 Root Causes of Food Insecurity

Over the last two decades, many resource-rich countries have faced extreme food crises, including Ethiopia, Bangladesh, Mali, and North Korea. As discussed in Chapter 7, Amartya Sen has demonstrated that hunger and famines are caused more by the economics of maldistribution than by food shortages (Sen 1999).

Sparsely settled Niger, bordering the Sahara Desert, ranked as one of the poorest countries in the world by the UN Human Development Index, is plagued with recurring droughts that frequently cause famines. The 2005 food crisis left 2.5 million people living in farming and grazing areas

(*continued*)

> **Box 8–2** Continued
>
> vulnerable to food insecurity, causing global acute malnutrition in over 15% of the affected population and elevated mortality among children under 5 (Centers for Disease Control and Prevention 2006c). The crisis was mostly blamed on locusts and drought, yet the 2004 crop yield was only 7% lower than previous years. The underlying cause was related to the Niger government's adherence to free market economic reforms: it eliminated critical regulations of the cereal market, which led to large price fluctuations (Share the World's Resources 2006). High food prices not only made food inaccessible, it diverted the meager incomes of poor farmers away from health expenditures. However, the government (backed by the EU, USAID, and UN) feared that too much food assistance would disturb the market and hamper long-term development. The Ministry of Health responded insufficiently by distributing small amounts of food and making some cereals available at subsidized prices. In effect, food was sold to the starving at prices few could afford (Tectonidis 2006). Feeding centers run by Médecins Sans Frontières admitted 63,000 children under 5 years old (Médecins Sans Frontières 2006). But supplementary feeding, medical treatment for malaria, respiratory illness, and diarrhea, and a vaccination campaign were only temporary measures. The underlying causes of the drought, and related food crisis, remained largely unaddressed. Tragically and ironically, Niger exported food during this time of food deficits.
>
> In southeast Africa, the country of Malawi has been able to turn around years of cyclical food insecurity. After the 2005 harvest ranked as the worst on record, with 5 million people requiring emergency food aid, the president vowed not to let it happen again. For years World Bank policy has been to pressure small countries to adhere to free market principles and eliminate fertilizer subsidies (despite the fact that many Western governments heavily subsidize their domestic farming industries). Breaking with World Bank policy, Malawi's president deepened fertilizer subsidies in 2005, reducing market prices (Dugger 2007). Since Malawi is landlocked, has no significant industry, and the economy is largely based on subsistence farming, the subsidies had a major impact. Small scale farmers have been able to increase their yields, and now Malawi is a net exporter of food.

Most of the large bilateral aid agencies are involved in food aid distribution. The UN World Food Programme and Food and Agricultural Organization provide emergency food assistance, daily food programs, and technical assistance in food and agricultural production and distribution. They deliver food aid to the *most vulnerable* groups, though this approach neglects *less vulnerable but still needy* groups. Their almost-exclusive reliance on food from donor countries (especially the United States), however, means that food aid is typically delayed and that farming in neighboring areas—which could far more readily provide a sustainable source of food—is undermined. The NGO CARE took the bold step in 2007 of declaring that it would no longer accept U.S. federal funding (US$45 million per year) to deliver American food aid to recipient countries, claiming that this funding was inefficiently disbursed and might ultimately be hurting the people it purports to help.

COMPLEX HUMANITARIAN EMERGENCIES: DEFINITION, CONTEXT, AND RESPONSE

Key Questions:

- What makes a disaster a CHE?
- What are the most pressing public health issues to address in a CHE?

Table 8-1 Famine Scale Based on Joint Criteria of Mortality, Malnutrition, and Food Security

Level	Phase Designation	Malnutrition and Mortality Indicators	Food Security Descriptors
0	Food security conditions	Crude mortality rate (CMR) <0.2/10,000/day and Wasting <2.3% of the population	Social system is cohesive; prices are stable; negligible use of coping strategies
1	Food insecurity conditions	CMR ≥0.2/10,000/day and/or Wasting ≥2.3%	Social system remains cohesive; price instability and seasonal shortage of key items; "reversible" coping strategies (e.g., mild food rationing) are employed
2	Food crisis conditions	CMR ≥0.5/10,000/day and/or Wasting >10%	Social system is significantly stressed but remains largely cohesive; dramatic rise in price of food; "reversible" coping strategies start to fail; increased adoption of "irreversible" coping strategies (e.g., selling livestock and land)
3	Famine conditions	CMR ≥1/10,000/day and/or Wasting ≥20%	Clear signs of social breakdown appear; markets begin to close or collapse; coping strategies exhausted; "survival strategies" are more common; affected populations identify food as the dominant problem at the onset of the crisis
4	Severe famine conditions	CMR ≥5/10,000/day and/or Wasting ≥40%	Widespread social breakdown; markets are closed or inaccessible to affected populations; "survival strategies" are widespread
5	Extreme famine conditions	CMR >15/10,000/day	Complete social breakdown; widespread mortality

Magnitude Category	Phase Designation	Mortality Range
A	Minor Famine	0–999
B	Moderate Famine	1,000–9,999
C	Major Famine	10,000–99,999
D	Great Famine	100,000–999,999
E	Catastrophic Famine	1,000,000 and over

Source: Howe and Devereux (2004).

- Where are the current hot spots for refugees and internally displaced persons?
- What are the political economy of health dimensions underlying CHEs?
- What are the key components of an effective public health response to mental health needs during a CHE?
- What are specific threats faced by women and children during wartime?

Civilian populations affected by conflict experience severe health consequences. CHE (complex humanitarian emergency) is the term used to describe a situation of

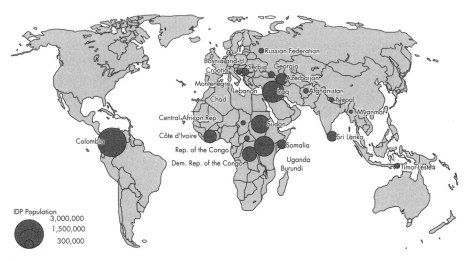

Figure 8–3 Map of complex humanitarian emergencies causing displacement.
Source: United Nations High Commissioner for Refugees (2006).

combined civil strife, food shortage, and population displacement that ultimately lead to excess mortality and morbidity (Noji and Toole 1997). This does not include "natural disasters," which are usually more short term and necessitate a qualitatively different response. By contrast, CHEs can last for years or even decades, such as the protracted wars in Sudan, Somalia, and the Democratic Republic of the Congo (DRC). Figure 8–3 shows the current places where CHEs are occurring.

History of CHEs

CHEs could describe thousands of conflicts in the past where large populations were affected by increased mortality. However, beginning in the 1970s, public health responses were systematized, spurred by the conflicts in Biafra (Nigeria) and Bangladesh, and during the flight of millions of refugees from Cambodia to Thailand during the 1975–1979 terror of the Khmer Rouge, and from Afghanistan to Pakistan during the 1979–1989 Soviet-Afghan war. The first technical guidelines on emergency nutrition were published in 1978, and the first textbook on refugee health care came out in 1983 (Simmonds, Vaughan, and Gunn 1983). Field manuals have also been published by NGOs that work predominantly in refugee health care settings, such as Oxfam, Save the Children, and Médecins Sans Frontières (MSF). The Pan American Health Organization (PAHO) includes an Area on Emergency Preparedness and Disaster Relief which conducts response activities in all member states. Its disaster assistance program is among the best in the world, conducting training, capacity building, and preparedness exercises for member states (PAHO 2007).

By 2000, a broad, informal coalition of humanitarian agencies and disaster experts cooperated to produce the *Sphere Project Handbook*, which outlined standards for the level of service to be attained in disaster response in six key areas (Waldman 2001a). The latest 2004 edition serves as a guide, but does not function as an on-the-spot handbook (The Sphere Project 2004). It proposes minimum standards in water supply and sanitation, nutrition, food aid, shelter and safe planning, and health services. A key section of the handbook is the Humanitarian Charter, which states that all people in all circumstances have the right to live with dignity and to protection and assistance as described in international humanitarian law. There are objections raised by some NGOs, however, that the handbook is too technical and that it places excessive emphasis on standards and not enough on the international community's obligation to provide protection. Indeed, "a vaccination card or a full belly does not protect against refoulement[1] or attack" (Terry 2000, p. 21). Other objections are that the standards will be taken too literally, without regard for the particular circumstances of each emergency.

Definition and Response

Traditionally, CHEs were defined as the doubling of the baseline CMR of a population. This was because refugees and IDPs have very high CMRs in the period immediately following their flight or migration, in some places as high as 60 times the baseline rate (e.g., in Goma, Zaire, 1994). But this doubling of the CMR threshold may be less helpful in settings of prolonged conflict affecting a large population over a large area. In 1990, Toole and Waldman proposed a quantitative CMR threshold of one death per 10,000 people per day to define the acute phase of a CHE (Toole and Waldman 1990). An objective indicator like this, in places where the previous mortality was unknown, allows for comparisons of different emergencies and for monitoring trends within an emergency.

The fact that in some situations measured mortality does not reach the threshold level should not preclude the use of the term CHE or the triggering of an emergency response (Salama, Buzard, and Spiegel 2001). Other triggers could be an increase in the incidence of a single disease, food insecurity, such as in a famine, large-scale displacement, deteriorating security, an increased level of mental health problems, or the deliberate targeting of a particular racial or ethnic group (such as the events that unfolded in the Kosovo conflict [1996–1999] or in East Timor [1975–1999]).

The health impact of CHEs has been the most severe in sub-Saharan Africa, South and Southeast Asia, and Central America, as the public health infrastructure in many of these settings is already tenuous. War, chronic food insecurity, intermittent droughts and floods, lack of an industrial base, unfair trade practices, and an imbalance of economic power (with a net extraction of wealth) have together result in a crumbling infrastructure unable to cope with massive influxes of people. The world's most pressing refugee health situations are located in developing world regions, as seen in Table 8–2.

Table 8-2 Main Sources of the World's Refugees, January 2005

Place of Origin	Estimated Persons	Main Country of Asylum
Afghanistan	2,001,000	Pakistan[a]/Iran/Germany/Netherlands/United Kingdom
Sudan	644,000	Chad/Uganda/Kenya/DRC/Ethiopia
Burundi	471,700	Tanzania/DRC/Rwanda/South Africa/Canada
DRC	371,000	Tanzania/Congo/Zambia/Burundi/Rwanda/Uganda
Somalia	303,000	Kenya/Yemen/United Kingdom/United States/Djibouti
Palestinian Territories	345,900[b]	Saudi Arabia/Egypt/Libya/Algeria
Iraq	144,000	Iran/Germany/Netherlands/United Kingdom/Sweden
Vietnam	343,300	China/Germany/United Status/France/Switzerland
Liberia	416,000	Guinea/Côte d'Ivoire/Sierra Leone/Ghana/United States
Azerbaijan	249,080	Armenia/Germany/United States/Netherlands/France

[a]UNHCR figures for Pakistan only include Afghan refugees living in camps. According to a 2005 government census, the latest estimates available, there were an additional 1.9 million Afghans living in urban areas in Pakistan, some of whom may be refugees.

[b]Palestinians under UNHCR mandate only.

Source: United Nations High Commissioner for Refugees (2006, p. 16).

The acute, or emergency, phase of the displacement and settlement of large numbers of people is usually characterized by the health priorities that cause the greatest amount of morbidity and mortality. This phase is addressed through: initial assessment, measles immunization, water and sanitation, food and nutrition, shelter and site planning, health care, control of communicable diseases (acute respiratory infections, measles, diarrhea, and malaria), surveillance, training, coordination, and camp management.

CHEs have direct and indirect effects on health, as the factors promoting disease transmission interact synergistically (Rowland et al. 1999; Reintjes et al. 2002).The most common causes of high mortality in CHEs are diarrheal diseases, acute respiratory infections, and malaria, frequently exacerbated by concomitant high rates of acute malnutrition. Measles was historically an important cause of death, but vaccination is now prioritized early in most contexts. With effective interventions, these diseases are all avoidable. Many countries affected by CHEs already have very high rates of under-5 mortality, and thus high rates of infectious disease should be expected (Salama et al. 2004).

Addressing common communicable diseases through vaccination is an essential component of a mortality and morbidity-reduction campaign during CHEs (Connolly et al. 2004). Measles vaccination coverage of 95% of the children under age five can decrease mortality by up to 20% to 30%, especially when it is administered with vitamin A.

Diarrheal disease can account for over 50% of the deaths during an acute phase of an emergency, mainly from inadequate quality and quantity of water, substandard sanitation facilities, overcrowding, poor hygiene, and a scarcity of soap. Clean water and sanitation for the prevention of waterborne diseases, oral rehydration salts for the management of fluid loss in young children with diarrhea, and the promotion of breast feeding should be mainstays of emergency response. Good case management of diarrhea and acute respiratory illness can save a large numbers of lives and prevent enormous outbreaks of cholera and shigella, unlike what was seen in Goma, Zaire, when 50,000 people died in the first month of the disaster (Goma Epidemiology Group 1995). Other interventions can also reduce the incidence of infectious diseases, such as the distribution of insecticide-treated bed nets, indoor residual spraying for malaria control, provision of clean delivery equipment, antenatal steroids, zinc treatment for diarrhea in children, nevirapine, and replacement feeding for HIV-infected mothers where appropriate.

During emergencies, tuberculosis and malaria require ongoing attention just as they do in a nonemergency setting (WHO 1997). The control of sexually transmitted diseases and HIV/AIDS is also a key component of CHE public health interventions, especially in sub-Saharan Africa (Khaw et al. 2000). New guidelines that promote an aggressive approach to the prevention, care, and treatment of people with HIV/AIDS during CHEs are now the standard of care (The Sphere Project 2004). Other areas that should be addressed, although less comprehensively, include reproductive health, psychosocial issues, and childhood immunizations for diphtheria, pertussis, and tetanus.

Security and protection have become even more pressing during the past 20 years, especially in CHEs where the major cause of morbidity and mortality is from violence, for example in Bosnia, Kosovo, Chechnya, and Rwanda. In Eastern Europe, injuries have been the major cause of mortality and chronic diseases the major cause of morbidity, in contrast to the infectious disease patterns during CHEs observed elsewhere.

Malnutrition

As with ecological disasters, malnutrition is a major complicating factor of many CHEs. Nutrition and food security have long been essential elements in any CHE response, and remain so. The understanding of nutritional problems in CHEs has evolved over the last decade from a narrow focus on marasmus to a more problem-solving approach, which has been termed "public nutrition" (Young 1999). This approach requires a situational analysis of nutritional risk and vulnerability, action-oriented strategies, and an assessment of nutritional outcomes. It emphasizes a range of interventions with programmatic links needed to address the underlying causes of malnutrition, as seen in Figure 8–4.

Three years of war in southern Sudan during the 1990s caused widespread food insecurity, with rural and nomadic tribes flocking to towns and cities. An estimated 78,000 people died during the crisis in 1998 alone (Deng 2002). Despite large-scale

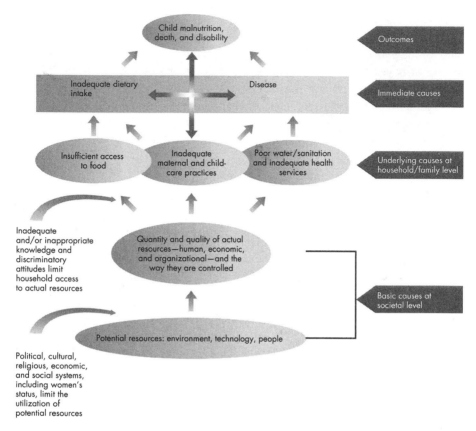

Figure 8–4 UNICEF framework for malnutrition.
Source: UNICEF (1998, p. 24).

humanitarian interventions and food drops, CMRs remained high. Responding agencies learned that not only were children at high risk of case fatality from acute malnutrition, but undernourished adolescents and adults were as well (Salama and Borrel 1998). The centralized distribution of food for children may have attracted people to places with poor sanitation and led to flourishing communicable disease. Humanitarian responses that focused on food-based interventions but neglected preventive health services (such as vaccination), were contributing factors to the measles outbreaks experienced during the Sudan emergency, as well as resultant excess mortality in the Ethiopian famine of 2000.

Mental Health during CHEs

During a CHE, the social, political, economic, and cultural infrastructure of the affected population is often destroyed, leading to social catastrophe (Toole and

Table 8–3 Prevalence of Mental Health Disorders in Adult
Populations Affected by Complex Emergencies

Complex Emergency Population	Posttraumatic Stress Disorder (%)	Depression (%)
Cambodian refugees in Thailand	37.2	67.9
Bosnian refugees in Croatia	26	39
Kosovar Albanians in Kosovo	17.1	N/A
Karenni (Burmese) refugees in Thailand	46	41.8
Cambodia (entire country)	28.4	N/A
Baseline U.S. population	1	6.4

Point prevalences in first four rows, lifetime prevalences thereafter. Different screening methods were used in these studies (see references for details).

Sources: Helzer, Robins, and McEvoy (1987); Kessler et al. (1995, 2003); Mollica
et al. (2004); Robins and Regier (1991). Reprinted with permission from Elsevier.

Waldman 1997). All kinds of health care services can be disrupted, including mental health services, if they exist at all. Although 90% of refugees and IDPs exhibit
tremendous resiliency during emergencies (Summerfield 2000; National Institute of
Mental Health 2002), the mental health consequences of CHEs range from acute
traumatic stress disorder to depression, anxiety, and over the long term, posttraumatic
stress disorder (PTSD). A major issue in addressing mental health needs is the lack
of culturally validated screening instruments and accurate population estimates of
mental health disorders (Mollica et al. 1992), as well as whether Western psychiatric categorizations are relevant cross-culturally. For example, should a refugee
Tibetan monk who goes into a trance as the Nechung Oracle be considered schizo-
phrenic? Studies that show the prevalence of mental health symptoms observed in
different CHEs are seen in Table 8–3.

In 2007 the Inter-Agency Standing Committee (IASC) Guidelines on Mental
Health and Psychosocial Support in Emergency Settings were released by
the heads of 27 UN and non-UN agencies (IASC 2007). These guidelines
recommend:

1. Coordination of mental health care into preexisting mental health services;
2. Assessment and monitoring based on the Sphere Project's standards;
3. Early intervention consisting of listening, conveying compassion, ensuring
   basic needs, mobilizing support from family, and protecting people from further harm (Leaning, Briggs, and Chen 1999);

4. Integration of the local mental health care system, involving culturally competent relief workers, primary care providers, and traditional healers who provide effective mental health services in a nonstigmatizing environment;

5. Training and education for local primary care practitioners, policy makers, teachers, and relief workers in mental health issues;

6. Cultural competence—including the use of locally appropriate terms for mental health distress such as *nervioso* in Latin America that may not have equivalent terms in Western psychiatry;

7. Community participation, particularly for large-scale interventions;

8. Self-care for relief workers, who are not immune to the negative mental health effects of CHEs (Antares Foundation 2002).

CHEs can be associated with a near complete destruction of society and its institutions. Restoring social cohesion and reducing hatred and revenge are central to post-conflict restoration. In the Balkans, feelings of revenge and hatred were common several years after the cessation of hostilities (Lopes Cardozo et al. 2003). The psychosocial approach to mental health care in CHEs focuses on marginalized and vulnerable groups and those with special needs in order to increase social cohesion. This approach assumes that people are affected in different ways in terms of particular human capacities (skills, knowledge, capabilities), social ecology (connectedness and networks), and culture and values (Psychosocial Working Group 2007). A more comprehensive mental health response plan should support the normalization of everyday life through the reduction of disease, reestablishment of sociocultural and economic activities, family reunification, and protection from violence (Mollica et al. 2004).

Figure 8–5 depicts the impact of a CHE on health and health services. Increased health needs due to casualties, displacement, and economic disruption have multifactoral influences, and can impact health service delivery on many levels. Organization, management, and economic support are all affected by the availability and distribution of resources during the emergency and post-conflict phases.

Gender-Based Violence

During the wars in Uganda, Liberia, Sierra Leone, and Bosnia in the early 1990s, women experienced widespread rape and abuse by soldiers and IDPs (Swiss and Giller 1993). The problem of sexual abuse and rape during war is hardly new. During World War II in the Pacific, Japanese troops abducted between 100,000 and 200,000 Korean, Chinese, Filipino, Indonesian, and Burmese women to serve as "comfort women" to the Japanese army (Ashford and Huet-Vaughn 1997). The women were seen as "war supplies," necessary to keep up the morale of the soldiers. In the end, only 10% of these female prisoners survived the end of the war, and few survived to receive Japan's formal apology for their treatment in 1993.

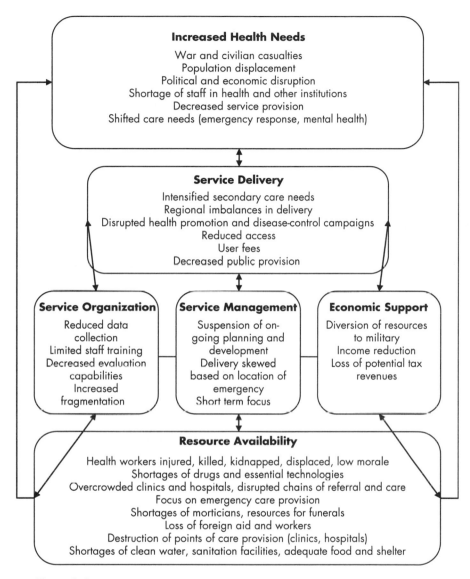

Figure 8–5 The impact of conflict and emergencies on health and health services.

Public rape is meant to terrorize an entire community during wartime, forcing the community to flee or submit to the will of the captors. During the 1994 Rwandan genocide, Hutu men were urged to rape Tutsi women as an expression of ethnic hatred. The trauma of this humiliation is magnified for many women who become pregnant as a result of the assault, or suffer from any number of sexually transmitted diseases including HIV. As well, the physical trauma of rape can lead to long-term reproductive health problems. Many women also suffer long-term psychological effects as a result of the fear and helplessness experienced in rape. For example, many of the "comfort women" held by the Japanese were never able to marry and raise a family due to the shame associated with sexual violation.

Social upheaval magnifies the everyday injustices that many women live with during times of relative peace. Women and young girls are exposed to cycles of abuse and can be caught in situations of sexual exploitation in camps and refugee settings. Sexual and gender-based abuse can range from harassment, domestic violence, female genital mutilation, withholding food for sex, rape, and death. Women and girls fail to get the same access to humanitarian assistance that men receive (UNHCR 2006).

Temporary housing and camps set up to assist displaced persons may not be safe havens for women. Separated from the security provided by family and friends, women and girls can become sexual prey for their fellow refugees as well as for camp guards and humanitarian relief workers. Poorly planned camps often ignore the security concerns of women and girls who may be forced to travel unprotected to areas in search of food, water, and firewood. Women in camps also receive less of everything, including water, food, and soap.

Prevention of sexual and gender-based abuse for IDPs and refugees is challenging for every humanitarian organization. In addition to being underreported, gender-based crimes are heavily stigmatized in most countries. Women and girls often remain silent due to shame and the fear of being shunned by their communities. These problems highlight the challenge of setting public health priorities in CHEs, particularly if cultural norms place certain groups (men) ahead of others (women) (Waldman 2001b).

Humanitarian aid organizations can mainstream camp management to reduce the incidence of gender-based abuse by:

1. distributing food supplies to women rather than men to ensure more even allocation within families;
2. visibly lighting latrines and other places visited at night time to reduce vulnerability of women;
3. instituting firewood programs;
4. involving women in decision making;
5. sensitizing staff to the issue of gender-based abuse; and
6. hiring local women for jobs in camps.

Effects of Violence and War on Children

UNICEF reports that since the mid 1990s conflicts have killed an estimated 2 million children and have left another 6 million disabled, 20 million homeless, and over 1 million separated from their parents (UNICEF 2005). The proliferation of newer and deadlier technologies of warfare such as landmines and small arms has also had dramatic consequences for morbidity and mortality among children (Fig. 8–6). In many conflict zones, for every child that dies from armed attacks, three times as many are left severely wounded or disabled. Subsequent to the loss and violence that many children experience in wartime, UNICEF estimates that some 10 million children have experienced psychological "trauma" or distress due to war (UNICEF 2005). For children, war represents not only acute risk of personal physical and psychological endangerment, but also extreme disruption to normal childhood development (Betancourt 2005).

War is characterized by the loss of security, predictability, and the structure of daily life. Some children experience infrastructure disruption and family separation; others may experience indirect violence by witnessing atrocities such rape or the killing of friends and family members; others may directly experience acts of violence from torture and rape to abduction or forced recruitment into fighting forces (Machel 1996; Macksoud et al. 1996).

The adverse consequences of children's exposure to war-related trauma are related to mental health distress (Sack, Him, and Dickason 1999; Kinzie et al. 2006). Some studies have indicated that younger children are particularly vulnerable to PTSD and that cumulative exposure to violent and nonviolent (relocation, lack of food, lack of shelter) stressors is associated with greater risk of mental health distress and PTSD symptoms (Allwood, Bell-Dolan, and Husain 2002).

It is currently estimated that some 250,000 "child soldiers" are active in conflicts around the globe, such as Afghanistan and Northern Uganda. Children conscripted with fighting forces take on a number of roles from forced combat positions to involvement in the commission of atrocities such as pillaging villages and mass rapes, to work as porters, cooks, servants, human shields, and/or sexual slaves

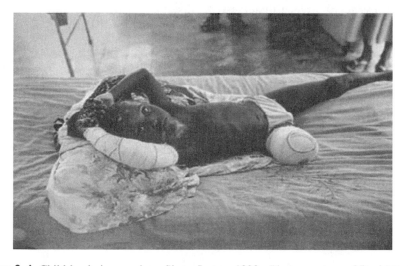

Figure 8–6 Child landmine survivor, Sierra Leone, 1990s. Photo courtesy of David Parker.

(Betancourt 2005). Child soldiers frequently face torture, forced use of substances, and persistent psychological threat from their captors (De Silva, Hobbs, and Hanks 2001). Girls also comprise a significant proportion of the children involved with armed groups globally. They are usually abducted and can face years of sexual violence, abuse, and unwanted pregnancy.

Research on the long-term social and emotional outcomes of child soldiering and forced abduction is limited, but the extreme situations faced by child soldiers likely have a significant impact on their psychological well-being (Goodwin and Cohn 1994). Few studies to date have assessed the effects of exposure to the full range of potential war traumas that may be experienced by child soldiers (Macksoud et al. 1996; Sack, Him, and Dickason 1999). Even fewer directly address the mental health of children recruited into fighting forces (McKay and Wessells 2004; Betancourt, Pochan, and de la Soudiere 2006). The stigma and discrimination experienced upon returning to their communities affects the mental health and adjustment of children formerly involved with fighting forces (Kohrt et al. 2008).

Constraints and New Approaches

The number of people not housed in camps who are affected by emergencies often greatly exceeds the number of camp-based refugees and IDPs (Salama et al. 2004). However, the medical care inside the camps may be better than that for local populations outside, as the UN and NGOs generally have more funds, affording camp-based residents greater access to health services. In long-established refugee camps, mortality rates are systematically lower than for the surrounding population (Spiegel et al. 2002). Although services for refugees sometimes benefit the surrounding community, most often this is not the case.

More research is needed to address the distal and underlying causes of CHEs, and thus to work at the primary and secondary intervention level (Lautze et al. 2004). Many emergencies occur as a result of failure in the political and diplomatic arena, and often flare up due to outside actors. Most CHEs that have occurred over the past 20 years are linked to civil wars (often protracted) occurring within the boundaries of sovereign states (Brennan and Nandy 2001). Many of these "internal" conflicts are caused by local and external forces in competition over lucrative resources, particularly over control of natural resources such as gold, diamonds, or coltan (used for consumer electronics). In these situations, civilians are increasingly recruited to kill, terrorize, or ethnically cleanse entire populations.

MILITARISM, WAR, AND PUBLIC HEALTH

Key Questions:

- What is the impact of militarism and war on public health?
- How should the lives of civilians be protected during war?

Militarism may be defined as the subordination of the ideals or policies of a nation's government or of its civil society to military goals or policies. It is a consistent feature of the rise of dominating nation states since the Roman Empire and has played a role in many of the world's current conflicts. In 2004, world military expenditures were estimated to be just over US$1 trillion, amounting to 2.6% of global GNP (Skon et al. 2005). There are variations between the major arms spenders, as can be seen in Figure 8–7, but spending has increased in both absolute and real terms since 1996.

The Unites States spends almost as much on arms and weapons as all other countries combined (46% of the world's total) (Stockholm International Peace Research Institute 2006). The U.S. President's 2008 budget called for nearly US$522 billion in military spending, 28% of the annual budget, versus just 0.07% of GDP (US$30 billion) toward nonmilitary international assistance (Global Issues 2007). This contrasts with Scandinavian countries such as Sweden or Denmark, which spend from 5% to 8% of their annual budget on the military, and 0.5% of GDP on international assistance (Global Issues 2007; U.S. Department of Commerce Bureau of Industry and Security 2007).

Weapons manufacture and sales are central to the economies of powerful countries. Eighty-eight percent of sales in arms are conducted by the five permanent members of the UN Security Council (China, France, the Russian Federation, the United Kingdom, and the United States) (Global Issues 2007). Militarism increases the amount of money spent on military research that could otherwise be used to improve quality of life. Some discoveries spill over into the civilian sector, such as the creation of the internet, the development of antimalaria insecticides, and advances in surgery and field medicine. However, increased funding for military contractors and agencies has caused a subtle brain drain of professionals away from nonmilitary research. World expenditures on weapons research exceeds the combined spending on developing new energy technology, increasing agricultural productivity, and controlling pollutants (Levy and Sidel 2007).

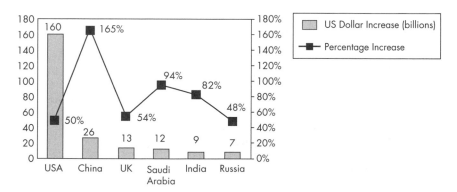

Figure 8–7 Military expenditures 1996–2005. *Sources*: Stockholm International Peace Research Institute (2006); Global Issues (2008). Reproduced by permission of Global Issues.

Although militarism is not identical to war, it is war's precursor, readying societ-ies logistically, technically, practically, politically, psychologically, and economi-cally. The causes of war are complex, relating to local and far larger struggles over power, long-standing animosities, political vacuums, repression, and colonial lega-cies. War is often fuelled when abundant resources are controlled by a few (Global Health Watch 2005).

Militarism and war harm public health in myriad ways. In addition to the deaths of thousands of soldiers, the civilian effects are much higher in locales where war takes place (for example, 50,000 Americans and more than 2 million Vietnamese died during the Vietnam War). Since the end of World War II, at least 23 million people have died in over 150 major conflicts—mostly from war's indirect effects of displaced populations, loss of social services, instable food sources, and loss of infrastructure (Garfield and Neugut 1997).

Globally, the impact of militarism is felt through its:

1. diversion of financial and human resources to arms, instead of improving the quality of life of people and communities;
2. development, production, and testing of nuclear and conventional weapons; and
3. promotion of the idea of violence as an acceptable way to resolve conflicts, contributing to increased violence worldwide (Levy and Sidel 2007).

In developing countries, the effects of militarism are particularly detrimental. First, there are human development costs to spending money on arms. For every dollar that is spent on weapons, there are nutrition, housing, education, and health services that are neglected or underfunded. Arms spending can disproportionately destabilize gov-ernments, as during the socially destructive wars in West Africa through the 1990s, in which the harvesting of raw diamonds paid for the weapons used in the fighting in turn fueling further conflict. In many developing countries, there are also long-term effects of landmines.

Box 8–3 Landmine Effects on Health

Landmines continue to kill hundreds of innocent men, women, and children years after the cessation of conflict. The ongoing effects incurred by landmines were not discussed until the late 1980s, when NGOs drew attention to their deadly ongoing effects in Afghanistan and Cambodia (Stover, Cobey, and Fine 1997). There continue to be undetonated landmines in over 88 countries. The true number is unknown, but there are likely more than 100,000 mines strewn across Angola, Mozambique, Ethiopia, Kuwait, Laos, Burma, Somalia, Sudan, Uganda, and the former Yugoslavia, killing approx-imately 10,000 people per year and injuring an unknown number (U.S. Department of State 2003). Landmines kill and maim indiscriminately. They are cheap, durable, easy to make, and effective (Coupland and Samnegaard 1999). Landmines are designed to kill or injure the victim. The blast and shrapnel cause traumatic wounds to the extremities, chest, genitals, and face of the unlucky soldier or civilian. Amputation of a limb is common, even among children (Fig. 8–6).

(continued)

Box 8-3 Continued

One of the tragedies of landmines is that they remain buried for years after hostilities cease (Keller et al. 1999). Farmers, civilians looking for firewood, and children playing can all activate the landmine mechanism. And these citizens are much more likely than soldiers to die in the field or on the way to medical care. Women are particularly subject to landmine injuries, as they are typically responsible for collecting water or firewood. When civilians do lose limbs, they have limited access to the proper prosthesis they need to once again be productive members of society. Amputees are often stigmatized and considered unemployable.

The only sure way to prevent casualties from landmines is to ban them. In contrast to other weapon systems, such as biological or chemical weapons, landmines have never been completely banned by all countries. In 1991, an international movement started by Physicians for Human Rights, Human Rights Watch, and other NGOs called for an unconditional ban on all landmines that detonate on contact. In 1992, U.S. and EU member states agreed to a 5-year moratorium on the sale, transfer, production, or export of antipersonnel mines (Cobey and Raymond 2001). As of 2007, 156 countries had ratified (or joined) the 1997 Mine Ban Treaty and over 350 international NGOs had signed on (Arms Control Association 2007). The United States, China, and Russia have not signed the ban. The number of mine-producing countries has dropped from 54 to 16. The United States remains one of the few countries that allows the production and export of antipersonnel mines to war zones around the world.

Deaths from War

Over time, as military weaponry has become more sophisticated and armies have grown, the number of military deaths has increased. The 20th century was the most deadly on record, with an estimated 45 million soldiers dying. Until World War II, more soldiers died from infectious diseases and war wounds than on the battlefield. The mortality rate from infectious diseases among soldiers fighting in the tropical environments of Southeast Asia and the South Pacific during World War II was 16 times higher than the mortality rate from battle wounds.

Defining what is a war-related injury or death is problematic. Although soldiers wounded or killed in battle are designated as killed in action (KIA) or wounded in action (WIA), no such designation exists for civilian casualties caused by military equipment. Civilians can be injured or can die from the disruption of existing food, housing, education, or medical care systems, but not necessarily be classified as a war-related injury or death. In addition, surveillance systems for the military usually operate out of the military medical system, but civilians treated in war clinics and hospital systems may not have their injuries counted.

The situation for civilians has become even worse. During the 18th and 19th centuries, civilian casualties were reported to be relatively low. As the number of civil wars and wars of national liberation increased during the 20th century, death rates among civilians rose dramatically. In the 20th century, an estimated 191 million people died as a result of conflict (more than half were civilians). During the Spanish Civil War, the Vietnam War, and the War in Croatia in 1991–1992, over half of all the deaths were among noncombatants. UNICEF has estimated that in the early 1990s civilian deaths from direct and indirect causes constituted 90% of all the deaths in war worldwide (UNICEF 1996).

During World War II, it was estimated that the Soviet Union lost 15% of its population—27 million people—1.2 million in the Leningrad blockade alone. Much of this was due to combat, but also due to starvation and exposure during the cold winter months. Poland lost 20% of its population, but Britain lost only 0.7% of its population and the United States even less (0.3%). Since World War II some wars have been just as deadly. Korea lost 10% of its population, and Vietnam lost 13%, in their respective wars (Sivard 1991). In the DRC almost 4 million have died since 1998, out of a total population of 57 million.

In addition to the direct effects of combat (bombing, etc.), the indirect effects of war can be just as dangerous for a fragile social system disrupted by conflict. Malnutrition, crowded housing conditions, poor sanitation, and lack of access to medical care all increase during wartime. This was especially true for the U.S.-supported wars in El Salvador and Nicaragua throughout the 1980s and into the early 1990s. Although called "low-intensity conflicts" by the U.S. government, these wars caused massive social disruption for the communities living through them. This was also the case in Mozambique and Angola in the 1980s, where the population suffered from destruction of national economic infrastructure, as well as widespread injury and disability and the psychological effects of violence.

NUCLEAR, CHEMICAL, AND BIOLOGIC WEAPONS

Key Questions:

- What are the potential effects on health of a nuclear war?
- Why should chemical and biological weapons be monitored?

Military, political, and corporate leaders in the major warring nations developed chemical weapons (CW) (e.g., mustard gas) that were responsible for the deaths of thousands of soldiers in World War I. Research on biological weapons (BW) proceeded at the same time although with only a few alleged cases of use during World War I. General revulsion against the horrific use of CW in World War I provided impetus for the Geneva Protocols of 1925 banning the use of chemical and biological weapons (CBW) in warfare. However, the Geneva Protocols did not prohibit the development, production, stockpiling, and transport of such armaments, and between the two world wars major military powers utilized this loophole to develop CBW programs. Table 8–4 shows the verified use of toxic and infective agents over the past 80 years.

World War II marked an expansion of BW programs, with the United States, Japan, and Great Britain weaponizing anthrax and other pathologic organisms, and culturing microorganisms and insect vectors. Plans to bomb numerous German

Table 8–4 Selected Antipersonnel Toxic and Infective Agents and Their Health Effects, Whose Hostile Use has Been Verified

Period	Agent	Used by/ Location	Health Effects
1919	Diphenylchloroarsine (sensory irritant)	U.K./Russia	• Eye and respiratory tract burning and blistering
1923–1926	Bromomethyl ethyl ketone (a tear gas)	Spain/Morocco	• Irritation to mucous membranes and skin
1919	Mustard gas	U.K./Russia	• Blistering of the skin and respiratory tract
1935–1940		Italy/Abyssinia	
1936–1937		USSR/China	• Carcinogenic
1937–1945		Japan/Manchuria	• Long-term damage, and higher rate of mortality
1982–1988		Iraq/Iran	
1988		Iraq/Kurds	• Increased vulnerability to infection
1937–1945	Hydrogen cyanide	Japan/Manchuria	• Rapid intoxication
			• Potentially fatal
1963–1967	Phosgene	Egypt/Yemen	• Irritation of mucous membranes
			• Damage to lung tissues
1965–1975	Agent CS/CS gas	U.S./Vietnam	• Irritation of skin and mucous membranes
1982–1988	Tabun (nerve gas)	Iraq/Iran	• Tremors
			• Death from lethal dose
1984	*Salmonella enteritidis* serotype *typhimurium*	Baghwan Shree Rajneesh/United States	• Gastrointestinal infection
1994–1995	Sarin (nerve gas)	Aum Shinrikyo/Japan	• Disrupts nervous system—loss of bodily functions
			• Potentially fatal
			• Long-term health effects
2001	Bacillus anthracis	Undetermined/United States	• Damage to skin, gastrointestinal tract or lungs, depending on route of exposure
			• Flu or rash-type symptoms
2002	Fentanyl	Russia/Moscow	• Confusion, inability to focus
			• Fatal in large doses

Source: Adapted from WHO (2004, p. 35).

cities with anthrax weapons failed to materialize, but Japan performed grisly experiments with biological agents on captured prisoners of war and civilians, and used chemical agents freely in the Manchurian war from 1937 to 1945. In addition, Japanese airplanes dropped various infectious agents, including plague bacteria, on numerous Chinese cities, with reported outbreaks of disease among the civilian population.

Box 8–4 War and the Environment

The first recorded use of a weapon of mass destruction was in Ypres, Belgium in 1915 during World War I. In order to make up for the shortage of explosives, Germany released 180 tonnes of liquid chlorine into the air. The resulting asphyxiation affected 15,000 allied solders—one-third of whom died (WHO 2004).

During World War II it was discovered that chemicals were as toxic to plants as the new nerve gases were to people. These new defoliant herbicides were used as weapons in several conflict areas of Africa and Southeast Asia during the period 1950–1975, sometimes targeted against food crops and sometimes against the forest vegetation that provided concealment (WHO 2004).

A notable example was the extensive spraying of the herbicide Agent Orange by U.S. forces in southern Vietnam during the Vietnam War (1961–1971). Agent Orange contains dioxin—one of the most toxic chemicals known, causing immune, reproductive, developmental, and nervous system damage; endocrine disruption; cancer; altered lipid metabolism; liver damage; birth defects; and skin lesions. Approximately 18 million gallons of Agent Orange were sprayed during the war, the largest dioxin contamination known to date. The environmental impact is still apparent, with elevated dioxin levels found in Vietnamese populations whose diet is fish based (Schecter et al. 2001).

More recently, U.S. and Colombian "war on drugs" programs have sprayed rural Colombian areas with glyphosate in attempts to eradicate coca production (the plant used to produce cocaine). While proponents claim that glyphosate is safe for humans, numerous environmental organizations argue that these sprayings are linked to human and livestock health problems (AIDA 2007).

Public Health Effects of Weapons of Mass Destruction (WMD)

Nuclear weapons directed at civilian or military populations have been used only once: by the United States against Japan in August 1945. The bombs, dropped on Hiroshima and Nagasaki, caused 118,000 deaths and 30,000 wounded in the first year alone, 95% of which were within a 1.3 mile radius of the explosions (Yokoro and Kamada 1997). The bombs caused not only the near complete destruction of the physical infrastructure and human communities of the two cities, but they also generated long-term health effects of radiation and psychological trauma among survivors and those who lost loved ones. Delayed effects included fetal deaths in 1946, elevated rates of leukemia in the 1950s, thyroid cancer in the 1960s, and breast and lung cancer in the 1970s.

Within a few years of the United States' bombings, the Soviets developed nuclear weapons, leading the two Cold War rivals to proliferate tens of thousands of nuclear warheads. Over time the horizontal proliferation of nuclear weapons programs has expanded beyond a core group of states (United States, Russia, the United Kingdom, France, and China) to now include Israel, India, Pakistan, and North Korea.

Control of WMD

Concerns among U.S. leaders about the potential spread of BW programs to non-nuclear weapons states led the Nixon Administration to propose a biological weapons convention (BWC) that called for the elimination of all biological weapons and offensive programs. It was signed in 1975 by 144 countries. However, the BWC allows continued stockpiles of biological agents for "defensive" purposes, such as vaccines and countermeasures. The U.S. government spurned a tentative global accord on a more vigorous BWC in 2001, due to a combination of pressure from the U.S. pharmaceutical industry raising concerns about loss of proprietary information, and U.S. desire to expand its own "biodefense" programs that are in potential violation of the BWC.

Similar concerns about CW, underscored by publicized use of such agents during the Iran–Iraq war of the 1980s, led to the ratification and entry-into-force of the chemical weapons convention (CWC) in 1997, with 175 current signatories. Enforcement of the CWC has been constrained by inadequate funding to carry out necessary inspections. Moreover, technical difficulties and related concerns around the safe destruction of stockpiles led to delayed deadlines for the elimination of the vast and dangerously deteriorating CW arsenals of the United States and Russia.

Most daunting have been global efforts to control and end the dangerous and ever-costly nuclear arms race, which in the United States alone cost over US$4.5 trillion (in 1998 dollars) from 1945 to 1996. The global nuclear weapons infrastructure has left massive amounts of toxic and radioactive waste that, on top of having already poisoned countless workers and communities, threatens public and environmental health for untold generations to come. The Nuclear Non-Proliferation Treaty (NPT) of 1968, currently having all but four nations as signatories, is aimed at curbing the global spread of nuclear weapons. The NPT has at its core an agreement that the nuclear weapons states should move speedily through disarmament toward the elimination of their nuclear weapons stockpiles. Toward this end, the Comprehensive Test Ban Treaty (CTBT), still not ratified by the United States, would end all nuclear weapons testing integral to the development of nuclear weapons. There is renewed attention to creating a Nuclear Weapons Convention that would extend the principles of the CWC and BWC to the nuclear realm, and lead to a renewed, concerted push to eliminate the scourge of all WMDs, given their fundamental threat to humanity.

CASE STUDIES OF CONFLICT AND PUBLIC HEALTH

Key Questions:

- What role can epidemiology play in assessing the impact on health from large-scale acts of violence?
- What are the public health effects of sanctions?

Epidemiology and other approaches in public health can provide valuable tools for eliciting and evaluating the assistance of health actors and agencies during times of crisis. In this section, we review several case studies of human-made crises (sanctions, war, and other forms of conflict), in order to explore how public health responses can aid in the assessment and monitoring of these events.

War in Iraq: The Politics of Epidemiology

Shortly after the Coalition Forces (mainly led by the United States and the United Kingdom) launched the Iraq War in March 2003, epidemiologists from Johns Hopkins Bloomberg School of Public Health and Columbia University School of Public Health undertook a classic household cluster sample survey to assess the impact of the war on civilian mortality compared to the period before the war started (Roberts et al. 2004). Thirty-three clusters of 30 households each were interviewed about births and deaths and about causes and circumstances of violent deaths. They found that the risk of death was 2.5 times greater after the invasion versus during the preinvasion period. After excluding the city of Fallujah, where many violent deaths took place, they estimated that there were approximately 98,000 more deaths (95% confidence interval 8,000–194,000 deaths) than expected after the invasion. Most of the victims of violent deaths were women and children. The risk of violent death was 58 times higher after the invasion than before.

The study showed that even during wartime and difficult circumstances, the collection of valid public health data was possible (albeit with limited precision as the authors noted). It also validated the fear that far more civilians were dying postinvasion than the Coalition Forces acknowledged. In fact, General Tommy Franks in charge of the operation was quoted as saying, "we don't do body counts." It was not clear to independent monitoring bodies how a military force could monitor the extent to which civilians are protected against violence without systematically conducting surveillance of their own.

In 2006 the same epidemiological team repeated their survey using a similar cluster sample survey method. In order to improve the precision of their mortality estimate, and therefore decrease the width of the confidence interval, they increased the sample size to 47 clusters, reaching a total of 1,849 households (Burnham et al. 2006). The researchers also used several techniques to verify the results of their first study, including sampling from similar clusters in the country to compare results, and including the time period from the first study in the second study. The study found that the preinvasion mortality rate was 5.5 per 1,000 per year (95% confidence interval 4.3–7.1), compared to 13.3 per 1,000 per year (95% confidence interval 10.9–16.1) in the 40 months after the invasion of Iraq. They estimated that by the time of the survey in July 2006, over 650,000 excess Iraqi deaths had occurred as a result of the war (92% due to violence). The study produced epidemiologic evidence that Iraqi civilians were dying at a rate more than two times higher than before the coalition invasion in March 2003, and that the coalition forces which were continuing to occupy the country were failing to protect Iraqi civilians. This was in violation of Convention IV, Part III, Section I, Article 27 of the Geneva Conventions, which states that "protected persons shall at all times be humanely treated, and shall be protected especially against all acts of violence or threats thereof and against insults and public curiosity."

9/11 and the Impact on Health

On September 11, 2001, a hijacked plane with 92 passengers and crew crashed into #1 World Trade Center (WTC) in New York City. A second airliner with 65 passengers and crew crashed into #2 WTC 15 minutes later. With help from rescue teams and civilians, thousands were guided to emergency exits, but the buildings quickly collapsed as a result of massive fires. The hijackers crashed a third airliner into the Pentagon in Arlington, Virginia and a fourth plane crashed in a Pennsylvania field after passengers battled the hijackers. In addition to the 19 hijackers, 2,973 people were listed as dead from the 9/11 attacks, with another 24 still missing and presumed dead. This toll includes airline passengers, rescue crewmembers, and people working in the buildings at the time of the attacks. Notwithstanding these deaths, widened stairwells, back-up power, and an emergency evacuation plan were credited with saving thousands of people from the WTC collapse.

The 9/11 attacks caused the single largest loss of civilian life from an act of terrorism. The sudden attack sent the New York City Department of Health (DOH) into an emergency response phase that lasted more than a month. Within days after the attack, priorities shifted to worker-injury surveillance and injury prevention, surveillance for bioterrorism, environmental health concerns due to building collapse and fires, ensuring food and water safety, rodent and vector control, and educating the public regarding the health implications of decomposing human remains and building collapse (Holtz et al. 2003).

The thousands of tons of WTC debris contained high levels of toxins, some known to be carcinogenic (dioxins, cadmium) and damaging to organs and the nervous system. Hundreds of emergency responders have either retired on disability leave or have chronic health problems as a result of their exposure at the scene. The long-term mental health effects on the residents of New York are unknown, but likely include elevated levels of PTSD, depression, and other psychological sequelae (Hoge, Pavlin, and Milliken 2002). A surveillance system has been set up to periodically monitor the mental and health effects of 71,437 people (enrolled in a specific registry) over a period of 20 years (Brackbill et al. 2006).

Sanctions and their Health Effects

Sanctions and embargoes have been used by wealthy, usually Western, nations to impose penalties on countries whose foreign and domestic policies they oppose. It was once believed that embargoes were the "safe" way to punish a country's leadership, but scholarship now shows that embargoes can have serious effects on the health and well-being of the recipient country's population. These effects can be partially modulated by the policies of the recipient country. Cuba, for example, has been under an economic and foreign policy embargo by the United States since the 1960s, which was tightened in 1992 to include even food and medicine (violating UN policy). Data from surveillance systems has shown declining nutritional levels, rising rates of infectious diseases, and increased violent death. The public health infrastructure has also deteriorated due to the sanctions. In the face of these challenges, Cuba instituted a policy that put women and children first for food rations, resulting in stable low mortality rates in those groups (Garfield 2000). Adult men and the elderly have shouldered much of the burden including an epidemic of optic neuropathy.

Economic sanctions and an embargo against Haiti between 1991 and 1994, and against Iraq in the lead-up to the 1991 Gulf War, resulted in very different effects on the population than in Cuba. The results in Haiti were devastating, with a decline in income, rising unemployment, worsened nutrition, a rise in child mortality, and a breakdown in the education system and family cohesion (Gibbons and Garfield 1999). Haitians coped by decreasing their caloric intake, moving in with relatives, selling domestic goods, taking children out of school to work or beg on the streets, and lending children to families as indentured servants. The impacts of the sanctions were felt in Haiti years after they were lifted. Much the same impact was felt in Iraq prior to the Gulf War. Embargo-related shortages of food, and the deterioration of the infrastructure increased child mortality, even after controlling for maternal and child characteristics (Ascherio et al. 1992; Garfield and Daponte 2000). Ultimately, the impact of sanctions was greatest on those least able to bear the burden.

Proxy War in El Salvador

El Salvador suffered a brutal civil conflict from 1980 to 1992, a war largely fueled by the U.S.'s support of an oppressive government. The "scorched earth" policy of the Salvadoran military resulted in the deaths of 80,000 people, and produced one million refugees and innumerable tortured and "disappeared" people in a country of only 6 million people. Massive aerial bombardment and use of napalm caused severe deforestation. The Salvadoran government was responsible for grievous violations of human rights, in place of its duty to protect the citizenry. During the conflict, the health budget was cut in half, and health posts were abandoned. NGO-trained community health workers became the backbone of health care, covering approximately one-third of the country. However, after the Peace Accords were signed in 1992, the Ministry of Health refused to hire them, arguing that they were communists and part of the insurgency. Over 15 years later, the effects of civil war are still felt in the country's health and social infrastructure.

Ongoing Conflict in the Palestinian Occupied Territories

The Palestinian Occupied Territories includes the West Bank, comprised of almost 2.5 million people dispersed over 6000 km², and the Gaza Strip, comprised of almost 1.5 million people concentrated in 365 km² (about twice the size of Washington, DC). The Israeli occupation of Palestine over the last five decades has resulted in the destruction of Palestinians' societal infrastructure and led to higher rates of physical and mental illness due to impeded access to vital health care (Palestinian Central Bureau of Statistics 2007).

A household survey reported that almost 50% of Palestinian households include at least one person suffering from a chronic illness or disability, and that more than two-thirds of Palestinians reported that they are depressed (Near East Consulting 2007). Among Palestinians, children are at even greater risk of depression and post-traumatic stress because of their life-long and generational exposure to the violence and effects of occupation. According to UNICEF, "one in ten children are stunted, one in two are anemic and 75 per cent of children under the age of five suffer from vitamin A deficiency" (UNICEF 2007).

Restrictions on the freedom of movement of Palestinians due to Israeli military checkpoints, closures, and blockades pose severe barriers to medical care. Many villages are cut off from major urban centers and related medical care, and ambulances are regularly stopped and detained at checkpoints resulting in numerous patient deaths including infants during childbirth (Near East Consulting 2007; UNICEF 2007).

Throughout the occupation, there have been issues with maintaining adequate quality and supplies of medicine, equipment, and health workers. Most hospitals experience recurrent drug shortages and diagnostic or life-supporting machines are nonfunctioning due to lack of access to spare parts or incapacity to repair the equipment.

Current political sanctions have also resulted in the government's inability to pay the salaries of workers. The Palestinian Authority employs 57% of all healthcare workers and provides nearly 65% of general health care to the Palestinian population (Palestinian Central Bureau of Statistics 2007). Its inability to maintain basic services, including dispensing medicines and employing health care workers, is having devastating effects: thousands of patients, some of whose lives are in danger, are unable to receive treatment.

Mortality from War in the Democratic Republic of Congo (Also Known as Second Congo War, or African World War)

Until November 1908, when King Léopold II of Belgium was forced to formally relinquish control of the Belgian Congo to the government of Belgium, the king considered the Congo Free State his personal property and ran an economic system based on forced labor. During the ensuing decades of economic and political exploitation, millions of Congolese died mining diamonds or harvesting palm oil for the king's personal estate (Hochschild 1998). It is estimated that during Léopold's rule, the population of the Congo dropped from 40 million to 20 million.

After a brutal struggle, Congo won its independence from Belgium in June 1960, with Patrice Lumumba as the first democratically elected prime minister. Shortly thereafter, Lieutenant-General Mobutu Sese Seko—backed by the United States as a Cold War ally—seized power, assassinated Lumumba, and installed himself as president of the country (then known as Zaire). As one of the world's most infamous dictators, he ruled the country for 32 years, pocketing billions of foreign aid dollars. He was overthrown in 1997 by Joseph Kabila. Since his overthrow, the world's deadliest conflict has been raging in eastern and southern Congo linked to Cold War alliances and factions, with local and international companies fighting over control of lucrative gold, diamonds, and coltan deposits.

Four surveys (including one with 19,500 households in 750 clusters) conducted in the DRC determined that 3.9 million people died due to the conflict between 1998 and 2006 (Roberts 2000; Roberts et al. 2001; Coghlan et al. 2006; International Rescue Committee and Burnet Institute 2007). Through cluster surveys, the International Rescue Committee (IRC) estimated that 1.7 million excess deaths occurred as a result of the fighting, with 34% in children younger than 5-years old. Outbreaks of shigella, cholera, and meningitis were reported by households, with little provision of medical care. In health zones reporting violence, both the CMR and under-5 mortality rate were nearly twice that of the rates in health zones not reporting violence (Table 8–5). The predominant causes of death were infectious diseases such as respiratory infections, diarrhea, and malaria. In addition to the 1.7 million direct deaths, researchers estimated that between 1998 and 2004, 2.2 million people had died indirectly as a result of the conflict and humanitarian crisis (Depoortere and Checchi 2006)

The conflict is now the deadliest since World War II, with a death toll far higher than other recent crises such as Bosnia (96,000 dead), Rwanda (800,000 dead),

Table 8–5 Comparison of Mortality in Violent and Nonviolent Zones in the Democratic Republic of Congo

	Crude Mortality Rate*	Under-5 Mortality Rate*
Health zones reporting violence	3.0	6.4
Health zones not reporting violence	1.7	3.1

* Mortality rates expressed as deaths per 1,000 per month.

Source: Reprinted from Coghlan et al. (2006) with permission from Elsevier.

Kosovo (12,000 dead) (Spiegel and Salama 2000), and Darfur, Sudan (200,000 dead) (Depoortere et al. 2004; U.S. Government Accountability Office 2006). Unfortunately, as in the Bosnian and Rwandan genocides, the international response to Congo's CHE has been abysmal. The need for simple yet life-saving interventions such as the provision of safe water, sanitation, vaccination, and access to effective medical care are not being met. This may be because although the DRC is rich in minerals and resources, it does not hold a place of military importance. Second, the area at war is large and unregulated, with vast tracks of undeveloped land, making it difficult to maintain supply chains. Thirdly, DRC is in Africa, where conflicts have historically attracted less attention on the world stage than have other conflicts in areas that are more accessible and politically strategic.

Role of Epidemiology and Public Health Response

Conflict-related mortality epidemiology has contributed greatly to public health efforts in CHEs. Retrospective mortality surveys demonstrate the deadly public health consequences of war, and have guided policy makers in their responses. Modern tools of epidemiology can also be used to gather data on mortality and human rights abuses in difficult situations. Using surveys, interviews, and Global Positioning System (GPS) locators in Haiti following a state coup, for example, Kolbe and colleagues estimated 8,000 murders and 35,000 sexual assaults occured in the Port-au-Prince area over 22 months. Criminals were the most identified perpetrators, but officers from the Haitian National Police and armed opposition groups accounted for 25% of the crimes (Kolbe and Hutson 2006). The household surveys demonstrated that systemic human rights abuses were rampant in the city, and led to a call for a better response by the UN and world community to address the problem.

REFUGEES AND IDPS: NUMBERS, TYPES, PLACES

Key Questions:

- How have the health needs of refugees and internally displaced persons changed over time?
- What are specific gender-based issues in refugee health settings?
- What dangers do humanitarian aid workers and staff face in the field?
- What role does the military play in providing humanitarian aid?

The United Nations High Commissioner for Refugees (UNHCR) is a UN agency charged with the protection of "persons of concern" (see http://www.unhcr.org). In 2005 there were approximately 19 million "persons of concern" around the world (Table 8–6). This number includes refugees, IDPs, the stateless, and asylum seekers. All told, the total number of people displaced or at risk of becoming displaced

Table 8–6 Total Population of Concern to UNHCR, January 2005

Region	Refugees	Asylum Seekers	Returned Refugees	IDPs of Concern	Others of Concern	Total Population of Concern
Africa	3,023,000	207,000	330,000	1,200,000	100,120	4,860,120
Asia	3,471,000	56,000	1,146,000	1,328,000	899,000	6,900,000
Europe	2,068,000	270,000	19,000	900,000	1,163,000	4,430,000
Latin America and the Caribbean	36,000	8,000	90	2,000,000	26,000	2,070,090
North America	562,000	291,000	—	—	—	853,000
Oceania	76,000	6,000	—	—	140	82,140
Total	9,236,000	838,000	1,495,090	146,000	2,188,260	19,195,350

Source: UNHCR (2006, p. 10).

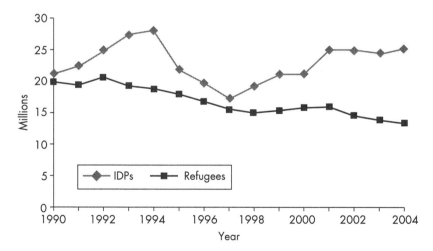

Figure 8–8 Number of IDPs and refugees, 1990–2004.
Source: UNHCR (2006, p. 154).

is estimated to be 30 million. Although there were 33 situations of conflict and protracted refugee exile involving 5.7 million people in 2004, there was a decline in the number of refugee "persons of concern" since the early 1990s (9 million refugees in 2004 vs. 18 million in 1992) (Fig. 8–8) due to fewer armed conflicts and several large repatriations, such as the return home of displaced Guatemalans from Mexico, Liberians from Ghana, and Hutus to Rwanda from DRC. Large-scale displacement camps such as Khao-I-Dang on the Cambodian–Thai border, where hundreds of thousands of displaced persons lived throughout the 1980s with high mortality rates from disease, no longer exist.

As the number of large conflicts has decreased, smaller conflicts are contributing more to refugee/IDP numbers. According to UNHCR, "the dominant trend is one of short-term, short-distance, repetitive dislocation rather than large-scale displacement into camps. It is often extremely difficult to distinguish between displaced and nondisplaced populations, or to differentiate movement as a coping mechanism from movement that is forced" (UNHCR 2006, p. 14). The largest current movement of displaced persons was caused by the protracted Iraq War (and "Coalition of the Willing" occupation) that began in 2003, with large numbers of refugees in Jordan and Syria. There are an estimated 1 million IDPs, with an additional 50,000 persons becoming displaced every month as of late 2008.

A large proportion of UNHCR's "persons of concern" are young people (nearly 50% are under 18 years old, and 13% are under age 5). Children and adolescents are just as (or more) vulnerable to separation from families, sexual exploitation, HIV/AIDS, forced labor, abuse and violence, recruitment into armed groups, trafficking, lack of access to education and basic assistance, and denial of access to asylum or family reunification. The most vulnerable are unaccompanied children, who have been separated from their parents during the process of war or refugee flight. Large reunification centers have been set up in large-scale displacements to reunite children with their families. According to UNCHR's 2003 data, among displaced persons, over one-third were living in camps, 15% were living in urban areas, and half were living dispersed in rural areas (UNHCR 2006).

The start of the 21st century has so far seen a continuation of the armed conflicts of the 1990s, resulting in large movements of peoples in Europe (the Balkans), Africa (Burundi, Rwanda, Somalia), and Asia (Burma, China). In recent years the Darfur region of Sudan has been an area of forced displacement, where violence by armed militias supported by the Sudanese government has driven hundreds of thousands of Sudanese villagers to flee to neighboring Chad (UNHCR 2006). A far greater number face displacement within Sudan itself, where attacks by the government-sponsored militia, known as the *janjaweed*, are a daily threat. The international community has learned little from its slow response to the genocides in the Balkans and Rwanda in the 1990s, and so far the protection offered the Sudanese refugees and IDPs has been minimal.

Environmental Refugees

In recent years there has been a surge in the number of environmental or climate refugees, stemming from the complex interplay among economic forces, human settlement patterns, and ecological change. For example, international demand for timber leads to excess logging and loss of forest cover, increasing flood magnitude along rivers, and provoking dislocation of entire communities from their homes. Christian Aid estimates that 1 billion people will be forced out of their homes over the next 50 years as a result of climate change and exploitation of land, water, and forests, resulting in uninhabitable environmental conditions (Christian Aid 2007).

Human Rights in Refugee Populations

Refugees suffer from high rates of human rights violations. Their vulnerability, created by being displaced from their known surroundings, makes their rights to food, housing, and proper medical care all the more pressing. Threats to the rights of refugees range from abuse in the hands of foreign authorities, theft, assault, domestic violence, child abuse, rape, and human trafficking. These threats can come from the local community itself, or from outside.

Armed groups within refugee flows threaten the population as they divert humanitarian aid from those who need it, often engage in recruitment of young men and boys, and increase armed attacks on refugee populations by opposing forces. However, identifying armed elements in mass influxes is especially difficult given the numbers of people involved. The local population, militants, errant military and police forces, and organized crime can also threaten refugees.

Armed refugees were a catalyst of violence in the Rwandan refugee camps in eastern Congo after the genocide in Rwanda. Hutu militias, known as the *inter-hamwe*, regrouped after their refugee flight into Congo and began to abuse their fellow refugees, who were mainly Tutsi. The resultant conflict in these camps led to the outbreak of fighting within the Congo itself, a protracted struggle that has been going on for nearly a decade and continues through 2008.

Shift from Response to Preparedness

The UN General Assembly declared the 1990s as the International Decade for National Disaster Risk Reduction to highlight the need to decrease vulnerabilities to disaster and increase preparedness and response capacity. Disaster risk reduction (also known as risk management or emergency preparedness) has two components: prevention and preparedness. Prevention refers to actions that reduce the chances of a disaster occurring. For example, aiding farmers to diversify their crops, livestock, and sources of income may prevent a famine from occurring. Preparedness includes activities that reduce the impact of the disaster when it happens (CARE 2001). For example, preparing a disaster plan, building seawalls and levees, and requiring new buildings to be earthquake-proof. Prepositioning food aid before the onset of the hungry season can reduce the impact of a famine. In the flood-prone regions of southern Nepal, CARE works to educate families about how to prepare for the annual monsoon flood waters and ameliorate the destruction of their possessions, crops, and livelihood (CARE Nepal 2007).

Usually, disaster prevention and preparedness are difficult for institutions to plan, fund, and implement because they blur the line between relief and development, sectors that are often siloed within organizations (Benson, Twigg, and Myers 2001). While individual institutions often develop their own protocols, much research and action is driven by regional and country level centers, such as the Coordination Center for National Disaster Prevention in Central America, and the Asian Disaster Preparedness Center. Early warning mechanisms and contingency planning processes provide situation specific preparedness at the national, regional and even local level (UNHCR 2006).

Early warning systems can cover a number of topics designed to prevent humanitarian emergencies. Surveillance systems for famine and hunger typically integrate variable indicators such as rainfall, crop production, and market prices. Systems can also include scenario based planning and mapping of priority zones and vulnerable groups. One of the most prominent early warning systems is FEWS NET (Famine Early Warning Systems Network), which was developed by USAID in the aftermath of the devastating famines in Ethiopia during the 1980s. Other systems for famine related disasters exist at the regional, local, and even organization specific levels. Following the devastating tsunami in 2004, the UN launched the International Early Warning Program to implement early warning for all types of "natural disasters."

Humanitarian Aid Workers

There is increasing recognition that humanitarian aid and relief workers face significant dangers when they enter conflict-stricken environments. Every year dozens of aid workers are intimidated, physically threatened, kidnapped, captured, or killed because they are carrying out their duties "in the line of fire" (Sheik et al. 2000). Sometimes they are specifically targeted because they represent the presence of the international peacekeeping or foreign interventional forces. As they are usually unarmed, aid workers are easy targets. Although humanitarian aid workers in war zones are themselves at risk, their presence can also discourage attacks on the displaced. The threats faced by relief workers have raised compelling questions about the role of security forces and the military in refugee protection.

Humanitarian aid NGOs have traditionally kept their distance from military forces during conflict, and are uneasy about being "strange bedfellows" in certain situations. The U.S. conflicts in Afghanistan and Iraq, with ongoing military intervention and political turmoil, are threatening the perceived neutrality of humanitarian aid workers. Tensions have arisen between human rights organizations (which are at times at odds with local authorities over the latter's alleged violations of international law) and humanitarian organizations that are dependent on cooperation from these same authorities (Rieff 2002).

In addition, humanitarian aid workers may experience some of the same mental health effects as survivors of mass violence in a CHE (WHO 2003). In the late 1990s in Kosovo, up to 14% of aid workers exhibited symptoms of depression and anxiety (Lopes Cardozo et al. 2005). Their colleagues, those who document human rights abuses in the field and collect stories of trauma and abuse, may also be susceptible to vicarious or "second-hand" traumatization (Holtz et al. 2002). These findings point to the need for comprehensive mental health care services for people working in humanitarian aid settings, either short-or long-term.

Politics of Humanitarian Aid

NGOs involved in humanitarian relief and development work have traditionally tried to avoid military relief campaigns, except for cooperation in the face of an acute crisis. There are examples of successful collaborations between humanitarian relief organizations and military relief operations, such as in Kurdistan after the first Gulf War and in Somalia during Operation Restore Hope. Military involvement has been important in past emergencies for security and logistical support to international relief organizations, including the UN, NGOs, and the International Federation of Red Cross and Red Crescent Societies. The lift-transport capacity of military and national guard forces are often the only agencies available to meet the reconnaissance, evacuation, and supply needs of an emergency response. Working with military forces, however, presents moral dilemmas for relief organizations.

In recent years the military forces of developing countries have played an increasing role in disease surveillance; for example Peruvian and Thai military health organizations work in partnership with the U.S. military's laboratory, communication, and epidemiologic resources (Chretien et al. 2007). This presents a conflict of interest between national governments' responsibility to serve and protect citizens and the military's security objectives. Moreover, it justifies the reallocation of health resources to military spending. In a related vein, humanitarian interventions often directly conflict with national security and foreign policy objectives. In these cases, the subordination of health concerns to foreign policy must be challenged head on "to avoid misuse of national authority" (Thieren 2007, p. 218).

In the past, relief organizations have maintained control and leadership over CHE responses by verifying their neutrality. Since the Balkan wars of the 1990s, however, military forces have become increasingly involved in community health and food programs during CHEs. Instead of improving security, however, increased military engagement potentially worsens it by blurring the line between civilian and military populations, eroding trust, and falsely associating relief organizations with military forces (Burkle and Noji 2004).

The U.S. Pentagon, for example, had a misbegotten foray into the aid business in Afghanistan. In 2002, as it launched its bombing campaign in Afghanistan, U.S. warplanes dropped food packages as well. But the food canisters had an almost identical yellow appearance to the cluster bombs that were also being dropped. As a result, an unknown number of persons were maimed or killed. After this was revealed, the Pentagon announced it would no longer drop cluster bombs and food packages in the same areas (CNN 2001; Human Rights Watch 2001).

On April 3, 2003, in an attempt to influence the U.S. President regarding humanitarian aid policies in the Iraq war, InterAction (a coordinating organization for 160 American humanitarian NGOs) issued a statement asserting that U.S. military coordination of relief efforts would undermine the impartiality and neutrality of humanitarian organizations, placing their workers under suspicion of being an arm of the military. Aid workers were already under pressure to provide relief in a society that was not yet adequately policed. However, in April 2003 InterAction was told that the government disaster and response teams would answer to the U.S. military and not to the U.S. State Department. Some of the largest U.S.-based NGOs (CARE, IRC, Save the Children, Mercy Corps, and World Vision) decided to coordinate with the U.S. military, hoping that there would not be too much interference by the military in their activities. European NGOs were also forced to coordinate activities with U.S. and U.K. military command. It marked the first time in history that the U.S. military interfered with civilian relief efforts (Burkle and Noji 2004).

Box 8–5 A Code of Conduct for Humanitarian Relief

The International Red Cross and Red Crescent Movement issued a code of conduct for humanitarian relief missions prior to the start of the current Iraq War. The code states that:

1. The humanitarian mission comes first.
2. Aid is given regardless of the race, creed, or nationality of the recipients and without adverse distinction of any kind. Priorities are calculated on the basis of need alone.
3. Aid will not be used to further a particular political or religious standpoint.
4. We shall endeavor not to act as instruments of government foreign policy.
5. We shall respect culture and custom.
6. We shall attempt to build disaster response on local capacities.
7. Ways shall be found to involve program beneficiaries in the management of relief aid.
8. Relief aid must strive to reduce future vulnerabilities to disaster as well as meeting basic needs.
9. We hold ourselves accountable to both those we seek to assist and those from whom we accept resources.
10. In our information, publicity, and advertising activities, we shall recognize disaster victims as dignified humans, not hopeless objects (Global Development Research Center 2007).

THE POLITICAL ECONOMY OF DISASTERS

The effects of Hurricane Mitch in Central America in 1998 illustrate the connections between political and ecological factors in causing large-scale death and destruction. Central America's vulnerability to hurricane-provoked mudslides has long-standing roots in political-economic domination by the North. Starting in the 19th century, much of the region was turned into profitable, U.S.-owned fruit plantations, stripping the land of indigenous flora. The U.S. military frequently invaded and occupied countries to protect plantations and other investments. For example, in 1954, after Guatemala's elected president Jacobo Arbenz seized U.S.-owned United Fruit Company land and redistributed it to peasants, the CIA orchestrated a coup against Arbenz and forced peasants to remain on overfarmed and deforested land. After the Cuban revolution, the United States continued supporting right-wing Central American dictators to stave off Cuban socialist influences. These dictators and their supporters sought to enrich themselves by pushing peasants off productive land, forcing them to take up residence on hillsides, where they cut down trees in order to be able to farm and overworked the land. In Nicaragua, the long-time dictator Anastasio Somoza himself owned 20% of farm land, while tens of thousands of peasants lived on river banks, which were routinely flooded by storms. The Nicaraguan Sandinistas, who attempted land reform in the 1980s, were driven out by the U.S.-backed Contra war.

In the 1980s and 1990s, structural adjustment programs hollowed out government social programs, depleting funding for evacuations, emergency supplies, vaccines, and secure housing. Public health prevention efforts were slashed, leaving much of the population of Central America exposed to the effects of annual storms. When Hurricane Mitch struck, bare hillsides could not withstand the storms, leading to destructive mudslides. The damage across Central America was devastating: 5,657 were killed and 8,052 went missing in Honduras; 2,863 were killed and 884 went missing in Nicaragua; 258 were killed and 120 went missing in Guatemala. Although not bearing the brunt of the storm, Costa Rica was relatively more prepared and only four people died and four went missing (Disaster Center 2007).

While political factors did not decide the timing or magnitude of Hurricane Mitch (though the intensity could have been linked to global warming, see Chapter 10), they played an instrumental role in determining the scale and extent of human and physical destruction (Cockburn, St. Clair, and Silverstein 1999). Tropical storms take place each year in the Caribbean (like monsoons in Asia). Public authorities can and should prepare for storms through zoning, infrastructure, secure housing, notification, and emergency supplies. Practicing disaster response on a community-wide scale is a key part of any preparedness plan. Indeed, many places, from south Florida to Japan, are usually able to minimize deaths due to preparedness planning.

Politics of Food Aid and Subsidies for Trade/Production

With one-sixth of the world chronically malnourished, one might think that there is a global deficit of food. In fact, nothing could be further from the truth. There is a surplus of food produced every year; however, it does not end up in the bellies of those who need it most. A great deal of food is traded on the world market to the highest bidder, and not necessarily delivered to countries in need. Food aid is also given to countries with food emergencies, although this process is often as much a political decision as a moral one.

Emergency food is distributed for free to food-insecure areas in times of crisis, war, or famine, usually by the World Food Programme (WFP) or by nonprofit organizations, or both. Emergency food aid means the distribution of food or food rations to nutritionally vulnerable groups. Project food aid is donated to support specific activities or projects, and is often related to promoting economic development, agricultural development, or security. These projects are also administered by the WFP or by NGOs (Kripke 2005).

Program food aid, however, is a different form of aid. This is a contribution of food produced in a rich country to the government of a poor country. A substantial proportion of this nonemergency food aid is now being "monetized" (i.e., sold in recipient country markets to generate cash). In 1990, roughly 10% of U.S. food aid was monetized. By 2001, this was up to 60% (Kripke 2005). In effect this means that most program food aid is not being donated as food at all, but rather is converted into cash. Although the cash can be used to fund antihunger projects, the fact is that food that is donated as aid is simply a heavily discounted cash contribution. Most U.S. program food aid is sold to recipient countries through concessional financing or export credit guarantees. The United States is almost the only country to "sell" food aid to recipients in this way (Kripke 2005). The U.S. law that oversees program food aid is known as Public Law 480. Most other countries give program food aid in grant form.

Food production, though owned and operated in the private sector, is heavily (publicly) subsidized in the United States, a source of controversy in many quarters. This system creates opportunities for private interests to benefit from the procurement, packaging, transport, and distribution of food aid. The U.S. government requests bids from a limited list of prequalified companies, and arranges for transport of these commodities on U.S.-flagged ships (U.S. law requires 75% of food aid be handled by U.S.-flagged ships). The bidding process results in expenses that are higher than market costs, and the usual companies that benefit from this process are the "Big 4" food transnationals—Cargill, Louis Dreyfus, Archer Daniels Midland/Farmland, and Kalama Export Company. Furthermore, this arrangement jeopardizes livelihoods of farmers in developing countries by flooding the market, and it does not expand overseas sales for their products (Barrett and Maxwell 2004).

In the 1990s, Guyanese rice producers penetrated an important neighboring market for rice exports in Jamaica, which produces very little rice. Rice exports from Guyana to Jamaica grew from 7,700 tons in 1994 to 57,700 tons in 1997. When U.S. food aid rice began pouring into Jamaica at subsidized prices, the competition forced Guyana to look elsewhere for export markets. Hundreds of small producers faced economic ruin because they could not compete. In effect, Public Law 480 was meant to boost food security and eliminate poverty; but while ending food insecurity in one place, it created it in another.

CONCLUSION

Learning Points:

- The ultimate magnitude of the human cost from deadly ecologic disasters such as hurricanes, tsunamis, and earthquakes depends just as much on human social organization and the political economy of prevention and response efforts as it does on the actual natural events.
- CHEs require a broad range of responses, including security measures, communicable disease prevention, mental health care, nutrition, and ongoing care of illness.
- Militarism drives global military expenditure and causes a great deal of death and suffering both directly and through diverting money from public health. Public health practitioners have a duty to confront militarism and the damage it causes.
- Nuclear weapons and other WMDs pose grave threats to public health, but preventing their use requires concerted social and political action.
- Refugees and IDPs are highly vulnerable to mental and physical trauma and illness. This vulnerability is heightened for women and children.
- The international causes of, and responses to, war and civil conflict are political and politicized, requiring both immediate response as well as critical preventive measures.

Disasters ("natural" or otherwise), CHEs, and war are important causes of morbidity, mortality, and disability worldwide. They affect significant numbers of people annually and have a large economic impact that can persist for years. The international health response to disasters has made tremendous strides over recent decades. Local and international public health agencies, such as PAHO, now regularly conduct preparedness exercises, and run trainings for public health professionals in developed and developing countries about how to handle casualties and deaths due to earthquakes, floods, and hurricanes. Unfortunately there is unlikely to be a reduction in the frequency of disasters in the coming years, so the focus on preparedness is a welcome one. Priority preventive interventions should be based on the models of primary health care and public health, with particular emphasis on health promotion and disease prevention. Women and children should be prioritized even in developed countries.

CHEs are one of the most visible, justified, and supported rationales for international health aid. Their consequences on health can be catastrophic, with high rates of infectious disease and malnutrition claiming more lives than the immediate situation the community is fleeing. The challenge in the coming decade will be how to prevent crises from turning into CHEs and, when this is not possible, how to reduce the long-term impact on health and safety. Organized and prioritized interventions, such as those laid out by the Sphere Standards and IASC Guidelines, may help alleviate suffering, even in the most underdeveloped countries. Bangladesh, a heavily populated and very low-income country lying mostly at sea level, suffers from annual flooding and loss of life and property. A combination of water control efforts, community education programs on how to deal with disasters, and a disaster preparedness plan have reduced the annual number of deaths from floods in this country (International Centre for Diarrhoeal Disease Research Bangladesh and Centre for Health and Population Research 2004).

Yet in many ways, such organized responses indicate a grand failure rather than success. Widespread mortality from ecological disasters as well as CHEs is largely due to poorly funded or nonexistent emergency response budgets in many developing countries, insufficient preparation and infrastructure, and a slow and disorganized response to calls for assistance. The inadequate public infrastructure and near collapse of public health systems in many underdeveloped countries lead to unnecessary loss of life when earthquakes or tsunamis strike. Exactly how many lives are lost, as we have seen in the examples in this chapter, is determined as much by how well government social and health programs have stood up to structural adjustment and to neoliberal globalization as by the magnitude of the actual events.

The disaster wrought by war continues to plague the human race. Refugees and IDPs are in continual need of assistance. Militarism must be fought against with as much vigor as the fight against poverty and disease. The best forms of prevention are those that promote peace building and conflict avoidance (MacQueen and Santa Barbara 2000), and that ensure an adequate social and physical infrastructure through fair and equitable development. This includes the promotion of nuclear disarmament and the destruction of biological and chemical weapons of mass destruction. Military conflicts—even civil wars—are almost always related to international exigencies such as institutional alliances and divisive colonial legacies, or most frequently, to the existence of commodities or land that have enormous value on the international market. In the end, peaceful ways of ending conflicts and preventing future ones will benefit the public health of all.

This is not to say that disasters and CHEs do not demand concerted and immediate attention when they occur, but simply that this should not sidetrack us from engaging in prevention efforts. As the examples in this chapter show, situations of health under crisis do not vary markedly. The international causes of, and responses to, conflict are political and politicized, requiring both immediate response as well as critical preventive measures.

NOTE

1. Refoulement means returning a refugee to a place where his/her life would be in danger, a practice which was forbidden under the 1951 Geneva Convention. This is known as a *jus cogens* (compelling law) in international law in which no exemption is ever permitted.

REFERENCES

AIDA. 2007. Environmental and health impacts. http://www.aida-americas.org/aida. php?page=plancolombia_enviroandhhdamages. Accessed August 8, 2007.

Allwood MA, Bell-Dolan B, and Husain SA. 2002. Children's trauma and adjustment reactions to violent and nonviolent war experiences. *Journal of the American Academy of Child and Adolescent Psychiatry* 41(4):450–457.

Antares Foundation. 2002. *Report of the Second Conference on Stress in Humanitarian Workers*. Amsterdam: Antares/Center for Disease Control.

Arms Control Association. 2007. *The Ottawa Convention at a glance.* http://www. armscontrol.org/factsheets/ottawa. Updated June 2008. Accessed December 29, 2007.

Ascherio A, Chase R, Cote T, Dehaes G, Hoskins E, Laaouej J, et al. 1992. Effect of the Gulf War on infant and child mortality in Iraq. *New England Journal of Medicine* 327(13):931–936.

Ashford M and Huet-Vaughn Y. 1997. The impact of war on women. In Levy BS and Sidel VW, Editors. *War and Public Health.* New York: Oxford University Press.

Barrett CB and Maxwell DG. 2004. *Policy Brief: Recasting Food Aid's Role.* Ithaca, NY: Cornell University.

Benson C, Twigg J, and Myers M. 2001. NGO Initiatives in risk reduction: An overview. *Disasters* 25 (3):199–215.

Bermejo PM. 2006. Preparation and response in case of natural disasters: Cuban programs and experience. *Journal of Public Health Policy* 27(1):13–21.

Betancourt T. 2005. Stressors, supports, and the social ecology of displacement: Psychosocial dimensions of an emergency education program for Chechen adolescents displaced in Ingushetia, Russia. *Culture, Medicine, and Psychiatry* 29(3):309–340.

Betancourt T, Pochan S, and de la Soudiere M. 2006. *Psychosocial Adjustment and Social Reintegration of Child Ex-Soldiers in Sierra Leone—Follow-up Analysis.* New York: International Rescue Committee.

Brackbill RM, Thorpe LE, DiGrande L, Perrin M, Sapp JH, Wu D, et al. 2006. Surveillance for World Trade Center disaster health effects among survivors of collapsed and damaged buildings. *Morbidity and Mortality Weekly Report Surveillance Summary* 55(2):1–18.

Brennan RJ. 2007. Personal communication, October 15.

Brennan RJ and Nandy R. 2001. Complex humanitarian emergencies: A major global health challenge. *Emergency Medicine* 13(2):147–156.

Brennan RJ and Waldman RJ. 2006. The South Asian earthquake six months later—an ongoing crisis. *New England Journal of Medicine* 354(17):1769–1771.

Brooks D. 2005. The storm after the storm. *New York Times*, A:23.

Burkle FM and Noji EK. 2004. Health and politics in the 2003 war with Iraq: Lessons learned. *Lancet* 364(9442):1371–1375.

Burnham G, Lafta R, Doocy S, and Roberts L. 2006. Mortality after the 2003 invasion of Iraq: A cross-sectional cluster sample survey. *Lancet* 368(9545):1421–1428.

CARE. 2001. *Emergency Preparedness Planning Guidelines.* Atlanta: CARE.

CARE Nepal. 2007. *Final Report on DIPECHO on CARE Nepal SAMADHAN Project: Community-based Disaster Risk Management.* Kathmandu: CARE.

Centers for Disease Control and Prevention. 2006a. Assessment of health-related needs after hurricanes Katrina and Rita—Orleans and Jefferson Parishes, New Orleans area, Louisiana, October 17–22, 2005. *Morbidity and Mortality Weekly Report* 55(2):38–41.

———. 2006b. Carbon monoxide poisonings after two major hurricanes—Alabama and Texas, August–October 2005. *Morbidity and Mortality Weekly Report* 55(9):236–239.

———. 2006c. Nutritional and health status of children during a food crisis— Niger, September 17-October 14, 2005. *Morbidity and Mortality Weekly Report* 55(43):1172–1176.

————. 2006d. Public health response to hurricanes Katrina and Rita—United States, 2005. *Morbidity and Mortality Weekly Report* 55(9):229–231.

Chretien J, Blazes DL, Coldren RL, Lewis MD, Gaywee J, Kana K, et al. 2007. The importance of militaries from developing countries in global infectious disease surveillance. *Bulletin of the World Health Organization* 85(3):174–180.

Christian Aid. 2007. *Human Tide: The Real Migration Crisis*. London, UK: Christian Aid.

CNN. 2001. Afghans warned over cluster bombs. http://archives.cnn.com/2001/US/10/29/ret.bomb.warnings/index.html. Updated October 30, 2001. Accessed September 16, 2007.

————. 2005. FEMA chief: Victims bear some responsibility. http://www.cnn.com/2005/WEATHER/09/01/katrina.fema.brown/index.html. Updated September 1, 2005. Accessed October 25, 2007.

Cobey JC and Raymond NA. 2001. Antipersonnel land mines: A vector for human suffering. *Annals of Internal Medicine* 134(5):421–422.

Cockburn A, St. Clair J, and Silverstein K. 1999. The politics of 'natural' disaster: Who made Mitch so bad? *International Journal of Health Services* 29(2):459–462.

Coghlan B, Brennan RJ, Ngoy P, Dofara D, Otto B, Clements M, and Stewart T. 2006. Mortality in the Democratic Republic of Congo: A nationwide survey. *Lancet* 367(9504):44–51.

Connolly MA, Gayer M, Ryan MJ, Salama P, Spiegel P, and Heymann DL. 2004. Communicable diseases in complex emergencies: Impact and challenges. *Lancet* 364(9449):1974–1983.

Coupland RM and Samnegaard HO. 1999. Effect of type and transfer of conventional weapons on civilian injuries: Analysis of prospective data from Red Cross hospitals. *British Medical Journal* 319:410–412.

De Silva H, Hobbs C, and Hanks H. 2001. Conscription of children in armed conflict—a form of child abuse: Study of 19 former child soldiers. *Child Abuse Review* 10(2):125–134.

De Ville de Goyet C. 2004. Epidemics caused by dead bodies: A disaster myth that does not want to die. *Pan American Journal of Public Health* 15(5):297–299.

Deng L. 2002. The Sudan famine of 1998: Unfolding the global dimensions. *Institute of Development Studies Bulletin* 33(4):28–38.

Depoortere E and Checchi F. 2006. Pre-emptive war epidemiology: Lessons from the Democratic Republic of Congo. *Lancet* 367(9504):7–9.

Depoortere E, Checchi F, Broillet F, Gerstl S, Minetti A, Gayraud O, et al. 2004. Violence and mortality in West Darfur, Sudan (2003–2004): Epidemiologic evidence from four surveys. *Lancet* 364(9442):1315–1320.

Disaster Center. 2007. Hurricane Mitch reports. http://www.disastercenter.com/hurricmr.htm. Accessed January 4, 2008.

Dugger C. 2007. Ending famine, simply by ignoring the experts. *New York Times*, December 2, 2007.

Editorial. 2005. Katrina reveals fatal weaknesses in US public health. *Lancet* 366(9489):867.

Feinstein International Center. 2006. *Annual Report 2006*. Boston, MA: Feinstein International Center, Tufts University.

Garfield R. 2000. The public health impact of sanctions: Contrasting responses of Iraq and Cuba. *Middle East Report* 215:16–19.

Garfield R and Daponte BO. 2000. The effect of economic sanctions on the mortality of Iraqi children prior to the 1991 Persian Gulf War. *American Journal of Public Health* 90(4):546–552.

Garfield RM and Neugut AI. 1997. The human consequences of war. In Levy BS and Sidel VW, Editors. *War and Public Health*. New York: Oxford University Press.

Gibbons E and Garfield R. 1999. The impact of economic sanctions on health and human rights in Haiti, 1991–1994. *American Journal of Public Health* 89(10):1499–1504.

Global Development Research Center. 2007. Code of conduct for NGOs in disaster relief. http://www.gdrc.org/ngo/codesofconduct/ifrc-codeconduct.html. Accessed August 15, 2007.

Global Health Watch. 2005. *Global Health Watch 2005–2006: An Alternative World Health Report*. London: Zed Books.

Global Issues. 2007. The arms trade is big business 2007. http://www.globalissues.org/Geopolitics/ArmsTrade/BigBusiness.asp. Updated October 30, 2007. Accessed October 15 2007.

———. 2008. World military spending. http://www.globalissues.org/Geopolitics/ArmsTrade/Spending.asp. Updated March 1, 2008. Accessed January 4, 2008.

Goma Epidemiology Group. 1995. Public health impact of Rwandan refugee crisis: What happened in Goma, Zaire, in July 1994? *Lancet* 345(8946):339–44.

Goodwin GS and Cohn I. 1994. *Child Soldiers: The Role of Children in Armed Conflict*. London: Oxford University Press.

Hartman C and Squires G. 2006. *There is No Such Thing as a Natural Disaster: Race, Class, and Hurricane Katrina*. New York: Routledge Press.

Helzer J, Robins LN, and McEvoy L. 1987. Post-traumatic stress disorder in the general population. Findings of the epidemiologic catchment area survey. *New England Journal of Medicine* 317(26):1630–1634.

Hochschild A. 1998. *King Leopold's Ghost: A Story of Greed, Terror, and Heroism in Colonial Africa*. New York: Houghton Mifflin Books.

Hoge CW, Pavlin JA, and Milliken CS. 2002. Psychological sequelae of September 11. *New England Journal of Medicine* 346(13):443–445.

Holtz TH, Leighton J, Balter S, Weiss D, Blank S, and Weisfuse I. 2003. The public health response to the World Trade Center disaster. In Levy BS and Sidel VW, Editors. *Terrorism and Public Health*. New York: Oxford University Press.

Holtz TH, Salama P, Lopes Cardozo B, and Gotway CA. 2002. Mental health status of human rights workers, Kosovo 2000. *Journal of Traumatic Stress* 15(5):389–395.

Howe P, and Devereux S. 2004. Famine intensity and magnitude scales: A proposal for an instrumental definition of famine. *Disasters* 28(4):353–372.

Human Rights Watch. 2001. Cluster bombs in Afghanistan: A human rights watch backgrounder. http://www.hrw.org/backgrounder/arms/cluster-bck1031.htm. Accessed September 15, 2007.

Inter-Agency Standing Committee. 2007. *IASC Guidelines on Mental Health and Psychosocial Support in Emergency Settings*. Geneva: Inter-Agency Standing Committee.

International Centre for Diarrhoeal Disease Research Bangladesh, and Centre for Health and Population Research. 2004. Documenting effects of the July-August floods of 2004 and ICDDRB's response. *Health and Science Bulletin* 2(3):1–11.

International Rescue Committee, and Burnet Institute. 2007. *Mortality in the Democratic Republic of Congo: An Ongoing Crisis*. New York: International Rescue Committee.

Keller AS, Horn SK, Sopheap S, and Otterman G. 1999. Human rights education for Cambodian health professionals. *Health and Human Rights* 1(3):256–271.

Kessler R, Sonnega A, Bromet E, Hughes M, and Nelson CB. 1995. Posttraumatic stress disorder in the national comorbidity survey. *Archives of General Psychiatry* 52:1048–1060.

Kessler R, Berglund P, Demler O, Jin R, Koretz D, Merikangas KR, Rush J, Walters EE, and Wang PS. 2003. The epidemiology of major depressive disorder: Results from the national co-morbidity survey replication (NCCS-R). *JAMA* 289(23):3095–4105.

Khaw A, Salama P, Burkholder B, and Dondero TJ. 2000. HIV risk and prevention in emergency-affected populations: A review. *Disasters* 24(3):181–197.

Kinzie J, Cheng K, Tsai J, and Riley C. 2006. Traumatized refugee children: The case for individualized diagnosis and treatment. *Journal of Nervous and Mental Disease* 194(7):534–537.

Kohrt BA, Jordans MJ, Tol WA, Speckman RA, Maharjan SM, Worthman CM, Komproe IH. 2008. Comparison of mental health between former child soldiers and children never conscripted by armed groups in Nepal. *JAMA* 300(6):691–702.

Kolbe AR and Hutson RA. 2006. Human rights abuse and other criminal violations in Port-au-Prince, Haiti: A random survey of households. *Lancet* 368(9538):864–873.

Kripke G. 2005. Food aid or hidden dumping? Separating the wheat from chaff. In *Oxfam Briefing Paper*. Oxford: OXFAM.

Krugman P. 2005. A Can't Do Government. *New York Times*, 19, September 2.

Landesman LY. 2005. *Public Health Management of Disasters: The Practice Guide, Second Edition*. Washington, DC: American Public Health Association.

Lautze S, Leaning J, Raven-Roberts A, Kent R, and Mazurana D. 2004. Assistance, protection, and governance networks in complex emergencies. *Lancet* 364(9451):2134–2141.

Leaning J, Briggs SM, and Chen LC. 1999. *Humanitarian Crises: The Medical and Public Health Response*. Cambridge: Harvard University Press.

Levy BS and Sidel VW. 2007. The impact of military activities on civilian populations. In Levy BS and Sidel VW, Editors. *War and Public Health, Second Edition*. New York: Oxford University Press.

Lopes Cardozo B, Holtz TH, Kaiser R, Gotway CA, Ghitis F, Toomey E, and Salama P. 2005. The mental health of expatriate and Kosovar Albanian humanitarian aid workers. *Disasters* 29 (2):152 170.

Lopes Cardozo B, Kaiser R, Gotway CA, and Agani F. 2003. Mental health, social functioning, and feelings of hatred and revenge of Kosovar Albanians one year after the war in Kosovo. *Journal of Traumatic Stress* 16(4):351–360.

Machel G. 1996. *Promotion and Protection of the Rights of Children: Impact of Armed Conflict on Children*. New York: United Nations.

Macksoud MS, Aber JL, Cohn I, Apfel RJ, and Simon B. 1996. Assessing the impact of war on children. In Apfel RJ and Simon B, Editors. *Minefields in their Hearts: The Mental Health of Children in War and Communal Violence*. New Haven, CT: Yale University Press.

MacQueen G and Santa Barbara J. 2000. Conflict and health: Peace building through health initiatives. *British Medical Journal* 321:293–296.

McKay S and Wessells MG. 2004. Post-traumatic stress in former Ugandan child soldiers. *Lancet* 363(9421):1646.

Médecins Sans Frontières. 2006. Niger: What to do next. http://www.doctorswithoutborders.org/publications/reports/2006/niger_2–2006.cfm. Accessed January 12, 2008.

Mollica RF, Caspi-Yavin Y, Bollini P, Truong T, Tor S, and Lavelle J. 1992. The Harvard Trauma Questionnaire: Validating a cross-cultural instrument for measuring torture, trauma, and posttraumatic stress disorder in Indochinese refugees. *Journal of Nervous and Mental Disease* 180(2):111–116.

Mollica RF, Lopes Cardozo B, Osofsky HJ, Raphael B, Ager A, and Salama P. 2004. Mental health in complex emergencies. *Lancet* 364(9450):2058–2067.

Morgan O, Tidball-Binz M, and Van Alphen D. 2006. *Management of Dead Bodies after Disasters: A Field Manual for First Responders*. Washington, DC: Pan American Health Organization.

National Institute of Mental Health. 2002. Mental health and mass violence: Evidence-based early psychological intervention for survivors/victims of mass violence. NIMH publication No. 02–5138. Washington, DC: US Government Printing Office.

Near East Consulting. 2007. Survey of Health in the Occupied Palestinian Territory. In collaboration with the Swiss Development Cooperation in Jerusalem. Berne: Swiss Agency for Development and Cooperation SDC.

Noji EK and Toole MJ . 1997. The historical development of public health responses to disaster. *Disasters* 21(4):366–376.

PAHO. 2007. Reducing vulnerability to disasters: A public health priority. http://www. paho.org/english/dd/ped/PED-about.htm. Accessed October 10, 2007.

Palestinian Central Bureau of Statistics. 2007. Population and demographic statistics. http:// www.pcbs.gov.ps/. Accessed September 10, 2007.

Psychosocial Working Group. 2007. *Psychosocial Intervention in Complex Emergencies: A Conceptual Framework*. Edinburgh, Scotland: Center for International Health Studies Queen Margaret University College.

Reintjes R, Dedushai I, Gjini A, Jorgensen TR, Cotter B, Lieftucht A, et al. 2002. Tuleramia outbreak investigation in Kosovo: Case control and environmental studies. *Emerging Infectious Disease* 8(1):69–73.

Relief Web. 2007. Summary of flash appeal expenditure by agency and country. http:// ocha.unog.ch/fts2/. Accessed July 30, 2007.

Rieff D. 2002. *A Bed for the Night: Humanitarianism in Crisis*. New York: Simon and Schuster.

Roberts L. 2000. *Mortality in Eastern DRC: Results from Five Mortality Surveys*. New York: International Rescue Committee.

Roberts L, Belyakdoumi F, Cobey I, Ondeko R, Despines M, and Keys J. 2001. *Mortality in Eastern Democratic Republic of Congo: Results from 11 Mortality Surveys*. New York: International Rescue Committee.

Roberts L, Lafta R, Garfield R, Khudhairi J, and Burnham G. 2004. Mortality before and after the 2003 invasion of Iraq: Cluster sample survey. *Lancet* 364(9448):1857–1864.

Robins L and Regier D. 1991. *Psychiatric Disorders in America: The Epidemiologic Catchment Area Study*. New York: The Free Press.

Rowland M, Munir A, Durrani N, Noyes H, and Reyburn H. 1999. An outbreak of cutaneous leishmaniasis in an Afghan refugee settlement in north/west Pakistan. *Transactions of the Royal Society of Tropical Medicine and Hygiene* 93(2):133–136.

Sack WH, Him C, and Dickason D. 1999. Twelve-year follow-up study of Khmer youths who suffered massive war trauma as children. *Journal of the American Academy of Child and Adolescent Psychiatry* 38(9):1173–1179.

Salama P and Borrel A. 1998. *Assessment of the Humanitarian Response during the Famine in Ajiep, Southern Sudan*. Dublin: Concern Worldwide.

Salama P, Buzard N, and Spiegel P. 2001. Improving standards in humanitarian response: The sphere project and beyond. *JAMA* 286(5):531–532.

Salama P, Spiegel P, Talley L, and Waldman R. 2004. Lessons learned from complex emergences over past decade. *Lancet* 364(9447):1801–1813.

Schecter A, Dai LC, Päpke O, Prange J, Constable JD, Matsuda M, et al. 2001. Recent dioxin contamination from Agent Orange in residents of a southern Vietnam city. *JAMA* 43(5):435–443.

Sen A. 1999. *Development as Freedom*. London: Oxford University Press.

Share the World's Resources. 2006. Free market famine 2006. http://www.stwr.net/content/ view/1230/37/. Updated October 27, 2006. Accessed January 12, 2008.

Sheik M, Gutierrez MI, Bolton P, Spiegel P, Thieren M, and Burnham G. 2000. Deaths among humanitarian aid workers. *British Medical Journal* 321(7254):166–168.

Simmonds S, Vaughan P, and Gunn W. 1983. *Refugee Community Health Care*. Oxford: Oxford University Press.

Sivard RL. 1991. *World Military and Social Expenditures 1991, Fourteenth Edition*. Washington, DC: World Priorities.

Skon E, Omitoogun W, Perdomo C, and Stalenheim P. 2005. *Stockholm International Peace Research Yearbook 2005*. Stockholm, Sweden: Stockholm International Peace Research Institute.

Spiegel P, Sheik M, Gotway-Crawford C, and Salama P. 2002. Health programmes and policies associated with decreased mortality in displaced persons in post-emergency phase camps: A retrospective study. *Lancet* 360(9349):1927–1934.

Spiegel PB. 2005. Differences in world responses to natural disasters and complex emergencies. *JAMA* 293(15):1915–1918.

Spiegel PB and Salama P. 2000. War and mortality in Kosovo, 1998–99: An epidemiological testimony. *Lancet* 355(9222):2204–2209.

Stockholm International Peace Research Institute. 2006. *Yearbook 2006: Armaments, Disarmament, and International Security*. Stockholm, Sweden: Stockholm International Peace Research Institute.

Stover E, Cobey JC, and Fine J. 1997. The public health effects of land mines: Long-term consequences for civilians. In Levy BS and Sidel VW, Editors. *War and Public Health*. New York: Oxford University Press.

Summerfield D. 2000. War and mental health: A brief overview. *British Medical Journal* 321:232–235.

Swiss S and Giller JE. 1993. Rape as a crime of war: A medical perspective. *JAMA* 270(5):612–615.

Tectonidis M. 2006. Crisis in Niger—outpatient care for severe acute malnutrition. *New England Journal of Medicine* 354(3):224–227.

Telford J and Cosgrave J. 2006. *Joint Evaluation of the International Response to the Indian Ocean Tsunami: Synthesis Report*. London: Tsunami Evaluation Coalition.

Terry F. 2000. The limits and risks of regulation mechanisms for humanitarian action. *Humanitarian Exchange Magazine* (17):20–21.

The Sphere Project. 2004. Humanitarian charter and minimum standards in disaster response. In *The Sphere Project, 2004*. Geneva: The Sphere Project.

Thieren M. 2007. Health and foreign policy in question: The case of humanitarian action. *Bulletin of the World Health Organization* 85(3):218–224.

Toole MJ and Waldman RJ. 1990. Prevention of excess mortality in refugee and displaced populations in developing countries. *JAMA* 263(24):3296–3302.

———. 1997. The public health aspects of complex emergencies and refugee situations. *Annual Review of Public Health* 18:283–312.

UNHCR. 2000. *Protecting Refugees: A Field Guide for NGOs*. Geneva: UNHCR.

———. 2006. *State of the World's Refugees: Human Displacement in the New Millennium*. Geneva: UNHCR.

———. 2007. *2006 Global Trends: Refugees, Asylum-Seekers, Returnees, Internally Displaced Persons*. UNHCR Division of Operational Services. Geneva: UNHCR.

UNICEF. 1996. *State of the World's Children*. New York: Oxford University Press.

———. 1998. *State of the World's Children*. New York: United Nations Childrens Fund.

———. 2005. *State of the World's Children*. New York: United Nations Childrens Fund.

UNICEF. 2007. Occupied Palestinian Territory. http://www.unicef.org/oPt/index.html. Accessed September 10, 2007.

U.S. Department of Commerce Bureau of Industry and Security. 2007. Sweden. http://www.bis.doc.gov/defenseindustrialbaseprograms/osies/exportmarketguides/european/sweden.pdf. Accessed February 7, 2008.

U.S. Department of State. 2003. The world's landmine problem and the U.S. humanitarian demining program: A timeline. Fact sheet. http://www.state.gov/t/pm/rls/fs/22182.htm. Updated July 2, 2003. Accessed December 29, 2007.

U.S. Government Accountability Office. 2006. Darfur Crisis: Death Estimates Demonstrate Severity of Crisis but Their Accuracy and Credibility Could Be Enhanced. Report # GAO-07-24. Washington, DC: U.S. Government Accountability Office.

van Griensven F, Chakkraband ML, Thienkrua W, Pengjuntr W, Lopes Cardozo B, Tantipiwatanaskul P, et al. and Thailand Post-Tsunami Mental Health Study Group. 2006. Mental health problems among adults in tsunami-affected areas in southern Thailand. *JAMA* 296(5):537–548.

Waldman RJ. 2001a. Prioritising health care in complex emergencies. *Lancet* 357(9266):1427–1429.

———. 2001b. Public health in times of war and famine. What can be cone? What should be done? *Journal of the American Medical Association* 286(5):588–590.

WHO. 1997. *Tuberculosis Control in Refugee Situations: An Inter-Agency Manual.* Geneva: WHO.

———. 2003. *Mental Health in Emergencies: Mental and Social Aspects of Health of Populations Exposed to Extreme Stressors.* Geneva: Department of Mental Health and Substance Dependence, WHO.

———. 2004. *Public Health Response to Biological and Chemical Weapons, second Edition.* Geneva: WHO.

Yokoro K and Kamada N. 1997. The public health effects of the use of nuclear weapons. In Levy BS and Sidel VW, Editors. *War and Public Health.* New York: Oxford University Press.

Young H. 1999. Public nutrition in emergencies: An overview of debates, dilemmas and decision-making. *Disasters* 23(4):277–291.

9

Globalization, Trade, Work, and Health

Idris is a 10-year-old boy growing up in Dhaka, Bangladesh. As portrayed in the documentary film "A Kind of Childhood," directed by Tareque and Catherine Masud, Idris works at a garment factory in order to support his family because his blind father is unemployed. When an international nongovernmental organization campaigns against child labor, however, Idris loses his job and the family its income. Local civic organizations, supported through international aid, help Idris and other former child laborers attend school with suspended fees. Because his family still needs money, Idris begins to work as a collector on a three-wheeled minibus, facing the triple perils of treacherous traffic, stress, and contaminated air. When the school schedule changes, he is forced to drop out and transforms his dream of education into one of minibus driver. Idris is involved in a minibus crash, and then faces respiratory problems. As the film progresses, we see Idris age before our eyes; when he becomes ill at the age of 14, he already seems to be an old man (Masud and Masud 2003). As this chapter will illustrate, the factors involved in Idris's plight, including poverty, child labor, and inadequate health, education, and social protections, are all linked to globalization processes and unsafe working conditions.

In recent years the term *globalization* has become omnipresent—used to describe new developments in arenas as diverse as communications and culture, technology, business, travel, and social movements. But what *is* globalization, what makes it new, and how does it affect health? This chapter explores the concept of globalization and outlines its implications for trade, work, and human health and well-being. We begin by discussing definitions of globalization, emphasizing a particular type of globalization called *neoliberal globalization.* Trade in goods, services, people, and capital is a key component of globalization, with the World Trade Organization (WTO) as the standard bearer of neoliberal economic principles and the main regulator of global trade. Then, we focus on the causal pathways that link neoliberal globalization with patterns of illness, death, or injury and provide concrete examples of the negative health impact of neo-liberal globalization. These pathways include trade liberalization, reorganization of labor, debt crisis and structural adjustment, financial liberalization, and environmental damage. The second half of the chapter will discuss work and occupational safety and health, as long-standing issues of primary importance and as problems linked to contemporary globalization processes. We will also discuss the effects that changing work patterns in a globalizing economy are having on worker health, as well as on women and children. The importance of international occupational safety policy and the role of the International Labour Organization (ILO) will be outlined. Following a theme in this book, we conclude with a discussion of existing alternatives to neoliberal globalization that serve to foster human health and well-being.

GLOBALIZATION AND ITS KEY FEATURES

Key Questions:

- What features of contemporary globalization are new?
- What is neoliberal globalization?

Generally speaking, globalization is the process whereby people (and the world writ large) are becoming more interconnected and interdependent via particular political–economic relations that work to compress time (everything is faster), space (geographic boundaries are less defined), and cognition (awareness of the world as a whole) (Labonte and Torgerson 2005). Globalization has been described as "a process of greater integration within the world economy through movements of goods and services, capital, technology, and (to a lesser extent) labor, which lead increasingly to economic decisions being influenced by global conditions" (Jenkins 2004, p. 1). Although societies have traded goods, ideas, and even people throughout human history, it is the speed at which current exchange is taking place, combined with the hegemonic (i.e., dominant and largely unquestioned) ideology underwriting this process, that marks globalization as a distinct historical phenomenon. As we will see, in the arena of international health, there have been globalization "winners" and "losers"; however, it is debatable whether globalization itself is inherently "good" or "bad"—perhaps it is merely a process to be expected in a world connected by telecommunications and rapid international transportation.

Historical Character and Definitions of Neoliberal Globalization

Globalization can be divided into several eras. Comparing the period between 1870 and 1914 to today, the late 19th century had a highly internationalized economy as measured by the sum of exports plus imports as a percentage of gross national product (GNP) (Hirst and Thompson 1996). This "globalization index" fell by the 1960s, then grew rapidly into the 1990s leading to the phenomenon we see today. Likewise, the mobility of capital (the international flow of money) was even higher in the 1890s than in the 1990s (Chernomas and Sepehri 2002). Methods of communication and transportation were also evolving rapidly during the late 19th century, as finance overtook labor in its ability to move across borders easily. In fact, many characteristics of 19th century globalization have persisted. The picture of child glass blowers in an Indiana factory taken by Lewis Hine typifies the working conditions of that era (Fig. 9–1). Yet we still witness similarly appalling working conditions for child workers in much of the world today, as seen in the contemporary photo of a child stone quarry worker in India (Fig. 9–2). In the 19th century, global economic expansion was promoted as the key to progress, shepherded by big businesses, trusts, and investors, especially in Europe and North America. At the same time, colonial domination facilitated the extraction of precious raw materials, exemplified by the exploitative relationship between the Belgian government and central Africa, including abusive treatment of slave holdings in what is now the Democratic Republic of Congo (Hochschild 1998).

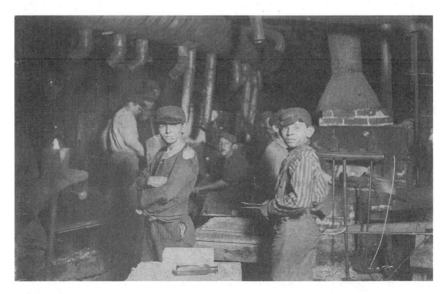

Figure 9–1 Child laborers at Indiana Glass Works, at midnight, 1908. Photograph by Lewis Hine. *Source*: http://www.loc.gov/rr/print/catalog.html.

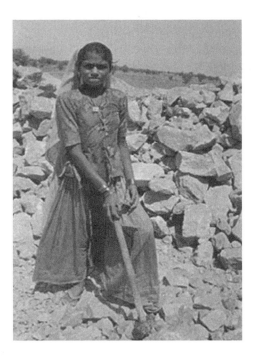

Figure 9–2 Child stone quarry worker, India. Photo courtesy of David Parker.

What are the dominant and increasingly prevalent political–economic relations that drive contemporary globalization? We suggest that they are part and parcel of the approach to economic relations described in greater detail in Chapter 4 as the *neoliberal economic model*. The main tenets of this model are that (a) unfettered free markets bring growth in annual per capita gross domestic product (GDP); (b) growth is synonymous with development; and (c) growth is necessary and sufficient to reduce poverty (Gershman and Irwin 2000). Neoliberal economists also accept that financial crises are an expected norm in between periods of growth, and that the state should do little to interfere. In fact, neoliberalism assumes that the state already plays too large a role in the economy and social policy, and that state interference prevents markets from acting efficiently. According to this view, protecting property rights and enforcing contractual agreements comprise the sole legitimate role of governments.

Neoliberal globalization's key elements are the promotion of "free markets" and the relaxation of trade barriers. In turn, these often result in the following:

- reduction of subsidies for the poor;
- cost recovery/user fees for essential services;
- privatization of public assets;
- weakened role of government;

- growing dominance of western-based transnational capital; and
- high military expenditures.

Defined by these neoliberal terms, the trade that occurs as part of globalization has multiple implications. To a currency trader, it might mean the lightning speed at which multimillion dollar transactions are completed anywhere in the world, at any time of day. To the poor farmer in rural Ethiopia, globalization might mean a new dirt road quickly linking him to the market to sell his crops, but also bringing low-priced competitor crops to town. To a garment factory worker in Honduras, it might mean a low-wage job to pay the rent, but one that lacks adequate safety precautions and the right to organize.

Neoliberal globalization has accelerated the growth of free trade zones in developing countries, "outsourcing" production that previously took place in developed countries. Free trade zones also shift employment patterns within developing countries and exempt multinational employers from laws safeguarding workers and the environment.

Consistent with neoliberal globalization, the political order is dominated by the logic of the market, and the benefits of a "shrinking" world have not been shared equally. In 1969 the World Bank's Pearson Commission on International Development reported that the gap between developed and developing countries would emerge as the central issue of our time. The situation has not improved, leading the United Nations Development Programme (UNDP) to declare at the turn of the century that "global inequalities in income and living standards have reached grotesque proportions" (UNDP 1999, p. 104). How globalization affects the health of people around the world depends on who controls the flow of capital, labor, and knowledge around the world, and who benefits from it. Therefore, power and politics are central to any assessment of the health effects of globalization.

The Global Trade Regime and the WTO

The WTO was formed in 1995 as a supranational trade body (see Chapter 3 for details). Distinct from other multilateral organizations, it includes a dispute resolution body that can impose fines or monetized trade concessions. WTO covers all forms of trade, including intellectual property, services, and goods, as well as environmental regulations because they are construed as barriers to international trade.

The main principles "underpinning all WTO agreements are: *national treatment* (foreign goods, investments or services are treated the same as domestic goods); *most favored nation* (whatever special preferences are given to one trading partner must be given to all WTO member nations); and *least trade restrictive practices* (whatever environmental or social regulations a country adopts domestically must be those that least impede trade)" (Global Health Watch 2005, p. 31).

On the surface, WTO rules may appear to treat all members equally, with the assumption that noninterference wins at the end of the day. However, the underlying motivations and processes of the WTO are more pernicious than meets the eye. With few exceptions, all WTO decisions to date have prioritized economic growth over social policies, and have ruled against labor and child labor rights when they have appeared to be in conflict with competition. Rulings on corporate taxation and the redistribution of corporate profits have been limited. Government procurement has been subject to trade restrictions in several cases, and pension policies have been made available for "open market access." In the end, commercial rights have almost always trumped public interest (e.g., cost-controls on health technologies), and public health policies (e.g., antismoking campaigns) have been deemed in violation of the "free market." In the experience of most low-income nations, free trade agreements grant more rights to investing corporations than to local populations and authorities.

The WTO's Doha Development Round of negotiations, which began in Qatar in 2001, has sought to further lower trade barriers, open markets, and expand intellectual property rights protection. Subsequent meetings in Cancun (2003) and Hong Kong (2005) stalled due to disagreements between developed nations (the United States, the European Union, and Japan) and developing countries (led by India, Brazil, South Africa, and China).

According to proponents of globalization, its effects on health are as follows: (a) economic integration and globalization raises incomes in poor countries; (b) assuming that the health of the poor improves as incomes rise, globalization improves the health of the poor; (c) despite certain negative consequences of economic integration on health, these problems can be addressed through health care and behavior change policies rather than through policies that regulate economic integration; and (d) despite the obstacles to access to medicines posed by intellectual property rights, these can be addressed through dual intellectual property rights regimes (one for rich countries and one for poor countries) (Dollar 2001). In the same vein, Richard Feacham (first executive director of the Global Fund to Fight AIDS, Tuberculosis and Malaria) argues that globalization increases the incomes of the poor, and that this overshadows any ill effects of rapid change. He asserts further that social and political benefits will accrue to poor and oppressed people who embrace the principles of economic integration (Feacham 2001). As yet, this promise is unrealized.

To the contrary, neoliberal globalization has been shown to negatively affect the economies of most poorer countries, in turn jeopardizing health. First, from 1980 to 2000, a period of rapid neoliberal globalization, economic growth was considerably slower than between 1960 and 1980 for countries at almost every level of GDP/ capita. Among the world's 17 poorest countries, the rate of growth from 1960 to 1980 was a healthy 1.9%, and the real per capita GDP was US$1,100 in 1980. During neoliberal globalization's surge between 1980 and 2000, involving economic integration and the imposition of loan conditionalities, among other measures, these same countries experienced net negative growth, and a lowering of the real per capita GDP

(Weisbrot et al. 2002). The slowdown in the rate of economic growth for most low- and middle-income countries over the past 25 years has been responsible for stalled health indicators in many settings, including a decrease in life expectancy progress, and stagnation or worsening of infant and child mortality rates (Weisbrot, Baker, and Rosnick 2006). Still, in recent years, the surge in global economic activity, especially trade in commodities, has led economic performance in some countries to improve. For example, in sub-Saharan Africa, *including* the oil exporting nations (Chad, Angola, Sudan, Nigeria, Gabon), economies grew at 5.6% per year between 1996 and 2003 (Biggeri 2007; United Nations Economic Commission for Africa 2008). But, as witnessed in late 2008, commodity-based growth is not sustainable over the long run.

Second, although globalization's advocates argue that increased trade and foreign investment leads to increased wealth and sustained investment in social services such as health care, sanitation, and education, in reality wealth has not been equitably distributed across populations. Indeed, most countries have experienced a marked deterioration in public social services over the past three decades. Vast numbers of people engaged in the global economy are no better off than they were in 1973 when the gold standard was abolished. The premise that liberalized trade, a key component of neoliberal globalization, levels the playing field for all does not stand up to scrutiny. As discussed in Chapter 4, when one excludes China the proportion of the world's people living on less than US$1/day as well as on less than US$2/day has changed very little since 1990.

Opponents of neoliberal globalization (such as many unions, small farmers, and social activists) decry globalization as an undemocratic process, with an unelected international authority—the WTO—favoring transnational corporations over national governments and human life. They point out that WTO rules have resulted in enormous losses to local industries and jobs (Shaffer et al. 2005).

Furthermore, countries held up as globalization success stories, such as India, Malaysia, and Thailand, began with more closed economies than the countries, mainly in sub-Saharan Africa, whose economic growth has stalled or declined (Dollar 2001). High performing "globalizers" such as South Korea, Taiwan, and Singapore, experienced much of their poverty-reducing growth before they began to open up their economies, reduce their import tariffs, and invite foreign investment. Their more recent but larger counterparts, namely India and China, have also grown despite import protection measures and strict controls over banking and investment.

According to development expert and former World Bank executive Nancy Birdsall, "globalization, as we know it today, is fundamentally asymmetric. In its benefits and its risks, it works less well for the currently poor countries and for poor households within developing countries" (Birdsall 2006, p. 1). In countries whose governments have been longtime adherents to the neoliberal model, for example in Central America and sub-Saharan Africa, poverty and inequality have increased, with consequent negative health effects, particularly on rural populations, the marginalized, women, and ethnic minorities. As a telling indicator, sub-Saharan Africa, home to roughly 12% of the world's population, only captures 1.5% of the world's share of trade (and exports are concentrated in a narrow range of commodities such as fuel) (Biggeri 2007).

While empirical research investigating globalization's direct health effects is difficult to conduct, most evidence suggests that the negative effects outweigh the positive for the vast majority of the world's population (Labonte and Torgerson 2005). Given the mixed effects of increased global trade, there needs to be greater democracy in its governance and far more equitable distribution of its benefits.

Because neoliberal globalization goes hand in hand with international trade rules that protect employers and owners from regulations, in recent years there has been a rise in the incidence of occupational health and safety problems and an increase in the number of workers exposed to potentially hazardous chemicals such as pesticides. There are other health problems linked to globalization, past and present. As discussed in Chapter 2, the spread of ailments such as bubonic plague, syphilis, and cholera was historically associated with increased trade, travel, and growing (and unsanitary) towns and cities. More recently, economic patterns associated with neoliberal globalization, such as migrant labor, rapid industrialization, travel, and urbanization (with inadequate housing, sanitation, etc.) have facilitated the emergence, or perpetuated the spread, of infectious diseases (e.g., SARS, HIV, TB). The global diffusion of political, social, and cultural conditions also underpins patterns of health and disease, including mental illness, diabetes, and stress-related ailments among others. To better understand how these complex relationships take place, and how globalization affects health, we present some key definitions in Table 9–1.

Table 9–1 Key Definitions Relating to Globalization, Trade, and Work

Free trade zones/ export processing zones	Areas of a country where tariffs and quotas are eliminated and regulations and labor protections are lowered in hopes of attracting new business and foreign direct investment. Most free trade zones are labor intensive manufacturing centers that involve the import of raw materials and the export of factory products.
Deregulation	Reduction of the role of the state in goods, services, and labor market.
Informal sector	Work carried out outside the official legal and social institutions of society.
Multinational and transnational corporations	Enterprises that own, manage, or oversee production and deliver goods and services in at least two countries.
Capital	Owners, investors, and financial and physical resources.
Labor	Work—or workers—and the sum total of the goods and services they produce.
Gross National Product (GNP)	A measure of national income and output that estimates the value of all goods and services produced in an economy. GNP includes personal and governmental expenditures, private domestic investment, exports minus imports, as well as net income from assets abroad. Gross domestic product (GDP), by contrast, does not include income from abroad, which for some countries can be substantial.

(continued)

Table 9-1 Continued

Protectionism	An economic policy of restraining trade between nations through tariffs on imported goods, restrictive quotas, and other governmental regulations that discourage imports.
Free trade	A market model in which trade in goods and services between and within countries flow unhindered by government-imposed restrictions. In reality, most "free trade" is not truly free, as the government creates regulations and loopholes that favor large enterprises at the expense of smaller businesses.
Currency devaluation	A reduction in the value of a currency with respect to other monetary units, as opposed to inflation, which implies a reduction in the value of a currency in terms of ability to obtain goods and services.
Foreign exchange market	A market that exists when one currency is traded for another by large banks, central banks, currency speculators, transnational corporations, governments, and other financial institutions.
Foreign direct investment	Investment made to acquire lasting interest in enterprises operating outside of the home country economy of the investor.
Liberalization	Policy that allows prices to be determined by market forces, including exchange rates, interest rates, real wages; lifts barriers to trade and investment such as tariff and non tariff barriers; "opens" economies; reduces the subsidies that keep the prices of some essential goods artificially low so that the "price is right," and reflects the actual value of the good in the market.
Subsidiary/foreign affiliate	A business entity that is controlled by another—often foreign—entity.
Privatization	Selling of government assets and state-owned enterprises.
Progressive taxation	A rate of taxation in which the effective tax rate increases as the amount to which the rate is applied increases. With regard to income taxes, people with a higher income would pay a higher percentage of that income in taxes.
Tariffs and duties	A tax on foreign goods upon importation. Tariffs can be a set amount or a percent of the total value of imports, or be set according to weight or volume.
Foreign reserves	The foreign currency deposits held by central banks and monetary authorities to safeguard against recession.
Subsidies	Governmental financial assistance, usually in the form of grants, tax breaks, or trade barriers, in order to encourage the production or purchase of goods.

HEALTH EFFECTS OF GLOBALIZATION

Key Questions:

- What are the major pathways through which globalization affects health?
- What would happen to health if the WTO did not exist?
- Which WTO Agreement has the greatest implications for public health?
- What are the positive and negative health effects of transnational corporate business activity in developing countries?
- What measures could make free trade zones safer, healthier places to work?

The causal pathways that link globalization with illness, death, or injury may be indirect, involving intervening variables and multiple determinants. Nonetheless, the connections are real and the influence on health is experienced in a comprehensive way. As discussed in Chapters 4 and 7, health is profoundly shaped by national and international economic and political factors—interacting with community level and individual conditions—that have long-lasting repercussions.

Pathways

Globalization influences health and generates health inequities through five major pathways (Labonte and Schrecker 2007) (Fig. 9–3):

1. Trade liberalization and the world trade regime (i.e., the WTO);
2. Global reorganization of production and labor markets;
3. Debt crisis and structural adjustment of developing country economies;
4. Environmental damage; and
5. Financial liberalization.

Trade liberalization changes employment patterns in a variety of ways. Some farmers are pushed out by agri-business, other workers are deindustrialized (i.e., lose factory jobs and must move to service sector jobs), while still others are industrialized and subjected to a system of social stratification that heightens exposure and susceptibility to disease. Trade liberalization disproportionately affects agricultural workers and small-scale entrepreneurs who have no safety net, women, and children. Jobs for these workers are usually in the informal economy and thus poorly regulated. At the same time, greater labor mobility of professionals (including health workers) has led to emigration from developing countries of needed professionals.

The global reorganization of production and labor markets has resulted in the exportation of jobs and entire industries to areas where regulation is lax. This has contributed to a "race to the bottom," in which jobs are lost from industrialized countries (leading to unemployment, stress, and poor health outcomes) and are relocated to poor countries where wages are inadequate and labor organizing is suppressed. Lastly, as commodification (i.e., the process of turning once nonmarketable or public goods, such as water, into market commodities) intensifies under neoliberalism, the environment has suffered. Under the pressures of neoliberal globalization, environmental regulation is unenforced or nonexistent in many locations. In this chapter we focus mostly on trade and labor aspects, whereas Chapter 10 elaborates on environmental health concerns.

Due to the debt crisis and the imposition of structural adjustment policies on many economies of the developing world, the ability of governments to invest in public health, education, water and sanitation, nutrition, and neighborhood improvement has been constrained. High debt-servicing payments limit public provision of

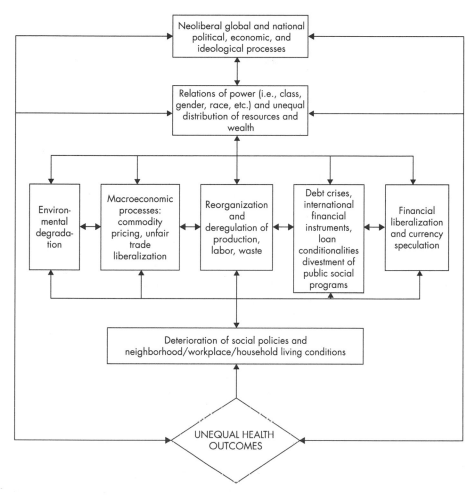

Figure 9–3 Pathways of neoliberal globalization and effects on health. *Source*: Adapted from Labonte and Schrecker (2007, p. 5).

these social goods, while loan conditionalities have stipulated decreased food subsidies, reduced state investment in social programs, and decreased public sector incomes, disproportionately affecting poor women and marginalized communities as a whole.

In turn, financial liberalization exposes national economies to the uncertainties created by large and volatile capital flows and intensifies the effects of inequality on the social determinants of health, as discussed in Chapter 7. The nearly US$2 trillion in daily currency transactions (which have soared since the mid-1980s) have caused enormous instability in many countries, with sudden currency devaluations evaporating purchasing power and undermining the livelihoods of hundreds of millions of people.

Trade Liberalization, the World Trade Regime, and Transnational Corporations

Health concerns resulting from changing patterns of trade and the global economy are slowly entering the debate about globalization and its benefits. Trade affects the determinants of health and disease in a variety of ways (Smith 2006). The increased fluidity of global production has facilitated the transfer of obsolete production technologies to poorer countries, posing hazards to both the newly unprotected employed population and to the overall population. Labor market "flexibility," as seen in export processing zones (EPZs), is often a pretense for minimal regulation, antiunion legislation, and unsafe working conditions (Brown 2005).

The increased movement of people and goods can lead to increased exposure to infectious diseases through rapid cross-border contamination, disruption of animal habitats through rapid urban growth (thus increasing exposure to diseases with animal hosts such as occurred with SARS), and unregulated food production and markets (as in the case of avian flu). Trade can also raise the probability of developing chronic diseases through the marketing of unhealthy products such as tobacco or alcohol, through the promotion of unhealthy behaviors, such as the consumption of trans-saturated fatty acids in fast food, and through increased environmental degradation. Trade can affect health by reducing the provision and distribution of health-related goods, services, and personnel. For example, extended patent protection may lead to decreased access to medical technologies, and trade treaties may restrict national governments from investing in or regulating health care. Lastly, relaxed trade rules can also result in the importation of insufficiently regulated or contaminated goods.

Health Implications of WTO Agreements

Several WTO agreements directly influence the health of the poor (see Table 9–2) (Labonte and Sanger 2006a, 2006b). Most prominent is the Agreement on Trade-Related Intellectual Property Rights (TRIPS), which protects patented pharmaceuticals, processes, and medical technologies (among other forms of intellectual property). Enacted in January 1995 (with a compliance deadline of 2000 for most developing countries), TRIPS stipulates that all WTO member states must abide by patents covering medicines and other technologies, wherever they are issued, for a minimum period of 20 years. This means that, within the period of patent protection, a pharmaceutical manufacturer can only produce patented drugs and technologies with a license (usually *very* costly) from the patent holder.

This regulation hurts the producers of generic medications in developing countries and the millions of people who cannot afford to purchase patented drugs, especially in settings with no domestic pharmaceutical production. The high prices charged by large pharmaceutical companies based in wealthy countries (Big Pharma—see Chapters 3 and 12), which are protected by TRIPS, drastically limit the availability of life-saving generic ARVs to millions of people with HIV/AIDS. The U.S. bilateral policy on patents, influenced by Big Pharma's quest to stave off generic competition, has pursued a similar or even more stringent policy through its own trade treaties (so-called "TRIPS-plus" provisions), such as the Central America Free Trade Agreement (CAFTA) and free trade agreements with Australia and Chile.

In 2001, opponents of the Doha Development Round charged that proposed new rules were bad for development and interfered with domestic policies—including access to generic drugs—that protect local economies. After intense lobbying, the Doha Declaration conceded that TRIPS should be implemented in a manner that supports the right of countries "to protect public health and, in particular, to promote access to medicines for all" (WTO 2001, p. 1) in times of emergency. The Declaration openly states: "we agree that the TRIPS agreement does not and should not prevent members from taking measures to protect public health" (ibid). Countries that declare public health emergencies can overcome patent barriers by granting compulsory licenses (for production of generic medicines), or through parallel imports of medicines if they do not have manufacturing capacity. The Doha Declaration also extended the deadline for TRIPS compliance for the 30 least developed countries until 2016. However, countries without manufacturing capacity are unable to grant compulsory licenses to improve access to medicines. A 2003 WTO ruling was supposed to ease the problems with parallel importing, but the process is so arcane that it has yet to be used as of mid-2008.

Several countries have used the "flexibilities" of the TRIPS Agreement to challenge the high cost of patent-protected drugs. Zimbabwe's government declared a national emergency in 2002, and issued compulsory licenses for import or local production of ARVs, leading to price reductions of 60% to over 90%. Mozambique followed suit (Mabika and Makombe 2006). Brazil, India (see ahead), Kenya, South Africa, and Thailand have also employed these provisions.

Yet TRIPS remains highly prejudicial against developing countries and all people of limited means. In providing unprecedented protection to large corporate pharmaceutical patent owners, TRIPS inhibits generic drug production. Generics help lower drug costs and ensure a constant and sufficient supply of medicines. As TRIPS blocks large producers of generics (Mexico, Brazil, India), the world's generic drug supply will be reduced or even disappear, jeopardizing the health of millions. In sum, TRIPS—like other WTO measures—enables profits to be prioritized over human well-being (Forman 2006).

Another WTO agreement, the Agreement on Sanitary and Phytosanitary Measures (SPS), allows each country to set its own standards for food and drug safety regulations but requires them to be based on a scientific risk assessment without discriminating between domestic and imported food products. For example, Canada, the United States, and Brazil launched a WTO dispute to compel the EU to permit imports of hormone-treated beef despite EU prohibitions on this product. The EU lost, but its member countries still do not allow these imports and must pay millions of euros per year in trade sanctions (Global Health Watch 2005). In effect, the SPS places free trade above human health and safety.

Table 9–2 Trade Treaties and Their Influence on Health

Agreement	Health Effects from Loss of Domestic Regulatory Space
Agreement on Trade-Related Intellectual Property Rights (TRIPS)	Extended patent protection limits access to essential medicines. Higher resulting cost of drugs drains money from PHC and other determinants of health.
Agreement on Sanitary and Phytosanitary Measures (SPS)	Requires scientific risk assessments even though foreign goods cannot be treated differently from domestic goods (i.e., there is no discrimination). Such assessments are costly and imperfect.
Technical Barriers to Trade Agreements (TBT)	Requires that any regulatory barrier to the free flow of goods be as "least trade restrictive as possible." Many trade disputes over domestic health and safety regulations have invoked this agreement.
Agreement on Trade Related Investment Measures	Prohibits governmental abilities to place domestic purchase requirements on foreign investment; such requirements can increase domestic employment, which can be important to improving population health.
Agreement on Government Procurement	Limits governmental abilities to use contracts or purchases for domestic economic development, regional equity, employment equity, or other social goals, all strongly linked to better population health.
Agreement on Agriculture	Allows continuation of export and producer subsidies by the United States, the EU, Japan, and Canada, which depress world prices, costing developing countries hundreds of millions of dollars in lost revenue that could fund PHC, education, and other health-promoting services. Subsidized food imports from wealthy countries undermine domestic growers' livelihoods. Market barriers to food products from developing countries persist and deny poorer countries trade-related earnings.
General Agreement on Trade in Services (GATS)	Locks in privatization levels in committed service sectors, several of which (health care, education, environmental services) are important in promoting public health, and are frequently prone to market failure (i.e., private provision often reduces access to services by poorer families and groups). Once a service sector is committed, there is no cost-free way to extend public provision of that service in the future.

Source: Adapted, with permission, from Labonte and Sanger (2006a).

Box 9–1 The Precautionary Principle and the WTO

A notable example of the WTO's conflict with public health principles has to do with the EU's concern over the agricultural use of genetically modified organisms (GMOs). Since the 1970s, the environmental health field has made growing use of the "precautionary principle" which calls on policymakers to take "preventive, anticipatory measures...when an activity raises threats of harm to the environment, wildlife, or human health, even if some cause-and-effect relationships are not fully established" (Smith 2000, p. 263) (see Chapter 10 for details). Invoking the precautionary principle and the need to protect health and the environment, the EU (and various European countries) banned the import of genetically modified foods in the early 1990s, arguing that they have not been proven safe. In contrast, the United States holds that in the absence of scientific evidence based on

(*continued*)

Box 9–1 Continued

"risk assessment" proving that GMOs harm human health, any limit on importing GMOs constitutes an unfair trade barrier.

In 2003 the U.S. government (with the support of Canada, Argentina, and other countries) brought the issue before the WTO, charging that the EU's use of the precautionary principle was inhibiting free trade and harming domestic farmers. In 2006, the WTO determined that the EU's 2003 prohibition on the import of GMOs created an unnecessary obstacle to international trade. As such, the EU has authorized traces of GMOs in its food imports for animal feed, but has not retracted its own ban on GMOs for human consumption. The EU maintains facilities across Europe that test imported products for traces of GMOs, particularly those intended for human consumption.

Despite the WTO's decision, in addition to the EU, various countries, including Japan, Mexico, and Venezuela, have moved to ban GMOs in the face of scientific uncertainty (and despite the possibility of generating trade disputes). Although the United States (by far the biggest GMO proponent and exporter) argues that banning GMOs hinders global efforts to address starvation and malnutrition, numerous developing countries facing problems with food insecurity (Malawi, Mozambique, Zambia, and Zimbabwe) have also moved to ban GMOs of their own accord (EurActiv.com 2007; Gaines and Palmer 2005).

The Technical Barriers to Trade Agreement (TBT) stipulates that all "like products" be treated alike, that all domestic regulations be "least trade restrictive," and that international standards be exceeded only if "justified on specific health grounds." Canada used the TBT to charge France's ban on asbestos products as being discriminatory since asbestos is a "like product" to glass fiber insulation (Global Health Watch 2005). Canada lost, in the only example to date of a WTO decision favoring health over trade.

The General Agreement on Trade in Services (GATS) is the most insidious of all WTO agreements. The agreement encourages private investment and deregulation of a wide spectrum of services. GATS in itself does not drive privatization, but it locks in existing levels of private provision of services, and indirectly creates incentives for foreign investors to lobby for privatization. GATS treats human services that are key social determinants of health as commodities subject to trade rules (Shaffer et al. 2005). This includes the opening to commercialization of health care and health insurance markets, the education sector, and even water and sanitation services. Any state subsidies for public services, including care for the poor, can be challenged by other countries and potentially barred. Moreover, services such as water, sanitation, and education can be (and have been) sold to the lowest bidder, resulting in increased costs and reduced coverage to those in need. Privatization of water has resulted in deleterious health outcomes in numerous communities and is a violation of health and human rights (WHO 2003).

Box 9–2 Water Privatization

The privatization of water rights in Latin America is an illustrative example of the effect of GATS on health. In an effort to remain in good standing with the World Bank, in 1997 the Bolivian government privatized water management (and other public enterprises) to foreign investors (including

(*continued*)

Box 9–2 Continued

the large U.S. transnational Bechtel). As the cost of access to water increased, eventually costing the equivalent of 6 months' earnings at minimum wage, consumers rebelled. A variety of citizens groups began to organize and protest the policy (Watson 2003). In 1999 the government was forced to terminate the contracts with foreign investors, leading Bechtel and other private water contractors to bring a law suit for breach of contract and violation of their trade rights (they did not win). Bechtel continues to be active in the privatization of water throughout the continent. In Guayaquil, Ecuador, residents organized against Bechtel in 2008 for cutting off water services to people who could not afford to pay, for dumping raw sewage into rivers, and for providing residents with contaminated water. A hepatitis A outbreak in 2005 that affected hundreds of residents was likely due to these practices (Food and Water Watch 2007).

These trade agreements include rules for dispute resolution between governments on matters of trade. At the WTO, trade charges must be brought by national governments, and undergo an internal panel ruling, endorsement or rejection by the WTO membership, and, under some circumstances, may be appealed. Ultimately, however, WTO decisions are binding, inflicting particular hardship on low-income countries. Bilateral and regional agreements, such as the North American Free Trade Agreement (NAFTA) among the United States, Canada, and Mexico, also use a dispute resolution mechanism. Under NAFTA's Chapter 11, governments are barred from maintaining policies that could lower the value of investors' property without compensation. NAFTA also confers standing before a trade tribunal to private investors, enabling them (rather than only national governments) to sue for compensation. This means that corporations have "investor's rights" and can bring enforcement claims directly against governments.

Transnational Corporations, Trade, and Health

A transnational corporation (TNC) is an economic entity—a business—that operates in two or more countries. It may be small or large in financial scale. It can operate any kind of business; examples include manufacturing, raw material extraction, agriculture, power generation, and services such as health care and insurance. The organizational structure of a TNC can vary greatly, ranging from a single company to a tightly or loosely knit set of companies bound by legal and financial ties. There may be various levels of authority or control, but ultimately the control of the TNC rests with its corporate executives and its shareholders. There are an estimated 35,000 TNCs operating globally, with 147,000 affiliates. The 500 largest corporations account for 70% of world trade alone.

TNCs assert that they advance economic development, which directly helps protect economic and social rights for the majority of a country's population, and indirectly promotes civil and political rights (Meyer 1996). TNCs also argue that they provide jobs and that their products can make life easier and more comfortable for those who can afford them. For example, corporate research and development contribute to technological advancements in diagnostic and medical treatments.

TNCs also maintain that the taxes they pay can help fund social programs, even though tax evasion is a major challenge in underdeveloped countries.

Although the benefits of TNC activities may be argued in terms of jobs or advancements in technology, medicine, and consumer products, it is imperative to analyze and act on the potential harmful impacts that TNC operations, including the political and financial systems that enable them, have on the environment and on the health and human rights of people worldwide.

TNCs benefit greatly from the new global trade rules, especially from GATS. Although there are some socially responsible TNCs, a large proportion of them are interested in taking advantage of free trade privileges, wages as low as 10 cents per hour, a near absence of unions, and the disinterest or corruption of unstable governments.

Box 9–3 Transnationals, the WTO, and Infant Formula: A Case Study of Unethical Practices

It is widely acknowledged that breast feeding is key to preventing diarrhea, respiratory infections, and infant mortality in developed and developing countries alike. WHO estimates that 1.5 million infants die each year because their mothers are encouraged to replace breast feeding with artificial breast-milk substitutes. The major cause of death in these infants is diarrhea, resulting from formula being mixed with contaminated water (there is often no other option). Formula can potentially be dangerous (if contaminated water is used) and expensive (because of the cost of fuel and the product itself). The current estimate is that only 45% of infants in the developing world (even less in the developed world) are breast-fed, as mothers are up against a constant barrage of ads promoting the benefits of infant formula.

During the 1960s, declining birthrates in the West led infant formula manufacturers to seek new markets for their products. Marketers dressed as nurses handed out free samples of formula to women giving birth in hospitals, encouraging them, during this most vulnerable time, to use formula instead of breast feeding. Several corporations were found responsible for promoting this practice, with Nestlé the most aggressive marketer. By the mid-1970s, health workers began seeing enormous growth in formula use in the developing world. A worldwide campaign against these unethical practices led to the 1981 World Health Assembly/UNICEF adoption of the International Code of Marketing of Breast-Milk Substitutes (only the United States opposed it until 1994) (WHO 1981). Although infant formula manufacturers temporarily stopped their most aggressive marketing practices, the International Baby Food Action Network has documented scores of examples from around the world that demonstrate that Nestlé and other TNCs continue to market infant formula with impunity in spite of the ban. The code is nonbinding, however, and, unlike WTO rules, is systematically ignored. International boycotts have intermittently put pressure on the infant formula manufacturers, but infant formula is a US$8 billion annual business.

The fight to safely promote breast feeding in Guatemala is a case in point. In an attempt to reduce its infant mortality rate, Guatemala passed a law in the 1980s to implement key elements of the WHO/UNICEF marketing code, which included prohibitions on the use of the words "humanized breast milk" and "equivalent to breast milk" as well as a ban on visual depictions of fat, healthy infants that promoted the use of bottle-feeding (Government of Guatemala 1983). The law also prohibited the free distribution of samples and the direct marketing of the product by sales personnel. All of the companies marketing formula in Guatemala abided by the new law, which resulted in a significant drop in the infant mortality rate, except one—U.S.-incorporated Gerber Products Company. Gerber continued to market its formula to new mothers, provided free samples to day-care centers, and refused to remove the pudgy infant—the "Gerber Baby"—from its label (Guatemalan Ministry of Health 1993). In 1992, Gerber submitted its packaging for approval by the Guatemalan

(continued)

Box 9–3 Continued

Food and Drug Registration Agency, which requested that Gerber remove the happy baby image, indicate the age for introduction of food into a baby's diet on the label, and add the words "breast milk is the best for baby." Gerber not only resisted these attempts to comply, it initiated legal action against the government despite a Guatemalan administrative tribunal decision that ruled in favor of the Ministry of Health in 1993. Arguing that the "Gerber Baby" is integral to their trademark, the company threatened action through the WTO and later won their case. Guatemala was forced to change its law so that imported baby food products would be exempt from the stringent infant food labeling policy (Wallach and Woodall 2004). In the end, Gerber not only remains able to promote its baby-milk substitute products in ways that violate the code in Guatemala, it continues to promote such practices elsewhere as well (e.g., in Malaysia, Mexico, and Egypt) (International Baby Food Action Network 2004).

TNC businesses exist for one purpose—to maximize profits for shareholders. They do this through many activities, such as cost-cutting, restructuring and downsizing workforces, reducing wages, cyclic mergers and divestitures, union busting, tax evading relocations, lobbying of lawmakers for exemptions from costly regulations (on tariffs, trade, labor rights, worker health and safety, and environmental protection), and noncompliance with or defiance of regulations intended to protect basic human rights, health, and the environment of local communities and ecosystems. These corporate activities can often violate economic, social, and cultural human rights, and, in turn, negatively affect the determinants of health.

These rights include the right to work, to earn a living by work freely chosen, to just and favorable working conditions, to fair wages and equal pay for equal work, to safe and healthy working conditions and the opportunity to be promoted, and to a reasonable limitation of working hours. These are all considered core labor rights. Other rights that are often violated include the right of children to be protected from economic and social exploitation; the right to education; the right to an adequate standard of living for individuals and their families; and the right of peoples to improvements in environmental protection and preservation. The Universal Declaration of Human Rights states that these economic, social, and cultural rights should not only be protected but also fulfilled by signatory states (Yamin 2005). The activities of many TNCs often involve child labor, sweatshop conditions, low wages, repression of citizen protest, and environmental pollution, which have had demonstrable adverse effects on human rights and health (Table 9–3).

In workplaces lacking adequate safety measures, production processes are directly harmful to workers and the local community environment. Without provision and enforcement of adequate labor laws that include protections for occupational safety and health, workers are often mistreated. Millions toil in sweatshops (i.e., in low wage, stressful, and usually unhealthy environments), and their efforts to organize independent unions and bargain collectively for basic rights are often brutally suppressed.

Table 9-3 Examples of Human Rights Violations Linked to Transnational Corporate
Activity

Issue	Year	Description
Child labor	1995	Young girls under the age of 15 were found working 70 hours per week in El Salvador at Mandarin International for 60 cents per hour. Mandarin is a major supplier of clothing to The Gap, a large U.S. retailer. After the stories were made public by the National Labor Committee (NLC), a U.S.-based labor rights group, The Gap threatened to pull out, but local activists demanded they stay and pay higher wages for fewer working hours (Seymour 1996).
Environmental contamination	1996	In southern Luzon, Philippines, 1.5 million cubic meters of toxic mine tailings spilled into the Boac river, killing all life in the 27 km river, contaminating surrounding water sources, and threatening the livelihood of 20 villages for years to come. The source of the spill was a mine owned by the Marcopper Mining Corporation, a TNC with revenues of US$7 billion in 1994 (Tauli-Corpuz 1996).
Low wages	1996	The U.S.'s Walt Disney Company was found to be paying 11 cents per hour to workers living in slums in Haiti to sew Mickey Mouse and Pocahontas pajamas while paying CEO Michael Eisner US$97,000 per hour (National Labor Committee 1996).
Child labor	1996– 1999	Following leads from fired workers, investigators found underpaid teenagers working in dingy sweatshops operated by subcontractors in Honduras and New York City making clothes for U.S. retail giant Wal-Mart under the name of Kathie Lee Gifford, a well-known TV show host. Gifford's clothing line reportedly earned her US$9 million in 1995. She initially denied any accountability when approached by the NLC, but when the scandal became public, Gifford transformed herself into a model crusader for the rights of child laborers (Press 1996). Yet in 1999, Gifford was again linked to poor working conditions at the Qin Shi factory in China, where workers were paid 13 cents per hour to produce her handbag line sold at Wal-Mart (National Labor Committee 2005).
Prison labor	1997	Sears and Levi Strauss were found to be subcontracting with Chinese prisons to produce consumer goods (Ross 1997).
Abetting atrocities, including crimes against humanity	1997– 2004	In 2007, a group of Colombian families sued Chiquita Brands International for making payments to the paramilitary group United Self-Defense Forces of Colombia (A.U.C.), reported to be responsible for the deaths of 387 people during the ongoing Colombian civil conflict. Chiquita acknowledged that a former subsidiary, Banadex, had illegally paid US$1.7 million to the A.U.C. from 1997 to 2004 (Associated Press 2007).
Villages razed to enable oil exploration	2000– 2004	Dozens of Sudanese villages in the oil-rich Malut Basin in Upper Nile State were leveled by Sudanese army forces and government sponsored Dinka militias in order to clear the way for oil exploration by Petrodar Operating Company Ltd. jointly owned by the China National Petroleum Company and oil companies from Malaysia, Sudan, and the United Arab Emirates (Wesselink and Weller 2006).

(*continued*)

Table 9–3 Continued

Repression of protesters and alluvial miners; threats to aboriginal lands and the environment	2007	Canadian-owned Barrick Gold, the world's largest gold mining company, was linked to the repression of dozens of alluvial miners (small-scale diggers) and antimining critics in Papua New Guinea, Tanzania, and Peru, as well as to thousands of forced evictions of small-scale miners and residents. Its heavy water use was shown to threaten supplies in water scarce areas in Australia and South America. Due to the negative track record of Barrick and other mining companies in desecrating sacred aboriginal lands and violating indigenous human rights, in March 2007 the UN Committee on the Elimination of Racial Discrimination called upon Canada to improve regulation and ensure accountability of its transnational mining corporations operating on indigenous lands abroad (CorpWatch 2007).
Workers' rights violations	2008	In the run-up to the 2008 Olympic Games in China, the Play Fair alliance documented horrendous working conditions in factories in China, India, Thailand, and Indonesia supplying sportswear for Olympic team sponsors such as Nike and Adidas. Although these and other sportswear companies adopted codes of conduct in the 1990s, they have continued to commit widespread workers' rights violations, including paying poverty level wages, imposing excessively long hours of underpaid overtime, engaging in exploitative terms of employment, sexual harassment, and physical and verbal abuse, and threatening health and safety due to high production quotas and exposure to toxic chemicals (Play Fair 2008).

Global Reorganization of Production and Labor Markets

The emergence of a global labor market (particularly through India and China) is a key element of globalization (Labonte and Schrecker 2007). (China has been one of the largest recipients of foreign investment since 2002, second only to the United States in some years.) Companies have reorganized production and service provision across national boundaries, fragmenting the creation of products, with outsourcing becoming the rule rather than the exception. Outsourcing to a globalized labor market limits governmental ability to implement labor standards, health and safety regulations, and redistributive social policy measures (Cox 1999). Despite the apparently global integration, the result has been economic and social inequalities, declining wages, poor working conditions, loss of jobs, increased workplace hazards, increased part-time and casual labor, and higher numbers of working hours. A sharp decline in the demand for, and wages of, low-skilled and semi-skilled workers has occurred with deindustrialization and outsourcing in developed nations, without any mirrored increase in wages in poor countries. This phenomenon is expected to continue.

Despite its belief in the panacea of the global marketplace, the World Bank has conceded that labor market changes are generating increased economic inequality in the countries with 85% of the world's poorest people. Unskilled workers are being left further and further behind (World Bank 2007), with consequent health deterioration. The impact of global economic changes on workplace health is explored in the second part of this chapter.

Labor markets draw TNCs to EPZs, also known as "free trade zones." EPZs are special areas set up to provide tariff-free production of primarily export-style goods. Textile and garment manufacturing and electronics assembly are the most common industries that have taken advantage of EPZs. Women are often the primary employees, as their fingers are more nimble for garment and assembly work, and employers can get away with paying them 60% to 80% of the wages that men would receive. In the end, EPZ jobs rarely improve the wage conditions of either women or men, and have been called "wage labor slavery." Where labor laws have been rolled back and unions suppressed, workers have faced unnecessary accidents and deaths on the job (La Botz 1994).

Mexico's *maquila* (factory) industrial belt along the U.S.-Mexico border is dominated by TNCs. Over one million Mexicans work in this EPZ near the U.S. border where prevailing local wages hover at US$1 per hour, housing is universally substandard, potable water is nonexistent, and high levels of pollution in the area contribute to excess morbidity and mortality (Hovell, Sipan, and Hofstetter 1988). Poverty level wages keep the poor living in slums despite the fact they work full-time jobs, preventing any sustainable development in these *maquila* communities (Moure-Eraso et al. 1994a, 1994b). Real technology transfer is rare. Apart from the jobs created, the EPZs have had virtually no impact on Mexico's overall development. Employment in Mexico's EPZs actually dropped from 1.3 to 1 million between 2000 and 2002. This was because some manufacturing shifted to China which has lower wages.

Human rights and health issues in the *maquila* sector center around fair wages, the right to organize, hazardous working conditions, the disclosure of hazardous waste, safety training, infrequent occupational inspections, occupational compensation for injury, sexual harassment, child labor, and housing conditions. Other more acute health issues include repetitive strain, noise pollution, solvent and toxic waste pollution, miscarriages, skin disorders, pulmonary disease/asthma, and mental health disorders like depression (La Botz 1994). In addition, there is concern that violence against women has increased due to the economic disruption in the region. Since 1993, over 450 women have been murdered or have disappeared in the border towns of Ciudad Juárez and Chihuahua (Amnesty International 2007).

Debt Crisis, "Poverty Reduction," and Health Effects of Economic Restructuring

The Bretton Woods institutions (the World Bank and International Monetary Fund), also known as international financial institutions (IFIs) are the chief multilateral agencies directing countries toward neoliberal economic reforms. Critics contend that International Monetary Fund (IMF) policies are just a means to protect international banks and to continue the exploitation of the South by the North. Others, including very sober senior officials within the financial system itself, have called for a basic rethinking of the Bretton Woods organizations, arguing that they require "tune-up" or complete overhaul after more than 50 years of operation (Stiglitz 2002). Joseph Stiglitz, a Nobel laureate economist, argues that the IMF in particular favors the rich over the poor, stifles development, undermines democracy, and promotes financial instability and crisis.

As discussed in Chapter 3, the adverse health effects of the debt crisis and resultant SAPs include: decreased funds for infrastructure development and maintenance, decreased supply, quality of, and access to health services, a decline in personal income, and increased unemployment with resultant deterioration in nutritional and health status particularly among the poorest groups. SAPs also result in reduced tax revenues and lowered budgets for social security, education, health services, and other government programs. Likewise, due to the increased costs of imports, health centers are less able to afford pharmaceuticals, medical supplies, vehicles, and gasoline.

According to several studies, government revenues and expenditures fell during the early stages of SAPs and economic reforms decreased the quality of health care and led to health care privatization in various countries. In Ecuador, for instance, when per capita Ministry of Health spending fell by more than half, the number of private clinics grew by 75%, and physicians in the private sector grew by 147%, leaving the growing poor population to face prohibitive payments or the overcrowded public sector (often with its own user fees). Large-scale child survival campaigns had to be mobilized to attenuate resultant alarming reversals in infant mortality rate declines and soaring disease problems in countries such as Chile (Peabody 1996).

Indeed, even the most generous analyses have found the effects of SAPs on health to be mixed. For example, while child mortality rates declined in some countries undergoing structural adjustment (e.g., Pakistan with a decline of 33%), in others (e.g., Brazil), rates were less pronounced and even stagnated or increased (e.g., Jamaica's IMR increased from 16 deaths/1,000 live births to 18/1,000 between 1980 and 1987) (WHO 2001).

In Zimbabwe, user fees implemented during structural adjustment led to reduced use of health services (even when people required care for disabling or fatal illnesses), an increase in IMR, and an increased incidence of malnutrition among rural children (Bijlmakers, Bassett, and Sanders 1996). In most South American countries that implemented SAPs, growth in average per capita income fell steadily between 1990 and 2001 (Morley and Vos 2004).

Such negative assessments have been extended to cover IFI policies as a whole. A recent study found that former communist countries that underwent IMF economic reform programs experienced significantly worse TB incidence and mortality than those that did not (Stuckler, King, and Basu 2008).

In 1999, the IMF and World Bank introduced the term "poverty reduction strategy" to replace SAPs, and made the preparation of poverty reduction strategy papers (PRSPs) a requirement for any low-income country wishing to borrow from the IMF and the World Bank (IMF 2008). Given that the World Bank and IMF boards must approve the PRSPs, governments typically write the PRSP with IFI approval in mind (Welch 2000). In the most recent review of PRSPs, the WHO concluded that:

> PRSPs do not systematically identify those health issues which are the biggest contributors to poverty or the greatest brake on economic growth...Nor do they look systematically at the health situation of the poor—beyond noting that they tend to have the worst health outcomes and are unable to afford health care fees...Finally, it is clear from the budgets presented in PRSPs...that PRSPs will not result in large increases in resources available for health (WHO 2004, p. 18).

The Heavily Indebted Poor Countries (HIPC) Initiative was first launched in 1996, to reduce debt to "sustainable levels" in countries with high debt burdens through debt forgiveness or reduction. To be eligible, each country must compile a PRSP and adhere to certain conditions and reforms decided by the IMF. The IMF asserts that spending on health, education, and other social services has increased by five-fold in countries that have undergone HIPC (IMF 2007). However, the initiative has been criticized for taking too narrow a focus on poverty reduction, as high levels of debt are often only one factor leading to poverty, and thus poorer health status in many countries and a focus on debt reduction may obscure the importance of broader societal development (Gautam 2003). In addition, the initiative places further conditionalities (reminiscent of SAPs) on participating countries, without following through on the promised debt relief commitments of international agencies and donor nations (Greenhill and Sisti 2003). The initiative has also been criticized for having a very short term focus, and for not actually creating conditions for long-term debt sustainability in participating countries (Pettifor, Thomas, and Telatin 2001).

Financial Liberalization and Crisis

Speculative finance has made some investors spectacularly rich while betting on currency devaluations. Communication technology now enables round-the-clock currency trading and finance capital exchanges to speed around the globe. On the whole, however, many developing countries have experienced "currency crises" nearly once per decade as financial institutions in developed nations have played on the global markets. Much of this capital flow is speculative, rather than reflective of hard investment in factories or productive capacity. These transactions dwarf the total foreign exchange reserves of many poor governments, and limit their ability to stabilize their economies and maintain fiscal discipline (UNDP 1999). Increased poverty and inequality occurs following each episode of insecurity, as health and social spending decreases.

Governments (and entire regions) that have followed the neoliberal global economic model have had socially disruptive economic crises in the past 10 years, including Mexico (1994–1995), South Asia (1997–1998), and Argentina (2001–2002). Although the origins of the crises in each region are different, they share the similarity of large-scale foreign investment, excessive bank lending, and currency speculation. These crises set back economies and undermined the livelihoods of hundreds of millions of people. Evidence from Asia shows that the financial crisis in Thailand, Indonesia, and Malaysia in the 1990s led to reductions in family income, which in turn led to reduced food intake, reduced health care utilization, and reduced expenditures on education (Hopkins 2006). In South Korea, there was substantially reduced health care utilization amidst increases in morbidity and mortality following the 1997 crisis, partially due to declining tax revenues and lower expenditures on health (Kim et al. 2003).

Environmental Damage and Health

Effects on health from neoliberal globalization and transnational corporate activity have extended beyond workplaces to shape local communities, natural habitats, and ecosystems, often in very costly or irreparable ways. Raw material extraction, chemical manufacturing, agri-business, and construction industries have been especially harmful to health and environments.

Between 1970 and 1990 Texaco discharged an estimated 16.8 million gallons of crude oil and 20 billion gallons of toxic waste into the vicinity surrounding its oil exploration activities in Ecuador (Kimerling 1994). This discharge has had deleterious effects on the environment, and has resulted in multiple adverse effects to the health of the surrounding community. In 1995, the company signed an agreement with the government of Ecuador to begin cleanup activities in return for immunity from any responsibility related to its oil operations. Despite the agreement, the "circle of poison" had already been put into place, and the mechanisms of differential exposure and differential susceptibility discussed above were already at work (Center for Economic and Social Rights 1994). Not only were the communities living in proximity to the oil exploration in Ecuador nutritionally and immunocompromised, they were exposed to toxic substances from oil drilling and its waste products (San Sebastián et al. 2001; Hurtig and San Sebastián 2004).

In the following years, multiple epidemiological studies documented the range of worsened health outcomes that could be directly linked to Texaco's oil operations, including adverse pregnancy outcomes and elevated rates of specific kinds of cancer (Hurtig and San Sebastián 2002a, 2002b; San Sebastián, Armstrong, and Stephens 2002). Due to the lasting damage wrought on their community, local Ecuadorians took Texaco to court. As of 2008, the case was still in litigation. The strategy of the TNC has included paying experts in health and epidemiology to discredit the epidemiological health assessments conducted for the plaintiffs, and to advertise their critiques in the public media (Breilh et al. 2005).

In Nigeria, the Niger River Delta remains one of the poorest regions of the country despite being richly endowed with natural resources. It contains 20 billion of Africa's 66 billion barrels of oil reserves and more than 3 trillion cubic meters of natural gas reserves. Oil and gas resources account for over 85% of the nation's GDP, largely from the Niger River Delta. Due to the ecologically unfriendly exploitation of this oil, largely driven by TNCs, the indigenous peoples of the delta have been stripped of their rights and left poor in the face of oil riches. The devastation incurred by TNC oil drilling has rendered farming and fishing, the main sources of income for local tribes, useless in many areas. The environmental degradation has left the local people in worse health and exacerbated their poverty (Aaron 2005).

Box 9–4 The Tragedy of Union Carbide in Bhopal

The chemical leak in Bhopal, India, on December 3, 1984 was one of the worst industrial disasters in history, with enormous human and environmental consequences. Within a 2-hour period more than 27 tons of deadly methyl isocyanate gas escaped out of a pesticide plant owned by the U.S.-based Union Carbide multinational corporation. An estimated 3,800 people died immediately, mostly residents of the plant's neighboring slum colonies, and tens of thousands more experienced serious health effects and premature death (Broughton 2005). More than two decades later, it is estimated that 50,000 people in the region continue to suffer from long-term health consequences due to the Bhopal disaster, ranging from chronic inflammation of the eyes and lungs to reproductive, genetic, and neurobehavioral problems. Increased rates of spontaneous abortion and an elevation in chromosomal and congenital abnormalities as well as cognitive impairments have also been connected to the methyl isocyanate gas leak (Dhara et al. 2002).

Union Carbide immediately sought to dissociate itself from the incident and deny legal responsibility, instead blaming local plant operators and Indian government regulators. Although a legal settlement was eventually achieved through the mediation of India's Supreme Court, and Union Carbide accepted "moral"—but not criminal—responsibility for the incident and paid US$470 million in compensation to victims and relatives, there remains heated debate about the company's relief efforts in Bhopal (Mehta et al. 1990). Even though operations at the Bhopal plant were discontinued, its remnants remain and the site continues to leak toxic chemicals and metals into the region's soil and groundwater (Sharma 2002). Though not intentional, the leak was both foreseeable and preventable: many local residents and international activists believe that Union Carbide (now owned by Dow Chemical) should be held criminally liable for the world's worst industrial disaster and held accountable for the persistent environmental and health consequences, but thus far the corporation has escaped punishment (Holtz 2000).

Shifts in perception about the destructive capacity of neoliberal globalization began after the Bhopal disaster in the 1980s. In the 1990s, human rights groups reported that numerous major oil, mining, and apparel/textile companies had clearly put profits before health and human rights principles in their business operations (Human Rights Watch 1997). Awareness is increasing that nonstate societal institutions, such as TNCs, "may strongly influence the capacity for realization of rights while at the same time eluding state control" (Mann et al. 1994, p. 19). TNCs have found themselves under greater scrutiny, but improvements in TNC practices are per force dependent on strong regulatory environments that conflict with free trade goals.

WORK AND OCCUPATIONAL HEALTH AND SAFETY IN DEVELOPING COUNTRIES

Key Questions:

• What makes the workplace a hazardous environment?
• What social forces are necessary to improve worker safety and health in developing countries?
• Where and how should hazardous waste be dumped?

Working conditions in developing countries for most workers have historically been poor, unsupervised, and difficult to regulate. Since the 1980s, neoliberal economic globalization has expanded the industrial workforce in developing countries yet, despite side agreements to trade treaties that have included occupational safety and health provisions, there has not been an overall improvement in working conditions. Protective legislation is also much weaker, and, compared to developed countries, there is less frequent enforcement of the laws on the books in developing countries. Working conditions affect health in a variety of ways—through poor wages, stress, bad environmental working conditions, toxic exposures, and the use of harmful substances. This section explores the relationship between work and health, as well as connections between workplace health conditions and processes of globalization.

According to the WHO, about 45% of the world's population (and 58% of the population over 10 years old) contribute to the global workforce. Although more men are registered in the workforce than women, these numbers do not include work at home or in the informal sector. Thus, health at work and healthy work environments (as laid out in the Universal Declaration of Human Rights) are among the most valuable assets that employers, communities, and governments can cultivate. Work can have positive and adverse effects on the health of workers and their families. Work provides income and material goods necessary for living. Positive work environments can contribute to improved work motivation, job satisfaction, and self-esteem, and to high overall well-being for individuals and families. On the other hand, poor work environments can lead to job stress, ill health, low living standards, and an overall poor quality of life.

The Workplace as a Hazardous Environment

In many settings the workplace is a hazardous environment, especially where occupational safety and health receive little attention. WHO estimates that from 33% to 50% of workers worldwide are exposed to serious physical, chemical, or biologic agents, or to unreasonably heavy loads that may be hazardous to health. Psychological overload can also contribute to stress and chronic physical complaints.

WHO estimates that as many as 250 million occupational accidents (with 330,000 fatalities) and over 70 million new episodes of occupational-related disease occur every year. Labor advocates estimate that there may be as many as 1 million fatalities and 1 billion accidents every year (Takala 2002). The direct and indirect costs of these illnesses can add up to 5% of a country's GNP (WHO 2007).

Workers in developing countries experience particularly high rates of workplace illness and death. There are five main reasons for this. First, the geography and natural resources of certain developing countries result in a different hazard profile. Where primary commodities and warmer climates are present, extractive industries and agriculture (which together make up the most hazardous jobs) figure prominently in the overall economic picture. Second, in many underdeveloped settings, work begins at an earlier age, is of longer duration, and is therefore more hazardous than in developed countries. Third, resources to control and prevent job injuries are scarce in many developing countries, as there are fewer experts, inspectors, and tools for health advocates to implement change, less safety and monitoring equipment, and fewer and less enforcement of labor laws. In many places unions are prohibited in the workplace. Fourthly, jobs requiring worker protection in developed countries with strongly enforced worker safety laws are often outsourced through subcontracting, subsidiaries, and trade to developing countries with weaker protections. Hazardous industries are increasingly relocated to underdeveloped countries. Lastly, and most importantly, in many developing countries there is weaker government enforcement of labor and occupational health and safety laws, reflecting greater exploitation of workers by the capitalist class, including country nationals, owners of TNCs, and foreign investors. Ultimately, high rates of occupational illness, injury, and death are the function of enormous inequalities in political power.

Working conditions in much of Africa, Eastern Europe, China, India, Pakistan, and Southeast Asia are abysmal. The protection of occupational health and safety in underdeveloped countries faces a range of challenges as seen in Table 9–4. Workers in developing countries face long work weeks with few breaks; consequently exposures to hazards may exceed acceptable levels of harm. Laboring in tropical climates when there is inadequate control of temperature and ventilation may lead to heat exhaustion. Equipment is frequently imported, often obsolete for use in the developed world, with few or no spare parts for maintenance. Most work takes place in small firms or the informal sector, which have lower use of safe technologies and modern safety equipment than larger counterparts. Neoliberal globalization has only exacerbated these already difficult conditions.

In many developed settings, the workforce is undereducated, has low literacy levels, and is also undernourished. For instance, some African workers have relatively high levels of enzyme deficiency, increasing susceptibility to some oxidizing chemicals. Some populations in Asia have high rates of hepatitis B viremia, which increases their susceptibility to hepatotoxins. Finally, shortages of

Table 9-4 Challenges for Occupational Health in Some Developing Countries

Challenges Related to Working Conditions

1. Long work weeks and work shifts; inadequate breaks
2. Inadequate safety measures in place against physical and chemical hazards
3. Unions not allowed and union activity threatened with retribution (including job loss and violence)
4. Inadequate control of climatic factors (insufficient heating, cooling, ventilation)
5. Nonadherence to ergonomic standards

Challenges Related to Political Conditions

1. Limited or no political representation of workers and workers' parties
2. Absence of an independent labor movement; little tradition of labor rights
3. Corruption that favors employers, including foreign-owned corporations
4. Inadequate legislation to protect workers, including workers' compensation and health insurance coverage
5. Limited enforcement or accountability of safety and protective measures

Challenges Related to Organization of Work

1. Preponderance of small firms
2. Large presence of multinational firms and subcontractors in some industries
3. Prominent role of the informal sector
4. Most machinery imported; modifications, replacement parts, and technical backup is difficult or unavailable
5. Technical alternatives, such as safer machinery, may be unavailable in local markets

Challenges Related to the Workforce

1. Low literacy rates
2. Low nutritional levels
3. Certain genetically linked enzyme disorders resulting in increased vulnerability to organophosphate chemicals and other pesticides

Human Resource Challenges

1. Insufficient industrial hygiene expertise
2. Poor training of employees in job safety
3. Inadequate expertise in epidemiology and occupational medicine and nursing

Source: Adapted from Frumkin (1999) with permission from Elsevier.

well-trained personnel can lead to workers performing jobs for which they are undertrained, in situations with limited, if any, industrial hygiene monitoring or standards enforcement. Most significantly, many countries lack independent labor movements or strong workers' parties to press for political change and advocate for safe environments.

Rates of occupational injury and illness in developing countries are extremely hard to quantify. Workers in extraction industries, forestry, construction, and agriculture are most likely to be injured or die on the job. Up to one-third of these workers may experience a work-related injury every year, leading to work-related

Box 9–5 The Organization of Work, Increased Risk of HIV, and Opportunities for Prevention

The organization of work can have profound implications on existing risk factors for disease. One example is the use of migrant and semi-migrant labor in the mining industry in southern Africa. The use of hostels containing large numbers of employed males, sometimes housed hundreds of miles from their families, increases their social vulnerability to HIV disease transmission.

In fact, it might be ethically imperative to consider HIV infection an occupational illness deserving of compensation (London and Kisting 2002). There are examples of how HIV testing policies at work have led to increased levels of discrimination and stigma. Therefore, initiatives to introduce workplace prevention, and voluntary counseling and testing, should take into account these considerations. The introduction of voluntary counseling and testing, as well as antiretroviral treatment programs at work are becoming more common, as employers realize that a healthy and fit workforce is essential to healthy production. Large employers in southern Africa, such as automobile production plants, have provided much of the initiative for the cost-effectiveness and operational efficiency of different models of ARV provision. Cooperation between labor, employers, and government in prevention and treatment is a crucial factor in expanding HIV care and support.

disability and sometimes to premature death. Less dramatic occupational health injuries occur in the service and retail industry, with psychological and ergonomic problems decreasing job satisfaction and affecting health and productivity.

Globalization and changes in trade rules have exacerbated hazardous working conditions, in both existing and new work sectors. As an example, pesticides are widely used throughout the developing world, and pesticide exposure during application remains a serious occupational health problem for workers, with millions of cases of acute poisoning and 40,000 deaths occurring annually worldwide. Several factors contribute to this problem, including unsafe working conditions, the introduction of hazardous powdered formulations of organophosphates and other harmful chemicals, and agricultural subsidies that encourage the use of pesticides (Frumkin 1999).

The liberalization of trade policies in east Africa has led to large increases in pesticide imports, an 80-fold proliferation of private pesticide retailers, and the recruitment of children in the retailing of pesticides (London and Kisting 2002). During structural adjustment in Zimbabwe, the annual increase in pesticide usage more than doubled in the early 1990s, exposing thousands of small farmers to neurotoxic chemicals. In Tanzania, most of these chemicals are used by small tract farmers who apply pesticides, insecticides, herbicides, and fungicides using hand-held tank sprayers or knapsack sprayers (Fig. 9–4). Few farmers are adequately trained in the use and application of pesticides, and most do not have proper protective equipment. Subsequent to the passage of free trade rules in Tanzania, there was a proliferation of private wholesalers and retailers that supply and distribute pesticides in the country. To this day, children can be seen selling pesticides on the streets or in open markets, in violation of the country's 1979 Pesticides Law.

An expansion of production in export-led sectors such as chemical, electronic, and biotechnology industries has added new hazards to those already prevalent in

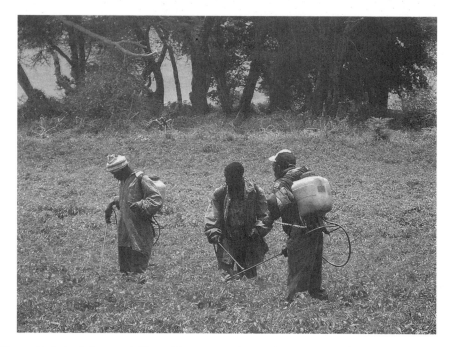

Figure 9–4 Applying pesticides without protective equipment, Tanzania. Photo courtesy of Vera Ngowi.

developing countries. Workers in computer chip manufacturing plants complain of exposure to solvents, glues, and heavy metals without adequate safety measures or supervision. Primary extractive industries such as mining are common in many developing countries, with many mines owned and operated by western-based TNCs. As discussed in Chapter 10, mining in particular is associated with high rates of workplace injury and illness. The tragic loss of 107 coal miners in a March 2007 explosion, occurring in a well-equipped, state-of-the-art mine in the Kemerovo region of Russia, is a case in point (CNN 2007). Pneumoconiosis (lung damage from heavy metals such as nickel and beryllium), chronic obstructive lung disease, and cancer are all common. Coal mining, still essential for power generation in many developing countries, results in "black lung disease," a chronic condition requiring supplemental oxygen and bronchodilators, rendering its victims incapacitated. The dangers of extractive industries are all compounded by inadequate engineering controls, lack of protective equipment and respirators, lack of proper medical surveillance, and a high prevalence of concurrent diseases like TB (especially true in the former Soviet Union and sub-Saharan Africa) (Frumkin 1999).

Lastly, the trend to outsource piecemeal and casual work locates the control of hazards largely in the realm of the private sector, which undermines trade unions' attempts to protect health. It may reduce production costs for employers, but it also shifts the responsibility of work safety onto unregulated contractors or the worker (who often lack the skills, knowledge, or political power to enact any changes) (London 2008). Outsourced jobs are frequently performed in cramped and unventilated conditions, with outdated machinery, and little in the form of personal protective equipment. The need to maximize output not only leads to increased exposure to physical and chemical hazards, but can lead to increased job stress and insecurity, and thus to poorer overall health status. What is clear is that workers in developing countries face hazards not seen for over a half a century in developed nations, and at levels that are accelerating alongside the pace of world trade.

Export of Hazard

The increasing trade and externalization of production characteristic of neoliberal globalization has led many labor advocates to call attention to the "export of hazard." This occurs when industries relocate plants to developing countries in order to lower labor costs, take advantage of lax regulatory requirements, and, in some cases, increase proximity to raw materials. Concomitant with the export of hazard is the downwards competition driven by neoliberal globalization and industrial migration, affecting worker safety and health in developing and developed nations.

During the negotiations for the North American and Central American Free Trade Agreements, among others, labor advocates argued that local governments in the U.S. and Canada would hesitate to enforce worker safety and environmental regulations for fear of pushing plants away to lower-wage areas. Moreover, workers, for fear of losing their jobs, would refrain from pressing for safer workplaces. Firms, including TNCs, would then play one locale against another, seeking the lowest possible costs and wages. In the end, according to this logic, standards and enforcement in developed nations would descend to those in developing nations, and threaten workers in both contexts.

Box 9–6 Export of Hazards: The Case of Canadian Asbestos Production

Asbestos is a naturally occurring mineral, found in numerous countries including Canada, Australia, Russia, China, Kazakhstan, Brazil, Zimbabwe, India, and South Africa. Because it is light, strong, durable, and noncombustible, asbestos was widely used in the building industry for the production of heat and acoustic insulation materials until the late 1970s. The dangers of all forms of asbestos have been recognized since the early 1920s, but it was only in 1963 that the link between asbestosis (scarring of the lung tissue caused by inhaling asbestos) and mesothelioma (a type of lung cancer) was demonstrated (Thomson 1963). Beginning in the 1970s, asbestos products were discontinued and asbestos abatement began.

Though use of asbestos was prohibited in Canada in 1973 under the *Hazardous Products Act*, Canada continues to be the world's second largest producer and exporter (after Russia) of chrysotile asbestos (the most common form of asbestos). Ninety-five percent of Canadian asbestos is exported

(continued)

Box 9–6 Continued

to developing countries that have not yet banned its use, including India, Thailand, Indonesia, and South Korea. Despite global consensus that all types of asbestos are carcinogenic and that all levels of exposure to asbestos are extremely toxic, the Canadian government—in concert with the asbestos industry—has repeatedly blocked global campaigns from adding chrysotile asbestos to the UN list of highly dangerous substances that cannot be exported to developing countries without their knowledge and agreement under the global right-to-know—"prior informed consent"—procedure of the 1998 Rotterdam Convention (Ban Asbestos Canada 2007). The Canadian government insists that chrysotile asbestos is safer than other kinds of asbestos and, when handled properly, can be used safely, a position clearly reflecting industrial self-interest rather than protecting the public's health. At the 2008 meeting of the Rotterdam Convention, Canada's position on chrysotile asbestos was allowed to stand.

Hazardous Waste Dumping

Waste dumping in poor countries or on the open ocean is an extremely difficult practice to monitor. Cargo ships that get turned back make the headlines, but many others successfully deliver their payloads to poor countries. As a striking illustrative example, in a 1991 leaked internal memorandum, then World Bank economist Lawrence Summers provided insight into the neoliberal logic behind this practice. In the memo, Summers argued for the transfer of waste and dirty industries from industrialized to developing countries:

> Just between you and me, shouldn't the World Bank be encouraging more migration of the dirty industries to the LDCs [less developing countries]? I can think of three reasons: 1) The measurements of the costs of health-impairing pollution depends on the foregone earnings from increased morbidity and mortality…I think the economic logic behind dumping a load of toxic waste in the lowest wage country is impeccable and we should face up to that. 2)…I've always thought that under-populated countries in Africa are vastly under-polluted, their air quality is probably vastly inefficiently low compared to Los Angeles or Mexico City. 3) The demand for a clean environment for aesthetic and health reasons is likely to have very high income elasticity (Summers cited in Editorial 1992, p. 99).

Summers later said the memo was meant to be ironic.

In one known case of dumping that harmed human health, 2,700 tons of toxic waste containing mercury and other heavy metals were shipped illegally from Taiwan to Cambodia in December 1998. The waste was transferred and dumped into an inland waste site, exposing approximately 2,000 residents of Sihanoukville either environmentally or occupationally. Six deaths and hundreds of illnesses were attributed to this one incident of toxic waste dumping, although no one was ever held accountable (Hess and Frumkin 2000). Other case studies of the export of hazards (such as asbestos, pesticides, hazardous waste, and industrial disasters such as Bhopal) are illustrated in Boxes 9–4 and 9–6.

One of the most notorious examples of global toxic waste dumping was the voyage of the ship the *Khian Sea,* which set sail from the United States in 1986 loaded with nearly 14,000 tons of toxic fly-ash from Philadelphia's municipal waste incinerator (Parayre 2006). After an unsuccessful attempt to dump the ash in the Bahamas, the ship sailed the Caribbean Sea in search of a port that would accept the waste. Over the next 16 months, the *Khian Sea* sought to offload its cargo in the Dominican Republic, Honduras, Panama, Bermuda, and the Dutch Antilles. All refused the waste, and the ship's attempt to return to Philadelphia was also blocked. Finally, the crew was authorized to unload the cargo in Haiti as "top-soil fertilizer," though it was far too toxic to be used for this purpose. When the true content of the cargo was revealed, the Haitian government ordered it removed and banned all waste imports. Nonetheless, an estimated 4,000 tons of ash was left on the beach adjacent to the Sedren wharf in Gonaives, Haiti, where it sat for 10 years leaking toxins into the local area. Eventually a deal was brokered with the United States for its safe removal. The rest of the ash remained on the ship for 27 months as the crew tried to dispose it of in Guinea-Bissau, the Philippines, Senegal, and Yugoslavia. The ash mysteriously disappeared from the ship in 1988. Six years later the ship's captain admitted to dumping more than 10,000 tons of the ash into the Atlantic and Indian Ocean. Although the owners of the *Khian Sea* were eventually convicted of perjury, they were never tried for the dumping in Haiti. Nor was the city of Philadelphia ever fined or punished, although it withheld payment to the company until the waste was disposed of permanently.

Notwithstanding the international outrage that ensued, 20 years later such illegal disposals continue. On August 19, 2006 a ship called the *Probo Koala* offloaded 500 tons of toxic waste sludge in Abidjan, Côte d'Ivoire, which was then illegally dumped at 12 municipal dumps throughout the city. The waste, an alkaline mix of water, gasoline, and soda, was believed to be releasing hazardous gases, including hydrogen sulfide. During subsequent weeks 10 deaths were associated with exposure to the waste, in addition to 23 hospitalizations and 40,000 visits for medical treatment, although no definitive link was established between the cause of death and the waste (IRIN 2007). It turned out that the *Probo Koala* was a Panamanian-registered tanker, owned by a Greek shipping company, chartered to a Dutch company, thus masking responsibility. Before it dumped the waste in Abidjan, it attempted to have the waste processed in Amsterdam but the contractor that agreed to dispose of the waste steeply raised prices immediately after delivery. In 2007 the Dutch company agreed to pay a US$198 million settlement to Côte d'Ivoire.

Not only do wealthier countries and populations pollute more and export their waste for reasons of political and economic expediency (Clapp 2001), but they are less affected by ecosystem degradation because of "their ability to import resources from, and displace health risks to, other geographical locations" (Corvalan, Hales, and McMichael 2005, p. 11).

Working Children and Child Laborers

According to ILO Convention 138, the term "child labor" refers to children below 12 years of age working in any economic activities, those aged 12 to 14 years engaged in harmful work, and all children engaged in the worst forms of child labor such as being enslaved, forcibly recruited, prostituted, trafficked, forced into illegal activities, and exposed to hazardous work (UNICEF 2006).

The ILO has estimated that there are 246 million "child laborers." They may be laboring long hours under poor working conditions, sacrificing time and energy that they might have spent at school or home at play, enjoying the formative experiences of childhood. Of those, approximately 210 million are under the age of 15, both boys and girls. Children this age are missing out on the vital role education plays in equipping them with knowledge, life skills, and the confidence to participate in the economic and social development of their family and community. In the worst cases, child workers are exposed to dangerous and physically and psychologically stressful work that strains their bodies and minds.

Children make up 11% of the workforce in Asia, 17% in Africa, and 25% in Latin America (LaDou 2003). They are the most exploited of all workers, are less able to defend themselves physically, emotionally, and legally, and are more subject to manipulation and disempowerment. Most child labor occurs in developing countries, where poverty and traditional modes of work prevent local and international efforts from stopping it. Nonenforcement of laws creates a vacuum in some societies that allows children to be held in near slave-like conditions, to be minimally paid or unpaid, and to be physically and sexually abused. The story of Idris at the beginning of this chapter is just one of thousands of accounts of children who are forced to work and who suffer from poor working conditions and a lack of proper education. Countless other children labor daily in carpet weaving factories, brick making, and vending.

Child labor is not new, but the changing patterns of work performed by children (like adults) is shaped by global economic and political forces. In many respects, the proportion of children who are child laborers (as opposed to children who work in and around their home assisting the family) is a measure of that society's adherence to norms of social justice. Many factors influence whether school-age children are required to be in the workforce instead of in school, including a country's economic growth, its distribution of wealth, the presence of SAPs, or the influence of the global trade regime. In a just society, no child under the age of 16 would have to work for a living. Not only are child laborers exposed to unsafe work environments, their future ability to flourish is jeopardized. Child workers are more likely to experience premature disability and death from their exposures at a young age.

Informal Sector

Much of the world's workforce is comprised of workers in the informal sector (LaDou 2003), which has grown since the onset of neoliberal globalization. In virtually every city in India and Africa thousands of people hawk goods on the street—selling garbage bags, candy, or radios to passing motorists, or making small meals to sell to pedestrians. The informal sector, which includes unofficial self-employed workers, independent contractors, and small family-run businesses is integral to the economies of many countries. In Mexico, over 18 million people work in the informal sector, and in India the bulk of the workforce is comprised of informal sector workers (Joshi and Smith 2002). While unemployment is generally seen as bad for one's health, so too is employment in the informal sector (London 2008), as lack of social security, extreme work conditions, and nonexistent labor protections result in higher rates of injury and disease. The informal sector generates little in taxes, leading governments to care little about the welfare of these workers.

Women and Work

In poor industrialized areas, women have higher rates of employment than men, but are paid lower wages. This leads to the feminization of poverty, wherein women work for lower wages and in worse conditions than men. Beyond wage labor, many women work in the home (e.g., child care, housekeeping, and food preparation) and, accordingly, girls are more likely than boys to be withdrawn from school to work or help at home (Rao and Loewenson 2000).

For example, with the expansion of international trade between North and Latin America, and between east Africa and Europe, the floriculture industry has seen a boom in production. This sector employs large numbers of women, but these are mainly dead-end jobs that reinforce their vulnerabilities. Employment in this sector is mainly limited to the recruitment of young women, for jobs that place them at high probability of exposure to neurotoxic and potentially endocrine disrupting pesticides and chemicals. Working under conditions of powerlessness and vulnerability, without freedom of association or union representation, they lack the ability to move beyond this level of work. High levels of violence and physical and sexual abuse of women have been reported as a major occupational hazard in this industry, where (mainly young) women have little legal power to fight back.

Trafficking of Women and Children

A common form of work exploitation that receives insufficient attention is human trafficking, specifically where women and children are forced to become slave laborers on plantations, in mines, factory sweatshops, domestic settings, and as commercial sex workers. While human trafficking has existed for thousands of years, it has become worse under neoliberal globalization, as dire economic conditions have forced more poor people into this form of exploitation, and deregulation has led to less government vigilance.

Women and children who are trafficked for bonded labor or commercial exploitation often come from or are sent to India. Boys from Bangladesh, Afghanistan, and Pakistan are also trafficked through India to the Gulf States for involuntary servitude as camel jockeys or houseboys. Indentured servitude is also practiced in northern Africa, where child slaves are openly sold in markets for transport and use in neighboring countries.

Trafficking also includes the prostitution of children, which involves offering the sexual services of a child (anyone younger than 18 years of age, as defined in the Convention on the Rights of the Child) or inducing a child to perform sexual acts for any form of financial or nonfinancial compensation (Willis and Levy 2002). Prostitution differs from sexual abuse in that it involves exploitation of a child's life for commercial gain. Both females and males are prostituted, some as young as 10 years old. Economic, cultural, and social factors—poverty, gender bias, discrimination, and low educational status—are the underlying causes of child prostitution. In some countries, males believe that children are less likely to be infected with HIV or other sexually transmitted diseases, or in some cases are thought to be protective or curative for these infections—and thus seek them out for unprotected sexual activity.

Estimates of the number of prostituted children worldwide range between 1 and 5 million (Table 9–5) (United Nations Economic and Social Commission for Asia and the Pacific 2007). The main prostitutors of children are local men; many children are also exploited by foreign pedophiles who pay for exclusive sex tours

Table 9–5 Estimated Number of Children Exploited through Prostitution (Worldwide)

Country	Estimated Number of Children Exploited through Prostitution
Bangladesh	10,000
Brazil	100,000
China	200,000
India	400,000
Nepal	40,000
Philippines	40,000
Russia	30,000
Thailand	200,000
United States	300,000
Venezuela	40,000
Zambia	70,000

Source: Reprinted from Willis and Levy (2002) with permission from Elsevier.

with young women and children. Organized criminal elements are commonly involved, often employing addictive drugs to control children and prevent escape. Poverty and the profitability of the practice drive its continuation. The sex industry generates roughly US$20 billion or more yearly, of which 25% is attributed to prostituted or exploited children (Editorial 1998). Children are often trapped by the earnings potential of sex work because they are obliged to provide remittances or other support to the families who sold them.

Prostituted children can have from 5 to 10 clients per day, which makes them vulnerable to morbidity and mortality, but is also a gross violation of their human rights (Willis and Levy 2002). Exploited children have a high likelihood of acquiring infectious diseases such as HIV, syphilis, and gonorrhea, and are at high risk of pregnancy and suffering complications from attempted abortions, mental illness, substance abuse, and violence. Health professionals can assist in the effort to provide medical care to prostituted children, but the ultimate challenge is to prevent the continuation of this illegal practice which has been called "slavery in our time" (Kristof 2006). Programs to rescue and provide services to children operate in most major countries, but they are understaffed and do not have sufficient resources to rescue all the children in need. Criminalizing sex tourism and enforcing local laws that prohibit the prostitution of children are the critical legal measures needed to end this horrendous practice.

Occupational Health Services

Access to occupational health services is very limited in most countries. Only 5% to 10% of workers in developing countries and 20% to 50% of workers in developed countries have access to modern occupational health services, treatment, and rehabilitation. Physicians and nurses trained in occupational health are rare in most poor countries. TNCs that operate production facilities or assembly plants rarely employ on-site occupational health workers. Workers who have lost digits or limbs can require months to years of occupational therapy to be able to rejoin the workforce, but frequently these kind of services are not available. For other chronic medical conditions, such as carpal tunnel syndrome, treatment, follow-up, and possibly pain-saving surgery are required. Usually workers who suffer from these injuries end up losing their jobs or working despite the pain, until they are no longer able to carry out their work.

Lastly, although 80% of the world's working population lives in developing countries, only 5% of occupational health research is conducted there (Rantanen, Lehtinen, and Mikheev 1993). "Brain drain" of occupational health professionals from developing to developed countries has also hampered progress toward improved work conditions for the majority of the world's working population. Occupational health is not a goal to be achieved in isolation (LaDou 2003). It should be part of institutional development and reform that reaches to every level of government in developed and developing countries. Occupational safety and health programs are linked to the overall economic success of a country.

INTERNATIONAL OCCUPATIONAL SAFETY AND HEALTH POLICY

Key Questions:

• How could the ILO be strengthened to improve occupational safety and health standards for low-income workers?
• What role does the WHO play in international occupational safety and health?

The *sine qua non* for successfully addressing global occupational health and safety concerns in the context of globalization revolves around the upward harmonization of health and safety standards set by policy, rather than the downward pressure to abandon health and safety that is increasingly seen in poor countries. Working conditions for the majority of the world's workers do not meet the basic minimum standards and guidelines set by the WHO and the ILO. In addition, it is estimated that only about 10% of the population in developing countries are covered by any occupational safety and health laws, omitting many dangerous occupations. Although occupational health is a recognized entity in most developed countries, bringing the field to developing countries is a painfully slow process, as many other issues in these poor countries compete for funding. Consequently, most countries defer responsibility to the UN, when in reality the UN has little or no accountability in the area of workplace health and safety. Importantly, while international standards obligate countries to pay for occupational injuries, inadequate detection and compensation make a mockery of these standards. Only 23 countries have ratified the ILO Employment Injury Benefits Convention adopted in 1964.

International Labor Standards

The ILO is an international coordinating body which was created by the Treaty of Versailles in 1919. It is a membership organization, just like the UN, and its conventions are binding to all signatory states. It is meant to guide all countries in the promotion of occupational safety and health. The ILO plays an important role in promoting uniform policies and standards, and is guided by both a core and a comprehensive set of conventions that member countries are directed to abide by as a condition of membership. The ILO sets minimum standards that have strong ethical and human rights components to them (some say the ILO was the first international human rights body) (Takala 2002). ILO conventions have legal standing in the ILO member countries where they have been ratified. More than half of the

184 conventions adopted by the ILO cover issues related to occupational safety and health, such as:

No. 81—labor inspection.
No. 87—freedom of association.
No. 98—freedom to organize and bargain collectively.
No. 105—freedom from forced labor (only one of 12 core conventions signed by the United States).
No. 155—occupational safety and health.
No. 161—occupational health services.
No. 174—prevention of major industrial accidents.

In addition to the conventions, the ILO also issues codes of practice and guidelines which are not compulsory. These are available online (see International Labour Organization 2005). Unfortunately, the ILO is understaffed and underfinanced, limiting its impact. Globally, few public health professionals seem to know of the ILO, even though it is an appropriate forum through which occupational health can be improved. Since the ILO has no enforcement authority, however, it is not enough (LaDou 2005).

The WHO is responsible for the technical aspects of occupational safety and health, such as the promotion of medical standards, medical examinations, and hygienic standards. A limited budget and staff, however, means it is unable to provide the required consultative services that are needed by so many developing nations. It is almost incomprehensible, but the WHO Program for Occupational Health supports a staff of only four to five people for the entire world! There are WHO Collaborating Centers in Occupational Health, but these regional offices have few trained specialists and have vague missions or purposes. There is clearly a lack of international scrutiny and accountability on behalf of the worlds' governments.

Since the Bhopal disaster in 1984 (Box 9–4), many of the world's TNCs have proclaimed that it is their company policy not to have international "double standards" in health, safety, and environmental protection in their global operations. Comparative analysis of the existence of these standards, however, proves otherwise (Castleman 1999). TNCs still take advantage of domestic hazardous industries, internal corruption, poor work practices, lack of regulation and enforcement of labor standards, and local workers' inability to claim compensation for illnesses and disabilities in order to maximize profits and cut costs.

There is much to be done in international occupational safety and health. Many industries and their workers can benefit from improved training in occupational safety standards. In this regard, international occupational health specialists, academics, and governments that are committed to the improvement of occupational health standards can provide technical assistance. There is a role for collaborative research as well, as the results from this work can be used for advocacy purposes by unions, civil service organizations, and governments.

SIGNS OF HOPE FOR THE FUTURE: GLOBALIZED EFFORTS IN THE NAME OF EQUALITY

Key Questions:

- What was the key to defeating the global trade treaty called the MAI?
- What are the main demands of the 50 Years is Enough Campaign?
- What have been the most effective efforts in challenging neoliberal globalization?

While neoliberal globalization has created gross inequalities in wealth and health, the increased worldwide connectedness brought about by globalization has also been employed to attenuate—and even reverse—some of the detrimental outcomes of neoliberal policies. It must be noted, however, that not all globalization is neoliberal globalization. There are some aspects of a globalized world that are beneficial for social justice and public health, such as the increased ability of public health activists to communicate via the internet to challenge neoliberal orthodoxy. In this section we highlight the myriad ways that the "global village" has challenged the prevailing political-economic order.

Governments Standing Up for Themselves and for Health

Notwithstanding the pressures of neoliberal globalization, a number of governments, bolstered by social movements, have taken concrete measures to protect the well-being of their populations. Various national governments have ensured access to generic drugs or to lower-priced patented drugs through legislation, standing up not only to Big Pharma but also to pressure from the U.S. government.

Before 2005, India recognized only process patents, not product patents, allowing its pharmaceutical companies to reproduce patented drugs inexpensively (Chatterjee 2005). India's upper house of parliament also blocked proposed government legislation conforming to the guidelines of the WTO (which India joined in 1995). Such legislation would have made essential drugs unaffordable for the poor and hurt small farmers by making the price of seeds prohibitively expensive. India has refused to have any changes in its patent laws dictated by the United States, emphasizing instead patent laws that suit their "best national interests" (Jayaraman 1997). As a result, many medicines in India are significantly cheaper than in many other countries, enabling access to medicines for millions of the country's poor (Loff and Heywood 2002). India has dealt with the pressures of compliance with TRIPS legislation as a matter of aligning international policy with domestic laws regarding patent eligibility.

In order to obtain a patent in India, companies must demonstrate a high standard of "novelty"—each new drug must bring significant efficacious benefit to patients beyond that of existing drugs—one of the most restrictive standards in the world. After pharmaceutical giant Novartis brought a patent denial case to the Indian High

Court, charging violation of the TRIPS Agreement, the Court ruled in 2007 that it had no jurisdiction over this issue, thus far leaving India's policies intact.

On the other side of the world, Brazil has fought to reduce drug prices through other means. Despite pressure from the U.S. government in the early 2000s, the Brazilian government interpreted the TRIPS Agreement quite liberally. Notably, its intellectual property law includes a provision that, unless locally manufactured, pharmaceutical products could be subject to compulsory licensing by the government. Drug companies were thus compelled to substantially lower prices of HIV/AIDS drugs, as discussed in Box 6–9 (Cohen 2006). Brazil has continued to make expert use of the limited flexibilities within the TRIPS Agreement, together with its own manufacturing capacity, to ensure access to patented pharmaceuticals for its population. It has used the compulsory licensing clause included in TRIPS as an effective tool on two fronts: first, by threatening the industry with issuing compulsory licenses, it has obtained price reductions of patented drugs; and second, by actually issuing a compulsory license (in 2007) to manufacture a patented ARV drug domestically. Brazil serves as an international role model of how to ensure that the pressures of globalization do not undercut domestic social policies.

Some countries have sought to resist foreign ownership of national resources in order to guarantee that local economies benefit from national industry. Bolivia's nationalization of its oil and gas industry to maintain control over its own resources is one example, ensuring resources for social investment in the country. Bolivian President Evo Morales brought the country's energy production under state control in 2006. This was regarded by the United States as a major threat to the region as well as U.S. national interests (West 2006). Nationalizing oil in Bolivia represented the fulfillment of Morales' campaign pledge and currently provides increased funding for social investment (Lettieri 2006).

Lastly, several countries have stood their ground against the Bretton Woods institutions and neoliberal orthodoxy. The Malaysian government under Prime Minister Datuk Seri Dr. Mahathir Mohamad strongly rejected the "neoliberal orthodoxy of liberalization and financial opening," and engaged in a "systematic counteroffensive designed to mitigate the influence of external economic forces and retain a degree of national policy autonomy" (Beeson 2000, p. 335). In order to achieve this, Malaysia used capital controls to support reflationary monetary policies instead of turning to the IMF when hit by the pressure of the East Asian financial crisis of 1997–1998. In doing so, the country averted the major adverse effects experienced by the surrounding countries of Thailand, South Korea, and Indonesia (Sundaram 2006). Likewise, Argentina set to follow a coherent strategy for negotiating with the IMF, allowing it to set its own terms and achieve much more than anticipated given its economic circumstances (Stiles 1987). Argentina (along with Brazil and Indonesia) repaid its debt to the IMF as a "declaration of independence" from the fund and its conditions (Griesgraber and Ugarteche 2006).

One lesson learned from the experiences above is that governments can change as a result of pressure from below. Public participation can and does play a role in setting public policy in democratic societies. The following example about the defeat of the Multilateral Agreement on Investment demonstrates the power of community organizing.

Multilateral Agreement on Investment and the Council of Canadians

One victory of community and civil society organizing over the power of transnational corporate business is the defeat of the Multilateral Agreement on Investment (MAI) in the 1990s. The 29 countries of the Organization for Economic Cooperation and Development (OECD) began secretly negotiating a global investment treaty that would have granted enormous rights to investors abroad, and would have solidified a set of global investment rules designed to impose tight restrictions on what national governments could and could not do in regulating their economies. Provisions of the OECD MAI agreement would have opened most economic sectors and natural resources to foreign ownership (not subject to environmental laws), required fair and equal treatment of foreign firms, removed restrictions against the movement of capital, and allowed individual firms to sue foreign governments before an international mediation panel (Council of Canadians 1998). In sum, the agreement would have allowed TNCs the unrestricted "right and freedom" to buy, sell, or move their operations whenever and wherever they wanted to around the world, unfettered by national governmental regulation (Council of Canadians 1998). Although TNCs would have had rights equal to nation states in this agreement, there were no corresponding obligations or responsibilities related to jobs, workers, consumers, or the environment. As this chapter has demonstrated, these changes would not have boded well for people's health.

NGO opposition to the MAI treaty was organized quickly, as community groups realized that they would have little say in this global investment treaty. Led by the Council of Canadians, community meetings were held worldwide, and protest marches were organized in opposition to the secret negotiations for the MAI. They produced educational handbooks, held hearings throughout Canada, and brought together a coalition of civil society groups, politicians, citizens, and unions. In the end, this protest was highly successful as the MAI negotiations stalled and eventually fizzled out.

Jubilee Movement

The Jubilee 2000 debt cancellation campaign began in the late 1990s to force the G7 countries "to cancel the unpayable debts of the poorest countries by the year 2000, under a fair and transparent process" (Jubilee Debt Campaign 2008). The campaign was based on readings from the Old Testament of the Bible, wherein a "jubilee" was declared when slaves were freed and debts were forgiven at the turn of every century. In total, by the time 2000 arrived there were 24 million signatories to a global petition and campaigns in over 60 countries that were staffed largely by local volunteers, consulting with citizens and campaigning within each country and around the world. Celebrities were included in the campaign, which relied on support from such world figures such as President Bill Clinton and UN Secretary General Kofi Annan. In the agreement reached at Gleneagles in 2005, US$110 billion in debt relief was declared for the 20 most highly indebted countries. This relief, however, was still accompanied by conditionalities. The Jubilee campaign continues to analyze data on debt and performs research on debt cancellation. There is now a global Jubilee Debt Campaign made up of many of the original members of Jubilee 2000, with a network of organizations in many countries. Similar groups have also joined the global move- ment against burdensome debt, such as the Halifax Initiative (Halifax Initiative 2007) and the Bretton Woods Project (Bretton Woods Project 2007).

50 Years Is Enough

The 50 Years is Enough Network was founded in 1994 during the 50th anniversary of the formation of the Bretton Woods institutions. The aim of the coalition is to radically transform World Bank and IMF policies and practices, to end the imposition of neoliberal economic policies, and to remake the system of loans to poor countries into a more democratic and transparent process. They do this primarily using grass- roots activities and community organizing through 65 country partner groups and 200 grassroots, solidarity, faith-based, economic justice, youth, labor, and development membership organizations (50 Years is Enough Network for Global Economic Justice 2007). The coalition principles call for broad stroke changes in the Bretton Woods organizations, including complete debt cancellation for the poorest countries, an end to SAPs and other conditionalities, transparency in decision processes, reparations for damage from past SAPs, reparations for social and ecological devastation (for dislo- cation, etc.) by World Bank projects, an end to aid to the private sector, and an eval- uation of the institutions by a "truth commission." 50 Years is Enough is a member of the organizing committee of the World Social Forum, and actively participates in public forum debates with leaders from the World Bank and IMF (Danaher 1994).

World Social Forum

The World Social Forum (WSF) was created in 2001 to counterbalance the effects of the Davos World Economic Forum, which meets every January in Switzerland. Using the slogan "Another World is Possible," the WSF challenges the neoliberal economic model as being outdated and harmful to poor people in developing coun- tries. From its humble beginnings in Porto Alegre, Brazil, the WSF has sponsored annual forums in Asia, the Mediterranean, and the United States. In January 2007, over 75,000 attendees were at the Nairobi conference, followed by the first ever

conference in the United States in Atlanta, Georgia. The fora are informed by the
WSF Charter of Principles. Popular grassroots movements make up most of the
membership. According to the organizers, the WSF is:

> an open meeting place where groups and movements of civil society opposed to
> neo-liberalism and a world dominated by capital or by any form of imperialism, but
> engaged in building a planetary society centred on the human person, come together to
> pursue their thinking, to debate ideas democratically, formulate proposals, share their
> experiences freely and network for effective action (World Social Forum 2008).

NGOs Working on Trade and Health

There are a number of organizations challenging the status quo on trade and
health issues. Global Trade Watch (GTW) was founded in 1995 as part of Public
Citizen (an organization founded by Ralph Nader in 1971) (Global Trade Watch
2008). GTW challenges the current mechanisms of globalization (as neither
based on free trade, nor inevitable), promotes government and corporate accountability, performs public education, and lobbies the U.S. Congress on behalf of
those affected by trade issues. GTW was a chief organizer of the opposition to
the WTO meeting in Seattle in 1999. The Center for Policy Analysis on Trade
and Health (CPATH) conducts research, policy analysis, and advocacy on trade
laws in the interest of improving the health of communities and populations.
CPATH is one of the few public health-oriented NGOs that studies trade laws,
analyzes their potential and real effects on public health, and educates the wider
community about the global trade regime (Center for Policy Analysis on Trade
and Health 2008). Their overall goal is to advance global economic policies that
are democratic, sustainable, and economically just. In addition, since the mid-
1990s numerous organizations have coalesced around social justice and health
issues regarding *maquiladora* factory work, sweatshop factory conditions, and
fair trade. Some examples include campaigns run by Global Exchange, No Sweat,
Corporate Watch, and Coop America.

The importance of these movements is illustrated in the issue of fair commodity pricing versus foreign aid. While foreign aid is touted by many international
development specialists as necessary to improve economic growth in developing
countries, there are various other mechanisms that affect economic conditions
more, and more permanently, than aid does, and without creating dependency (see
Chapter 4). For example, in 2004 UNCTAD estimated that subsidies to cotton producers in developed countries resulted in a loss of US$300 million to producers in
Africa—more than the US$230 million in aid provided by the World Bank and the
IMF to cotton producing countries in Africa. The same report noted that coffee-
producing countries earned just US$5.5 billion of the US$70 billion generated from
the retail sale of coffee—illustrating the low returns to primary producers who face

the unpredictability of the commodity market. If trade relations were fair, foreign aid would be unnecessary (UNCTAD 2004).

CONCLUSION

Learning Points:

- Globalization, including financial integration, faster communication, and an internationally mobile labor force, has the potential both to benefit and harm population health.
- Trade liberalization, labor market reorganization, structural adjustment, financial liberalization, and assaults on the environment can all act to harm public health and damage communities.
- Transnational corporations provide employment, but can also harm communities through exploitation of workers, contamination of the environment, and undemocratic political influence.
- International occupational health and safety is a critically neglected area in international health, and one that has not been substantially improved with an increasingly globalized economy.
- Community organizing and advocacy can and have confronted undemocratic and unaccountable global financial and trade institutions and catalyzed change for the better.

Neoliberal globalization, as defined in this chapter, is associated with unregulated markets and policies that favor growth over economic equity, profit over people, and "free trade" over "fair trade." Governments have become weakened as global trade pacts have been pushed onto the rest of the world by the dominant economies, with transnational corporations as their allies. The global economy has resulted in an increased number of absolute poor and near-poor, although its proponents argue that this is a necessary process in order to "lift all boats." Data demonstrate that those economies that have undergone neoliberal structural adjustment have fared equal or worse to those who have not, much to the detriment of the health of those countries.

Globalization affects countries to varying degrees, but is fundamentally unequal and has direct relevance to health inputs in many regions. This chapter discussed the four major pathways through which globalization affects health, and the specific mechanisms through which these take place. First, trade liberalization has not resulted in economic benefits to all trading partners. Freer markets have led, however, to increased exposure to infectious disease, a reduction in available generic medications, an inability of governments to regulate harmful products and food, and increased foreign ownership of essential services for public health (e.g., water/sanitation). The WTO and its agreements (TRIPS, SPS, TBT, GATS) all have potentially undemocratic and deleterious effects on public health, limiting the control that poor nations have over their own public health services, laws, and regulations. Despite the protections for public health in the Doha Declaration, countries' ability to determine their own health and social services is under threat. Transnational corporations play a role in increasing this threat, as evidenced by their involvement in the privatization of public water services in poor communities. TNCs often place market share, trade, and profits before health concerns, and their activities can violate essential human rights that have a direct and indirect effect on health.

Second, TNCs play a large role in global labor markets. The reorganization of labor has led to an increase in low-skilled and poorly paid jobs in developing countries with poor occupational health standards and increased exposure to harmful substances and waste products in the workplace and surrounding community. The health problems in the *maquiladora* industrial belt along the United States–Mexico border are a prime example of the problems created by "free trade zones." Environmental damage, some of which is due to transnational corporate activity, has resulted in communities facing harmful chemicals, waste products, and other substances that have directly impacted their health.

Third, countries that have undergone structural adjustment reforms dictated by the World Bank and IMF have reduced government expenditures on education and health, increased user fees for the poor, and decreased workplace and social protections. The HIPC Initiative (aimed at debt reduction for some of the poorest countries—see Chapter 3) has not been shown to improve health and social outcomes. Fourth, financial liberalization and currency speculation has led to economic crisis in many countries, with resultant worse health indicators especially in Asia and Latin America.

Occupational health and safety has been profoundly affected by the processes of globalization. In some communities standards have improved, but in many others working conditions are no better than those in the developed world 100 years ago. These conditions include child labor, exposure to pathogenic chemicals, and lax occupational health standards. Occupational health services are largely absent for hundreds of millions of the world's working population in developing countries. International labor standards, as advocated by the ILO, are well established international norms. The monitoring and evaluation of adherence to these standards need to be strengthened. Lastly, incentives to export hazardous materials to, and dump waste products in, poor countries have not been eliminated. Rigorous international regulation is required to monitor and prevent this harmful practice.

Challenging the primacy of the neoliberal economic model is possible: communities around the world have organized around health concerns specific to their setting in order to resist and counter unilateral decisions made by undemocratic and unaccountable global institutions such as the WTO, World Bank, and IMF. A world with accountable representation at the trade table, more equal trade relationships, and adequate occupational health and safety measures will undoubtedly change health for the better.

REFERENCES

50 Years is Enough US Network for Global Economic Justice. 2007. About Us. http://www.50years.org/about. Accessed June 30, 2007.

Aaron KK. 2005. Perspective: Big oil, rural poverty, and environmental degradation in the Niger Delta region of Nigeria. *Journal of Agricultural Safety and Health* 11(2):127–134.

Amnesty International. 2007. Violence against women: Demand justice for the women and girls of Ciudad Juárez and Chihuahua, México. http://www.amnestyusa.org/women/juarez. Accessed January 15, 2008.

Associated Press. 2007. Victims of Colombian conflict sue Chiquita Brands, *New York Times*, November 15.

Ban Asbestos Canada. 2007. Who we are. http://www.bacanada.org/main.html. Accessed August 17, 2007.

Beeson M. 2000. Mahathir and the markets: Globalisation and the pursuit of economic autonomy in Malaysia. *Pacific Affairs* 73(3):335–351.

Biggeri M. 2007. The 'resurgence' of globalisation into sub-Saharan Africa: Economic impact and policy implications for human development. Annual Conference on Development and Change, Cape Town, South Africa. December 9–11, 2007.

Bijlmakers L, Bassett M, and Sanders D. 1996. Health and structural adjustment in rural and urban Zimbabwe. Uppsala, Sweden: Nordiska Afrikainstitutet.

Birdsall N. 2006. *Stormy Days on an Open Field: Asymmetries in the Global Economy*. Helsinki: UNU-World Institute for Development Economics Research.

Breilh J, Castelo Branco J, Castelman BI, Cherniak M, Christiani DC, and Cicolella A. 2005. Texaco and its consultants. *International Journal of Occupational and Environmental Health* 11(2):217–220.

Bretton Woods Project. 2007. http://www.brettonwoodsproject.org/. Accessed December 15, 2007.

Broughton E. 2005. The Bhopal disaster and its aftermath: A review. *Environmental Health* 4(1):6.

Brown G. 2005. Protecting workers' health and safety in the globalizing economy through international trade treaties. *International Journal of Occupational and Environmental Health* 11:207–209.

Castleman BI. 1999. Global corporate policies and international "double standards" in occupational and environmental health. *International Journal of Occupational and Environmental Health* 5(1):61–64.

Center for Economic and Social Rights. 1994. Rights violations in the Ecuadorian Amazon: The human consequences of oil development. *Health and Human Rights* 1(1):82–100.

Center for Policy Analysis on Trade and Health. 2008. Globalization and health resource center—Oveview. http://www.cpath.org/id2.html. Accessed January 15, 2008.

Chatterjee P. 2005. India's new patent laws may still hurt generic drug supplies. *Lancet* 365(9468):1378.

Chernomas R, and Sepehri A. 2002. Is globalization a reality, a tendency or a rationale for neoliberal economic policies? *Globalization* 2(2):1–27.

Clapp J. 2001. *Toxic Exports: The Transfer of Hazardous Wastes and Technologies from Rich to Poor Countries*. Ithaca, NY: Cornell University Press.

CNN. 2007. Searchers look for Russian miners. http://www.cnn.com/2007/WORLD/europe/03/20/russia.mine/index.html. Accessed March 20, 2007.

Cohen J. 2006. Expanding drug access in Brazil—Lessons for Latin America and Canada. *Canadian Journal of Public Health* 97(6):I15–I18.

CorpWatch. 2007. *Barrick's dirty secrets: Communities Worldwide Respond to Gold Mining's Impacts. An Alternative Annual Report*. Oakland, CA: CorpWatch.

Corvalan C, Hales S, and McMichael A. 2005. Ecosystems and human well-being: Health synthesis. *A Report of the Millennium Eco-System Assessment*. Geneva: WHO.

Council of Canadians. 1998. The MAI: It could crush Canada—Final report of citizen's inquiry into the MAI. http://www.canadians.org/archive/MAI.html. Accessed October 15, 2007.

Cox RW. 1999. Civil society at the turn of the millennium: Prospects for an alternative world order. *Review of International Studies* 25:3–28.

Danaher K, Editor. 1994. *50 Years is Enough: The Case against the World Bank and the International Monetary Fund*. Boston, MA: South End Press.

Dhara VR, Dhara R, Acquilla SD, and Cullinan P. 2002. Personal exposure and long-term health effects in survivors of the Union Carbide disaster at Bhopal. *Environmental Health Perspectives* 110(5):487–500.

Dollar D. 2001. Is globalization good for your health? *Bulletin of the World Health Organization* 79:827–833.

Editorial. 1992. Let them eat pollution. *Economist* 322 (7745):66.

———. 1998. The sex industry giving the customer what he wants. *Economist* 346(8055):21–23.

EurActiv.com. 2007. EU GMO ban was illegal, WTO rules. http://www.euractiv.com/en/trade/eu-gmo-ban-illegal-wto-rules/article-155197. Accessed September 12, 2007.

Feacham R. 2001. Globalisation is good for your health, mostly. *British Medical Journal* 323:504–506.

Food and Water Watch. 2007. Bechtel profits from dirty water in Guayaquil, Ecuador. http://www.foodandwaterwatch.org/world/latin-america/water-privatization/ecuador. Accessed January 15, 2008.

Forman L. 2006. Trading health for profit: The impact of bilateral and regional free trade agreements on domestic intellectual property rules on pharmaceuticals. In Cohen JC, Illingworth P, and Schuklenk U, Editors. *The Power of Pills: Social, Ethical, and Legal Issues in Drug Development, Marketing, and Pricing*. London: Pluto Press.

Frumkin H. 1999. Across the water and down the ladder: Occupational health in the global economy. *Occupational Medicine* 14(3):637–663.

Gaines J and Palmer K. 2005. Genetically modified organisms and WTO trade rules. *Aussenwirtschaft* 60(1):7–24.

Gautam M. 2003. *Debt Relief for the Poorest: An OED Review of the HIPC Initiative*. Washington, DC: World Bank.

Gershman J, and Irwin A. 2000. Getting a grip on the global economy. In Kim JY, Millen JV, Irwin A, and Gershman J, Editors. *Dying for Growth: Global Inequality and the Health of the Poor*. Monroe, Maine: Common Courage Press.

Global Health Watch. 2005. *Global Health Watch 2005–2006: Alternative World Health Report*. London: Zed Books.

Global Trade Watch. 2008. Global Trade Watch: Promoting democracy by challenging corporate globalization. http://www.citizen.org/trade/. Accessed January 24, 2008.

Government of Guatemala. 1983. Law on the Marketing of Breast-milk Substitutes: Guatemalan Presidential Decree 68–83.

Greenhill R and Sisti E. 2003. *Real Progress Report on HIPC*. London: Jubilee Research.

Griesgraber JM and Ugarteche O. 2006. The IMF today and tomorrow: Some civil society perspectives. *Global Governance* 12(4):351–359.

Guatemalan Ministry of Health. 1993. Memo related to Gerber's Alleged Violations of Guatemalan Presidential Decree 68–83, cited in Wallach L and Woodall P. 2004. *Whose Trade Organization? A Comprehensive Guide to the WTO*. New York: The New Press.

Halifax Initiative. 2007. http://www.halifaxinitiative.org/. Accessed December 16, 2007.

Hess J and Frumkin H. 2000. The international trade in toxic waste: The case of Sihanoukville, Cambodia. *International Journal of Occupational and Environmental Health* 6(4):331–344.

Hirst P and Thompson G. 1996. *Globalization in Question: The International Economy and the Possibilities of Governance*. Cambridge: Polity Press.

Hochschild A. 1998. *King Leopold's Ghost: A Story of Greed, Terror, and Heroism in Colonial Africa*. New York: Houghton Mifflin Company.

Holtz TH. 2000. Tragedy without end, the 1984 Bhopal gas disaster: A narrative of exploitation, fear, and suffering. In Kim JY, Millen JV, Irwin A, and Gershman J, Editors. *Dying for Growth: Global Inequality and the Health of the Poor*. Monroe, Maine: Common Courage Press.

Hopkins S. 2006. Economic stability and health status: Evidence from East Asia before and after the 1990s economic crisis. *Health Policy* 75(3):347–357.

Hovell MF, Sipan C, and Hofstetter R. 1988. Occupational health risks for Mexican women: The case of the maquiladora along the Mexican-U.S. border. *International Journal of Health Services* 18:617–627.

Human Rights Watch. 1997. *Human Rights Watch World Report 1997: Events of 1996*. New York: Human Rights Watch.

Hurtig AK and San Sebastián M. 2002a. Gynecologic and breast malignancies in the Amazon basin of Ecuador, 1985–1998. *International Journal of Gynecology and Obstetrics* 76:199–201.

———. 2002b. Geographical differences in cancer incidence in the Amazon basin of Ecuador in relation to residence near oil fields. *International Journal of Epidemiology* 31:1021–1027.

———. 2004. Incidence of childhood leukemia and oil exploitation in the Amazon basin of Ecuador. *International Journal of Occupational and Environmental Health* 10:245–250.

International Baby Food Action Network. 2004. *Breaking the Rules, Stretching the Rules: Evidence of Violations of the International Code of Marketing of Breast-milk Substitutes and Subsequent Resolutions*. Penang, Malaysia: International Baby Food Action Network.

International Labour Organization. 2005. SafeWork: Codes of practice. http://www.ilo.org/public/english/protection/safework/cops/english/index.htm. Accessed October 10, 2007.

International Monetary Fund (IMF). 2007. Debt relief under the Heavily Indebted Poor Countries (HIPC) initiative. http://www.imf.org/external/np/exr/facts/hipc.htm. Accessed May 12, 2007.

———. 2008. Poverty reduction strategy papers. http://www.imf.org/external/np/exr/facts/prsp.htm. Accessed July 10, 2008.

IRIN. 2007. Côte D'Ivoire: Company settles over toxic waste scandal. http://www.irinnews.org/Report.aspx?ReportId=70185. Accessed March 3, 2008.

Jayaraman KS. 1997. US threat to end science agreement with India over patent law. *Nature* 387(6633):540.

Jenkins R. 2004. Globalization, production, employment and poverty: Debates and evidence. *Journal of International Development* 16(1):1–12.

Joshi TK and Smith K. 2002. Occupational health in India. *Occupational Medicine* 17(3):371–389.

Jubilee Debt Campaign. 2008. http://www.jubileedebtcampaign.org.uk/. Accessed January 15, 2008.

Kim H, Chung WJ, Song YJ, Kang DR, Yi JJ, and Nam CM. 2003. Changes in morbidity and medical care utilization after the recent economic crisis in the Republic of Korea. *Bulletin of the World Health Organization* 81:567–572.

Kimerling J. 1994. The environmental audit of Texaco's Amazon oil fields: Justice or business as usual? *Harvard Human Rights Journal* 7:199–224.

Kristof N. 2006. Slavery in our time. *New York Times*, January 22.

La Botz D. 1994. Manufacturing poverty: The maquiladorization of Mexico. *International Journal of Health Services* 24(3):403–408.

Labonte R and Sanger M. 2006a. Glossary of the World Trade Organisation and public health: Part 1. *Journal of Epidemiology and Community Health* 60(8):665–661.

———. 2006b. Glossary of the World Trade Organisation and public health: Part 2. *Journal of Epidemiology and Community Health* 60(9):738–744.

Labonte R and Schrecker T. 2007. Globalization and social determinants of health: The role of the global marketplace. *Globalization and Health* 3:6, doi:10.1186/1744–8603-3–6.

Labonte R and Torgerson R. 2005. Interrogating globalization, health, and development: Towards a comprehensive framework for research, policy, and political action. *Critical Public Health* 15(2):157–179.

LaDou J. 2003. International occupational health. *International Journal of Hygiene and Environmental Health* 206(4–5):303–313.

———. 2005. World Trade Organization, ILO conventions, and workers' compensation. *International Journal of Occupational and Environmental Health* 11(2):210–211.

Lettieri M. 2006. Bolivia's gas nationalization: Morales does the unthinkable—he carries out his campaign pledge. http://www.coha.org/NEW_PRESS_RELEASES/New_Press_Releases_2006/06.27_Morales_Nationalization.html. Accessed February 20, 2008.

Loff B and Heywood M. 2002. Patents on drugs: Manufacturing scarcity or advancing health? *Journal of Law, Medicine, and Ethics* 30(4):621–631.

London L. 2008. Worker health and safety: International issues. In Heggenhougen H, Editor. *Encyclopedia of Public Health*. Oxford: Elsevier Publishers.

London L and Kisting S. 2002. Ethical concerns in international occupational health. *Occupational Medicine* 17(4):587–600.

Mabika A and Makombe P. 2006. Claiming our space: Using the flexibilities in the TRIPS agreement to protect access to medicines. Policy Series No. 16. Harare, Zimbabwe: EQUINET and SEATINI.

Mann J, Gostin L, Gruskin S, Brennan T, Lazzarini Z, and Fineberg HV. 1994. Health and human rights. *Health and Human Rights* 1(1):6–23.

Masud T and Masud C, Directors. 2003. A Kind of Childhood. A Xingu Films/Audiovision Production in association with TV Ontario.

Mehta PS, Mehta AS, Mehta SJ, and Makhijani AB. 1990. Bhopal tragedy's health effects: A review of methyl isocyanate toxicity. *Journal of the American Medical Association* 264(21):2781–2787.

Meyer WH. 1996. Human rights and MNCs: Theory versus quantitative analysis. *Human Rights Quarterly* 18(2):368–397.

Morley S and Vos R. 2004. *Bad Luck or Wrong Policies? External Shocks, Domestic Adjustment, and the Growth Slowdown in Latin America and the Caribbean.* Working Paper Series No. 398. The Hague: Institute of Social Studies.

Moure-Eraso R, Wilcox M, Punnett L, Copeland L, and Levenstein C. 1994a. Back to the future: Sweatshop conditions on the Mexican-U.S. border. I. Community health impact of maquiladora industrial activity. *American Journal of Industrial Medicine* 25(3):311–324.

Moure-Eraso R, Wilcox M, Punnett L, MacDonald L, and Levenstein C. 1994b. Back to the future: Sweatshop conditions on the Mexican-U.S. border. II. Occupational health impact of maquiladora industrial activity. *American Journal of Industrial Medicine* 31(5):587–599.

National Labor Committee. 1996. *The U.S. in Haiti: How to Get Rich on 11 Cents an Hour.* New York: National Labor Committee Education Fund.

———. 2005. Wal-Mart dungeon in China. http://www.nlcnet.org/campaigns/archive/report00/walmart.shtml. Accessed January 8, 2005.

Parayre C. 2006. World dumps toxic waste in Africa. http://health.iafrica.com/features/211720.htm. Accessed September 26, 2006.

Peabody JW. 1996. Economic reform and health sector policy: Lessons from structural adjustment programs. *Social Science and Medicine* 43(5):823–835.

Pettifor A, Thomas B, and Telatin M. 2001. *HIPC: Flogging a Dead Process.* London: Jubilee Research.

Play Fair 2008 Campaign. 2008. Clearing the hurdles: STEPS to improving wages and working conditions in the global sportswear industry. http://www.playfair2008.org/docs/Clearing_the_Hurdles.pdf. Accessed September 15, 2008.

Press E. 1996. No sweat: The fashion industry patches its image. *The Progressive* 60(9):30–32.

Rantanen J, Lehtinen S, and Mikheev M. 1993. Health protection and health promotion in small-scale enterprises: Proceedings of the Joint ILO/WHO Task Group, November 1 3. Helsinki: Finnish Institute of Occupational Health.

Rao M and Loewenson R. 2000. *The Political Economy of the Assault on Health. People's Health Assembly Background Papers.* Dhaka, Bangladesh: People's Health Assembly.

Ross A, Editor. 1997. *No Sweat: Fashion, Free Trade, and the Rights of Garment Workers.* New York: Verso.

San Sebastián M, Armstrong B, Cordoba JA, and Stephens C. 2001. Exposures and cancer incidence near oil fields in the Amazon basin of Ecuador. *Journal of Occupational and Environmental Medicine* 58(4):517–522.

San Sebastián M, Armstrong B, and Stephens C. 2002. Outcomes of pregnancy among women living in the proximity of oil fields in the Amazon basin of Ecuador. *International Journal of Occupational and Environmental Health* 8(4):312–319.

Seymour C. 1996. Independent monitoring in El Salvador. *The Progressive* 60(10):13.

Shaffer ER, Waitzkin H, Brenner J, and Jasso-Aguilar R. 2005. Global trade and public health. *American Journal of Public Health* 95(1):23–34.

Sharma D. 2002. Bhopal's health disaster continues to unfold. *Lancet* 360(9336):859.

Smith C. 2000. The precautionary principle and environmental policy: Science, uncertainty, and sustainability. *International Journal of Occupational and Environmental Health* 6(3):263–265.

Smith RD. 2006. Trade and public health: Facing the challenges of globalisation. *Journal of Epidemiology Community Health* 60(8):650–651.

Stiglitz J. 2002. *Globalization and its Discontents.* New York: W.W. Norton and Co.

Stiles KW. 1987. Argentina's bargaining with the IMF. *Journal of Interamerican Studies and World Affairs* 29(3):55–85.

Stuckler D, King LP, and Basu S. 2008. International Monetary Fund programs and tuberculosis outcomes in post-communist countries. *PLoS Medicine* 5(7):e143.

Sundaram JK. 2006. Pathways through financial crisis: Malaysia. *Global Governance* 12 (4):489–505.

Takala J. 2002. Life and health are fundamental rights for workers. *Labour Education.* 126(1).

Tauli-Corpuz V. 1996. The Marcopper toxic mine disaster. *Third World Resurgence* 69:2. http://www.twnside.org.sg/title/toxic-ch.htm. Accessed September 20, 2008.

Thomson JG. 1963. Exposure to asbestos dust and diffuse pleural mesotheliomas. *British Medical Journal* 1(5323):123.

UNDP. 1999. *Human Development Report 1999: Globalization with a Human Face.* New York: Oxford University Press for the UNDP.

UNCTAD. 2004. *Least Developed Countries Report 2004: Linking International Trade with Poverty Reduction.* New York: United Nations.

UNICEF. 2006. Child protection from violence, exploitation, and abuse: Child labour. http://www.unicef.org/protection/index_childlabour.html. Accessed October 15, 2007.

United Nations Economic and Social Commission for Asia and the Pacific. 2007. Commercial sexual exploitation of children. http://www.unescap.org/esid/gad/issues/csec/index.asp. Accessed May 27, 2007.

United Nations Economic Commission for Africa. 2008. Economic Commission for Africa. http://www.uneca.org/. Accessed February 25, 2008.

Wallach L and Woodall P. 2004. *Whose Trade Organization? A Comprehensive Guide to the WTO.* New York: The New Press.

Watson C. 2003. *Sell the Rain: How the Privatization of Water caused Riots in Cochabamba.* Bolivia. CBC Radio report. February 4, 2003.

Weisbrot M, Baker D, Kraev E, and Chen J. 2002. The scorecard on globalization 1980–2000: Its consequences for economic and social well-being. *International Journal of Health Services* 32(2):229–253.

Weisbrot M, Baker D, and Rosnick D. 2006. The scorecard on development: 25 years of diminished progress. *International Journal of Health Services* 36(2):211–234.

Welch C. 2000. Structural adjustment programs and poverty reduction strategy. *Foreign Policy in Focus* 5(14).

Wesselink E and Weller E. 2006. Oil and violence in Sudan: Drilling, poverty and death in Upper Nile state. http://www.multinationalmonitor.org/mm2006/052006/wesselink.html. Accessed September 15, 2008.

West L. 2006. Bolivian president seizes oil and natural gas fields. http://environment.about.com/b/2006/05/03/bolivian-president-seizes-oil-and-natural-gas-fields.htm. Accessed February 20, 2008.

Willis BM and Levy BS. 2002. Child prostitution: Global health burden, research needs and interventions. *The Lancet* 359(9315):1417–1422.

World Bank. 2007. *Global Economic Prospects 2007: Managing the Next Wave of Globalization.* Washington, DC: World Bank.

World Health Organization. 1981. International Code of Marketing of Breast-milk Substitute. Geneva: WHO.

———. 2001. Commission on Macroeconomics and Health. Anna Breman and Carolyn Shelton. Structural Adjustment and Health: A literature review of the debate, its role-players and presented empirical evidence Working Paper WG6: 6. Geneva: WHO.

———. 2003. *The Right to Water.* Geneva: WHO.

———. 2004. *PRSPs: Their Significance for Health: Second Synthesis Report.* Geneva: WHO.

———. 2007. Occupational health. http://www.who.int/occupational_health/en/. Accessed October 15, 2007.

World Social Forum 2008. January 26, 2008—Act Together for Another World! http://wsf2008.net/. Accessed February 20, 2008.

World Trade Organization. 2001. Declaration on the TRIPS agreement and public health http://www.wto.org/English/thewto_e/minist_e/min01_e/mindecl_trips_e.htm. Accessed December 10, 2007

Yamin AE. 2005. The future in the mirror: Incorporating strategies for the defense and promotion of economic, social and cultural rights into the mainstream human rights agenda. *Human Rights Quarterly* 27(4):1200–1244.

10

Health and the Environment

Worldwide environmental conditions have changed more rapidly in the past half-century than at any other time in human history, shaped and strained by economic, social, and military exploits. Increases in agricultural output have been accompanied by pollution from fertilizers, pesticides, and excessive irrigation. Wars have displaced millions of people, with weapons producing dangerous radiation and chemical toxins. Continuing to this day, manufacture of high-demand disposable electronics generates harmful waste; oil drilling and spills challenge ecosystems, and destroy bird and fish habitats; coal mining denudes mountainsides and its by-products threaten water and wildlife; and the burning of fossil fuels contaminates and heats the earth's atmosphere.

Yet environmental degradation—and its harm to health—is not inevitable: it is provoked by a range of human activities, including industrial production, energy extraction and use, transportation, consumption, conflict, migration, and urbanization. Looming as they may seem, environmental health problems and their driving forces can be mitigated, and even reversed, through concerted, collective efforts at community, national, and global levels.

The term environment refers not just to our natural surroundings and resources, but also to built conditions—that is, the constructed spaces of work, home, transport, and recreation, from planned cityscapes, to jerrybuilt dwellings, to industrial sprawl. The context of social relations may also be understood in environmental

---

Box 10–1 Definitions

Natural Environment

• Physical, chemical, and biological factors and processes external to people, though potentially of their making.

(*continued*)

Box 10–1 Continued

Built Environment

- Human-made settings, such as buildings, housing, sanitation, and transportation systems, whether part of large cityscapes, roadways, or small settlements.

Social Environment

- Conditions within which people live and work, as shaped by cultural, historical, social, economic, and political relations and factors.

Ecology

- Study of the relationships and interactions between living organisms and their environment.

Ecosystem

- System formed by the interaction of a community of organisms and their natural environment, usually geographically defined.

Political ecology

- Understanding of the relationship and tensions between natural (environmental) and anthropogenic (human-led) change.

Sources: Evans (2002); Prüss-Üstün and Corvalán (2006).

---

terms; since we have covered social perspectives in depth in Chapter 7, here we focus on the natural and built environment.

This chapter explores the most pressing environmental health concerns facing communities and countries across the globe and the many issues that go beyond borders. We begin with a historical overview of human interaction with the environment. Next, we develop an explanatory framework for understanding the political, social, and ecological variables involved in environmental change, the consequent human health implications, and the varied levels at which these problems can be addressed, together with tools for analyzing different approaches to environmental health. This framework is applied to the situation of global warming. We then turn to the causes and impact on health of the overuse and misuse of the most important natural resources—air, water, soil, and forests—and the implications of these patterns for the built environment. Finally, we discuss a range of policies and practices at global, national, local, and individual levels that seek to address environmental health problems.

POLITICAL ECOLOGY IN THE PAST: INTERACTION OF HUMANS WITH THE NATURAL AND BUILT ENVIRONMENTS

Long-term survival has historically depended on maintaining the assets of the natural environment. During most of the 150,000 years that *Homo sapiens* are known to have existed, they lived as hunter-gatherer societies—small nomadic communities that made tools and obtained food and supplies within the limits of their local environments, moving to nearby lands as needed. Collective human efforts to control nature began some 10,000 to 15,000 years ago, as the domestication of plant and animal species initiated a gradual transition to agriculturalism. Stable settlements began several millennia later in the fertile crescent of the Middle East. Thus, for well over 90% of human history, humans minimally affected their surroundings (McMichael 2001).

The advent of agriculture transformed social and economic relations, with accompanying effects on the built and natural environments. As settlements grew, land productivity increased and crop surpluses were generated. Water began to be irrigated and more and more land was cleared. Approximately 5,000 years ago, cities arose, first in the Middle East and North Africa, then in Asia and the Americas, later in Europe. Gradually, societies became stratified by wealth and power, and local leaders began to fight over territory and resources. To accumulate further wealth, rivals captured and enslaved agricultural workers (or tied peasants to the land as serfs) and began to build monuments and cities and acquire precious metals and minerals as testaments to their power. Quarries and mines were constructed and early systems of commerce developed.

By the Middle Ages (900–1500), extractive industries had become an important source of trade and wealth. With the growth of towns, the clearing of forests, and the development of small industries, particularly in Europe, the Middle East, and Asia, energy use began to rise, and mined coal became a necessary counterpart to wood-burning. As cities and industries grew, so did rat populations. Urban filth, combined with growing trade, facilitated the largest pandemic ever: the 300-year long Black Death (plague), which killed an estimated 85 million people, approximately one-third of the European and Central Asian populations at that time.

The exploitation of natural resources rose rapidly during the transition from feudalism to capitalism and with the rise of colonialism, starting in the 16th century. After European kingdoms were consolidated, monarchs—backed by noblemen and a growing merchant class—turned to more distant lands for resources, labor, wealth, and power. The military conquest and political subjugation of peoples across the Americas, Africa, Asia, and the Pacific was also an environmental occupation. Colonial administrators strained local environments through forest clearing, mining, and the building of transport routes, with deleterious health effects on local populations and millions of slaves and forced laborers.

In colonial Mexico, for example, sanitary and living conditions, and their associated gastrointestinal, respiratory, and vector-borne mortality, worsened markedly due to environmental changes. Traditionally, through regular refuse collection and extensive sanitary and hygienic measures, the Mexica (Aztecs) kept the streets, markets, and plazas of their capital Tenochtitlán conspicuously clean. Moreover, waste water was carefully separated from the clean sources of Lake Texcoco which surrounded the city (Soustelle 1970; Ortiz de Montellano 1990). But after Tenochtitlán was destroyed and rebuilt as Mexico City under Spanish rule, Lake Texcoco was transformed into a giant cesspool: swampy landfill projects, heavy canal commerce, and inadequate sewage disposal generated frequent flooding, contamination, and mosquito breeding sites, with enormous negative health consequences (Cooper 1965).

While all civilizations—including Chinese, Egyptian, Greek, Roman, and Inca—subsumed nature in their quest for progress (Dauvergne 2005a), the scale and character of the European imperial enterprise made its environmental impact far larger. By 1800, mercantilism (the creation of a colonial market system based on sale and circulation of labor and products) was yielding huge profits. This commercial impetus, together with scientific and technical advances (in production, then transport and communications) and social policies pushing peasants off the land, gave rise to a new economic order—capitalism—based on the private ownership of enterprise and free market economic principles.

With the advent of the Industrial Revolution, vastly expanded energy use and urban immiseration caused enormous environmental damage, initially concentrated in Europe. Filthy emanations from factory smokestacks, including sulfur, chlorine, ammonia, and methane, blackened the air of countless towns and the lungs of their residents, as commemorated in William Blake's 1804 poetic reference to "dark satanic mills" and their destruction of nature. Rivers thick with industrial, human, and animal waste (the Thames River in London was infamously known as "Monster Soup") supplied drinking water in tenement cities and also downstream, causing countless deaths from ingesting toxins. Contaminated water elevated rates of infant and child mortality due to cholera, diarrhea, and other gastrointestinal ailments in both town and countryside. The deadly mix of environmental contamination and dangerous occupational and living conditions led death rates to rise across the industrial belt.

Worker struggles against noxious working and living conditions in the 19th and early 20th centuries served as precursors to modern environmental movements. Still, industrial production, urban degradation, and the large-scale depletion and contamination of life's essentials—air, groundwater, forests, and soil—have continued. Indeed, the magnitude of environmental change since 1900 is almost unfathomable. According to Tony McMichael, one of the world's leading environmental health specialists:

During the twentieth century we humans doubled our average life expectancy, quadrupled the size of our population, increased the global food yield six fold, water consumption six fold, the production of carbon dioxide twelve fold, and the overall level of economic activity twenty fold. In so doing we had, by the turn of the century, exceeded the planet's carrying capacity by approximately 30%. That is, we are now operating in ecological deficit. These rates of change in human demography, economic activity, and environmental conditions are unprecedented in history (McMichael 2001, p. 319).

Of late, environmental health problems in developing countries have become even worse than in developed countries, as the economic processes of recent decades have accelerated industrialization, commerce, migration, exploitation, and extraction in Asia, Latin America, and Africa.

POLITICAL ECONOMY OF ENVIRONMENTAL HEALTH: DETERMINANTS, EFFECTS, AND RESPONSES

Key Questions:

- What are the most pressing environmental issues in your neighborhood and country?
- What is creating and exacerbating these problems?
- What is being done or could be done to address them?

As far back as the 5th century BCE, Hippocrates observed the influence of climate on disease patterns in ancient Greece. His *Airs, Waters, Places* began:

> Whoever wishes to investigate medicine properly should proceed thus: First, he ought to consider what effects each season of the year can produce; for the seasons are not at all alike, but differ widely both in themselves and at their changes. The next point is the hot winds and the cold, especially those that are universal but also those that are peculiar to each particular region... for with the seasons, men's diseases, like their digestive organs, suffer change (Hippocrates 1868).

Today we count on large-scale data collection and scientific research to provide evidence regarding the relationship between health and the environment. As presented in Figure 10–1, an understanding that human activity is at the core of environmental health problems requires us to transcend analysis of individual behavior. The forces driving the global economy—industrial and agricultural production, resource exploitation and contamination, energy extraction and use, transportation and building patterns, militarism, inadequate regulation, and market-driven consumption patterns—place mounting pressure on the built and natural environments. The changes experienced in, to use Hippocrates's term, "airs, waters, and places" include damage/depletion of ozone, wetlands, coastal reefs, forests, land, plant, and animal species, and living spaces. These ecosystem and built environment alterations generate a range of direct, mediated, and indirect human health consequences. Fortunately, as we will discuss later in the chapter, this is not the end of the story: sustained political and organized responses can help mitigate or reverse underlying forces and pressures, environmental changes, and health consequences at household, municipal, ecosystem, and larger political levels.

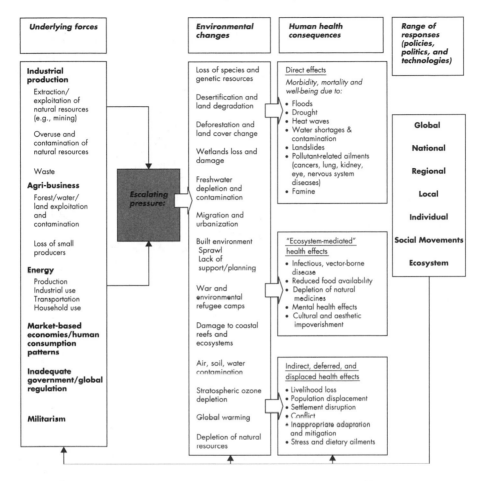

Figure 10–1 Political economy of environmental health determinants, effects, and responses. *Sources*: Adapted from WHO (2005); and UNEP (2007b).

Applying the Framework to Climate Change

How might our political economy of environmental health framework explain a particular environmental problem? Here we start with climate change—its existence, its underlying forces, its health implications, and the responses necessary to stem the problem.

The Underlying Forces

In recent years, the phenomenon of global warming has been splayed across the media with doomsday predictions of the decreasing livability of the earth. Climate records date only to the 19th century, but geological evidence suggests that temperature rises over the last century have exceeded those of every other century in the last millennium (Dauvergne 2005a), with the 1990s as the warmest decade on record (IPCC 2001). There is now overwhelming scientific consensus from over 2,000 scientists in 100 countries—the United Nations (UN) Intergovernmental Panel on Climate Change (IPCC)—that global warming is taking place and that it is related to human activities, mainly the burning of fossil fuels. Global warming's ecological and human health effects include melting polar icecaps, rising sea levels, severe storms, new diseases, and droughts (IPCC 2007a; UNFCCC 2007).

How has this happened? The earth's temperature is warmed, rendering the earth habitable through the "greenhouse effect," whereby naturally occurring gases trap the heat of the sun and raise the temperature of the atmosphere. However, the greenhouse effect has been magnified over recent centuries through the increasing emission of "greenhouse gases" generated by human activities. Over the last 30 years alone, the earth's temperature is estimated to have risen by 1°C and is projected to rise by between 2°C and 10°C by 2100 in the absence of concerted efforts to control emissions.

Global concentrations of the three main greenhouse gases (carbon dioxide [CO_2], methane [CH_4], and nitrous oxide [N_2O]) have increased markedly since 1750 and now greatly exceed preindustrial levels. These gases arise from electricity generation, factory-based production, motor vehicle use, agriculture and land-use changes, and forest clearing, all of which constitute core activities in modern economies (Clapp and Dauvergne 2005b). Between 1973 and 1998 total consumption of goods doubled, and there has been a fourfold rise in energy consumption since 1950. Fossil-fuel combustion accounts for 75% to 85% of the rise in atmospheric CO_2 concentration, with deforestation accounting for the remaining 15% to 25% (Bierbaum et al. 2007).

Some argue that population increase is the prime causal factor of global warming. However, the regions with the largest per capita fossil fuel emissions have smaller populations and lower population increases than other regions. Combined, North America and Western Europe, with fewer than 12% of the world's population, account for over 60% of total private energy consumption, and the United States alone consumes 30% of the world's energy resources (see Table 10–1). South Asia and sub-Saharan Africa, by contrast, have one-third of the world's population and account for a mere 3.2% of world energy consumption (Dauvergne 2005a).

As such, population per se is far less of a driving force in fossil fuel emissions than are the industrial and market forces that frame production and consumption patterns. Of course, virtually every industry in every country releases greenhouse gases, and most people use at least some of these products, travel in vehicles, and employ energy from the burning of fossil fuels. But contribution to the problem differs between countries—by level of development and marketization of the economy—and within countries, by social class and other factors.

In 2004, underdeveloped countries (over 80% of the world's population) and OECD nations emitted roughly equal quantities of CO_2, meaning per capita energy

Table 10–1 World CO_2 Emissions (Billion Metric Tons) by Region

Region	1990	2004
North America	11.4	13.5
Northern and Western Europe	5.8	6.9
Japan and South Korea	4.1	4.4
Former Soviet Union	1.5	2.2
Asia	9.8	13.5
Middle East	0.7	1.3
Africa	0.6	0.9
Central and South America	0.7	1.0
Total	21.2	26.9

Source: Adapted from U.S. Department of Energy (2007, p. 74).

consumption (and emissions) were 3.5 times higher in wealthy (OECD) than in poorer nations (U.S. Department of Energy 2007). India, with 16% of the world's population, accounted for approximately 4% of global CO_2 emissions, whereas the United States, one-fourth the size of India, generated 25% of world emissions (Global Health Watch 2005). Rapidly growing economies—most notably China and India—are increasing polluters due to booming industrial development, soaring energy use for production and transportation, urbanization, and higher consumption levels stemming from income increases among urban middle and upper classes. Still, per capita emissions levels trail those of high-income OECD nations. For example, China is soon expected to surpass the United States as the world's single biggest polluter, although per capita emissions in the United States remain more than three times higher than China's.

Health Consequences of Climate Change

Like other environmental changes outlined in Figure 10–1, global warming has led to, and is likely to further exacerbate, a range of human health problems, including seasonal malnutrition due to drought-induced food shortages and the loss of millions of hectares of habitable and arable land (see Box 10–2). Such changes are already provoking enormous ecological disruptions, with direct and indirect health effects. For example, during the 2003 European heat wave, temperatures were 10°C above the 30-year average, resulting in 21,000–35,000 deaths (Epstein 2005). In Niger, children born in drought years in the early 2000s were 72% more likely to be stunted (UNDP 2007).

Persistent temperature changes over the last decades have also led to altered patterns of precipitation. Arid and semi-arid regions are becoming drier, while other areas are becoming wetter. Polar ice caps are melting, and there has been a disproportionate increase in the frequency of heavy storms. As a consequence, ocean levels rose by an average of 10 to 20 cm during the 20th century (Dauvergne 2005b).

Weather-related changes, in turn, may cause the proliferation of water- and air-borne pathogens (WHO 2002b). Longer rainy seasons result in indoor crowding, and increased interpersonal contact encourages the spread of measles, lower respiratory tract infections, and diarrhea. Likewise, desertification or deforestation can displace mosquito or rodent populations, thereby altering patterns of vector-borne diseases (Corvalán, Hales, and McMichael 2005).

Mosquitoes, which transmit malaria, yellow fever, dengue, and other diseases, are also very sensitive to temperature changes. Rain and stagnant water create ideal breeding sites, while warmer weather:

> boosts their rates of reproduction and the number of blood meals they take, prolongs their breeding season, and shortens the maturation period for the microbes they disperse. In highland regions, as permafrost thaws and glaciers retreat, mosquitoes and plant communities are migrating to higher ground (Epstein 2005, p. 1435).

Climate shifts may lead other vector-borne diseases, such as schistosomiasis, to spread and new diseases to emerge. According to the WHO, 30 new diseases appeared between 1976 and 1996, including Ebola and West Nile virus; many are linked to climate change.

Given that two-thirds of the world's population lives within 60 km of the sea line, rising sea levels could displace millions of people, greatly diminish availability of arable land, and damage fresh water aquifers and fisheries (McMichael 2001; Smith et al. 2003; IPCC 2007b). These changes could provoke loss of livelihood, malnutrition, childhood stunting, and increased susceptibility to disease.

Box 10–2 Climate Change and Human Development

The UNDP identifies five main mechanisms through which climate change (an increase in temperature by 2°C or more) may stall and/or reverse human development (UNDP 2007):

1. Reduced agricultural production and food security.
2. Water stress and water insecurity.
3. Rising sea levels and exposure to climate disasters.
4. Ecosystems and biodiversity.
5. Human health.

Responses to Climate Change

The scientific consensus on the role of fossil fuel burning in global warming is an important initial step in developing responses. After all, powerful industrial interests, together with their political allies (and some scientists), have long contested both the existence of climate change and the causative role of emissions. But recognition does not automatically lead to change.

To cite just one contributor to greenhouse emissions, there are 800 million road vehicles worldwide, which account for nearly half of all global oil consumption (Dauvergne 2005a). At the local and personal levels, development and use of affordable and comprehensive subway and rail systems and extensive (and safe) bike and walking paths can help to reduce vehicle emissions. But building and using alternate forms of transportation are only part of the story. The oil, automobile, and road construction industries wield enormous power and are formidable opponents of collective transport in the United States and many other places. As well, numerous features of the built environment—such as unplanned and unregulated commercial, industrial, and urban growth—shape automobile overuse.

Certainly the consequences of global warming go "beyond the lifetimes of politicians and business leaders." More importantly, lowering "greenhouse gas emissions will require significant changes to global economic production and consumption patterns. It will require, too, governmental, corporate, and personal sacrifices" (Dauvergne 2005a, p. 390). Of course, global warming is just one of a multitude of environmental health concerns that extend to natural resource contamination and depletion, industrial and consumer waste, unsafe housing, and exposure to chemical toxins.

As we will explore further in the last section of the chapter, the political economy perspective means that household and community actions, valuable as they are, must be combined with national and global efforts to address the underlying determinants of environmental problems.

Environmental Worldviews and Ecological Footprints

There are four main ways of understanding environmental concerns:

Box 10–3 Four Environmental Worldviews, as Identified by Jennifer Clapp and Peter Dauvergne

Market Liberals: As proponents of neoliberal economics, market liberals hold that "economic growth and high per capita incomes are essential for human welfare and the maintenance of sustainable development" (Clapp and Dauvergne 2005, p. 6). Conversely, they believe that the main causes of environmental degradation "are lack of economic growth, poverty, distortions and failures of the market, and bad policies" (ibid). Advocates of market liberalism, such as the WTO and the World Business Council for Sustainable Development, hold that voluntary corporate efforts—together with market pressures—will ultimately improve environmental management, although inequalities may worsen in the short run. Rejecting the catastrophic urgency of environmental degradation, market liberals emphasize scientific approaches to environmental problems based on ingenuity, technology, and cooperation.

Institutionalists: Sharing market liberal assumptions regarding economic growth, trade, foreign investment, and technology, institutionalists "emphasize the need for stronger global institutions

(continued)

Box 10–3 Continued

and norms as well as sufficient state and local capacity to constrain and direct the global political economy" (Clapp and Dauvergne 2005, p. 9). Institutionalists believe that improved global governance and consensus-building offer effective means of enhancing environmental cooperation and management. Institutionalists support the diffusion of knowledge and resources from developed to developing countries, as well as collective action, to forestall further environmental deterioration.

Bioenvironmentalists: Often scientific activists, bioenvironmentalists emphasize that humans—due to population growth and patterns of consumption—consume far too much of the planet's finite and fragile resources, and that the earth's capacity to sustain this level of consumption has already been or will soon be surpassed. Holding that "we must respect the biophysical limits to growth: both for people and economies" (Clapp and Dauvergne 2005, p. 10), bioenvironmentalists view limits to economic growth, curbs on immigration to high-consumption countries, individual approaches to lowered consumption, and family planning as key solutions to environmental degradation.

Social Greens: Social greens draw on radical social and economic theories that consider political, economic, and environmental problems to be inseparable. Like bioenvironmentalists, social greens believe that there are physical limits to economic growth and that overconsumption in industrialized countries is at least partially to blame. However, social greens reject bioenvironmentalist positions on population growth (and control) as an assault on the rights of women and marginalized peoples around the world. Instead, social greens call for a major overhaul of the global economic system to reduce social inequalities, and many advocate the abandonment of industrial and capitalist life for self-reliant, small-scale economic communities (Clapp and Dauvergne 2005).

A useful concept to assess the impact of human actions on the natural environment is the "ecological footprint" (developed by Canadian ecologists Bill Rees and Mathis Wackernagle in 1996), which translates human consumption of renewable natural resources into hectares of average biologically productive land (Dauvergne 2005a). An *individual's* ecological footprint is the total area in productive hectares required to sustain his or her way of life including use of food, water, energy, household materials, and other goods and services. The *global* ecological footprint changes with average consumption per person, resource efficiency, and population size.

Ecological footprints are also used to gauge the rate at which consumption patterns compare to the natural environment's ability to renew itself. In 2001, the World Wildlife Fund estimated that the global ecological footprint was 13.5 billion global hectares, or 2.2 global hectares per person, while globally the biologically productive area was 11.3 billion hectares or 1.8 hectares per person; thus, consumption patterns require over 20% more ecological productivity per person than the earth's biocapacity can sustain (Loh and Wackernagel 2004).

There is considerable regional variation in the magnitude of ecological footprints (Fig. 10–2). Though the *global* average ecological footprint was 2.3 hectares per person in 2003, the ecological footprint of someone in the United States—with the largest national footprint—was 9.6 hectares. By contrast, in Malawi, the average person's ecological footprint was 0.6 hectares per year (Schaefer et al. 2006).

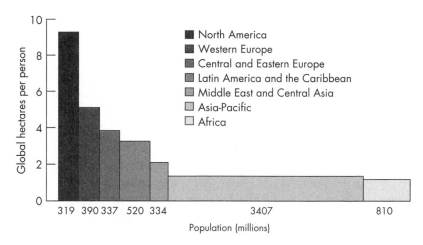

Figure 10–2 Ecological footprints: A global snapshot.
Source: Courtesy of Global Footprint Network (2006).

Carbon footprints (measuring greenhouse gas production) for U.S. cities are almost twice as high as in large European cities, reflecting more urban sprawl, less public transport, and higher consumption rates (Beatley 2000).

While ecological footprints offer a useful snapshot of the environmental effects of consumption, they do not disaggregate the environmental effects of production versus consumption (nor of different population groups within countries) or the ways in which consumption is framed by the global system of market economics. As such, footprints reflect an almost purely bioenvironmentalist view that puts human consumption and behavior change at the center of its environmental strategy.

HEALTH PROBLEMS ARISING FROM ENVIRONMENTAL CONDITIONS

In 2006, the WHO estimated that almost *one-fourth of all* diseases and deaths were caused by modifiable environmental factors (see Table 10–2) (Prüss-Üstün and Corvalán 2006). While all people are affected by unhealthy environmental conditions, those living in poverty experience a disproportionate amount of mortality and morbidity arising from depletion and contamination of natural resources and from unhealthy effects of the built environment. Marginalized populations also face greater exposure to the hazardous by-products of resource extraction, manufacturing, and other industrial processes (Doyal 1979; Howard and Newby 2004) and to displacement and destruction caused by war.

The differential impact of environmental factors within or across countries arises from varying levels of exposure to contaminants and from differing underlying

Table 10–2 The Impact of Environmental Problems and Conditions on Health

Problematic Environmental Practices and Conditions	Health Impact
Inadequate supplies of clean water and sanitation access	• 1.5 million deaths annually (Prüss-Üstün and Corvalán 2006) • 88% of all cases of diarrhea (WHO 2006b)
Household use of biomass fuels and coal	• 1.6 million deaths annually due to respiratory disease (WHO 2006a)
Deforestation and other policies regarding land use, house design, water management	• 42% of annual malaria cases (Prüss-Üstün and Corvalán 2006) • Malnutrition
Urban ambient air pollution in developing countries	• 130,000 premature deaths annually (WHO EURO 2006)

social and political conditions, which affect susceptibility and resistance to, access to prevention and treatment for, and regulation of environmental problems (see Fig. 10–3). For example, in Africa, Asia, and Latin America, between one-fourth and one-half of the population lives in informal settlements or on the outskirts of cities with little or no access to clean water, sanitation, and other public services and no effective regulation of pollution or ecosystem degradation (Corvalán, Hales, and McMichael 2005).

In this section we outline an important array of environmental health problems, including industrial and military contaminants and waste, air pollution, and the overuse and misuse of water, land, and forests, all interacting with the spaces and places where people work and live.

It is important to reiterate that the environment does not simply refer to natural resources and the need to conserve and protect them but also to the built environment, which directly affects health and facilitates or mitigates resource use and degradation. The built environment refers to commercial, public, and industrial buildings, dwellings, transportation, roads, and other infrastructure, as well as policies relating to land use, zoning, and community design (or lack thereof). The health effects of the built environment include both indoor and outdoor (ambient) factors. The larger features of the built environment influence health, for example, via the distances and nature of travel to work and to obtain needed services and food, the safety and conditions of neighborhoods (abandoned "slums" as opposed to continuously designed areas with services and upkeep), and the existence of green space. Built structures may generate health dangers through their very construction, such as through poor ventilation systems, use of toxic building materials, and inadequate structural protection against floods, landslides, storms, and other disasters (see Chapter 8).

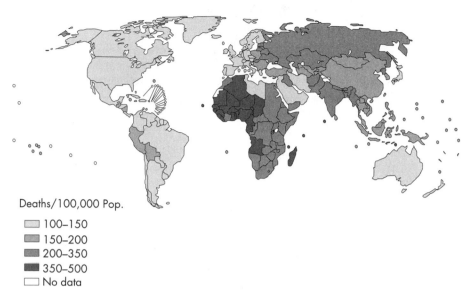

Deaths/100,000 Pop.
- 100–150
- 150–200
- 200–350
- 350–500
- No data

Figure 10–3 Environmental disease burden by WHO subregion, 2002.
Source: Prüss-Üstün and Corvalán (2006, p. 10).

Table 10–3 provides an overview of important agents of environmental health problems that enter the air, water, soil, food chain, and built environment, thus making their way to humans.

Box 10–4 Child Health and the Environment

The WHO attributes over one-third of childhood deaths (under the age of 14) to environmental causes, with rates 12 times higher in developing than in developed countries (Prüss-Üstün and Corvalán 2006). Children are vulnerable to environmental factors for both biological and developmental reasons. From a physiological perspective, children eat, breathe, and drink proportionally more than adults, thus taking in far higher concentrations of the toxins in our environment (Hjertaas and Taylor 2002). Children are particularly susceptible to toxins at young ages, when their tendency to explore and put objects and hands in their mouths exacerbates exposure. Small doses of certain toxins (such as lead, mercury, and pesticides) can cause permanent developmental abnormalities, including learning disabilities, reproductive problems, endocrine disruption, cognitive deficits, and cancer (Daniels, Olshan, and Savitz 1997; Schwartz and Chance 1999; Basrur 2002). Conditions of poverty further increase children's vulnerability due to immunological fragility and higher presence of contaminants in soil, air, water, and foods.

Industry and Environmental Health

Because of the chemical and physical manipulation involved in manufacturing and energy production, modern industry generates extremely toxic by-products, which pose enormous human health and disposal problems. Industrial toxins include PCBs,

Table 10–3 Agents of Environmental Health Problems

Agent	Use/Exposure/Conditions	Health Effect
Water Contamination		
Vibrio cholerae	• Ingestion of feces-contaminated water or raw food	• Cholera (diarrhea, dehydration, 50% case fatality rate if untreated)
Giardia intestinalis	• Feces-contaminated water, food, soil	• Giardia (diarrhea)
Dracunculus medinensis	• Unfiltered water containing small crustaceans	• Guinea worm disease (intestinal infection, skin ulcers/lesions)
Chemical contamination	• Main contaminants: aluminum, arsenic, fluoride, lead, pesticides, radon, disinfection by-products	• Cancers, adverse reproductive outcomes, cardiovascular disease, neurological disease
Vector-Borne Diseases		
Mosquitoes	• Breeding sites include stagnant water, swamps, ditches; exacerbated by some agricultural and development projects, absence of sanitation	• Malaria, yellow fever, dengue, West Nile virus, viral hemorrhagic fever
Fleas/flies/rodents	• Inadequate waste collection; filth; overcrowding; ecologic change	• Hantavirus, plague, tularemia, trachoma
Waste/Sewage		
Hazardous waste	• Origins: industry, mining, households, health care • Dumped on land, into water, stored in ponds, incinerated	• Cancers, neurological effects, miscarriage, birth defects, reproductive disorders • Infection and injury
Human waste	• Nonexistent or poorly maintained sewage systems contaminate water and soil	• Diarrheal, helminthic, other infectious diseases
Nuclear waste	• Heavy water, spent fuel, dismantled weapons • May be improperly disposed of, leaching into groundwater/soil or in dump sites with human presence (e.g., through scavenging)	• Radiation poisoning/syndrome: seizures/coma, skin, hair, immune system damage, some cancers
Air Contaminants		
Polycyclic aromatic hydrocarbons (PAHs)	• Incomplete burning of coal, oil, gas, garbage, tobacco, meat, and other organic substances • Manufactured in dyes, plastics, and pesticides • Exposure through contaminated air; grilled or charred meats, contaminated or pickled foods; contaminated water, milk	• Most links to health have been shown in animal testing: lowered fertility, higher rates of birth defects, and damage to immune systems • Long-term exposure may cause cancer
Ozone	• Chemical reaction of air pollutants	• Respiratory impairments and eye irritation
Nitrogen dioxide, carbon monoxide	• Combustion of gasoline and fossil fuels	• Damage to lungs and respiratory system • Reduced oxygen in blood, leading to learning disabilities
Particulate matter	• Burning wood and diesel fuels	• Respiratory irritation, lung damage

(continued)

Table 10–3 Continued

Agent	Use/Exposure/Conditions	Health Effect
Physical Agents		
Heat	• Temperature change • Melting polar ice caps, rising sea levels, increased storms, droughts, flooding	• Death, disease, and displacement from ecological disasters and heat waves • Malnutrition • Increased vector-borne diseases
Ionizing radiation	• Produced in nuclear facilities and testing sites, as well as by x-rays, CT scans, MRIs, and cancer treatments/radon	• Carcinogenic (lung, breast, thyroid), especially in rapidly dividing cells (skin, bone marrow, blood cells, sperm cells)
Nonionizing radiation	• Ultraviolet radiation: from the sun • Extremely low frequency radiation: exposure through extensive work with power sources, power lines, cell phones, radar, including exposure experienced by airline pilots and crew	• Sunburn, immune system damage, cataracts, skin cancer • Ocular damage, some cancers; many findings are inconclusive
Toxic Pesticides and Organic Chemicals		
Pesticides (DDT, organophosphates, heptachlor)	• Pesticides, insecticides, fungicides, herbicides, defoliants • Bioaccumulation in humans and animals • Exposure via ingesting contaminated foods, breathing contaminated air, skin absorption through handling, and via breast milk	• Pesticide poisoning—potentially fatal • In large doses causes tremors, nausea, and other nervous system effects • Carcinogenic: lymphoma • Long-term exposure may damage liver
Persistent organic pollutants (POPs): dioxin, polychlorinated biphenyls (PCBs)	• Coolants and lubricants in electrical equipment • Formed during combustion processes, production of herbicides and paper • Bioaccumulation in wildlife and humans • Exposure through using old electrical appliances and eating contaminated meat/fish • Spraying of defoliants (e.g., Agent Orange) and herbicides (e.g., in cotton fields)	• Damage to skin, kidneys, and liver • Carcinogenic • Fatal in high doses • Reproductive disorders • Impedes immunological development and response
Disinfection by-products (chloroform, bromate)	• Reaction of organic and inorganic compounds with water disinfection practices (e.g., chlorine) • Exposure through inhalation or ingesting contaminated food or water	• Continued exposure may cause kidney and liver damage • Some association with bladder and anal cancers and reproductive damage
Benzene	• Plastics, resins, synthetic fibers, rubbers, lubricants, dyes, detergents, drugs, pesticides, crude oil, gasoline, and cigarette smoke • Exposure at workplace and via inhalation	• In high doses, affects bone marrow and may lead to anemia and leukemia • Fatal in very high doses

(continued)

Table 10–3 Continued

Agent	Use/Exposure/Conditions	Health Effect
Toxic Metals		
Lead	• Batteries, aluminum, metal products, x-ray products, cans, glazes, leaded gasoline • Some paints and construction materials • Exposure via ingestion	• Toxic to all organ and nervous systems • May permanently damage brain and kidneys • Retards physical and mental development • Miscarriage and decreased fertility
Arsenic	• Wood preservative and pesticide • At workplaces, near hazardous waste sites • Drinking water, especially in Bangladesh	• Skin and blood vessel damage, nausea • Elevated incidence of certain cancers • Fatal in high doses
Mercury	• Used to make chlorine gas (as disinfectant; weapon), thermometers (if mercury is aerosolized), dental fillings, batteries, some creams and ointments • Some agricultural fungicides • Contaminated fish	• Short-term exposure causes nervous system disorders and nausea • Can permanently damage the brain (Minimata disease), kidneys, and fetus
Cadmium	• Extracted in production of zinc, lead, copper • Used in batteries, dyes, pigments, and plastics • Ingested in workplace and via contaminated food, water, soil, and inhaled cigarette smoke	• Repeated exposure may cause kidney disease, lung damage, and fragile bones • Fatal in high doses
Food Agents		
Campylobacter bacteria	• Ingestion of undercooked meat, unpasteurized dairy products, contaminated water	• Most common causative agent of diarrhea; may be fatal in young children
Escherichia coli (toxigenic)	• Undercooked meat, proximity to livestock, petting zoos, feces, unpasteurized beverages, and contaminated produce • Also found in contaminated water	• Diarrhea, dehydration, may be fatal • Possible kidney failure, anemia, neurological damage in 10% of cases
Salmonella	• Ingestion of contaminated food of animal origin or food contaminated with manure	• Fever, diarrhea, vomiting, may be fatal
Shigella	• Transmitted in contaminated water and food (e.g., shellfish, dairy products, poultry)	• Diarrhea, vomiting, rarely fatal
Genetically modified and irradiated food	• Unknown	• Should undergo further, rigorous testing

Sources: Agency for Toxic Substances and Disease Registry (2007); Hilgenkamp (2006); Friis (2007); WHO (2002a).

dioxins, asbestos, heavy metals, and certain plastics used in modern office equipment, housing and building materials, and home appliances. Though routinely used, (the health consequences of) these substances typically generate public attention only at times of horrifying incidents, such as the 1984 gas leak at the Union Carbide pesticide plant in Bhopal, which killed over 3,000 people in one night, 30,000 since then, and continues to affect the health of hundreds of thousands more.

Since World War II, roughly 80,000 new chemicals have been manufactured and released into the environment. Accordingly, the sheer magnitude of potentially dangerous substances makes testing for toxicity enormously complicated: of the 15,000 chemicals commonly used today, only a minute fraction have been individually assessed and none have been tested in combination (ICEH 2007).

The health effects of physical agents, including ionizing radiation generated by nuclear weapons and nuclear reactors are still being documented. The U.S. bombings of the Japanese cities of Hiroshima and Nagasaki in 1945 caused more than 100,000 immediate deaths from burns and debris, but over 60 years later, elevated levels of leukemia and solid tumor cancers are still being documented. The Chernobyl (Ukraine, former Soviet Union) nuclear power plant explosions in 1986 killed 31 people immediately, but also exposed millions more to dangerous levels of radiation. Because of delayed carcinogenic effects, elevated rates of cancer and congenital birth anomalies are only now being observed.

Production processes have particularly damaging effects on workers and nearby populations and locales. Farmers, factory workers, miners, and construction workers, together with people who work in certain service occupations (including cleaners, firefighters, data clerks, and garbage collectors) experience extremely high job-related illness and death. Of the 30 most polluted places in the world, as documented by the Blacksmith Institute, six are mining sites (Table 10–4).

As industrialization has shifted eastward and southward from Western Europe and North America, contamination has followed: ten of the world's most polluted places are in Eastern Europe and Central Asia; six are in China; six in Latin America; five in South Asia; two in Africa; and one in the Pacific. In older industrial settings such as Western Europe and North America, concerted environmental efforts have led to the clean up of many contaminated sites. For decades, industrial and household waste contaminated Europe's leading waterway, the Rhine River. In 1986, a chemical plant fire in Switzerland released tons of toxic pesticides, sparking a movement for regulation and regional cooperation with Germany, France, and the Netherlands. More than 20 years later, fish are only now starting to live in the river. There have also been incipient cleanup efforts in the former USSR and in India at industrial sites with radioactive materials, mercury, lead, and groundwater contamination (Blacksmith Institute 2007).

In the United States, 450,000 brownfields—former industrial or commercial facilities since abandoned or idle—leak hazardous contaminants or pollutants into the environment, often in areas redeveloped for housing. In the 1970s,

Table 10–4 Selected Pollution Hotspots

Site Name and Location	Major Pollutants and Sources	Human Health Impact	Cleanup Status as of 2007
Linfen, China	Particulates and gases from coal-based industry and transportation	Worst air quality in China—high prevalence of respiratory and skin diseases and incidence of lung cancer	Plans to replace 200 plants
La Oroya, Peru	Lead and other heavy metals from mining and metal processing	Blood lead levels for children are triple the limits set by the WHO	No major activity
Dzerzhinsk, Russia	Chemicals, toxic by-products, lead, chemical weapons (was a Cold War era manufacturing site)	Due to contaminated water supplies, life expectancy is shorter and the death rate is higher than elsewhere in Russia	No major activity
Chernobyl, Ukraine	Radioactive materials due to the explosion of the nuclear reactor	Thousands of cancer deaths, respiratory ear, nose, and throat diseases	Most residents have moved; some cleanup has occurred

Source: Blacksmith Institute (2007, p. 7).

an environmental movement around this issue was galvanized by a discovery that the Hooker Chemical Company had buried toxin-filled barrels near Niagara Falls several decades before, resulting in soaring birth defects and illnesses. The U.S. Environmental Protection Agency established a Superfund program in 1980 to monitor and clean up the most hazardous of such sites. While initially effective—with over 750 sites remediated—Superfund has lost both funding and momentum (Sapien 2007), showing the importance of ongoing pressure and monitoring to ensure environmental health improvements.

Of particular concern is the export of toxic industrial waste. An estimated 440 million metric tons of toxic waste were generated annually in the 1990s. In various developed country settings, public mobilization regarding the harmful effects of toxic waste has led to growing resistance to landfills and increased regulations over industrial disposal. Unfortunately, these efforts have displaced rather than ended toxic dumping. From 1980 to 1988, the cost of dumping hazardous waste jumped by over 1,600%, leading the United States and other countries to export more and more waste to developing countries with less stringent environmental regulations.

As a result, while 95% of the world's hazardous waste is produced by industrialized countries, the developing world's volume of toxic wastes, much of it imported, is rapidly rising (Clapp and Princen 2003). The 1992 Basel Convention on the Control of Transboundary Movements of Hazardous Wastes and their Disposal was designed to end such practices but has little enforcement capacity. Indeed, India has recently offered itself as a global waste destination—contrary to the Convention provisions.

For years, much of North America's "e-waste"—old computers and electronic equipment—has been dumped in Chinese and Indian landfills, with lead, mercury, cadmium, and other heavy metals and organic acids leaching into soil and groundwater and exposing waste pickers and local populations to dangerous toxins (Clapp and Princen 2003; Chopra 2007).

Because of these problems, many municipal recycling programs have developed provisions for disposing of batteries, e-waste, and other hazardous materials, with varying effectiveness. A more successful approach has been adopted in Europe, where electronics manufacturers are required to properly recycle their own products. Switzerland, for example, has a long-standing collective "takeback" system for electrical and electronic consumer products, involving detoxification, shredding, and refining.

Notwithstanding solid and mounting evidence, it can be difficult to establish precise causal connections between the environment and health because effects may be indirect and multifactoral (Corvalán, Hales, and McMichael 2005). Moreover, epidemiology and toxicology are not well equipped to trace the effects of long-term, low-level exposure to hazardous substances or the dangers posed by chemical interactions (Brown, Kroll-Smith, and Gunter 2000). A growing number of experts believe the precautionary principle (see ahead) should be applied to potentially dangerous substances and processes: rather than assuming that all processes and substances are safe until proven otherwise, the principle calls for precautions (limits to or suspensions of use) to be taken in the face of uncertainty, thus protecting population health against unknown hazards.

Box 10–5 Environmental Racism

The concept "environmental racism" was coined by U.S. activists and scholars to address the effects of racial discrimination stemming from differential enforcement of environmental policies and regulations. These practices include targeting of racial minorities for the placement of polluting industries, such as chemical plants or toxic waste disposals. Environmental racism also refers to the international context, where racial and ethnic minorities—and marginalized populations—are disproportionately compelled to live on polluted land and near "dirty" industries because the land is cheaper and laws less stringent for slum dwellers and industry alike. The concept also refers to the exclusion of racialized groups from decision-making processes and environmental justice initiatives.

The study *Toxic Wastes and Race at Twenty: 1987–2007. Grassroots Struggles to Dismantle Environmental Racism in the United States* found that ethnicity (more than income, education, and other factors) continues to be the variable most closely correlated with the location of commercial hazardous waste facilities; African-Americans, Latinos, Native Americans, Asians, and Pacific Islanders comprise majority populations (59%) in neighborhoods with commercial hazardous waste facilities. The study also found that racial minorities have been afforded little government protection or remediation from environmental hazards, even with land use and health and environmental laws in place (Bullard et al. 2007). While patterns of environmental racism have thus far been documented most extensively in the United States, they also apply globally.

Air Contamination and Health

Outdoor Air Pollution

Air pollution is one of the most pervasive problems of modern societies, linked to industrial contamination, power plants, and household fuel use, and auto exhaust. Among the most infamous air pollution episodes was the London Smog of December 1952, which killed an estimated 4,000 people within a week, mainly children, the elderly, and persons with respiratory illnesses (WHO 2002b; Goldstein and Goldstein 2002). The London Smog became a potent political issue, resulting in some of the world's earliest emissions regulations (McMichael 2001). The adoption of air pollution standards, and the subsequent introduction of unleaded gas and cleaner engines have been effective at controlling pollution levels in some settings (WHO 2002b). One region that notoriously overlooked air pollution was the former Soviet Union: after its dissolution in 1991, contamination was believed to rival levels during the worst years of the Industrial Revolution.

Today, urban air pollution is experienced across the world, with 1.3 billion city dwellers breathing in unsafe air. The problem is worse in developing countries due to generally fewer controls on vehicular and industrial emissions, garbage burning, and household fuels; little rail-based public transport; and wide industrial use of inexpensive high sulfur fuels, such as brown coal. From Shanghai to São Paulo, air pollution has risen to deadly levels, with rates of respiratory disorders rising far higher than in Western Europe (Goldstein and Goldstein 2002). Just breathing Mumbai's air is the equivalent of smoking two-and-one-half packs of cigarettes per day (WHO 2007).

Air pollution is linked to an array of acute and chronic health problems depending on the size and nature of the pollution's constituents. Scientists have consistently and independently demonstrated that fine particulate pollution has the most severe health consequences, including lung cancer and cardiopulmonary diseases. Other constituents of air pollution, such as lead and ozone, have been associated with asthma, decreased cognitive function, and upper respiratory ailments, including bronchitis. Combustion pollutants—particles, lead, and ozone—form an increasing share of global greenhouse gases (WHO 2002b). Air pollution is also a primary factor in the formation of acid rain—precipitation carrying acidic compounds formed when components of air pollution (sulfur dioxide and nitrogen oxides) interact with water, oxygen, and oxidants. When acid rain settles on the earth it creates abnormally high levels of acidity that harms forests, certain species of fish, and human health.

Particulate matter (PM) is a mixture of fine solid particles including dirt, dust, mold, and soot, with aerosols formed through combustion by-products, such as sulfur dioxide and nitrogen oxides. Particles are emitted by vehicle exhaust, solid-fuel and waste burning, factory smokestacks, pavement erosion from road traffic, abrasion of brakes and tires, and excavated mines (WHO EURO 2005). PM inhalation increases respiratory deaths in infants under 1 year, affects lung development, aggravates asthma and chronic obstructive pulmonary disease (including emphysema and bronchitis), and is associated with lung cancer and other respiratory ailments.

Mexico City is one of the world's largest (21 million people) and most polluted cities, the latter mostly due to the exhaust from over 4 million vehicles, many of which are old, diesel-based, and noncompliant with emissions standards. Exposure to PM causes 1,000–3,000 deaths and 10,000 cases of chronic bronchitis annually (Stevens, Wilson, and Hammitt 2005). Mexico City's ozone levels exceed WHO standards more than 200 days a year, facilitated by an inversion layer created by polluted air trapped just above the Mexico City Valley, which is encircled by mountains. While transportation policies to address Mexico's pollution have led to declines in several key contaminants, they have also had some reverse consequences: the phasing in of unleaded gas in 1998 led to increased photochemical smog due to new additives; and a mandatory one rest day per week for every car has increased rather than reduced the number of cars circulating, as many people have turned to taxis (not affected by the restrictions) or have acquired additional, often older and highly polluting, vehicles to use on their primary car's rest day.

In East and South Asia, there has been a three to fourfold increase in the number of motor vehicles over the past two decades, with heavy reliance on highly polluting gasoline-based two-stroke engines (mopeds and three-wheelers) (see Figs. 10–4 and 10–5). Cities that are phasing out these vehicles, such as Bangkok and Dhaka, have experienced some abatement in PM concentration (Potera 2004).

Although concentrated urban air pollution is most severe in the cities of developing countries, it is important to remember that per capita emissions of CO_2 and other air contaminants are far higher in industrialized countries. In addition to auto and industrial emissions, a prime factor is aircraft exhaust, the fastest growing source of greenhouse gases and a leading cause of air pollution and ozone alteration. The main component of jet fuel is kerosene, which through combustion produces carbon monoxide and other oxygenated organic compounds (Civil Aviation Authority 2007). The European Union (EU) has proposed placing heavy taxes on air travel, but so far it is only accelerating, especially in North America and Europe.

Box 10–6 Lead Contamination

Lead is present in small quantities in the earth's crust but its ambient levels have risen markedly through mining, manufacturing, and the burning of fossil fuels. The advent of motor vehicles caused substantial increases in contamination because of the addition of lead to petrol to increase engine power. Lead has also been used in an array of common products including batteries, ammunition, paint, x-ray shields, cosmetics, crayons, toys, pottery, and cables. Due to these multiple uses, and to limited regulations and uneven enforcement, lead is widely present in the air, dust, soil, and water.

Lead enters the body mainly through ingestion or inhalation and affects multiple organ systems, causing increased blood pressure, cognitive deficits, and other developmental problems. People with acute lead poisoning may suffer from gastrointestinal symptoms, kidney problems, anemia, high blood pressure, and neurological damage. Elevated concentrations of blood lead are associated with significant and sustained intelligence quotient (IQ) reductions.

(continued)

Box 10–6 Continued

In the late 1960s scientific evidence of its various and often subtle adverse health effects led to lead's abolition as a petrol and paint additive in many industrialized countries (McMichael 2001). Although the world is gradually converting to unleaded petrol, chronic exposure to low levels of lead remains a significant public health issue, particularly among disadvantaged groups—those who live in substandard housing (where lead abatement has not been carried out) or near polluting industry or heavy traffic (WHO 2006b). Cognitive impairments due to lead exposure are estimated to be nearly 30 times higher in regions where leaded gasoline is still being used, as compared to places where it has been phased out (Prüss-Üstün and Corvalán 2006).

In industrialized countries, acute occupational lead poisoning has been significantly reduced through manufacturing and workplace regulations, but it continues to be a major problem in many developing countries due to exposure from mining, paint, smelting, and battery factories. In the United States and other developed countries, the most common sources of lead exposure among young children are ingested paint chips and water from corroded lead pipes. In developing countries, where 97% of children affected by lead poisoning live, exposure routes are more varied (WHO 2002a), making it a far graver environmental health challenge.

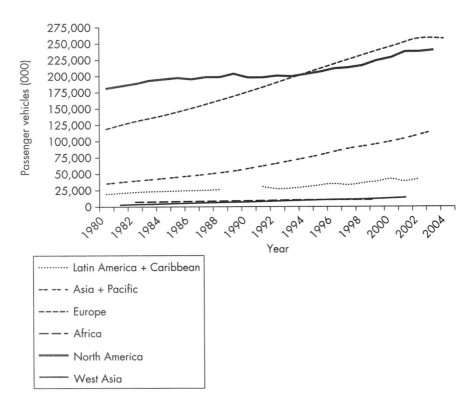

Figure 10–4 Number of passenger vehicles by region.
Source: GEO Data Portal http://geodata.grid.unep.ch.

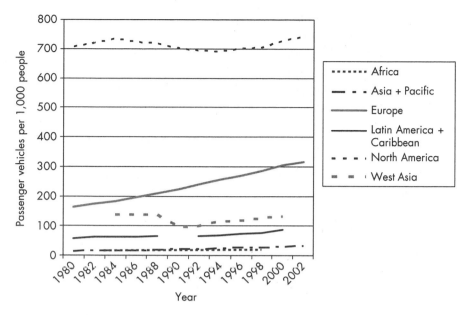

Figure 10-5 Passenger vehicles as a proportion of population by region.
Source: GEO Data Portal http://geodata.grid.unep.ch.

Indoor Air Pollution

Each year, indoor air pollution is responsible for 1.6 million deaths due to pneumonia, chronic respiratory disease, and lung cancer: the main culprit is indoor use of biomass fuels in open, poorly ventilated stoves. More than half of the world's population uses biomass, including animal dung, wood and logging waste, crop waste or coal as their main source of energy for cooking, heating, and repelling insects (Ezzati 2005; WHO 2006a).

Because biomass fuels do not burn completely, small particles, sulfur dioxide, nitrous oxide, and other chemical contaminants are present in indoor smoke, causing inflammation of the eyes, airways and lungs, and impaired immune response, and leading to cardiovascular disease, COPD, asthma, conjunctivitis, reproductive problems, laryngeal cancer, and tuberculosis. As well, carbon monoxide can cause fatal poisoning and reduces the oxygen-carrying capacity of the blood (WHO 2006a). Women, children, and the elderly living in poor households are especially subject to indoor inhalation of smoke and gases due to their cooking and other social roles, which keep them inside for long periods of the day.

Less damaging alternatives to the use of biomass for energy include electricity and kerosene, together with cleaner stoves. While improved living conditions and income generally enable the switch to safer fuels and stoves, the transition to cleaner energy sources is also related to public policies. For example, due to massive infrastructural growth, China now has near-universal access to electricity, but 80% of households continue to use biomass fuels as their main energy source because of electricity's high price (Ezzati 2005).

Indoor air pollution is also linked to "building-related illness" from chemical contaminants used in construction, furnishings, and poor ventilation. Multiple chemical sensitivity provokes respiratory disorders from exposure to indoor biological and chemical contaminants. The exact etiology of these ailments remains little known. Americans, for example, use 28.5 million kg of pesticides and 126.6 million kg of antimicrobials and disinfectants each year in their quest to be free of insects and germs (Kroll-Smith, Brown, and Gunter 2000), but the safety of the vast majority of these chemicals has not been tested. Moreover, many chemicals banned in the United States are exported for use in developing countries.

Box 10–7 Asthma and Air Pollution

An increasingly prevalent ailment linked to airborne contaminants is asthma, the chronic irritation and inflammation of the lung passages. During an asthma attack, the lining of the airways swells, mucus is secreted, and muscles tighten, impeding airflow and obstructing breathing. Asthma rates worldwide are rising on average by 50% each decade. Between 100 and 150 million people suffer from asthma, and deaths associated with asthma have reached over 180,000 annually. Most diagnosed cases are in industrialized countries, but over 80% of asthma deaths occur in low- and lower-middle-income countries (WHO 2006a).

Although the exact reasons for the rise in asthma rates are unknown, asthma has been connected to indoor allergens (such as cockroaches and domestic mites in bedding, carpets, and furniture), tobacco smoke, and the chemical irritants of outdoor air pollution, including diesel exhaust. In New York City, high ambient levels of desiccated rat feces in neighborhoods with infrequent garbage collection (and thus large rat populations) have also been associated with increases in asthma (Perry et al. 2003).

Water

Fresh water—essential for fulfilling basic human needs, including hydration, food preparation, and personal, home, and community hygiene—is plagued by intertwined problems of scarcity, unequal access, and contamination. Although two-thirds of the earth's surface is water, only 2.5% is fresh water suitable for human consumption, and only 11% of this is available for human use (with most of the remainder trapped in glaciers or inaccessible groundwater). The 20th century rate of water withdrawal exceeded population growth by a factor of 2.5 (Shiva 2002), suggesting that *how* water is used is key to its conservation. Agricultural irrigation is the biggest single use of water worldwide, accounting for two-thirds of water consumption (Arthurton et al. 2007). Large sprinklers used by most agri-businesses to maximize crop output not only waste large quantities of water from evaporation, they spread more contaminants than root-based irrigation systems that deliver water through the earth using soil as a filter.

Box 10–8 The Aral Sea Crisis

The Aral Sea crisis has become emblematic of human-made water disasters. Once the fourth largest inland sea in the world, the Aral Sea has been drying up due to mismanagement and overuse of its river water supplies for agriculture (Black 2004). The saline lake—located between Uzbekistan and Kazakhstan (both former republics of the Soviet Union)—began shrinking in the 1960s, a process which accelerated after 1991. To date, half the sea has dried up, leaving behind a half dozen smaller lakes/seas and generating respiratory illnesses and cancer from widespread dust and salt left behind (see Fig. 10–6).

The area around the sea is heavily polluted due to industrial contamination, bioweapons testing and dumping, and fertilizer runoff occurring both before and after the breakup of the Soviet Union. Approximately 150,000 tons of toxic chemicals are believed to have entered the lake's feeder, the Amu-Darya River, in the last 10 years alone. Because of heavy application of insecticides, herbicides, and defoliants in surrounding areas, and the use of Aral Sea water for irrigation, the entire region is highly contaminated, with the population chronically exposed to toxic chemicals and bearing significant health problems including cancer, birth defects, and cognitive problems.

In recent years, dams and dykes have been built to divide the smaller North Aral Sea (in Kazakhstan) from the sea to the south, enabling the former to expand (with water piped in from Siberia) and reopen fisheries (Fletcher 2007). However, the much larger South Aral Sea benefits little from this division. Uzbekistan wants to explore the south seabed for oil and use tributary water for agricultural purposes rather than refill the sea, leaving few prospects for recovery (Greenberg 2006; Fairless 2007).

Almost half of the world's population lacks a household connection to piped water and faces some level of water shortage (WHO and UNICEF 2008): literally billions of people must use contaminated water to meet their daily survival needs. Ingestion of contaminated water and poor hygiene due to inadequate water availability can lead to a variety of bacterial illnesses such as cholera, typhoid, and salmonella; skin infections; cryptosporidium and other parasitic diseases; dysentery; and food-borne pathogens. Even households with access to some water may have to reuse it for multiple ends, inevitably leading to contamination. Many people in lower-income settings use contaminated rivers, streams, lakes, and reservoirs because they have no clean water options. Others use rainwater accumulated in leftover industrial barrels, which may be contaminated with toxic chemicals. People without household plumbing often resort to storing water in open containers, creating ideal breeding sites for mosquitoes. In 2006, 95% of dengue fever was attributable to environmental causes (Prüss-Üstün and Corvalán 2006), almost entirely preventable by eliminating breeding sites for the disease's vector, *Aedes aegypti*.

Waterborne diseases kill up to 3 million people each year, accounting for approximately 6% of all deaths globally. Hardest struck are infants and malnourished young children, more than 1.5 million of whom die each year from dysentery and diarrhea (Global Health Watch 2005). The accompanying malnutrition places millions more at greater susceptibility to death from other diseases. As well, toxins entering water supplies from industrial and agricultural runoff can cause acute poisonings and a variety of cancers.

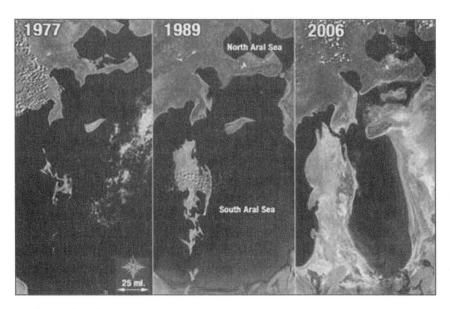

Figure 10–6 Aral Sea shrinkage.
Source: Earth Observatory NASA, http://earthobservatory.nasa.gov/Newsroom/NewImages/
images.php3?img_id=16277.

The UN estimates that since 1990 over 1 billion people have gained access to
"improved water sources." However, it is important to read between the lines.
"Improved" means access to a household connection, public standpipe, borehole,
protected well, protected spring, or rainwater collection tank—often for a fee—*not*
regular, easy, reliable, affordable, or household access. Some 1.1 billion people—
one-sixth of the world's population—remain without any clean water access what-
soever, and 2.6 billion people lack basic sanitation (without even pit latrine access)
(see Figs. 10–7 and 10–8) (UNDP 2006). Charges for community latrines in Ghana
and other settings can reach up to 10% of daily earnings, forcing many to use forests, fields, and alleys, despite problems of disease and violence.

The lowest water coverage rates are in sub-Saharan Africa (58%) and in the
Pacific (52%), but the largest numbers of people lacking water access are in Asia.
The majority of people lacking adequate water and sanitation live in growing peri-
urban slums or rural areas of developing countries. In slums, water services are
prohibitively expensive or frequently interrupted due to shortages. In rural areas,
water and sanitation infrastructure is minimal. At the same time, large consumers
from industrial and agribusiness sectors are adept at capturing public water supplies
at discounted rates (Global Health Watch 2005).

Water and sewage access constitute a political problem of resource allocation
rather than a technical one—after all, Roman aqueducts were built thousands of
years ago, and modern engineering of waterworks and sanitation systems developed before 1900. In order to be safe for human consumption, water must undergo

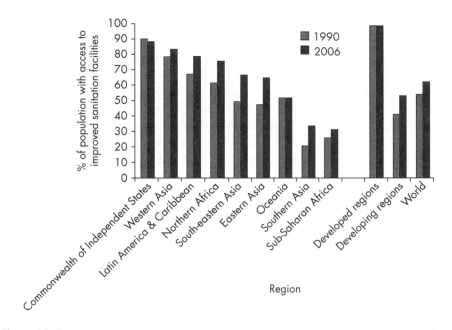

Figure 10–7 Percentage of population with access to "improved sanitation," 1990 and 2006. "Improved sanitation" includes connection to public sewers or septic systems, or access to pour-flush latrines, simple pit latrines, and ventilated pit latrines.
Source: WHO and UNICEF (2008).

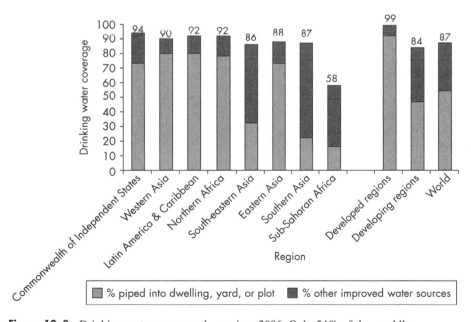

Figure 10–8 Drinking water coverage by region, 2006. Only 54% of the world's population has water piped into their dwelling or land plot.
Source: WHO and UNICEF (2008).

treatment and filtration (either at a plant or at the community/household level) and be routinely monitored for toxins and pathogens.

The interaction of deregulation, escalating water prices, and water contamination can have deadly consequences. When water was privatized in KwaZulu-Natal, South Africa in 2000, 106,000 cases of cholera were reported over a 6 month period—representing more than half the number of reported cases worldwide for that year (WHO EURO 2003)—and over 3,000 people died. Previously, water had been provided free of charge, and South Africa's postapartheid constitution guaranteed the rights of citizens to live in a safe and healthy environment with access to water as a basic human necessity. However, in 1998, pressured by the World Bank and the IMF, the South African government adopted "cost recovery" measures for public services. Private mega-companies contracted to provide water imposed a connection fee of 51 rands (then US$7), an amount categorically "unaffordable for thousands of people" (Bond 2004, p. 128). Just weeks after instituting this fee, local authorities began shutting off water services to residents who were unable to pay their bills, and cholera broke out as thousands resorted to using polluted river water.

Inadequate water access goes hand in hand with inadequate sanitary facilities and waste disposal (discussed ahead). While donor agencies have long refused to support the public provision of water and sanitation systems because they (erroneously) perceive them to be too costly, a simple calculation of the benefits in life, time, and health within just a few years shows the shortsightedness of this position (see Chapter 11). At the same time, the excess use and waste of water on the part of agri-industry and the world's wealthiest populations have met with inadequate regulatory strategies. In sum, the failure to provide universal access to clean water and sanitation is bad economics, bad health policy, and bad environmental policy.

Box 10–9 Food Safety

Maintaining food safety through regulation, inspection, and education is a central environmental health responsibility at local and national levels but also extends to the rapidly expanding global food production and distribution system. In recent years there has been an increase in reported food-borne diseases, such as *E. coli*, cholera outbreaks, adulterated oil, alcohol poisonings, and the discovery of chemical contaminants, raising concerns that regulation and inspection in the United States, China, the United Kingdom, and other countries are severely deficient.

Food safety includes preventing the following substances from entering the food supply (Friis 2007):

Microbiological hazards:

• bacteria, parasites, fungi, viruses, prions, worms.

(continued)

Box 10–9 Continued

Chemical hazards:

- heavy metals (e.g., mercury), pesticides, chemical preservatives and additives (to increase the shelf-life of goods), antibiotic residues (used to keep penned animals, such as chickens, from getting sick).
- packaging, including waxes, plastic, and other materials that may leach into food.
- debris, cleaning chemicals.

Physical hazards:

- foreign objects: glass, metal, stones, bones, radioactive materials.

Nutritional hazards:

- foods with excess or deficiency of nutrients.

Other safety concerns have to do with inadequate data regarding growing practices, such as irradiation of food and genetically modified (GM) foods.

The most important sources of food-borne illness are Campylobacters, *E. coli*, Salmonella, and Shigella, all prime causes of diarrheal death among children living in poverty. While food contamination may occur in the household, particularly where clean water is deficient, it is common at other points in the food chain due to business cost-cutting measures, such as use of contaminated water, inadequate refrigeration, poor working conditions, and poor hygienic facilities for workers.

Raising commercial livestock also poses health risks, as animals in overcrowded pens spread diseases to one another and to humans (zoonoses), the prime route of emerging diseases and potential new epidemics, such as Nipah virus and H5N1 influenza. Several well-known (and preventable) zoonoses can be transmitted to humans through food (brucellosis, tuberculosis) or food contamination (hydatidosis). These problems go hand in hand with inadequate inspections of farms, food plants, stores, restaurants, and street vendors.

The growing use of genetically modified organisms (GMOs) to increase resistance to pests or drought and increase nutritional content (or food irradiation to destroy microorganisms) has raised new concerns related to food safety (allergenicity) and the environment (loss of seed varieties; transfer of genes from plants to other plants and to humans). While GM foods have thus far not demonstrated negative health effects, the WHO, EU, and various African countries have invoked the precautionary principle in limiting GMO use until the effects are rigorously assessed (WHO 2002b).

The Codex Alimentarius was jointly developed by the WHO and FAO in 1963 to set nonbinding international foods standards, with the (sometimes contradictory) purpose of protecting health and facilitating trade. However, it has no enforcement capacity. As such, in all countries, surveillance systems and impartial public regulations are the key to maintaining food safety.

Land and Forests

Arable land, which covers less than 10% of the earth's surface, has been grossly overworked in recent decades. Between 20,000 km^2 and 50,000 km^2 of soil is lost annually through degradation, with soil erosion rates up to six times higher in developing compared to developed countries (Dent et al. 2007). Land degradation stems from soil erosion and rising salinity levels due to deforestation, climate change, excess water use, and agricultural practices including overgrazing, poor irrigation, overcultivation, mono-crop production, and pesticide and defoliant use and contamination (CIDA 2007; USDA NRCS 2007). Land degradation affects approximately 1 billion people whose livelihoods depend upon farming and who may be subject to food shortages and forced migration. In a cyclical relationship, "crop failure may lead desperate people to put further pressure on the land, resulting in a downward spiral of increasing poverty and further degradation" (Corvalán, Hales, and McMichael 2005, p. 11). Land degradation is thus intimately linked to food insecurity: the inability to maintain continuous access to nutritionally and culturally acceptable quantity and quality of food leaves over 860 million people, almost 15% of the planet's population, undernourished (FAO 2006).

The intensive use of synthetic products, such as chemical pesticides and fertilizers, and the toxic runoff they generate, is a large factor in land degradation, together with overuse and weather-related erosion. Farmers in the United States now employ more than 1 billion pounds of pesticides each year, a 20-fold increase since the 1940s (Clapp and Dauvergne 2005). While large agri-businesses are responsible for much of the problem, poor global regulation of chemical products also plays a key role. The export of pesticides banned for commercial use in the United States and Europe has increased by nearly 50% in recent years, with a large volume likely unreported.

From Ecuador to Kenya to Thailand, toxic pesticides are routinely used because they are inexpensive and effective. Those administering pesticides are rarely protected from them (Cole, Crissman, and Orozco 2006), resulting in millions of poisonings and 40,000 fatalities each year (ILO 2006). Toxic pesticides also enter the food supply, water sources, and waste systems.

Farming has become the world's most dangerous occupation, claiming half of the 335,000 fatal workplace accidents every year. In addition to poisonings, falls, drownings, and tool injuries, morbidity and mortality stem from respiratory ailments (from toxic dust and gases), zoonotic diseases, increased incidence of non-Hodgkin's lymphoma, gastric, bronchial, and other cancers, hearing deficits, musculoskeletal problems, numerous skin conditions, as well as poor water quality, sanitation, nutrition, and other features of impoverished living and working circumstances (ILO 2000; Batchelder 2001).

Mining

Mining is one of the most lucrative—and destructive—industries on earth. In 2006, the 40 largest companies in the mining industry (representing 80% of the market) brought in US$249 billion in revenues (PricewaterhouseCoopers 2007). Mining involves surface techniques (strip mining or quarrying in open pits) and underground extraction (drilling holes, tunnels, and shafts in order to reach valuable ore) to recover a range of minerals and metals, including diamonds and other precious stones, gold, silver, copper, iron, nickel, tin, lead, and bauxite. Coal and oil shale are mined as energy sources; uranium for nuclear reactors, military ammunition, and shields; and limestone as a building material. Past and present, competition for minerals has caused destructive wars, including the ongoing conflict over gold riches in the Democratic Republic of Congo, which has killed almost 4 million people over the last decade.

Mining, especially coal mining, causes extremely high occupational mortality. Due to poor ventilation in underground shafts, miners are exposed to harmful gases, dust, toxins, and heat, leading to silicosis and other lung diseases, heat stroke, and cancer. Underground explosions of methane and other gases trap and kill thousands of miners every year, with under-regulated Chinese mines currently leading the death toll.

In mineral-rich Russia, mining has become the country's leading industry, with 14% of world extraction in recent years. A boon for investors, mining is devastating to the environment and human health, contaminating air, water, and grazing lands. For example, uranium miners face elevated levels of lung cancer, silicosis, and, together with the surrounding population, are exposed to radiation, causing birth defects, immune impairment, and cancer. Uranium mine runoff also threatens fish stocks, animal livestock, and wildlife. The numerous mines built in the Soviet era are poorly maintained and are among the most dangerous in the world, with hundreds killed in recent years due to explosions and collapses (Kylychbekova 2007).

Mining operations typically leave behind hundreds of acres of open pits; seepage of heavy metals, acids, and other toxic by-products into the land and rivers destroys forests and kills nearby wildlife. Restoring vegetation to mining areas is difficult because the mining process causes organic matter, nutrients, and water to become either too acidic or too alkaline for plant growth (Walker and Powell 2001).

Box 10–10 Biodiversity and Human Health

Biodiversity refers to the variation of existing life forms and is often used as an indicator of ecosystem health. In the early 1990s, 50,000 species were believed to be lost each year (Wilson 1992). It remains impossible to comprehend the full scope and impact of current biodiversity loss because only an estimated 10% of the total number of species thought to be in existence (1.7 million species) have been classified. Because humans rely on a diversity of species and ecosystems (Gunter 2004), many environmentalists believe that biodiversity loss threatens the future of human existence.

Crop diversity, for example, ensures greater resilience to pests, such as the potato blight which afflicted Ireland in the 1840s, following the introduction of single species reliance. Over centuries, Indian farmers evolved 200,000 varieties of rice through conserving and sharing seeds, some of which could even be cultivated in coastal saline waters (Shiva 2000). However, global agri-business has shrunk these resources: presently, 10 corporations control 32% of the commercial-seed market, leading to a loss of local varieties. The majority of traded seeds are more vulnerable to pests than local seeds and are dependent on synthetic pesticides and fertilizers that are environmentally dangerous (Altieri 2000; Shiva 2000).

Deforestation

Close to 50% of the earth's original forests are now gone. Intensive logging and the clear cutting of forests for construction materials, fuel, and the expansion of living and agricultural space have caused massive deforestation. Destructive forest fires—up to 90% of which are caused or exacerbated by poor planning, careless-ness, drought, and inadequate fire fighting—have worsened the situation. From 1990 to 2005, the global forest area shrank by 0.2% per year, with a loss of 350 million hectares in 2000 alone. This loss disproportionately affects developing countries (FAO 2007; Dent et al. 2007).

Deforestation has many negative health effects, including displacement of dis-ease-bearing insects, loss of natural carbon and rain production processes—leading to excess CO_2 levels—, land degradation, disruption of animal habitats, and loss of biodiversity.

Haiti has experienced an unparalleled level of deforestation. A combination of inadequate regulation and human desperation has caused Haiti's forests to shrink from about 75% of land mass during the colonial era to less than 1% in 2003. This has led to the erosion of rich topsoil needed for agriculture. Each year, 36 million tons of topsoil are lost as rains and floods wash nutrient-rich dirt into the Caribbean Sea. Not only is arable land shrinking (at least one-fifth of food supplies must now be imported), but topsoil runoff is damaging Haitian fisheries (Erikson 2004).

The destruction of forests and fragmentation of wildlife habitats has generated new human-microbial interactions and the introduction of previously unknown (or the reemergence of disappeared) infectious diseases in human beings, such as Nipah virus in Malaysia, hemorrhagic dengue, and other fevers in Latin America. Deforestation also jeopardizes health by worsening the effects of floods, landslides, tidal waves, and hurricanes.

Box 10–11 Deforestation of the Amazon

The Amazon is the world's largest rainforest in terms of size and biodiversity. Because it produces much of the world's oxygen, it has often been described as the earth's lungs. Intense deforestation began in the mid-20th century with aggressive economic development activities by the eight South American countries it traverses. Brazil, with 60% of the rainforest, has experienced massive forest clearing through burning or logging, mostly for agricultural use (especially soy production), as well as cattle ranching, timber, mining, and oil drilling. It is now estimated that 12% of the Amazon rainforest has been lost during the last half century, with varying rates of deforestation by country.

Of global concern are the increases in atmospheric CO_2 caused by deforestation. As the Amazon forest shrinks, its ability to absorb and filter CO_2 (via photosynthesis, yielding oxygen) is reduced. When forests burn, the carbon matter in trees (released in the form of CO_2) further pollutes the atmosphere (PAHO 1994). Greenpeace (2007a) estimates that 75% of Brazil's CO_2 emissions are the result of deforestation. In addition, deforestation reduces the water cycling services provided by trees.

Deforestation also endangers environmental health by intensifying the effects of floods and land-slides. Deforestation in tropical rainforests is associated with increased exposure to malaria and other vector-borne diseases: as the habitats of mosquito, tick, and rodent populations are displaced, they move closer to human settlements (Corvalán, Hales, and McMichael 2005).

In 2006, the President of Brazil issued a decree protecting 2% of Brazil's Amazon forest from logging. Around the same time, deforestation rates fell slightly, although market demand for biofuels may reverse this trend (Roach 2007). For the most part, the Amazon's profitability continues to pre-vail over long-term environmental policies.

Sanitation and Garbage

Industrialization inaugurated the era of waste. Previously, most edible garbage was used as farm feed, and human and animal excrement were recycled as fertilizer. The small volume of material goods no longer reusable was buried or burned, sullying air and soil to be sure, but to a comparatively minor degree. Human and industrial waste rose concomitantly with the rise of cities and factories. Early urban transport systems—horses and donkeys—littered streets with great volumes of manure, attracting flies (handy spreaders of trachoma, diarrhea, and dysentery), and causing severe disposal problems. Before the advent of routine waste collection and sewage disposal, garbage, excrement, and animal carcasses were summarily dumped into rivers, lakes, and makeshift landfills, contaminating human water supplies, and animal habitats. What remained behind accumulated along unpaved streets and back alleys mixed with mud and stagnant water, generating foul stenches and cesspools of disease. Until the late 19th century, pigs ran wild in the streets of New York helping diminish the piles of garbage, but leaving behind further muck and noxious gases. More than a century later, waste disposal continues to be a vexing problem around the world, with billions of tons of garbage produced each year (excluding industrial waste).

Garbage disposal is illustrative of the interdependent relationship among the natural and built environments, social policies, patterns of consumption, and human health. North Americans generate the most garbage—over 2 kg per person per day, almost twice as much as Chinese city dwellers, who in turn exceed the volume of waste produced in lower-income countries. Where waste management systems are in place, solid waste undergoes five logistically complex processes: collection, composting, recycling, land filling, and combustion (Friis 2007). In cities, garbage is typically collected by large, diesel-run trucks that contribute to air pollution and congestion. Composting of organic waste (household and garden) may be undertaken at the household or government level (e.g., in Toronto, Canada and the Greek island of Crete). Recycling may be informal (waste pickers who rescue and resell garbage from Latin American dumpsites) or municipally organized. In places with strong policies, most notably the EU, up to three-quarters of packaging is recycled; elsewhere recycling may not reach even half this rate.

Garbage that is not composted or recycled ends up dumped either haphazardly or in a large landfill. Landfills that are not well sealed may leak toxic metals (from batteries, electronics, and other manufactured products) and chemicals into the land and groundwater, destroying fish, bird, and plant habitats, and contaminating rivers and lakes. Landfills also generate methane and other gases, which are fire risks, greenhouse gas contributors, and carcinogens. In many settings, incineration is the main method of waste disposal, adding to air pollution. In rural areas, this may take place household by household; in numerous cities incineration processes double as an energy source. Incineration plants emit harmful toxins that can only be partially mitigated through scrubber and filter technologies (Friis 2007).

Liquid sewage—industrial and household waste water and human excreta—is the counterpart of solid waste. Without proper sewers, wastewater ends up in, and contaminates, groundwater, rivers, and other potential drinking water sources. Even cities and towns with sewage systems may dump untreated sewage into waterways or the open ocean. Inadequate disposal of human excreta exacerbates the oral–fecal transmission of pathogens and spreads parasitic worm diseases. Pit latrines and dug sewers are promoted as cheap alternatives to the longer-term (yet cost-effective) commitment to building water and sewage systems, but the former, short-term solutions are more likely to result in groundwater contamination.

Modern sewage plants are able to remove sludge, counter microbes, and return water to waterways or even for reuse as drinking water. Biological treatment, filters, UV radiation, and other forms of disinfection remove bacteria, nitrates, and phosphates, but other toxins may remain in water, making vigilance of hazardous waste dumping especially important (Friis 2007).

The generation of nonbiodegradable consumer and industrial garbage remains an aesthetic, ecological, and health problem throughout the world. Some years ago, bright blooms began to dot the landscape of sub-Saharan Africa. These "desert flowers" are not flora at all but ubiquitous one-time-use plastic bags for carrying drinks and other small purchases. Tossed away—as in countless settings—plastic bags damage the health of birds and other wildlife that ingest or become entangled in them, block drains, and create breeding sites for malaria-bearing mosquitoes, all poignant reminders of the fragility of ecosystems. This is a global problem: hundreds of billions of plastic bags are dispensed and then discarded each year, contributing to greenhouse gases (as petroleum-based products) and marring natural beauty. Most end up as litter in landfills (estimated to take up to 1,000 years to disintegrate), leaching toxins into soil and waterways, and threatening marine life and other animals.

Dilemmas of Development

Schemes for farming, mining, irrigation, and water extraction from subterranean aquifers are some of the economic activities that have affected forests, watersheds, lakes, and river systems. Agricultural development schemes (e.g., the Green Revolution, see Chapter 4) have been hailed by economists for expanding the global food supply, but their social and environmental costs have been substantial. In relying on hybridized high-yield seeds, these schemes have displaced drought-resistant local crop varieties. The new water-guzzling crops deplete water supplies in areas where water is scarce. Sadly, previous water extraction methods based on low volume, minimally disruptive indigenous irrigation technologies were deemed "inefficient" because they used human or animal energy. Instead, these were "replaced by oil engines and electric pumps that extracted water faster than nature's cycles could replenish the groundwater" (Shiva 2002, p. 10).

A related problem is the draining of wetlands to open space for agriculture, housing development, and oil extraction. Wetlands—marshes, swamps, bayous, bogs, and fens—are an important habitat for wildlife (birds, fish, and reptiles) and plants. Most fisheries rely on wetlands, which filter water pollutants, protect coastlines, and serve as a buffer against flooding. Wetland loss threatens human livelihoods as well as one-fifth of endangered species.

Dams

Of all large-scale environmental engineering programs, major dams are the most dramatic. Dams, canals, and diversions now disrupt almost 60% of the world's large rivers (Clapp and Dauvergne 2005). Where topography permits and rainfall is abundant, dams provide large amounts of relatively cheap electric power. Dams also help with flood control and distribution of water on the downstream side, although they may cause flooding of adjoining lands. Upstream, impounded water can be used for fisheries and recreation.

Large-scale dams—many financed by international banks—have been constructed on the great rivers of Africa, Asia, and Latin America. For each of these, tens of thousands of people have been relocated, with numerous attendant problems. The building of the Akosombo Dam across the Volta River in Ghana from 1961 to 1964, primarily to provide electric power to an enormous aluminum smelter, destroyed 739 villages, home to 80,000 persons, mostly subsistence farmers. Resettlement sites around newly filled Lake Volta were inadequately prepared, and the lake itself posed a severe health problem to surrounding residents. Rates of schistosomiasis soared, with the prevalence among schoolchildren in some localities going from 5% before the dam was built to 90% a few years after formation of the lake.

Dams, particularly those that divert the course of rivers over long stretches, are harmful to humans and the natural environment. Consequences include large-scale forced migration, the displacement or deterioration of wildlife habitats, water runoff, and replenishment disruptions. The World Commission on Dams estimates that between 40 and 80 million people have been displaced by dam projects around the world, including 1.3 million people for a single project: the Three Gorges Dam in China's Yangtze River Valley, designed to produce energy and control centuries of flooding (Shiva 2002; Clapp and Dauvergne 2005; Yardley 2007).

Completed in 2003, Three Gorges is the largest dam in the world: 660 km long, submerging 632 km^2 of land, with an eventual hydroelectric generating capacity of over 18 gigawatts. While the dam's energy output will reduce coal consumption by up to 30 million tons per year (with concomitant reductions in greenhouse gases), it is provoking other environmental problems. The Chinese government recognizes that the dam may cause landslides and that the submergence of hundreds of factories, mines, and waste dumps, and the presence of massive industrial centers upstream are creating extensive pollution problems in the reservoir and the tributaries of the Yangtze (Yardley 2007). The dam is also affecting one of the world's biggest fisheries, in the East China Sea, with declines in fresh water and accumulated sediment reducing annual catches by 1 million tons.

Dam projects have generated significant resistance movements that have challenged the supposition that dams are the best means of providing water and energy. In the 1980s, Narmada Bachao Andolan (Save the Narmada Movement) was formed to protest the building of 30 large and hundreds of smaller dams along the Narmada River in central India, arguing that the displacement of population would lead to human suffering, loss of livelihood, deepened inequality, and environmental problems. The movement formed an international coalition of supporters, took out full-page advertisements in the *New York Times*, and in 1993 pressured the World Bank to rescind its funding for Sardar Sarovar, the largest of the dams. Construction was halted, but in 1999/2000 the Indian Supreme Court ruled that dam building could resume on the condition that thousands of displaced families be rehabilitated. These terms have yet to be met and protests continue (Narmada 2006).

WHAT IS TO BE DONE? MULTIPLE LEVELS OF CHANGE

Key Questions:

- Does "reduce, reuse, and recycle" work?
- Whose responsibility is it to ensure the viability of natural resources and the protection of environmental health?
  - Is it consumers of the North or the West?
  - Is it multinational corporations?
  - Is it international trade organizations?
  - Is it local or national governments?
- Which policy examples cited here demonstrate use of the precautionary principle?

Markets, Government, and the Environment: Making the Links

Although most environmental health problems originate with a specific issue in a particular locality, environmental abuse and its health consequences—whether greenhouse gas emissions, toxic chemical use, or forest clearing—ultimately transcend place, affecting us all (Corvalán, Hales, and McMichael 2005). Many cultural and social factors combine to influence the forces driving environmental change, but one stands out: political economy. Massive market-driven industrial growth, especially since World War II, has generated increased demand for all sorts of goods, a demand that agriculture, industry, and government combine to promote as well as meet. Increased production and consumption have given rise to an infinity of mechanical, chemical, and electrical devices that have altered the built and natural environment of almost every human being. While Soviet communism was also marked by industrial production and environmental disruption, this resulted more from orienting much of its economy to the Cold War's arms race and technological competition with the West than from the logic of its economic system.

As Soviet power waned, the global capitalist model began to consolidate through accelerated economic and financial integration, growth of multinational firms, deregulation, and privatization. The increasing collective power of private corporate interests vis-à-vis the masses of workers and small farmers explains why the tools and institutions of global governance focus "on the needs of capitalism and national security rather than on the safety" of vulnerable populations or the protection of the environment (Dauvergne 2005b, p. 36). Regional and international free trade agreements, and in recent years the WTO, are particularly responsible for putting "downward pressure on environmental standards" (Dauvergne 2005a, p. 384), as governments are convinced to loosen environmental protections in order to become more competitive in global markets.

These features of neoliberal globalization not only increase demands on the natural environment but also lengthen the distance between consumption and the consequences of production, which once stood side by side. Nowadays purchasers of cut-price electronic goods or clothing in, for example, Barcelona or Baltimore do not witness the human and environmental effects of production processes in Bangkok or Bangalore. It may be harder for people to gauge or even be aware of the chemical waste, air, land, and water contamination, and human damage involved in producing these goods. The prices of commodities rarely "reflect the full environmental and social costs of production—the value, for example, of an old-growth tree as a source of biodiversity—leaving consumer prices far too low and consumption far too high for global sustainability" (Dauvergne 2005a, p. 384).

Box 10–12 Exxon Valdez Oil Spill

Legally, governments are responsible for setting and monitoring environmental regulations, but local and national regulatory abilities are also influenced by global economic forces. Environmental laws and standards have been vigorously resisted by corporate interests (and through the WTO) as impediments to private enterprise (see Chapter 9 for details). For example, multinational oil and gas company Exxon has funded researchers skeptical of global warming, and the company has been at the forefront of efforts opposing the raising of emissions standards.

Indeed, one of the most blatant environmental cases of corporate impunity involved Exxon. On March 23, 1989, one of Exxon's largest oil tankers, the Valdez, struck a reef and emptied 11 million gallons of crude oil into Alaska's Prince William Sound. This was the world's most environmentally destructive oil spill, killing thousands of birds and causing untold ecosystem damage along 1,200 miles of coastline. Exxon's cleanup response was slow, but it quickly offered 11,000 local residents US$300 million in compensation (Editorial 2003). Nonetheless, 33,000 plaintiffs harmed by the oil spill, including commercial fishers, Alaska natives, cannery workers, and landowners, brought

(continued)

Box 10–12 Continued

a lawsuit against the company, and in 1994 an Alaska jury found Exxon liable for US$5 billion in punitive damages. Exxon (now merged into ExxonMobil as the world's largest company with record profits of almost US$40 billion in 2006) pursued a long-term appeals process to delay or avoid payment (Mokhiber 1999). In 2006, the company managed to get a federal appeals court to halve the award to US$2.5 billion (Greenhouse 2007).

At the time of writing, ExxonMobil was appealing the decision to the U.S. Supreme Court, claiming that this largest-ever punitive award is excessive, and that the US$3 billion it says it has paid in cleanup costs, compensation, and fines should be sufficient. After almost two decades, the plaintiffs (20% of whom have since died) have yet to receive any payment, and outstanding claims for environmental cleanup remain (Barringer 2006). Exxon's prolonged refusal to accept responsibility for the oil spill demonstrates the need for laws (and enforcement) that hold industries accountable for the environmental consequences of their activities.

In sum, we are now at a crucial crossroads. The solutions to our present environmental challenges are complex and difficult but doable. They will involve clever ideas, cooperation, and intense political struggle (Beatley 2000; McKibben 2003). The market liberal approach laid out earlier in the chapter is clearly insufficient: market strategies to environmental improvement are based on profitability (Evans 2002), almost inevitably at cross-purposes with environmental benefits.

What other approaches might be pursued? Bioenvironmentalists have drawn attention to the depletion and contamination of natural resources as exemplified in former U.S. Vice President Albert Gore's film "An Inconvenient Truth," which helped earn him the 2007 Nobel Peace Prize. Disappointing to many viewers is the finale of the film, which calls for greater personal responsibility for lowering one's ecological footprint, rather than for structural approaches to lowered greenhouse gas emissions, such as industrial limits on hazardous wastes and emissions or the development of public transport systems.

As we will explore in the next section, the institutionalist approach, emphasizing global agreements on emissions, biodiversity, and other concerns, has gained ground in recent years. For global governance to succeed, however, national compliance must not be jeopardized by corporate interests. We will also examine the proposals and actions of social greens, who argue that concerted human action is capable of addressing environmental problems (Tilly 2004; Brown and Zavestoski 2005) but not solely, or even largely, through individual actions. Political mobilization strategies (such as bona fide democratic participation in decision making and social movements) give citizens the collective power to shape environmental, economic, social, and health policies.

The array of responses is considerable, ranging from purely technological (e.g., lower-emission vehicles), to behavioral (e.g., recycling and bicycling), to managerial (e.g., altered farm practices), to policy-based (e.g., planning incentives). As

Table 10–5 Actions to Confront Environmental Hazards

Sphere of Action	Examples	Advantages	Disadvantages
Global and Regional	• Kyoto Protocol • Agenda 21 • Ban on asbestos • CFC phaseout • Debt swaps • Corporate responsibility • Precautionary principle • Bilateral agency efforts (e.g., Canada's International Development Research Centre)	• Involves multiple actors • Sets international targets on global environmental issues	• Targets are usually nonbinding and nonenforceable • Goals are made within a global market paradigm
National (Government) or Regional Authority (i.e., state, province)	• Environmental Impact Assessment • National regulations (e.g., on pesticide use, toxic waste disposal) • Green taxes and incentives • Waste regulation	• Is legitimate body to collect taxes, set policies and regulatory standards, etc. • Has broad purview • Can integrate population needs and protection	• Sovereignty of national governments may be curtailed by economic treaties (e.g., WTO) • Governing and legislative processes may lack transparency and legitimacy • Concern for economic development often privileges corporate interests over public welfare
Local (Government or Community)	• Public transportation policies • Eco-housing • Green city design • Local food production • Supportive infrastructure	• Generates high levels of public interest and participation • Can address/plan for multiple issues at once	• Does not address large-scale industrial regulations and policies • May require national support/counterparts to succeed
Individual (Household)	• Green consumer efforts • Ecologically friendly behavior change (e.g., turning lights off, thermostat down; buying energy-efficient appliances, low-pressure shower heads, low-flush toilets)	• Some success in mobilization and education for environmental protection	• Focus on individual/consumer as agent of change, rather than on structural issues • Individual behavior contributes but is not the prime motor of environmental degradation

(continued)

Table 10–5 Continued

Sphere of Action	Example	Advantages	Disadvantages
Social Movements (May be Local, National, or International)	• Informal (e.g., urban agriculture, RUAF) • Gender-environment (e.g., the Greenbelt Movement) • Occupational (e.g., plantation workers' lawsuit against transnational corporations) • Human rights (e.g., People's Health Movement) • Monitoring (e.g., Pesticide Action Network) • IDRC • Natural resource protection (e.g., Rainforest Action Network)	• Long term outlook • Address underlying determinants of environmental health • Community support • International solidarity • Integrated scientific and social approaches • Broad understanding of environment and health • Strong community involvement/visible efforts at local level	• Gains may be slow in coming • Activists may be targeted for harassment and sometimes assassinated • May be hard to maintain adequate resources • May be hard to mobilize and regulate all relevant stakeholders • May not address economic forces pressuring environment • Once gains are institutionalized (at local, national, or global levels), movement may disband

outlined in Table 10–5, confronting environmental health problems demands attention at household, community, national, and international levels.

Global and Regional Responses

It was not until the 1960s that concern for the environment was transformed into a transcendent global issue, a transformation that took place within the context of social and political movements for economic justice, peace, and gender equality. A pivotal moment was publication in the United States of Rachel Carson's *Silent Spring* (1962) which detailed how chemical pesticides entered the food chain, affecting flora, fauna, and human health. The book's focus on the effects of the anti-mosquito pesticide DDT (used in the global malaria campaign) on birds led to its ban in numerous countries. Almost simultaneously, local protests in India, Africa, and Latin America against the environmental effects of large-scale development projects garnered international attention, while social movements in Eastern and Western Europe railed against the environmental implications of nuclear weapons production and warfare. This worldwide environmental awakening spurred numerous international conferences and reports, which reached a crescendo in the 1990s.

Box 10–13 Key International Environmental Conferences and Agreements

Stockholm Conference (1972): For the first time national governments reported on the state of their environments in an international venue. While industrialized countries were concerned with preventing pollution, controlling "overpopulation," and conserving natural resources, underdeveloped nations expressed concern about widespread hunger, disease, poverty, and the environmental effects of growing industrialization. The United Nations Environment Programme (UNEP) was established to monitor changes in the physical and biological resources of the Earth, and the WHO developed environmental health criteria to review and document the relationship between environmental factors and human health.

Montreal Protocol (1987): The world's first environmental agreement, initially signed by delegates from 24 nations and the EU. Signatories committed to decreasing CFC production by 50% by 2000. It was followed by the 1989 Helsinki Declaration on the Protection of the Ozone Layer, which called for the complete phase-out of CFCs by 2000, and the London (1990), Copenhagen (1992), Beijing (1999) and other amendments, which accelerated and expanded the phase-out to cover related substances and provided support to developing countries for compliance. To date the protocol has been signed by 191 countries. See Box 10–14 for further details.

The Rio Earth Summit (1992): The UN Framework Convention on Climate Change (UNFCCC) was agreed to in Rio de Janeiro, Brazil and ratified by 189 countries. This convention calls on parties to: "protect the climate system for the benefit of present and future generations of humankind, on the basis of equity and in accordance with their common but differentiated responsibilities and respective capabilities. Accordingly, the developed country Parties should take the lead in combating climate change and the adverse affects thereof" (UN 1992).

The Convention on Biological Diversity (opened for signature in 1992—adopted at Rio summit; entered into force in 1993): Calls for conservation and sustainable use of biodiversity and fair sharing of the benefits of genetic resources; signed by 168 countries as of 2007. In 2000 the Cartagena Protocol on Biosafety was adopted (entered into force in 2003) as the first international treaty to employ the precautionary principle for biological resources protection (Secretariat of the Convention on Biological Diversity 2004).

Kyoto Protocol (1997): See text for details. The follow-up 2007 Bali meeting called for its renewal and expansion, with special attention to issues of deforestation and climate change adaptation.

World Summit on Sustainable Development Johannesburg (2002): Declaration called for "a collective responsibility to advance and strengthen the interdependent and mutually reinforcing pillars of sustainable development—economic development, social development and environmental protection—at the local, national, regional and global levels" (World Summit on Sustainable Development 2002, p. 1).

Agenda 21: Blueprint for Action for Sustainable Development

An important outcome of the 1992 Rio Earth Summit was the commitment of more than 178 governments to Agenda 21—a set of sustainable development strategies to guide actions by governments, UN organizations, development agencies, NGOs, municipalities, commerce, and industry in every area in which human activity affects the environment (MacArthur 2002). Although accompanied by moral exhortation,

Agenda 21 is not binding. Still, at the local level, Agenda 21 has inspired thousands of projects, making advances only in areas where municipalities have implementation responsibility such as solid waste management and water pollution.

Agenda 21 also motivated the European Union's Biofuels Directive, adopted in 2003 to reduce greenhouse gas emissions and increase the security of fuel supply through greater biofuel production and use. Biogas, one of the biofuels, entails fermentation of biodegradable waste (including manure, feed, sewage, solid waste) under anaerobic conditions to form methane and CO_2, which can be used for electricity production, heating, or as a substitute for natural gas in cars. However, if not properly contained, the methane in biogas can explode and cause high greenhouse gas emissions. Thousands of biogas plants now operate across Europe (particularly in Germany, where farmer-run plants meet over 5% of total energy needs). Another biofuel, biodiesel, made from processed rapeseed oil and other vegetable oils, is used in European diesel engines. The world's most common biofuel, bioethanol, is made from starch and sugar crops, and is increasingly used in Sweden, France, and other countries (UNESCO 2007).

The United States, Brazil, China, Canada, and India are also relying to a greater extent on corn-based ethanol (with the United States and Brazil supplying most of the world's ethanol), less as an environmental strategy than as a cheaper fuel source. Indeed, experts now consider biofuels a threat to global warming. Ethanol production requires enormous quantities of water and energy (producing only 20% more energy than it takes to process it) and may pollute even more than petroleum does. Moreover, expanding ethanol production means extra land must be cleared to produce food, leading to a massive release of CO_2, a prime greenhouse gas (Eilperin 2008). Higher demand for maize has caused severe hardship in Mexico, where the cost of corn doubled at the end of 2006 and thousands took to the streets (Runge and Senauer 2007). Diversion of palm oil, wheat, and other staples to profitable biofuels has led to steep food price increases in numerous countries. In 2007 and into 2008, food shortages and price hikes—due to insufficient supplies and soaring energy costs—provoked protests in Italy, Morocco, Guinea, Yemen, Haiti, Egypt, Madagascar, Indonesia, Mauritania, the Philippines, Cameroun, Senegal, Uzbekistan, and elsewhere. The prospecting of other biofuel sources—such as cassava (also known as manioc and yucca), a hardy staple crop in Latin America, Asia, and Africa—has further dire implications for food security and sovereignty.

The Kyoto Protocol on Climate Change

The 1997 Kyoto Protocol is the core global agreement on addressing climate change. It requires 36 developed countries to reduce emissions of six greenhouse gases by an average of 5% below 1990 levels between 2008 and 2012. If achieved, emissions levels in 2010 would be about 20% lower than without the Protocol (Dauvergne 2005a). As of October 2008, a total of 183 countries had ratified the agreement (UNFCCC 2008). Countries that fail to meet the Kyoto targets will have to submit 1.3 emissions allowances for every ton of greenhouse gases emitted. Emissions allowances require a country to purchase other countries' emissions allowances, export products that emit greenhouse gases rather than using them domestically, or use environmental features—such as carbon sinks—that purportedly compensate for emissions.

The Kyoto Protocol has been critiqued by bioenvironmentalists and social greens on several grounds: emissions targets are inadequate and nonbinding; so-called flexible mechanisms counteract potential gains and commodify the atmosphere for trading within a market system; and reporting/accountability mechanisms are too weak (Global Health Watch 2005). Two of the biggest polluters in the world, the United States and Canada, have, respectively, rejected the Kyoto Protocol or stated that they would not meet targets. Meanwhile, developing countries that have ratified the Protocol, including India and China, are not required to reduce their carbon emissions. Critics also argue that the Kyoto Protocol does not address the power imbalances that have resulted in the overuse and unequal use of the atmosphere (Lohmann 2001).

The Kyoto Protocol has also been undermined by the Asia-Pacific Partnership on Clean Development and Climate (AP6), a voluntary agreement created by six countries (the United States, Australia, Japan, China, India, and South Korea, since joined by Canada) that together account for half of the world's energy consumption. Contrary to Kyoto, AP6 members set their own (minimal) targets which are significantly lower than Kyoto targets.

Still, many environmental activists believe Kyoto is a promising step in the right direction. The EU has proposed extensive regional responses to global warming: the intergovernmental European Environment Agency monitors the region's caps on CO_2 emissions, and ESPACE (European Spatial Planning: Adapting to Climate Events) is a 4-year project aimed at ensuring the implementation of public, organizational, and transnational climate change strategies.

At the Social Forum on Climate Change held in Moscow in 2003, more than 250 civil society representatives from 33 countries called on their governments to urgently enforce the Kyoto Protocol (Environmental Defense Fund 2003, 2007). To date these calls have been little heeded (including in Russia), yet advocacy efforts continue.

Box 10–14 Environmental Health Cooperation and Chlorofluorocarbons (CFCs)

A landmark effort of environmental cooperation has been the reduction of chlorofluorocarbons (CFCs) released into the atmosphere. Invented in 1928, CFCs quickly found broad industrial use as propellants (in aerosols), refrigerants, flame retardants (in insulation), and solvents. In 1974, three scientists (from Mexico, the Netherlands, and the United States) recognized that CFCs were drifting into the atmosphere, breaking apart, releasing chlorine, and reacting to deplete the ozone layer. The ozone layer provides a protective shield from the harmful effects of ultraviolet-B radiation from the sun (which can contribute to skin cancer, cataracts, decreased immunity, and lower plant productivity), and it also screens out lethal UV-C radiation (Dauvergne 2005a). The three scientists received the Nobel Prize for Chemistry in 1995 for their pioneering work.

(continued)

Box 10–14 Continued

Efforts to reduce use of CFCs gained momentum in 1985 when a thinning of the ozone layer over a wide area (referred to as a "hole") was discovered over the Antarctic. This finding generated swift action. The Montreal Protocol on Substances that Deplete the Ozone Layer was adopted in 1987, setting mandatory targets to reduce the production of human-made chlorines, including CFCs, halons, and other significant ozone-depleting substances (Dauvergne 2005a). A CFC Multilateral Fund was established in 1992, raising more than US$2.3 billion to help developing countries implement the protocol. Worldwide production of CFCs was rapidly reduced by 1996; all told, since 1987 there has been a 95% decrease in worldwide use of CFCs and other ozone-depleting chemicals.

The international effort to eliminate the use of CFCs is an environmental success story. There has been near-universal participation of countries and, following initial resistance, support from industry—due to the relatively slow phase-out process and the development of alternative technologies. Moreover, because CFCs were produced by only 21 firms, 88% of which were based in industrialized countries, enforcement was feasible. The coordinated political response was also bolstered by widespread public support in developed countries (Clapp and Dauvergne 2005). Scientists have recently argued that CFC phase-out has also slowed global warming.

Notwithstanding the almost complete phase-out of CFCs (production of new stocks ceased in most countries as of 1994), the ozone layer over Antarctica is still less than half of its thickness before 1980 and, according to the UNEP, will likely not be fully replenished until 2050 due to black-market trading, increasing air conditioning use, and because "old" CFC emissions are still drifting upward, rising into the stratosphere (Kuylenstierna et al. 2007).

Debt Swaps, Cancellation, and Relief

"Debt-for-nature" swaps are another international solution. A debt swap involves purchasing foreign debt at a discount, converting the debt into the local currency, and using the proceeds to fund local conservation initiatives. In a *bilateral* debt-for-nature swap, the creditor government cancels the debt owned by a debtor government in exchange for the latter's commitment to environmental protection spending. Under a *commercial* debt-for-nature swap, a private organization, such as the World Wildlife Fund, solicits individual debt donations or purchases discount debt from a creditor. The organization then negotiates with the debtor government, offering to cancel debt in exchange for conservation project funding. While proceeds from swaps have the advantage of staying in the debtor country, thus far they have entailed minimal transactions. For example, in 2002, the Peru debt-for-nature swap cancelled just US$14.3 million of its US$28 billion international debt; still, this effort enabled Peruvian NGOs to fund conservation efforts in Peru's Amazon forest (World Wildlife Fund 2007).

National Level Responses and Efforts

While international efforts can spur national laws and policies, national governments remain the prime regulatory and decision-making bodies. With the exception of trade treaties (which employ sanctions and other punitive measures), most international agreements are nonbinding and nonenforceable. As we have seen, the

Kyoto Protocol is only effective insofar as signatories abide by their promised emissions targets. As such, the nation-state, with its broad purview over economic and industrial policy, land use, and social protection, is potentially the most important player in protecting environmental health. While some governments have passed and enforced effective legislation that protects natural resources, curtails hazardous industrial processes and substances, and regulates growth and construction patterns, many others have shirked this role.

Depending on the integrity and representativeness of democratic institutions and decision-making processes, government policy is shaped by, to use the two largest categories, the interests of corporations and the interests of workers. Virtually every government measure reflects a struggle on some level between these two sets of interests. Of course, government decisions are also influenced by larger geopolitics and by particular industries, events, advocacy groups, and other forces. As examined in Chapter 9, the exigencies of market competition and enormous corporate power mean that governments often privilege economic needs over social and environmental ones. Nonetheless, as we explore here, there are also many instances of governments responding to collective demands to protect environmental health.

Regulations and Standards

Environmental health protection involves numerous measures, ranging from elimination of hazardous materials and waste in industrial settings, to land conservation and zoning laws. Workers and occupational health advocates have struggled for centuries to improve factory and living conditions, but most laws that protect natural resources and monitor emissions are more recent. In the 1970s, many governments began to pass legislation to regulate discharge of toxins in the air and water, protect endangered species, and limit the use of—and exposure to—hazardous substances in industrial settings and the built environment. Permanent agencies, such as the U.S. Environmental Protection Agency (established in 1970) and counterparts elsewhere, set regulations and standards and may be charged with enforcing the "polluter pays" principle. Notwithstanding these formal missions, enforcement ability may wax or wane depending on budget allocations, reporting requirements, number and training of inspectors, and other activities affected by political decisions.

Bans on harmful products and chemicals are another growing environmental health measure. In 2007, the Australian government announced the first-ever ban on traditional light bulbs, to be replaced with more sustainable fluorescent bulbs. The ban is expected to cut Australia's carbon emissions by 800,000 tons by 2012 and reduce household electricity bills. Numerous countries have prohibited particular toxins, polluting engines, and dangerous materials, although accelerated trade patterns sometimes inhibit monitoring and enforcement. For example, 39 countries and the EU have banned the use, export, and import of asbestos. In 2002, Zambia, following the precautionary principle, refused aid or trade of products made with GMOs.

Box 10-15 Environmental Protection and Health Promotion: EIA, HIA, and the Precautionary Principle

Environmental Impact Assessment (EIA) is an assessment tool used to determine the effects of human activities on the environment (and on health). The purpose of the assessment is to ensure that decision makers consider environmental impact before deciding whether to proceed with new projects.

Since 1991 the World Bank—pushed by activist movements—employs EIA as a mandatory feature of all of its project proposals (Clapp and Dauvergne 2005). World Bank assistance for postwar reconstruction in Lebanon, for example, has been subject to EIA, and in 1993 Lebanon's first Ministry of Environment was created. However, a lack of infrastructure, limited political commitment, continuing instability, and inadequate resources have left environmental concerns secondary to economic goals in rebuilding the country (El-Fadel, Zeinati, and Jamali 2000).

A related and similar concept to EIA is Health Impact Assessment (HIA, see Chapter 5), which is used to describe and estimate the effects of a proposed policy or project on human health (Renewable Energy Access 2005). HIA has been applied by public health departments, policymakers, community groups, and NGOs at the local, regional, and national levels to evaluate the health effects of a wide range of policy interventions. In London, HIA was recently used to analyze the effects of urban development and transport in a marginalized neighborhood, but the findings were challenged by various stakeholders (Collins and Taylor 2007). In Tuscany, HIA had wider political support, leading to ecosystem and wetland revitalization (Siliquini, Nante, and Ricciardi 2007)

In sum, HIA can be helpful but suffers, like any estimation, from uncertainty. As Nobel prize-winning physicist Neils Bohr once joked, "prediction is difficult—especially about the future." Moreover, impact assessments are inevitably embedded in political processes. Critics argue that EIA and HIA are limited by their exclusive focus on new policies—ignoring those already in place—and that they may not lead to meaningful participation by all stakeholders. As well, potentially costly HIAs may be wasted as "evidence of impacts is only one of many factors affecting implementation of policies" (Krieger et al. 2003, p. 661).

Precautionary Principle
Another approach to addressing the health and environmental impact of human activities is the Precautionary Principle, which advocates that precautionary measures be taken even if cause and effect relationships have not been fully established through scientific inquiry. The term, translated from the German *vorsorge*, meaning foresight, originated in the 1970s and became a tenet of the 1992 Rio Declaration.

Unlike EIA or HIA, the precautionary principle shifts the burden of proof to the proponents of an activity. It calls for preventive action under conditions of uncertainty and until an activity has been demonstrated to be safe. Rather than calculating potential levels of risk and their significance, the precautionary principle assesses whether the substance or intervention is needed at all (Kriebel and Tickner 2001).

Green Taxes and Incentives

Green taxes on carbon emissions, car purchases, household waste, groundwater withdrawal, and water pollutants are intended to reduce pollution levels through levies on industries, companies, and individuals. Several European countries have adopted carbon and other eco-taxes to encourage more sustainable use of land and water and ecosystem balance. High gasoline taxes are meant to lower automobile use, increase funding for and use of collective transportation, and (somewhat ironically) subsidize road construction. Green policies also include subsidies and incentives for green investments. For example, the Dutch government reimburses (tax-free) companies that pay employees to use public transport. Developing countries, such as Trinidad and Tobago, have also implemented green sales taxes. The Gambia taxes second-hand goods that may contain environmental pollutants; and Brazilian states can apply a portion of income taxes to conservation (UNEP 2007a).

These strategies have generally helped to reduce waste and promote ecologically sustainable energy sources. Still, such approaches emphasize consumer behavior over industrial accountability.

Waste Minimization and Recycling

Many national and municipal governments have implemented source reduction policies, which involve a "change in the design, manufacture, purchase, or use of materials or products (including packaging) to reduce their volume or toxicity before they become municipal solid waste" (U.S. Environmental Protection Agency 2006), and are far less expensive and damaging than garbage collection. A 1991 German packaging law, for example, requires companies either to directly take back their packaging waste or to make arrangements for its collection and reuse, resulting in over 70% reduction of waste. In an uncoordinated but rapidly spreading effort, countries as distinct as Ireland, China, and Tanzania—as well as numerous municipalities in South Asia, the United Kingdom, and North America— have either placed a steep tax on plastic bags or banned them outright.

A growing number of localities from Toronto to Tokyo encourage or require recycling (through depots or regular collection) of reusable products, including paper, plastics, metals, and organic waste, coupled in some cases with a monetary incentive or threat of fines. At least half of consumer waste is estimated to be recyclable. Household and community composting are also encouraged to minimize yard waste, protect against water loss, and return essential nutrients back to topsoil. In the absence of regular refuse collection, environmental waste is particularly problematic. Rwanda has a community cleanup effort one Saturday a month requiring all those not working to either clear trash or plant a tree.

Corporate Accountability

Market liberals and institutionalists have promoted the idea of environmentalism as marketable through schemes to trade carbon emissions, environmentally friendly production processes (such as making timber from sustainable sources), and voluntary corporate stewardship (Clapp and Dauvergne 2005). Corporate social responsibility—the stated commitment made by businesses to enhance the public good—is likewise portrayed as good for the environment, for marketing and public relations, and, ultimately, for profits (Hirschhorn 2004; Crowther and Rayman-Bacchus 2004). Voluntary agreements between industry and governments have played a small role in some environmental policies, such as vehicle emissions standards and source reduction. However, in contrast to mandatory measures, these agreements have not achieved significant emissions reductions (IPCC 2007c) because they do not incorporate enforcement and accountability mechanisms. Moreover, despite the self-serving publicity surrounding corporate social responsibility, the environmental repercussions of most past and present business activities remain unaddressed.

Most important, corporations are legally bound to make profits for their shareholders, making impediments to profit-making subject to shareholder scrutiny, objection, or legal action. As such, "goodwill" or voluntary measures are patently insufficient protection for environmental health. As Nobel-winning economist Milton Friedman puts it, *"asking a corporation to be socially responsible makes no more sense than asking a building to be"* (Friedman 2006).

Sustainable Technologies

Environmentally friendly technologies offer some promising prospects. The most advanced building designs provide emissions-free cooling and heating and greatly reduce energy and water demands. Replacing biomass cooking and heating fuels (including agricultural residues and animal dung burned in inefficient stoves) with cleaner sources—and better stoves—can reduce the production of black soot and other contaminants and improve the health of women and children exposed to high indoor air pollution.

Cleaner engines and waste processing, development of renewable energy sources, and other technologies also have an important role to play in improving environmental conditions (see Table 10–6 and Box 10–16), but regulation and policies that prioritize collective human and environmental health (including working and living conditions) are fundamental. Technologies themselves, while potentially helpful, do not address the root causes of environmental injustice. Nevertheless, environmentally friendly technologies can be highly effective if framed through political efforts that regulate industrial waste and emissions, subsidize public transportation rather than the auto industry, and redistribute income, enabling poor families to better their housing conditions (including through improved ventilation, stoves, and fuels).

Box 10–16 Alternative Energy Sources

Solar Power: Solar power has been in use for decades. Energy from the sun is absorbed through windows, panels, walls, etc., which slowly release the sun's heat; collectors, pumps, and valves can also be used to transfer energy from the sun to a storage place, such as a battery. Depending on the size of the panels and battery, and available light, solar energy can be used to power a light bulb for a few hours or partially heat a building. Even without a battery solar energy can be used directly, for example, to power a water pump.

(continued)

Box 10–16 Continued

Wind Power: Windmills for pumping water and grinding grain date back to at least the Middle Ages (Hilgenkamp 2006). Today, windmills are no longer quaint wooden structures, instead resembling aerodynamic airplane propellers made from fiberglass. Air slows down as it passes through the blades, causing them to turn and produce energy that can be transmitted as electricity onto a grid. Wind turbines are often clustered together in wind farms. Unlike solar power, wind systems also produce energy at night. Wind is both efficient and far less costly than coal or nuclear energy. Areas most suited for wind machines are free of obstructions—open plains, tablelands, hilltops, ridges, and even bays and inlets. While wind power is not yet widely used due to these topographic requisites and high start-up costs (which quickly dissipate through energy savings), Denmark obtains 20% of its total energy from wind (American Wind Energy Association 2007), and Spain's wind energy use is growing by over 30% annually (Renewable Energy Access 2005).

Local Response and Efforts

Although national government measures have a larger reach, "the meaningful implementation of many policies...conducive to ecologically sustainable living (such as the development of environmentally friendly transport systems, or the production of 'organic' food) work best through local communities at a sub-national level" (McMichael 2001, p. 348). Local settings tend to be more shaped by direct democracy, have considerable decision-making agency, and may face fewer market-constructing pressures than national governments.

Green Cities and Ecological Design

Cities are central to the global agenda of sustainability for several reasons. First, urbanization is accelerating: more than 50% of the world's population now lives in cities. Second, local governance is closest to the population and usually the most effective at working with community stakeholders—a prerequisite for many environmental health initiatives. Third, cities have sizeable ecological footprints.

Making urban environments healthy remains a great challenge: the built and natural environments interact through use of resources and space, yet in developing and developed countries alike there is insufficient support for ecological design and planning. Economic development priorities typically trump environmental concerns, and most governing authorities lack the political and social values necessary to plan and build a healthy city. In many U.S. cities, the quantity of land consumed by urban development far exceeds population growth, generating habitat losses, destruction of productive farmland and forestlands, and huge infrastructure spending. Urban growth patterns impede public transport and walking or bicycling, leading to high CO_2 emissions, excessive energy and resource use, and proliferation of waste (Beatley 2000). Still, a few examples go a long way.

Table 10–6 Technologies and Practices to Improve Environmental Conditions

Sector	Technology	Policies
Energy	• Renewable heat and power (hydro-power, solar, wind, and bioenergy)	• Reduction of fossil fuel subsidies • Taxes or carbon charges on fossil fuels • Producer subsidies for renewable energy technologies • Phasing out coal
Transportation	• Fuel efficient vehicles, hybrid vehicles, biofuels	• Modal shifts from road to rail transport • Subsidies for public transportation (buses, trains, electric streetcars, bike lanes, sidewalks) • High fuel taxes • Mandatory fuel efficient cars
Buildings	• More efficient lighting, electrical appliances, and heating and cooling devices (solar energy) • Improved stoves, insulation • Alternative refrigeration fluids	• Eco-taxes, appliance rebates, exchanges, standards, and labeling • Building codes and certification • Eco-housing
Industry	• More efficient end-use electrical equipment • Heat and power recovery • Recycling • Clean production • Control of gas emissions • Carbon sequestration	• Carbon taxes • Regulations on chemicals and materials produced • Performance standards • Subsidies and tax credits • Tradable permits
Agriculture	• Improved (crop and grazing) land management techniques to increase soil carbon storage • Restoration of degraded lands • Low water-use rice cultivation techniques • Livestock and manure management to reduce CH_4 emissions • Improved nitrogen fertilizer application techniques to reduce N_2O emissions • Dedicated energy crops to replace fossil fuel use; improved energy efficiency	• Subsidies and incentives for increased organic and local agricultural production • Regulated and mandated reductions in pesticide and chemical use • Financial incentives and regulation for improved land management, maintaining soil carbon content, efficient use of fertilizers, irrigation, and energy
Waste	• Landfill methane recovery • Waste incineration with energy recovery • Composting of organic waste • Controlled waste water treatment • Recycling and waste minimization	• Hazardous and household waste taxes • Composting and recycling collection and processing systems

Source: IPCC (2007c).

Box 10–17 Curitiba, Brazil—"The Green City"

Curitiba, Brazil's seventh largest city, with a population of 1.6 million, is a world-recognized model of ecological and planning practices. Starting in the late 1950s, Curitiba's population doubled every decade, threatening to overwhelm its services. Attempting to accommodate the city's population growth, planners focused on environmental solutions to urban challenges (Macedo 2004). They restricted high-density growth in favor of several corridors radiating from the city center, connected through a highly efficient public transportation system. At the same time, city leaders encouraged community self-sufficiency and decentralized education, health care, recreation, and park services. One of the city's first successes was Curitiba Industrial City, a model green industrial park for non-polluting industries (largely textile, electronics, and biotechnology companies), which included vast green spaces, schools, and housing (Herbst 1992).

Beginning in the mid-1960s, city officials organized what is considered one of the world's most efficient and heavily used bus systems (BRT), based on above-ground buses connected through an "integrated network" that eliminates gridlock (see Fig. 10–9) (Macedo 2004). Passengers can use all BRT services on a single fare, with daily expenditures on transport reduced to approximately 10% of income—much below the national average. In 2007, 2.3 million people (including residents of the larger metropolitan region) used the bus system every day (Lubow 2007). A 1991 study found that 28% of BRT riders previously traveled by car and that the BRT generated a reduction of approximately 27 million auto trips per year, saving 27 million liters of fuel. Although it has one of the highest car-ownership rates in Brazil, Curitiba uses approximately 30% less fuel per capita than other Brazilian cities of its size, resulting in one of the country's lowest levels of ambient air pollution (Herbst 1992; Parasram 2003; Goodman, Laube, and Schwenk 2006).

Curitiba also has an extensive recycling system, anchored by a promotional scheme that appeals to children—green trucks with bells that collect recyclables from neighborhoods on a weekly basis. Roughly one-fifth of the city's waste is recycled in a local facility that itself makes use of recycled equipment; some 95% of Curitiba's residents now separate their garbage (Lubow 2007). However, as in many Brazilian cities, urban slums (*favelas*) are expanding, with the city struggling to keep up with sanitation and other needs (Macedo 2004).

Ecological design, as employed in Scandinavia and elsewhere, seeks to minimize environmental harm while integrating "green spaces" and strategies into the urban environment. Because 40% of the world's energy consumption results from the construction and operation of buildings and dwellings, ecological housing and "green" commercial buildings emphasize high-energy conservation, low water usage, and minimal need for cars (thanks to bike racks and proximity to public transport). Most use sustainable and recycled building materials (Beatley 2000).

Other ecological housing features may include solar energy, green roofs, organic gardens, grey water (recycled household and drainage water for watering gardens, sanitation, etc.), rainwater retrieval systems, high-efficiency natural gas furnaces, reused concrete in the foundation, and the installation of water-conserving taps, showerheads, and toilets. Eco-roofs enable local vegetable production, offer visual appeal, protect against UV rays, extend roof life, cool the urban environment, sequester CO_2, and provide a habitat for plants, invertebrates, and birds (Beatley 2000). Notwithstanding these benefits, ecological design has not been widely implemented due to high up-front costs, complex logistics, and little institutional support from most municipal authorities.

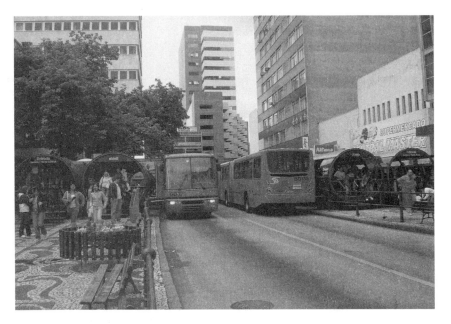

Figure 10–9 Curitiba transit stop, Estação Central.
Source: Photo courtesy of Vera Marques.

Local Transportation

An important element of urban environmental health is the implementation of convenient, safe, low pollution, affordable public transportation systems (Litman 2003). Other policies to reduce automobile use include safe and abundant cycling and walking paths, and limits on the growth of low-density suburbs and out of-town shopping centers. Car-centered North American cities, for example Atlanta, have notoriously defied such strategies, using road expansion as a prime solution to transport problems, in turn generating pollution problems and economic isolation of those without cars. This is not simply a question of cultural preference: the oil, rubber, road building, car manufacturing, sales and repairs, and advertising industries have fought hard in favor of dependence on automobiles. After World War II, General Motors bought the public transportation system of Los Angeles. Rather than making promised expansions, the company all but dismantled the transport network (a minuscule subway system was opened only in the 1990s), laying the ground for the largest automobile market in the world (McMichael 2001). Even amidst mounting concerns regarding toxic CO_2 emissions, most U.S. cities invest little in public transport: only 2% of urban trips in the United States are on public transport, compared to 10% in Western Europe (National Research Council 2001). Instead, many U.S. states provide tax incentives for hybrid cars that combine a gasoline engine with a battery-powered electric motor, with little impact on automobile use or emissions levels.

By contrast there are numerous creative actions that can be taken to restrict, discourage, or "calm" automobile traffic. Many cities have discontinued public subsidies for road building and have instead implemented road and bridge tolls, channeled increasing tax monies and subsidies to subway, tramway, and light rail expansion and use, and otherwise increased the costs and penalties of city driving and parking. In Oslo, a system of electronic charges for cars entering the city center has been in place since the early 1990s and collects daily tolls from about 230,000 vehicles (Beatley 2000). London, Paris, Singapore, Stockholm, Santiago, and Oregon have followed suit, often channeling toll revenues to public transport systems. In Bogotá, the city center is car-free on Sundays, with plans to expand to weekdays as infrastructure improves.

Other cities have developed creative car-sharing schemes that make cars available at certain collective depots and allow them to be dropped off at other sites after use, thus eliminating the need for private automobile ownership. Speed bumps, curb and sidewalk extensions, physical barriers of all types, placement of trees in streets, and fewer parking lots have been effective in reducing car traffic in the Netherlands. One town even uses sheep as a way of slowing traffic (Beatley 2000).

Box 10–18 Principles of Sustainable Cities

A Healthy City is: "One that is continually creating and strengthening those community resources which enable people to mutually support each other in performing all the functions of life and achieving their maximum potential" (Hancock and Duhl 1988, p. 24). Trevor Hancock, originator of the concept of healthy cities, argues that the built environment has almost become the "natural" environment in urban settings, as the population spends more time indoors and in built spaces (Hancock 2002).

Local Management: refers to the political process of local planning and accountability, which requires a range of tools to address environmental, social, and economic concerns in order to provide the necessary basis for integration.

Policy Integration: involves intersectoral collaboration and coordination based on the concept of shared responsibility.

Ecosystems Thinking (for cities): emphasizes the city as a complex system that is characterized by continuous processes of change and development. It incorporates aspects such as energy, natural resources, and waste production as chains of activities that require maintenance, restoration, stimulation, and closure in order to contribute to sustainable development.

Cooperation and Partnership: Holds that sustainability is a shared responsibility with cooperation and partnership among different levels, organizations, and interests as crucial elements.

Source: Beatley (2000).

Cycling: Low-Tech Eco-Transport

Perhaps the best alternative to car-based transport is cycling, which though both environmentally sustainable and health promoting, is often a missing link in urban transport planning. Local policies that promote cycling range from eco-taxes on car use and parking, city-run bike-sharing systems (as in Paris, Amsterdam, Vancouver, Barcelona, and Helsinki), bicycle trails, painted bicycle lanes, and protective barriers for bike lanes. Other incentives include secure bike parking and equipping public transportation with bike racks, employer incentive schemes, and employer mileage allowances for bike use (Batterbury 2003).

Environmental Budgets and Charters

Local environmental budgeting entails the preparation of ecological budgets to accompany yearly or semi-yearly spending plans, together with a clear accounting of environmental spending (i.e., the cost of pollution, resource use), which must stay within certain limits or targets. Porto Alegre, Brazil's participatory planning process, in place since 1989, has channeled taxes to improve piped water coverage, which now reaches 99.5% of residents and has additional salutary effects on the environment (see Chapter 13 for details) (Global Health Watch 2005).

Consumer Efforts

Consumer efforts are an important first step towards addressing environmental depletion and contamination and may raise awareness among children and wide swaths of the citizenry. These measures include:

- using eco-friendly and recycled products (cleaning solutions, bags, clothing, food, paper);
- composting/vegetable gardening/ rainwater collection;
- expanded use of public transit, biking, walking;
- using reusable containers and coffee mugs;
- using energy efficient appliances, bulbs;
- using appliances during nonpeak hours;
- installing low-flush toilets;
- sealing cracks, installing new windows, insulation, roofs;
- lowering thermostats (in the winter) and water heater temperature;
- lowering or eliminating air-conditioner use;
- ensuring better ventilation;
- employing solar cookers; and
- limiting idling and auto use.

Of course, the consumer approach assumes that people have the time, access, resources, and education or need to "change their lifestyles," and thus consumer efforts are far more relevant to middle- to high-income residents of middle- to high-income countries than to members of the working class or people in underdeveloped settings with far lower levels of consumption overall. If combined with municipal subsidies, producer and retailer taxes, and incentives, these measures might have wider reach.

Still, it is essential to emphasize that policies aimed at consumption and individual behavior are insufficient to address the main forces driving environmental health problems because: (a) individual level solutions do not affect structural determinants, including energy, industrial, and military production processes that are based on a market logic that prioritizes profits over human and environmental health; (b) consumers are seen as the agents of change, thereby encouraging more consumerism; and (c) there is a limit to what individual consumers can do in the absence of larger measures.

Instead, efforts to improve environmental health need to draw from multiple levels (local, national, global) of regulation and reduction of the overuse and misuse of natural resources and the built environment.

Social Movements

In addition to documenting and addressing environmental health hazards, and improving ecosystem planning, the advancement of environmental health has resulted from hundreds of environmental health and justice movements that pursue collective social, philosophical, political, and ethical approaches (Cole et al. 1999; Brown 2007). Here we discuss a sample of informal, local, transnational, gender-based, occupationally-oriented, and other social movements that have raised awareness and spurred the development of policies to improve environmental (health) conditions, some working downstream (where environmental hazards and improvements are experienced first hand); others working upstream, addressing the underlying economic and political forces that affect environmental health.

Chipko (meaning "to cling/embrace" in Hindi) began spontaneously in 1973 when Indian villagers, mainly women, began to hug trees that were destined to be cut down. In 1980, as a result of these actions, the government of Uttar Pradesh imposed a 15-year ban on logging in the Himalayan region. Chipko movements, which are based on Gandhi's principle of *satyagraha* (nonviolent resistance), are generally autonomous and have since extended to the protection of water and other resources (Ekins 2005).

Kenya's Greenbelt Movement, led by Wangari Maathai (the 2004 Nobel Peace Prize winner), combines women's empowerment with environmental projects. Local women help reforest by planting indigenous tree species, enabling small-scale farmers to become foresters. Through these efforts, women are able to earn income by selling seedlings, as well as reduce the burdens of traveling long distances to collect firewood and increase their decision-making power. The Greenbelt Movement, which has spread from Kenya to Congo and other countries, also seeks to reduce migration from small communities to cities.

The People's Health Movement (also discussed in Chapter 14) promotes environmental health as a human right through efforts to reclaim knowledge and science for the public good and "end imperialist [and corporate] control of the earth's natural resources" (PHM 2005). Among its causes are a worldwide campaign for a UN Treaty on the Right to Water to prevent and reverse "commodification and privatization of this vital resource"; a moratorium on extractive mining and petroleum exploration/extraction; and a ban on nanotechnology research and the development and use of all biochemical weapons (PHM 2005).

Various movements address occupational health and environmental health jointly. The Movimiento Agroecológico para América Latina y el Caribe (MAELA), made up of 150 Latin American partners, focuses on sustainable agricultural practices, biodiversity, ecological trade, and preserving indigenous knowledge.

Although not constituting a formal movement, a series of lawsuits brought by Latin American and U.S. lawyers on behalf of farm workers across the region have garnered widespread attention. Several cases involve poisonings by the hazardous pesticide Nemagon, which was banned in the United States but is still used widely on U.S.-owned banana plantations in Central America and elsewhere. Results include a 1997 out-of-court settlement, and a 2002 case in which the transnational corporations Dow, Shell, and Dole were ordered to pay US$490 million in compensation to 583 Nicaraguan banana workers who were sterilized by Nemagon (Ling and Jarocki 2003).

La Via Campesina, founded in 1993 in Belgium, is an international movement of peasants, small- and medium-sized producers, landless people, rural women, indigenous groups, rural youth, and agricultural workers. La Via Campesina works for preservation of land, water, seeds, and other natural resources; food sovereignty; sustainable agriculture; gender and equity; and fair economic relations. Its efforts on economic and food sovereignty and social justice make it as much (or more) an environmental health actor as explicitly environmentally focused international agencies.

Urban agriculture has become a leading component of food security in many settings, and its practitioners form an informal environmental movement. Resource Centres on Urban Agriculture and Food Security (RUAF) is an international network of poverty reduction and urban development organizations that promotes urban garden plots at home, on rented or reclaimed plots (e.g., in parks or along waterways), or in semi-public areas (hospital or school grounds) as a form of food and economic security and nutritional enhancement. Typically raised by poor urbanites, schoolteachers, and women (who combine urban agriculture with other household tasks) in rapidly urbanizing areas, produce and animal products are both sold and consumed by agriculturalists. In Dakar and Shanghai, for example, up to 60% of vegetables and poultry (and over 90% of Shanghai's milk and eggs) are cultivated by urban farmers. These activities constitute anywhere from 10% to 100% of household earnings and help generate other enterprises (e.g., delivery, street vending) (RUAF 2007). Ecological benefits include the productive use of food waste as compost and fertilizers and the creation of "green zones." However, using human waste and untreated wastewater can cause health problems: urban soil may be toxic, and urban farmlands may be hazardous worksites. Moreover, despite the benefits, the proliferation of urban agriculture precludes easy health and safety inspection (Mougeot 2006).

Monitoring contamination is an important activity of local environmental health groups and larger networks. The Indonesian NGO Yayasan Duta Awam has been monitoring a World Bank "integrated swamps development" project since 1997, training local farmers to monitor their own health and the general use of toxic pesticides. The group showed that there was increased use of hazardous pesticides without proper training regarding handling (with women excluded from training), project corruption, and that the project's pesticides were being sold in local markets. Yayasan Duta Awam developed connections with other national groups and with the Pesticide Action Network (an international network of grassroots organizations) and in 1998 presented the World Bank and government officials with a list of reforms. These efforts pressured the project to suspend use of chemical pesticides and train farmers in alternative forms of ecological pest management (Ishii-Eiteman 2000).

Environmental organizations and movements (such as the Center for Health, Environment and Justice and the Toxics Action Center) in the United States and elsewhere have also been shaped by "popular epidemiology" (Brown, Kroll-Smith, and Gunter 2000) in which nonexperts (lay people) mobilize to identify and assess environmental hazards. For example, starting in the 1970s in Woburn, Massachusetts, local residents noticed unusually high occurrence of childhood leukemia and began to conduct their own research, eventually forging partnerships with professional researchers to show that elevated leukemia rates were linked to toxic emissions and by-products from local industries (Brown and Mikkelsen 1990). These efforts culminated in a successful lawsuit against a local industry for dumping chemicals (Arksey 1998).

Other longstanding environmental efforts have moved in the opposite direction, joining forces with corporate interests in recent years. For example, the Environmental Defense Fund, based in Washington, DC, is a scientific advocacy group founded in the 1960s that successfully fought for a DDT ban in the United States, helped secure the passage of the 1974 U.S. Safe Drinking Water Act, and ensured protection for 75,000 sq. miles of ocean. But more recently it has addressed environmental problems through corporate partnerships, leading to watered-down measures such as market mechanisms to buy and sell emissions rights (Environmental Defense Fund 2007).

Mining Watch (Canada) also straddles corporate and environmental interests. In monitoring the activities of mining companies to ensure that their practices are sustainable and ecological, it helps "prevent the development of projects that would adversely affect areas of ecological, economic and cultural significance," and advocates for policies to reduce the human and environmental hazards of mineral development (Mining Watch 2006).

A number of North American environmental movements have been active for almost half a century. Greenpeace began in 1971 in Vancouver to "bear witness" to U.S. nuclear testing off the coast of Alaska. The publicity Greenpeace generated around the dangers nuclear testing posed to wildlife pressured the U.S. government to suspend testing in that region and create a bird sanctuary. Today Greenpeace has approximately 2.8 million supporters and 41 offices around the world. Its victories have included the phasing out of the use of dangerous chemicals in apple products, a switch from nuclear to renewable energy plants in five European countries, a nine-country ban on the use of phthalates in toys, and a variety of measures to protect oceans. Greenpeace is often engaged in high-profile stunts to draw media attention, but the largest was not of its own making: in 1985, French secret service agents sank Greenpeace ship, "The Rainbow Warrior," in New Zealand, where it was based to protest nuclear testing in the South Pacific (Greenpeace 2007b).

CONCLUSION

Learning Points:

- The political economy of environmental health analyzes the interaction of humans with the natural and built environments. It traces the role and pressure of underlying economic and political forces on environmental change, on the creation and spread of damaging agents, and on ensuing health consequences, as well as the interaction of policies, politics, technologies, and human actions with each of these factors.
- Every society and economic order disrupts the environment to a greater or lesser extent. However, since the rise of industrial capitalism in the 19th century, and especially in the last 50 years, there have been persistent detrimental changes to the climate, land, forests, water, air, wildlife, and the ecosystem writ large, on a far greater scale than ever before.
- Environmental degradation and the means to redress it are simultaneously local and global: regional variations may be understood within the logic of global capitalism.
- Ameliorating and preventing damage to the environment and to human health requires actions at household, community, national, and global levels; social and political movements play a key role in ensuring passage of protective legislation and industrial regulation.

When all is said and done, what are the best means of improving environmental health and reducing the impact of human activity on particular ecosystems and the globe as a whole? Undoubtedly, a single strategy is insufficient. Certainly many effective local and individual activities play a vital educational role and help to improve local environmental conditions. But in the end, efforts must focus on national and transnational companies and industries, which are the largest users of energy and resources, and, ultimately, the shapers of consumption, transport, and other patterns of use and abuse of the built and natural environments. Does this mean that industry should be regulated through incentives or penalties? Will prioritizing the health of the natural and built environments return us to simple living, or will eco-building enable an integration of new technologies and environmental protection? And how will these changes affect and engage with the governance of societies?

While these are momentous problems that may appear intractable, understanding the political-economy basis of environmental health is a critical first step in generating lasting change. Stopgap solutions may avert disaster in the short term, but constructive change in the long term will require transformations to the very structures of society. Of course, health and environmentally friendly decision-making capacity rests on economic and political sovereignty and equity, struggles which are still in the making. Both current and future generations will need to wrestle with and resolve these vital issues.

REFERENCES

Agency for Toxic Substances and Disease Registry. 2007. ToxFAQs: Frequently asked questions about contaminants found at hazardous waste sites. http://www.atsdr.cdc.gov/toxfaq.html. Accessed September 24, 2007.

Altieri MA. 2000. Ecological impacts of industrial agriculture and the possibilities for sustainable farming. In Magdoff F, Foster J, and Buttel F, Editors. *Hungry for Profit: The Agribusiness Threat to Farmers, Food and the Environment.* New York: Monthly Review Press.

American Wind Energy Association. 2007. Wind energy potential. http://www.awea.org/faq/wwt_potential.html. Accessed August 28, 2007.

Arksey H. 1998. *RSI and the Experts: The Construction of Medical Knowledge.* London: UCL Press.

Arthurton R, Barker S, Rast W, Huber M, Alder J, Chilton J, Gaddis E, Pietersen K, and Zockler C. 2007. Water. In *Global Environment Outlook: Environment for Development, GEO 4.* Nairobi, Kenya: UNEP.

Barringer F. 2006. $92 million more is sought for Exxon Valdez cleanup. *New York Times,* June 2.

Basrur S. 2002. *Lawn and Garden Pesticides: A Review of Human Exposure & Health Effects Research.* Toronto, Canada: Toronto Public Health.

Batchelder T. 2001. Agrochemicals and health: An anthropological perspective. *Townsend Letter for Doctors and Patients* 210:38–41.

Batterbury S. 2003. Environmental activism and social networks: Campaigning for bicycles and alternative transport in West London. *The Annals of the American Academy of Political and Social Science* 590(1):150–169.

Beatley T. 2000. *Green Urbanism: Learning from European Cities.* Washington, DC: Island Press.

Bierbaum R, Holdren JP, MacCracken M, Moss RH, and Raven PH, Editors. 2007. *Confronting Climate Change: Avoiding the Unmanageable and Managing the Unavoidable.* Scientific Expert Group Report on Climate Change and Sustainable Development. Prepared for the United Nations Commission on Sustainable Development. Research Triangle Park, NC: Sigma Xi Foundation; Washington, DC: The United Nations Foundation.

Black M. 2004. *The No-Nonsense Guide to Water.* London: Verso Books.

Blacksmith Institute. 2007. *The World's Worst Polluted Places: The Top Ten of the Dirty Thirty.* New York: Blacksmith Institute.

Bond P. 2004. The political roots of South Africa's cholera epidemic. In Fort M, Mercer M and Gish O, Editors. *Sickness and Wealth: The Corporate Assault on Global Health.* Cambridge, MA: South End Press.

Brown P. 2007. *Toxic Exposures: Contested Illnesses and the Environmental Health Movement.* New York: Columbia University Press.

Brown P, Kroll-Smith S, and Gunter V. 2000. Knowledge, citizens and organizations: An overview of environments, diseases and social conflict. In Kroll-Smith S, Brown P, and Gunter V, Editors. *Illness and the Environment: A Reader in Contested Medicine.* New York: New York University Press.

Brown P and Mikkelsen EJ. 1990. *No Safe Place: Toxic Waste, Leukemia and Community Action.* Berkeley, CA: University of California Press.

Brown P and Zavestoski S. 2005. Social movements in health: An introduction. In Brown P and Zavestoski S, Editors. *Social Movements in Health.* Oxford: Blackwell Publishing.

Bullard R, Mohai P, Saha R, and Wright B. 2007. *Toxic Wastes and Race at Twenty: 1987—2007. Grassroots Struggles to Dismantle Environmental Racism in the United States.* A Report Prepared for the United Church of Christ Justice & Witness Ministries. Cleveland, OH: United Church of Christ.

Carson R. 1962. *Silent Spring.* Boston, MA: Houghton Mifflin.

Chopra A. 2007. Developing countries are awash in e-waste. Basel Action Network homepage. http://www.ban.org/ban_news/2007/070330_awash_in_ewaste.html. Accessed September 24, 2007.

CIDA. 2007. Land degradation. http://www.acdi-cida.gc.ca/CIDAWEB/acdicida.nsf/En/JUD-121164957-TLW. Accessed November 23, 2007.

Civil Aviation Authority. 2007. Aircraft emissions and climate change. http://www.caa.co.uk/default.aspx?catid=68&pagetype=90&pageid=52. Accessed October 23, 2007.

Clapp J and Dauvergne P. 2005. *Paths to a Green World: The Political Economy of the Global Environment.* Cambridge, MA: MIT Press.

Clapp J and Princen T. 2003. Out of sight, out of mind: Cross-border traffic in waste obscures the problem of consumption. *Alternatives Journal* 29(3):39–41.

Cole DC, Crissman CC, and Fadya Orozco A. 2006. Canada's International Development Research Centre's Eco-health projects with Latin Americans: Origins, development and challenges. *Canadian Journal of Public Health* 97(6):8–14.

Cole DC, Eyles J, Gibson BL, and Ross N. 1999. Links between humans and ecosystems: The implications of framing for health promotion strategies. *Health Promotion International* 14(1):65–72.

Collins K and Taylor L. 2007. A large-scale urban development HIA: Focusing on vulnerable groups in London, England. In Wismar M, Blau J, Ernst K, and Figueras J, Editors. *The Effectiveness of Health Impact Assessment: Scope and Limitations of Supporting Decision-Making in Europe.* Brussels: European Observatory on Health Systems and Policies.

Cooper DB. 1965. *Epidemic Disease in Mexico City, 1716–1813: An Administrative, Social, and Medical Study.* Austin, TX: University of Texas Press.

Corvalán C, Hales S, and McMichael A. 2005. *Ecosystems and Human Well-Being: Health Synthesis. A Report of the Millennium Eco-System Assessment.* Geneva: WHO.

Crowther D and Rayman-Bacchus L. 2004. *Perspectives on Corporate Social Responsibility.* Aldershot, England: Ashgate.

Daniels JL, Olshan AF, and Savitz DA. 1997. Pesticides and childhood cancers. *Environmental Health Perspectives* 105(10):1068–1077.

Dauvergne P. 2005a. Globalization and the environment. In Ravenhill J, Editor. *Global Political Economy*. Oxford: Oxford University Press.

————. 2005b. Dying of consumption: Accidents or sacrifices of global morality? *Global Environmental Politics* 5(3):35–47.

Dent D, Asfary AF, Giri C, Govil K, Hartemink A, Holmgren P, et al. 2007. Land. *Global Environment Outlook: Environment for Development,GEO-4*, UNEP, Editor. Nairobi, Kenya: UNEP.

Doyal L. 1979. *The Political Economy of Health*. London: Pluto Press.

Editorial. 2003. Court is ordered to reconsider award in Exxon Valdez spill. *New York Times*, August 23.

Eilperin J. 2008. Studies say clearing land for biofuels will aid warming. *Washington Post,* February 8, A05.

Ekins P. 2005. Environmental regeneration. In Amoore L, Editor. *The Global Resistance Reader*. New York: Routledge.

El-Fadel M, Zeinati M, and Jamali D. 2000. Framework for environmental impact assessment in Lebanon. *Environmental Impact Assessment Review* 20(5):579–604.

Environmental Defense Fund. 2003. Social forum urges Putin to ratify Kyoto protocol. http://www.environmentaldefense.org/article.cfm?contentid=3066. Accessed August 28, 2007.

————. 2007. About Us. http://www.edf.org/home.cfm. Accessed November 28, 2007.

Epstein, PR. 2005. Climate change and human health. *New England Journal of Medicine* 353(14):1433–1436.

Erikson D. 2004. The Haiti dilemma. *The Brown Journal of World Affairs* 10(2): 285–297.

Evans P. 2002. Introduction: Looking for agents of urban livability in a globalized political economy. In Evans P, Editor. *Livable Cities? Urban Struggles for Livelihood and Sustainability*. Berkeley, CA: University of California Press.

Ezzati M. 2005. Indoor air pollution and health in developing countries. *Lancet* 366(9480): 104–106.

Fairless D. 2007. Northern Aral Sea recovering. *Naturenews*, April 12.

FAO (Food and Agriculture Organization). 2006. *The State of Food Insecurity in the World 2006*. Rome: FAO.

————. 2007. *Fire Management Global Assessment 2006*. Rome: FAO.

Fletcher M. 2007. The return of the sea. *Times Online*, June 23.

Friedman M. 2006. theCorporation.com. http://www.thecorporation.com/index.cfm?page_id=3. Accessed December 5, 2007.

Friis RH. 2007. *Essentials of Environmental Health*. Sudbury, MA: Jones & Bartlett Publishers.

Global Footprint Network. 2006. *National Footprint Accounts, 2006 Edition*. Oakland, CA.

Global Health Watch. 2005. *Global Health Watch 2005–2006: An Alternative World Health Report*. London: Zed Books.

Goldstein, IF and Goldstein M. 2002. *How Much Risk? A Guide to Understanding Environmental Health Hazards*. New York: Oxford University Press.

Goodman J, Laube M, and Schwenk J. 2006. Curitiba's bus system is model for rapid transit. *Race, Poverty and the Environment: A Journal for Social and Environmental Justice* 12(1): 75–76.

Greenberg I. 2006. A vanished sea reclaims its form in Central Asia. *International Herald Tribute*, April 7.

Greenhouse L. 2007. Justices to hear Exxon's challenge to punitive damages. *New York Times*, October 30.

Greenpeace. 2007a. Agreement on acknowledging the value of the Amazon forest and ending deforestation. Translated from the original Portuguese text: 'Pacto pela Valorização de Floresta e pelo Fim do Desmantamento na Amazônia. http://www.greenpeace.org/raw/content/international/press/reports/amazon-deforestation-agreement.pdf. Accessed December 12, 2007.

————. 2007b. Greenpeace victories. http://www.greenpeace.org/international/about/ victories. Accessed December 5, 2007.

Gunter, MM. 2004. *Building the Next Ark: How NGOs Work to Protect Biodiversity.* Lebanon, NH: University Press of New England.

Hancock, T. 2002. Indicators of environmental health in the urban setting. *Canadian Journal of Public Health* 93(Supp 1):S45–S51.

Hancock T and Duhl L. 1988. Healthy cities: Promoting health in the urban context. Healthy Cities Papers No. 1. Denmark: WHO EURO.

Herbst K. 1992. Brazil's model city. *Planning* 58(9):24–27.

Hilgenkamp K. 2006. *Environmental Health: Ecological Perspectives.* Sudbury, MA: Jones & Bartlett Publishers.

Hippocrates. 1868. *Airs, waters, places.* In Jones WHS, Translator and Editor. Hippocrates Collected Works I. Cambridge, MA: Harvard University Press. http://www.chlt.org/ sandbox/dh/HippocratesLoeb1/page.103.a.php?size=240x320. Accessed December 11, 2007.

Hirschhorn N. 2004. Corporate social responsibility and the tobacco industry: Hope or hype? *Tobacco Control* 13:447–453.

Hjertaas P and Taylor Al. 2002. Chemical warfare in the school zones: Concerned parents are working to replace poisons in the schools with safer, child-friendly alternatives. *Briarpatch* September.

Howard CV and Newby JA. 2004. Could the increase in cancer incidence be related to recent environmental changes? In Nicolopoulou-Stamati P, Hens L, Howard V, and Van Larebeke N, Editors. *Cancer as an Environmental Disease.* Dordrecht, The Netherlands: Kluwer Academic Publishers.

ICEH (Institute for Children's Environmental Health). 2007. National learning and development disabilities advocacy groups analyze body burden studies. www.iceh.org/ pdfs/LDDI/bodyburdenbriefLDDI.pdf. Accessed August 17, 2007.

ILO. 2000. Top on the agenda: Health and safety in agriculture. *Labour Education* 1–2 (118–119).

————. 2006. Safety and health in agriculture. http://www.ilo.org/public/english/dialogue/ sector/sectors/agri/safety.htm. Accessed December 4, 2007.

IPCC. 2001. *Climate Change 2001: Synthesis Report Summary of Policy Makers.* London: UN Intergovernmental Panel on Climate Change.

————. 2007a. *Climate Change 2007: Impacts, Adaptation and Vulnerability.* Geneva: UN Intergovernmental Panel on Climate Change.

————. 2007b. *IPCC WGI fourth Assessment Report: The Physical Science Basis.* Geneva: IPCC Secretariat.

————. 2007c. *Mitigation of Climate Change.* Bangkok, Thailand: UN Intergovernmental Panel on Climate Change.

Ishii-Eiteman M. 2000. Countering corporate influence at the World Bank: The mobilization of transnational coalitions. http://www.panna.org/campaigns/docsWorldBank/ docsWorldBank_001201.dv.html. Accessed November 27, 2007.

Kriebel D and Tickner J. 2001. The precautionary principle and public health: Re-energizing public health through precaution. *American Journal of Public Health* 91(9):1351–1355.

Krieger N, Northridge M, Gruskin S, Quinn M, Kriebel D, Davey Smith G et al. and the "HIA promise and pitfalls" conference group. 2003. Assessing health impact assessment: Multidisciplinary and international perspectives. *Journal of Epidemiology and Community Health* 57(9):659–662.

Kroll-Smith S, Brown P, and Gunter V. 2000. Environments and diseases in a postnatural world. In *Illness and the Environment: A Reader in Contested Medicine*. New York: New York University Press.

Kuylenstierna JCI, Panwar TS, Ashmore M, Brack D, Eerents H, Feresu S, et al. 2007. Atmosphere. In *GEO-4*. Nairobi, Kenya: UNEP.

Kylychbekova M. 2007. Russia's worst mining tragedy. http://www.pacificenvironment.org/article.php?id=2289. Accessed September 24, 2007.

Ling A and Jarocki MO. 2003. Pesticide justice. (The Front). *Multinational Monitor* 24(1-2).

Litman T. 2003. *Reinventing Transportation: Exploring the Paradigm Shift Needed to Reconcile Transportation and Sustainability Objectives*. Victoria, BC: Victoria Transport Policy Institute.

Loh J and Wackernagel M, Editors. 2004. *Living Planet Report 2004*. Gland, Switzerland: WWF.

Lohmann L. 2001. Democracy or Carbocracy? Intellectual Corruption and the Future of the Climate Debate. *Corner House Briefing*, October 24.

Lubow A. 2007. The road to Curitiba. *New York Times*, May 20.

MacArthur ID. 2002. Local environmental health planning: Guidance for local and national authorities. London: WHO Regional Publications European Series.

Macedo J. 2004. City profile: Curitiba. *Cities* 21(6):537–549.

McKibben B. 2003. *Enough: Staying Human in an Engineered Age*. New York: Holt Paperbacks.

McMichael AJ. 2001. *Human Frontiers, Environments and Disease: Past Patterns, Uncertain Futures*. Cambridge: Cambridge University Press.

Mining Watch. 2006. Mining watch. http://www.miningwatch.ca/index.php. Accessed November 27, 2007.

Mokhiber R. 1999. Exxon: Mean and stupid. *Multinational Monitor* 20(3).

Mougeot LJA. 2006. *Growing Better Cities*. Ottawa, ON: International Development Research Centre.

Narmada. 2006. The Sardar Sarovar dam: A brief introduction. http://www.narmada.org/sardarsarovar.html. Accessed December 4, 2007.

National Research Council. 2001. *Making Transit Work: Insights from Western Europe, Canada, and the United States. Special Report 257*. Committee for an International Comparison of National Policies and Expectations Affecting Public Transit. Washington, DC: The National Academies Press.

Ortiz de Montellano B. 1990. *Aztec Medicine, Health, and Nutrition*. New Brunswick, NJ: Rutgers University Press.

PAHO. 1994. *A World Safe from Natural Disasters. The Journey of Latin America and the Caribbean*. Washington, DC: PAHO.

Parasram V 2003. Efficient transportation for successful urban planning in Curitiba. http://www.solutions-site.org/artman/publish/article_62.shtml. Accessed July 15, 2007.

Perry T, Matsui E, Merriman B, Duong T, and Eggleston PJ. 2003. The prevalence of rat allergen in inner-city homes and its relationship to sensitization and asthma morbidity. *Allergy and Clinical Immunology* 112(2):346–352.

PHM. 2005. The Cuenca declaration. http://www.phmovement.org/pha2/papers/cuencadec3.php. Accessed November 27, 2007.

Potera C. 2004. Air pollution: Asia's two-stroke engine dilemma. *Environmental Health Perspectives* 112(11):A613.

PricewaterhouseCoopers. 2007. *Mine: Riding the Wave. Metals and Mining: Review of Global Trends in the Mining Industry.* Johannesburg: PricewaterhouseCoopers.

Prüss-Üstün A and Corvalán C. 2006. *Preventing Disease through Healthy Environments: Towards an Estimate of the Environmental Burden of Diseases.* Geneva: WHO.

Renewable Energy Access. 2005. Spain's wind power industry on a roll. http://www. renewableenergyaccess.com/rea/news/story?id=35745. Accessed September 24, 2007.

Roach J. 2007. Amazon deforestation drops 25 percent, Brazil says. http://news. nationalgeographic.com/news/2007/08/070814-amazon-brazil.html. Accessed November 24, 2007.

RUAF (Resource Centres on Urban Agriculture & Food Security). 2007. Why is urban agriculture important? http://www.ruaf.org/node/513. Accessed November 27, 2007.

Runge CF and Senauer B. 2007. How biofuels could starve the poor. *Foreign Affairs* 86(3).

Sapien J. 2007. Massive undertaking to clean up hazardous waste sites has lost both momentum and funding. http://projects.publicintegrity.org/superfund/report. aspx?aid=851. Accessed October 23, 2007.

Schaefer F, Luksch U, Steinbach N, Cabeca J, and Hanauer J. 2006. *Ecological Footprint and Biocapacity: The World's Ability to Regenerate Resources and Absorb Waste in a Limited Time Period.* Luxembourg: European Communities.

Schwartz S and Chance GW. 1999. Children first. *Alternatives Journal* 25(3):20–25.

Secretariat of the Convention on Biological Diversity. 2004. *CBD News: The Convention on Biological Diversity: From Conception to Implementation.* Montreal: SCBD.

Shiva V. 2000. *Stolen Harvest: The Hijacking of the Global Food Supply.* Cambridge, MA: South End Press.

———. 2002. *Water Wars: Privatization, Pollution, and Profit.* Cambridge, MA: South End Press.

Siliquini R, Nante N, and Ricciardi W. 2007. Ecosystem revitalization: community empowerment through HIA in Tuscany, Italy. In Wismar M, Blau J, Ernst K and Figueras J, Editors. *The Effectiveness of Health Impact Assessment: Scope and Limitations of Supporting Decision-Making in Europe.* Copenhagen: European Observatory on Health Systems and Policies.

Smith RD, Beaglehole R, Woodward D, and Drager N, Editors. 2003. *Global Public Goods for Health: Health Economic and Public Health Perspectives.* New York: Oxford University Press.

Soustelle J. 1970. *Daily Life of the Aztecs on the Eve of the Spanish Conquest.* Palo Alto, CA: Stanford University Press.

Stevens G, Wilson A, and Hammitt JK. 2005. A benefit–cost analysis of retrofitting diesel vehicles with particulate filters in the Mexico City metropolitan area. *Society for Risk Analysis* 25(4):883–899.

Tilly C. 2004. *Social Movements, 1768–2004.* Boulder, CO: Paradigm Publishers.

UN. 1992. United Nations Framework Convention on Climate Change. http://www. undocuments.net/unfccc.htm. Accessed August 2007.

UNDP. 2006. *Human Development Report 2006: Beyond Scarcity: Power, Poverty and the Global Water Crisis.* New York: UNDP.

———. 2007. *Human Development Report 2007: Fighting Climate Change: Human Solidarity in a Divided World.* New York: UNDP.

UNEP. 2007a. Economic instruments to promote compliance. http://www.unep.org/dec/
    onlinemanual/Enforcement/InstitutionalFrameworks/EconomicInstruments/tabid/88/
    Default.aspx. Accessed October 23, 2007.
———. 2007b. *Global Environment Outlook: Environment for Development, GEO 4.*
    Nairobi, Kenya: UNEP.
UNESCO. 2007. The European Union biofuels directive. http://webapps01.un.org/dsd/
    caseStudy/public/displayDetailsAction.do?code=245. Accessed August 17, 2007.
United Nations Framework Convention on Climate Change (UNFCCC). 2008. Kyoto
    protocol: Status of ratification. http://unfccc.int/kyoto_protocol/
    status_of_ratification/items/2613.php. Accessed November 19, 2008.
———. 2007. UNFCCC Executive Secretary calls for speedy and decisive international
    action on climate change. http://unfccc.int/files/press/news_room/press_releases_and_
    advisories/application/pdf/070202press_rel_paris_en.pdf. Accessed August 2007.
U.S. Department of Energy. 2007. *International Energy Outlook.* Washington, DC: Energy
    Information Administration, U.S. Department of Energy.
U.S. Environmental Protection Agency. 2006. Source reduction and reuse. http://www.epa.
    gov/msw/sourcred.htm. Accessed December 5, 2007.
USDA NRCS. 2007. Land degradation and desertification. United States Department
    of Agriculture, Natural Resource Conservation Service. http://soils.usda.gov/use/
    worldsoils/landdeg/. Accessed November 23, 2007.
Walker LR and Powell EA. 2001. Soil water retention on gold mine surfaces in the Mojave
    Desert. *Restoration Ecology* 9(1):95–103.
WHO. 2002a. *WHO Global Strategy for Food Safety: Safer Food for Better Health.*
    Geneva: WHO.
———. 2002b. *World Health Report 2002: Reducing Risks, Promoting Healthy Life.*
    Geneva: WHO.
———. 2005. *Ecosystems and Human Well-Being: Health Synthesis. A Report of the
    Millennium Ecosystem Assessment.* Geneva: WHO.
———. 2006a. Chronic respiratory diseases. http://www.who.int/respiratory/en/. Accessed
    July 28, 2006.
———. 2006b. Water related diseases. http://www.who.int/water_sanitation_health/
    diseases. Accessed October 12, 2006.
———. 2007. Facts: Urban settings as a social determinant of health. http://www.who.int/
    social_determinants/features/en/index.html. Accessed March 13, 2007.
WHO EURO. 2003. *Healthy Cities Around the World: An Overview of the Healthy Cities
    Movement in the Six WHO Regions.* Copenhagen: WHO Europe.
———. 2005. *Particulate Matter Air Pollution: How it Harms Health.* Fact sheet. Berlin,
    Copenhagen, Rome: WHO Europe.
———. 2006. Healthy cities and urban governance. http://www.euro.who.int/healthy-cities/
    introducing/20050202_2. Accessed October 12, 2006.
WHO and UNICEF. 2008. *World Health Organization and United Nations Children's
    Fund Joint Monitoring Programme for Water Supply and Sanitation. Progress on
    Drinking Water and Sanitation: Special Focus on Sanitation.* New York: UNICEF;
    Geneva: WHO.
Wilson, EO. 1992. *The Diversity of Life.* New York: WW Norton.
World Wildlife Fund. 2007. Bilateral debt-for-nature swaps by creditor: Summary
    table. http://www.worldwildlife.org/what/howwedoit/conservationfinance/
    WWFBinaryitem7089.pdf. Accessed March 13, 2007.

World Summit on Sustainable Development. 2002. *Johannesburg Declaration on Sustainable Development: From Our Origins to the Future.* Johannesburg, South Africa: United Nations.

Yardley J. 2007. Chinese dam projects criticized for their human costs. *New York Times*, November 19.

11

Health Economics and the Economics of Health

Global spending on health is immense but inequitable. The WHO estimates that in 2004, US$4.1 trillion was spent on the health sector—both public and private (WHO 2007b)—totaling over 10% of world income (see Table 11–1). Some consider health care to be the world's largest industry. As such, one of the key concerns of both international and national health policy making is determining how to allocate and spend available resources in an appropriate and effective way in order to achieve particular health-related goals and objectives. The field of economics can help in providing a road map to this end. The main issue in health economics is not simply minimizing costs, but obtaining the greatest value from an efficient use of resources. For a specific health problem, health economics attempts to calculate how to accomplish a better outcome for the same cost, the same outcome at a lower cost, or ideally, a better outcome at a lower cost. In broad terms, health economics may be defined as the:

> application of the theories, concepts and techniques of economics to the institutions, actors and activities that affect health. It is concerned with such matters as the allocation of resources between various health-promoting activities; the quantity of resources used in health service delivery; the organization, funding, and behavior of health services institutions and providers; the efficiency with which resources are used for health purposes; and the effects of disease and health interventions on individuals, households, and society (Mills 1997, p. 964).

As national governments and international agencies increasingly emphasize prudent health spending, health economics is playing a growing role in health system planning and program implementation. While many economists regard health spending largely in terms of medical treatment and individual preventative measures, others understand health investments at the societal level *apropos* the underlying determinants of health, including education, safe housing and employment,

537

Table 11–1 Spending on Health: Some Examples of the Extent of Inequities (in US$)

Total global expenditure on health	$4.1 trillion
Per capita expenditure globally	$639
Country with highest per capita expenditure	United States ($6,103)
Country with lowest per capita expenditure	Burundi ($2.90)
WHO estimate of minimum needed expenditure per capita	$35–$50
Number of WHO member countries spending less than $20 per capita	30

Source: Adapted from WHO (2007b).

water and sanitation, and environmental protection. Though health economics is essential to understanding patterns of global health care spending and decision making, it is important to remember the difference between investing in health—which involves multiple layers of determinants—and investing in health care, just one particular determinant of health.

The World Bank and other proponents of orthodox (neoclassical) health economics support targeted low-cost interventions for developing countries (Jamison 2006), though not for high-income nations. This advice is based on evidence of health improvements that are usually measured by short-term drops in specific disease rates. According to this approach, allocation decisions must prioritize resources and interventions that have the greatest impact at the lowest cost because health resources are considered to be scarce.

Proponents of health and social justice approaches, by contrast, argue that technical cost analyses favor short-term, narrowly focused approaches to health improvement rather than overall health gains in the long run (Kim et al. 2005). Instead, progressive health economists stress the importance of comprehensive means of improving health that integrate primary health care-oriented universal health systems with social and political investment and redistribution on a broad scale. They also emphasize that income distribution is a key determinant of the supply of health services, of health outcomes, and of economic growth (Chernomas 1999).

Ideally, health economics can help assess the fairness and equity of health-oriented investments, though these concerns often remain at a rhetorical level. Even the most technically elaborate economic analyses of health policies are not neutral, but are in fact based on value judgments and decisions. The way in which priorities are set in the health system clearly illustrate that social objectives and factors other than empirical evidence continue to play a large role in determining resource allocation (Jan, Dommers, and Mooney 2003). This is true whether one examines priority-setting for reproductive health services in Ghana, where donor interests are highly influential (Reichenbach 2002), or amongst regional health authorities in

Canada, where local politics and historical patterns are more influential than health economics in setting priorities for resource allocation (Mitton and Donaldson 2002). A further problem with technocratic priority-setting mechanisms is that most reflect Western values on decision-making processes yet are applied widely with little regard for local social, historical, cultural, and political contexts.

Box 11-1 Georgia's Experiences with Changes in Health Financing

Georgia became independent from the Soviet Union in 1991. Under the Soviet system, Georgia enjoyed high health status indicators: in 1991, the maternal mortality ratio was 37 maternal deaths/100,000 live births, life expectancy at birth was 73, and there were low rates of infectious disease, in part thanks to extensive social welfare infrastructure, including a state-run universal health system. The civil unrest and deteriorated economic conditions following independence—and an end to reliance on Moscow for health system funding—led Georgia's new government to abandon its universal health care system. This move was backed by the World Bank and IMF, which viewed the former Soviet system as inefficient and pushed for health reform with more private sector involvement.

In 1993, Georgia switched to a social insurance model that included only a select basket of services, with out-of-pocket payments required for all other services. Because roughly 65% of the Georgian population is employed in the informal sector, the tax base for public services is small, but virtually no effort was made to regularize employment conditions. Cost-effectiveness analysis was employed in this reform process, and there was some continued public funding for certain services covered previously, such as inpatient psychiatric care and drugs for terminally ill patients. In the end, the reform left most health care needs abandoned by the public sector.

In 2002, 50% of the Georgian population had nominal access to health care services, though in reality the majority had virtually no access due to high costs of care and an inequitable distribution of resources. At the same time, health workers became increasingly impoverished, as user fees were insufficient to cover their salaries. Georgia has one of the highest rates of out-of-pocket health care spending in the world, at 83% of all expenditures (UNDP 2000, Gamkrelidze et al. 2002; Collins 2006).

Since Georgia's independence, equity, quality, and access to health services have all deteriorated, contributing—together with a range of social and political determinants—to an increase in infant mortality and infectious diseases. Life expectancy declined by 3 years beginning in 1992, and only reached 73 again in 2003 (WHO EURO 2007). The maternal mortality ratio reached a high of 70 deaths/100,000 births in 1997 (World Bank 2005), somewhat declining by 2005 to 66/100,000 (WHOSIS 2008). TB rates climbed, from 28.8 cases/100,000 in 1990 to 86.6 cases/100,000 in 1998. Although rates slightly improved to 84 cases/100,000 in 2006, they are still markedly higher than under the Soviet regime (WHO 2007c).

This chapter presents an overview and critique of health economics and health system financing, covering the aims, assumptions, and uses of the main tools of health economics. This lens will also, consistent with the textbook as a whole, understand health to be determined by many factors that lie outside of health care services and systems. Income, education, housing, water and sanitation, social security systems, nutrition, and transport are as important, if not far more important than, medical care. Economic factors outside of the traditional realm of health care services also have a significant impact upon health, such as school fees, housing costs, and food prices and a household's ability to pay for those needs. For that reason, government subsidies for food, price controls, and unemployment benefits may have a greater effect on health status than funding health services. This chapter will deal only with the economics of the formal, allopathic medical sector. Traditional healers will be discussed in Chapter 12.

ECONOMIC APPROACHES TO PUBLIC HEALTH AND MEDICAL SPENDING

Key Questions:

- What is the relationship between health and the economy?
- What are the underlying assumptions of markets?
- How does health differ from other goods/services?
- Why are markets incapable of equitably providing health services?

As evidenced by measures as varied as Roman aqueducts and Aztec street cleaning, recognition of the societal merits of health investments is far from new. With the 19th century Industrial Revolution, the productivity of workers (and by association, their health) became an ever-higher public priority. Unionized workers and social reformers struggled to improve working and living conditions, including sanitation and housing conditions. Although merchants, manufacturers, and colonial authorities were reluctant to pay for municipal improvements (which were ultimately shouldered by taxpayers), by the early 20th century employers became concerned with maintaining the health of workers, particularly skilled laborers, as a means of improving productivity, decreasing absenteeism and training costs, and staving off unrest. Physical exams became a prerequisite for employment, as well as military service, in these years. Meanwhile, unionized workers fought for rights such as social insurance, workers' compensation, and an 8-hour workday, and began an ongoing struggle for occupational safety and health measures.[1] Notwithstanding the widely recognized value of health care services for society-at-large, and the role of collective planning and organization of health services delivery, many orthodox health economists continue to portray and favor health system organization as the fruition of individual consumer choices.

How (Health Care) Markets Work (and Their Limits)

Neoclassical economic theory holds that the price of a good or service is determined by demand for that good/service (i.e., how many people are willing and able to pay for it), as well as its supply (the amount that has been produced/exists); because many goods are finite, the market provides a forum for consumers to compete for them. This school of thought argues that the extent of scarcity of an item, combined with the level of competition, determines its price. In particular, as supply becomes limited, and competition more fierce, the price of a product is driven up. As the price climbs, people begin to be "priced out" of the market: meaning they no longer desire the product at that price. Conversely, as a product becomes more abundant, its price falls and demand increases, as those who previously deemed the product to be too expensive now find it affordable.

For example, if there are 20 schoolbags produced in a given year at $10/schoolbag and 40 people wanting to buy schoolbags, some individuals may be willing to pay more to ensure they obtain the product. The schoolbag manufacturer (and/or seller) can test this scenario by increasing the market price. The price increase may continue until enough people have been "priced out" of the market and the supply of schoolbags matches the demand. However, if there are 40 schoolbags produced, but only 20 people interested in purchasing the product at $10, the producer/seller may lower the price until the number of people willing to buy a schoolbag matches the number available on the market. Further, if the schoolbags are found to be defective or of extremely low quality, people may stop buying them and the price will drop significantly. If the sellers can find new (typically very low-income) buyers and can continue to make profits at the lower prices, the defective bags will remain on the market; otherwise they will be withdrawn.

This line of reasoning rests on two assumptions: (1) all players participate voluntarily in the market and can choose to leave (i.e., no longer make, sell, or purchase a product) at any time, or are able to select an alternative product, at a more desirable price; and (2) all players (both suppliers and purchasers of a product) have equal access to information regarding price, demand, and availability. Notably, true need is left out of this calculus: only supply and demand are taken into consideration in a market-based system.

Health care markets, however, differ from other kinds of markets.[2] Consequently, the classic supply and demand curve—whereby the relationship between supply and demand is mediated by price—does not apply to the health care market. Instead, suppliers (providers, principally doctors and facilities) create their own demand, so that as supply goes up so does demand, in a (theoretically) limitless fashion. In economic terms, "producer sovereignty" overshadows "consumer sovereignty," meaning producers have vastly greater information and decision-making capacity than do consumers. As well, there is a conflict of interest between producer and consumer; doctors act as agents for their patients' consumption of health services, but their interests and motivations vary (physicians, for example, may prioritize alleviation of suffering, understanding etiology, furthering knowledge, and disease control rather differently from patients), making for a complicated and imperfect relationship.

Why Do Health Care Markets Differ from Other Markets?

First, the "health care market" operates differently from the more familiar market of goods and services. For personal medical care in particular, the patient (i.e., the consumer) cannot control when or how he/she will spend money on care. While a schoolbag can be purchased now or delayed, with little consequence (not a life and death matter), an injury or illness may require immediate health care services. Once the decision has been made by, or for, a person to enter the health system, that person is no longer in charge of further expenditure decisions. In most countries, physicians maintain control over medical decisions due to specialized knowledge and legal privilege through licensure (although decisions are increasingly mediated by payer restrictions and incentives—see ahead). Decisions regarding diagnostic tests, surgery, medicines, return visits, and many other costly "purchases," are either heavily influenced by the recommendations of a physician, or are made by the physician directly, not by the patient. Moreover, the choice of grade, size, quality, or cost per item, usually available to the consumer in a market economy, is also absent. Not only are patients essentially powerless to control expenditures, they are likely unaware of the need for a particular item. In contrast to other markets, health services include a structural asymmetry of information amongst the parties.

In order for market economics to apply even partially to the health sector, virtually everyone in a given society would have to suffer from Munchausen's syndrome—the feigning of symptoms in order to garner medical attention—and have the wherewithal to repeatedly purchase services. The view that health system users generate boundless demand for health care unless somehow reigned in is clearly incorrect: providers—and the economic interests often surrounding them—influence most decisions about what constitutes disease and the use of health care services, including norms and inducements regarding routine preventive care and advice on when symptoms require medical attention. Doctors thereby generate most of the demand for health care.

Second, the money spent or allocated by the physician may be third-party money from an insurance company or a government program. According to insurance companies, separating clinical decisions from financial considerations means physicians have little incentive to save. In fact, they may have strong motivations for overuse and "to provide the maximum level of services." The policies of the impersonal third-party payer are therefore important in controlling direct expenditures. However, as we shall see in the discussion on managed care, the incentive is to minimize the "medical loss ratio" rather than to reduce administrative costs and profits. Of course, health professionals may also benefit directly from prescribing a particular drug (e.g., in parts of Asia, where doctors earn profits by dispensing medications) or service to a patient (e.g., if the doctor owns shares in a diagnostic clinic), which may influence decision making. As well, under various payment schemes the health provider may have an incentive to increase his/her income by giving unneeded or questionable services, or conversely, by limiting those services.

Insurance companies argue that the coverage they provide leads to "moral hazard" in the form of a limitless demand for health care: the patient does not worry about generating health expenditures because it "doesn't cost me anything." Although this idea is popular in economics circles, it is a myth. Unlike in other sectors, more health care does not provide automatic gratification. Certainly medical care may ameliorate illness, as well as provide comfort and understanding to the sick. Yet medicine remains painful, scary, and downright dangerous, and few people needlessly demand care. As such, other than 1% or so of expenditures driven by patient demand, the vast majority of medical expenditures occur once the patient is already in the door and under the decision-making watch of the provider.

Third, varying amounts of money charged for health services may go to purposes having no health benefit. Some medical procedures are patently useless; others positively dangerous. The evidence-based medicine movement of recent years clearly demonstrates that more is not necessarily better: for example, U.S. heart attack patients are almost eight times as likely to undergo coronary-artery bypass surgery compared to their Canadian counterparts, with no difference in long-term outcomes (Tu et al. 1997). If unnecessary surgeries were reduced, resources would be freed up for other services, such as universal health insurance or preventive services.

Moreover, high incomes, fancy facilities, premiums for malpractice insurance, corruption and profits, error, inefficiency, and large bureaucracies all absorb substantial amounts of health sector funds in different countries. In the United States, overhead and administration use up to one-fourth of health expenditures, and the practice of "defensive medicine" to avoid potential accusations of malpractice leads to a surfeit of diagnostic and therapeutic procedures.

Fourth, money is not the only consideration when analyzing health markets. Health (or its absence) underpins virtually every human activity and is thus different from almost all other goods or services. It may be far better *not* to need health services than to need them. The special nature of health care also derives from human vulnerability at times of illness, pain, or impending death.

Fifth, health services reflect the characteristics and values of the societies of which they are a part. As such, the use of health resources is shaped more by political and cultural factors than by "rational" allocation based on consumer decisions. The myriad differences between health services and other markets are outlined in Table 11–2.

Perhaps the most compelling argument as to why health should not be viewed in market terms is that most people around the world deem health to be a universal human right that should not be determined by an individual's ability to pay or by market forces (Global Health Watch 2005). Framing health as a marketable good based on supply and demand undermines this right. If access to health care is viewed as a human right, then it should be funded as a public good.

Because of the insuperable problems with providing health services through market systems, most countries have—to a greater or lesser degree—turned to regulation and nonmarket provision of health services as a means of protecting health as a

Table 11-2 How the Health Care Sector Differs from Markets

Typical Market Assumptions	Using Health Care Services
Buyers and sellers freely enter and exit the market at any time	Most people use health care services due to an emergency or chronic condition that requires long-term care, or to comply with school, workplace, or government regulations. Health care providers usually decide what services are needed and when they should be discontinued.
Buyers use personal resources to purchase goods and services	In many societies, governments, employers, or privately-run insurance companies purchase health care services, with consumers paying indirectly through taxes, premiums, and/or coinsurance. People without insurance may not have the resources to purchase health care services at all.
Buyers are free to choose which good/service they wish to purchase, if any	Health plans typically provide limited choice to "buyers" (with private insurance also restricting choice). In countries with underdeveloped health systems, or for people living in very remote areas, there is usually no choice in health services or providers.
	Consumers may prioritize accessibility and availability of health services over choice of services or providers.
	Some health services are essential to prolonging, or saving, a life and not purchasing that good/service could be fatal.
	Health decisions may be made for the patient by health care providers or by family members.
Buyers and sellers have equal access to information from which to make rational decisions	Due to asymmetric information between providers and consumers, patients are often unaware of which health good/service is needed, if any, or which is most effective or cost-effective. Conversely, patients may not always disclose vital health information to providers.

public good (or human right). Nonetheless, the dominant international health actors insist on a market approach to health services, especially in low-income settings where donors are instrumental in health financing.

HEALTH SYSTEM FINANCING

Key Questions:

- How are decisions made regarding health financing?
- What is the role of international institutions in shaping health system financing policies?

Chapter 12 will examine health system organization in depth. Here, health financing is examined as a question of health economic models and their assumptions, rather than on the political processes of policy making. There are three main means of financing health care:

1. Revenues gathered by national or local governments through taxation;
2. Tax-based or salary-deducted contributions to public insurance systems; and
3. Private payment to private insurance schemes or out-of-pocket expenditure at the point of health care provision (Wagstaff and van Doorsaler 1998).

It is important to recognize that although these mechanisms differ greatly, households and businesses are almost always the primary funders of a health system, through corporate, income, and payroll taxes, or out-of-pocket expenditures (Fuchs 1998). Health system financing mechanisms are characterized by how progressive (fair distribution of funding by income and health status) or regressive (the poor and sick bear a disproportionate financial burden) they are. As health systems become more progressive, they generally also become more equitable, and fewer persons face impoverishment as a result of health care expenditures. Still, as we will see, equity and access are determined by health system organization as well as by health financing policy.

Different types of health system financing yield different levels of progressivity (fairness): (a) financing through general taxation is most progressive, especially taxation generated from progressive personal and corporate income taxes, and not taxes on goods and services; (b) depending on how contribution rates are established, mandatory health insurance—especially in high-income countries—can be regressive if there are income ceilings on contribution requirements or if there is a single premium, and, especially, if it operates largely in the private sector; (c) private voluntary health insurance is more regressive than mandatory health insurance since "risk"—and therefore premium rates—is usually evaluated at the individual rather than the community level; and (d) out-of-pocket payments are the most regressive form of health financing, as people with the lowest incomes generally also have the highest health care costs. The ways in which countries organize health care financing can also influence the economy, and in turn health status, through effects on tax structures, savings rates, and poverty levels (Hsiao and Heller 2007).

Inadequate health financing is an important cause of poverty and insecurity in many underdeveloped countries without universal health insurance, and, as we shall see, it was a prime motivator of the Commission on Macroeconomics and Health. In the United States, health care debts are the leading cause of personal bankruptcy (Himmelstein et al. 2005), but the United States is an exception to a general trend of countries moving toward publicly funded health insurance systems as they become wealthier (Jamison 2006).

Box 11–2 Covered Health Care Services and the Limits to Access in South Africa

Public coverage of health services according to a limited basket of interventions means that some people will not receive needed medical care. In South Africa, a case (Soobramoney v. Minister of Health, Case 32/1997) was brought against the state in 1997 by a patient who was refused renal dialysis treatment by a public hospital. Soobramoney argued that the South African Constitution ensured his right to emergency medical treatment and that the public hospital was denying him that right. The Constitutional Court found in favor of the state, arguing that since the patient had a chronic, rather than acute, condition, he did not qualify for emergency treatment. The judge further ruled that an application in terms of the right to health care, which is also a constitutional mandate, would not have succeeded either, as the hospital was able to show why, given its limited resources, it was only able to provide care to patients with particular clinical profiles, which did not include patients with chronic kidney disease (Brand 1998).

The Health Insurance Model

Health insurance in one form or another has been around for centuries. In the Middle Ages, guilds and other groups began mutual aid societies to help one another through periods of ill health and impairment that prevented wage earning. By the late 19th century these "friendly societies" became common throughout industrialized settings and among immigrants to the Americas. In countries where public social insurance has been slow to develop, such as the United States and Canada, private insurance companies organized health insurance as a profit-making enterprise, often in conjunction with employers.

If health outcomes were certain, many individuals would make specific arrangements to either prevent or guarantee them. Some might plan in advance in order to be able to afford medical care. However, injuries or illnesses can—and often do—occur unexpectedly. Insurance plans (public or private) hold the promise that funding for health care will be available when it is needed by the individual. The key element of health insurance is the expectation of certain health events based on the illness, disability, or mortality patterns of large pools of individuals. Many pay premiums into a common pool, from which any one individual may withdraw funds when needed; this is known as *risk pooling*. The risk pool becomes larger as more households are included; when 100% of households are included in an insurance scheme, it is universal (Murray et al. 2003). Universal social health insurance provided by the state covers all legal residents (sometimes after a waiting period), but private risk-pooling mechanisms often exclude those who are most in need of coverage.

Private insurers may select who they will provide coverage for, or may decide to delay or reduce benefits paid. This is known as *risk selection*. In contrast with private insurance, publicly funded insurance programs do not select individuals on the basis of risk and are therefore far more equitable. In countries where health insurance is compulsory, governments may implement a public insurance plan, or they may regulate the private insurance industry, requiring level premiums and universal coverage, regardless of risk.

Uniform premiums and benefits for a pool of associated people, regardless of health status, is called "community rating." Premiums or benefits may be adjusted based on age, family size, and so on. This ensures that insurers do not "cherry pick" the young and healthy, or charge higher premiums to unhealthy or elderly persons. Based on past data, the insurer averages all the individual risks over the entire pool of policyholders to come up with the expected number of payouts in any time period. The amount each individual should contribute to the insurance scheme is then calculated. In private insurance schemes, higher premiums are often charged to people with an increased "risk" of illness or death; private insurance premiums are also calculated to include profits for the insurer.

To discourage excessive use, and purportedly to save money for all taxpayers, policyholders, or health plan members, the insurer may require some form of cost sharing such as a copayment or fee at each visit. The insurer may also place limits on certain types of claims, or only insure for limited periods of time with frequent renewability requirements for coverage. Yet, aside from race car drivers and others involved in "extreme sports," it is improbable that people will intentionally pursue dangerous activities just because they have health insurance.

Another form of social insurance is community-based health insurance, which arose in the wake of the 1978 Alma-Ata primary health care conference, and which brings together geographic, ethnic, or occupational groups into small non-profit, insurance schemes (Ekman 2004; Carrin, Waelkens, and Criel 2005). These schemes are growing across Africa, with local population coverage ranging from 1% in some settings to over 90% in one Senegalese town (Carrin, Waelkens, and Criel 2005). Undoubtedly, community-based health insurance offers financial protection against health care costs in countries without other forms of social health insurance, but it does not distribute health financing equitably across the population. Thus, while providing community control and increased access to care for those able to afford premiums, community health insurance can do little for the poorest populations.

U.S. and Canadian Health Financing Models Compared

Several Canadian health economists reviewed the two different health insurance models—that of a single-payer public system (employed in Canada) and multi-payer private–public insurance system (United States) in terms of equity and efficiency (Evans 2003). Despite frequent claims that the single-payer system was more costly, Evans found: "universal comprehensive coverage was not more expensive than the previous fragmented mix of public and private insurance coverage and out-of-pocket payment. Consolidation of expenditures in the hands of a single payer made possible the control of rates of escalation through a variety of different mechanisms" (Evans 2003, p. 5).

With respect to equity, Chernomas and Sepehri found that the single-payer health system was more likely to distribute resources according to need, whilst the multi-payer system distributed services according to ability to pay. In addition, for-profit hospitals were less likely to provide services for economically disadvantaged individuals or

Table 11–3 Organization and Effects of Single-Payer and Multiple-Payer Systems Compared

Single-Payer Public Health System	Multiple-Payer Private Health System
• Raises funds, administers claims, and shares costs across the population more efficiently and equitably	• Overhead costs can be upwards of 10 times higher among private insurers compared to a public single payer
• One authority with an incentive and the capacity to contain costs	• Administrative costs over three times higher in United States compared to Canada
• No marketing expenses	• The larger the share of private health care financing, the more difficult it is to control expenditures (e.g., for-profit hospitals are 3% to 11% more expensive than nonprofit hospitals)
• No need to estimate risks to establish differentiated premiums	• Employer-provided health insurance is a disincentive for labor mobility and hence negatively affects the allocation of labor
• No profits paid to shareholders	• As the cost of health insurance increases, so do costs to employers who provide health insurance, resulting in fewer salary increases, cuts in benefits, decreased employment levels, and more costs passed on to employees through higher premiums and copayments and limits on coverage
	• Premiums for those with chronic conditions are typically larger—placing a higher financial burden on the sick
	• For-profit hospitals provide minimal care for the poor, leaving nonprofits with a disproportionate financial responsibility

Sources: Chernomas (2005); Sepehri and Chernomas (2004).

24-hour emergency services, as they are usually unprofitable (Chernomas and Sepehri 1998). Overall, these comparisons show that a single-payer system is more equitable and less costly than a multipayer insurance scheme (see Table 11–3).

User Fees and Out-of-Pocket Spending

In the late 1980s, World Bank analysts began to promote user fees as a cost-recovery/cost-sharing mechanism for chronically underfunded health systems. The Bank's short 1987 report *Financing Health Services in Developing Countries: An Agenda for Reform* argued that people were willing to pay for health care and that free services impeded government revenue collection. Thanks to market-level user fees, the pamphlet asserted, health system revenues would be generated, improving access, efficiency, and quality of care. In addition, resources would shift from expensive inpatient treatment to more affordable primary health care services (World Bank 1987). In sum, if patients paid for services, according to this reasoning, they would use health resources more rationally.

It turned out that the Bank's report was based more on ideology than evidence. Although it recommended that user fees be accompanied by vouchers or exemptions

---

Box 11-3 The Bamako Initiative

The Bamako Initiative (BI) was adopted in 1987 in Mali by African Ministers of Health, originally envisioned as a mechanism for the rapid implementation of the Health for All strategy of the WHO. At the time, African countries were experiencing severe disruptions in health care services largely due to heavy debt loads and structural adjustment (SAP) cutbacks. Employment levels, social service provisions, and health status indicators were worsening, with impoverished rural populations disproportionately affected (Coll 1990). Focused on strengthening district health systems (particularly in rural areas), the BI used revolving funds to ensure payment for and distribution of health services, bolstered by US$8 million raised by WHO and UNICEF for the procurement of essential drugs (WHO AFRO 1997). The BI is perhaps best known for formalizing "cost recovery" from users as a legitimate means of health sector financing.

Eventually implemented in 33 countries, the BI combined government subsidies, external and community financing, and user fees in an attempt to improve health care access, particularly for rural residents. Governments typically paid local health care worker salaries, and external donors helped financed infrastructure and prepayment for drug and vaccine stocks. Certain interventions were subsidized (such as immunization and oral rehydration therapy), and the poorest households could be (in principle) exempt from payment. User fees were pooled with other revenues at the local level for community reinvestment

A 5-year WHO/AFRO review credited the BI with making a significant contribution to strengthening community involvement in health care (WHO AFRO 1994), and various World Bank assessors found dramatic health status improvements and widespread popularity of the initiative (Soucat et al. 1997; Knippenberg et al. 2003).

Other evaluations showed that cost recovery was popular mainly because it was the only way to obtain health care in many settings. Sustainability was rarely achieved, in large part because the region was flooded with unnecessary pharmaceuticals (Gertler and Hammer 1997, cited in Kim, Shakow, and Bayona 2000). Moreover, the rhetoric of community-based care was translated into little decision-making involvement by women and other key local groups despite the extra time burden necessitated by the Bamako strategy (McPake, Hanson, and Mills 1993).

There is wide agreement that implementation of the Bamako Initiative was uneven and left many of those who it sought to assist—namely, poor, rural populations—no better off. People who were already on the margins of survival due to loss of services and low earning capacity had no means of paying for health care out of pocket. Fifteen years later, many of the poorest households remained unable to access needed services, suffering increased inequities due to community financing strategies (Gilson et al. 2001). Uzochukwu et al. (2004), using data from southeast Nigeria, found that poor and less educated groups had a limited understanding of the fee exemption policies and consequently used health centers less frequently than more affluent groups. Conversely, the termination of user fees in Uganda in 2001, after their initiation 8 years previously, led to a doubling of health services usage within 2 years (Gilson and McIntyre 2005).

---

for the poorest populations, both in-house and external reviews showed that user fees resulted in significant barriers to care:

- People were far less willing or able to pay for care than had been posited, and income levels were closely correlated with demand (Gertler and van der Gaag 1990).
- Few countries actually implemented protective or exemption policies for low-income groups. Where such policies did exist, their implementation was impeded by numerous constraints (Russell and Gilson 1997).

- User fee policies in underdeveloped countries have proven inequitable, as they deter health services utilization by those least able to pay; their health suffers accordingly (Palmer et al. 2004).
- Where user fees have been introduced, there is a demonstrated 40% to 50% decrease in health services utilization, particularly where exemption policies are either not in place or the administrative systems are not adequate to implement such policies (Save the Children 2005).
- User fees have a negative impact on adherence to treatment for chronic or long-term health conditions, most notably HIV/AIDS (James et al. 2006).

Due to the negative repercussions of user fees on health equity, many governments and international agencies have called for their abolition, particularly in low- and middle-income countries (Global Health Watch 2005; James et al. 2006). However, World Bank analysts continue to argue that free services do not "constitute the most promising approach to meeting the needs of disadvantaged population groups" (Gwatkin 2005, p. 9).

The World Bank now recommends that any decisions to implement user fees take the local context into account and that services be provided free of charge when:

- the benefits are widely diffused (e.g., sanitation, pest control);
- the cost of services is minimal; and
- the services are disproportionately used by the poor, unlikely to be delivered adequately without user fees, and unlikely to be overused (e.g., low-cost primary health care, antenatal care, immunization, low-cost treatment for priority diseases) (World Bank 2004).

Of course, user fees make up only one aspect of health financing strategies.

COST ANALYSES IN THE HEALTH SECTOR

Key Questions:

- What are cost-effectiveness analysis and cost–benefit analysis?
- Why are they used and how do they differ?
- What are their respective limitations?

Cost–Benefit Analysis

In 1873 Max von Pettenkofer, Munich's health officer and Professor of Hygiene, attempted to demonstrate "the value of health to a city" through a rational economic calculation. Seeking to understand why London's death rate was so much lower than that of Munich, he found that the difference was not due to better medical care or hospitals but, rather, stemmed from London's better sanitation, housing, and nutritional conditions. Pettenkofer carried out a cost–benefit analysis (CBA) of Munich's lower health status, based on lost earnings due to sickness. Calculating that the city experienced 3.4 million days of sickness per year and consequently lost 3.4 million florins annually due to work absence, he interpreted the city's failure to invest in public health as a kind of feudal tax that impeded economic growth. Pettenkofer estimated that an investment in municipal health would see profitable returns, with gains far outstripping the costs. He estimated that a reduction in work absences related to a drop in the mortality rate from 33/1000 to 30/1000 would save almost 350,000 florins per year. In order to earn an equivalent sum on the capital market (at a rate of 5%), 7 million florins would need to be invested. In sum, Pettenkofer concluded, spending 7 million florins on a comprehensive water and sewerage system was a highly profitable business move (Pettenkofer 1941).

This was one of the earliest cost–benefit analyses ever carried out. At the simplest level, CBA is a cost-accounting mechanism that calculates the benefits of a particular activity (or initiative), its costs, and whether the benefits outweigh the costs (i.e., Benefits − Costs = Net Benefits). If they do—that is, if the net benefits exceed zero—then the activity is deemed worth carrying out. It all sounds simple enough. The complexity arises when we try to decide what counts as costs, what counts as benefits, and how to take into account the future benefits and costs in addition to the current ones. The most problematic issue of all is trying to place a monetary amount on the value of a life.

Economists frequently use the concept of the margin—the magnitude of the benefit that will accrue from a given additional expenditure—for decision-making purposes. Moreover, those responsible for planning and financing any project want to know the return that they may expect on their investment. Implicit in their decision making is the idea that costs and benefits can be measured, or at least estimated and projected. The business investor can usually tell just how much profit (or loss) has accrued from a transaction, as costs and benefits are stated in monetary terms. Investments in health cannot always furnish such exact figures because resources are used today in the hope of avoiding future losses from illness, disability, and death, and the medical expenses that these would have incurred. While immediate costs can be stated easily, the future savings are difficult to demonstrate with accuracy. The nonmonetary benefits of better health, such as increased well-being and longevity past one's years of economic productivity, are even harder to quantify.

Measures that avert future costs altogether seem the best way to spend on health. Such programs are most valuable but, paradoxically, least visible because nothing happens. Parents do not notice when their child does not get hepatitis or diphtheria or is not paralyzed by polio, nor do they recognize the "extra" money that was saved as a result.

Although various prevention activities have been demonstrated to be relatively cost-beneficial, it may be difficult to guarantee continued political will for, as an example, an immunization campaign. If an immunization program has reduced the incidence of measles by 95%, the absence of big outbreaks may suggest to government officials that measles is no longer a concern, and they may decide to spend their money on other pressing and politically salient issues. However, it is precisely at this point that continued control is needed. If control work is stopped for reasons of politics or false calculations of cost savings, measles could return in an epidemic wave and the previous investment in measles control would have been wasted. In fact, the eventual cost of such an epidemic is likely to be much greater than continued preventative efforts over a long period.

Calculating future costs and savings according to standard business investment models is central to CBA. Future benefits must be "discounted" by a certain percentage (sometimes set at central bank interest rates) because one euro or yuan today is valued at more than the same amount next year due to inflation and to the opportunity costs from not investing in another arena. In other words, future savings are worth less than present savings. The amount of benefits and costs after discounting is called the net present value. According to CBA, only if the net present value of future benefits and costs is positive should a project or intervention be carried out.

For example, the WHO's worldwide campaign against smallpox (discussed in Chapter 13) is estimated to have cost US$100 million in 1967 dollars (Barrett 2004), almost US$1 billion today. D.A. Henderson, the former director of the smallpox campaign, calculated that the eradication of smallpox saves the world's governments more than US$1 billion annually, indefinitely, in reduced productivity losses and medical care costs (Fenner et al. 1988), augmented by indirect savings from averted deaths, blindness, and other disabilities. This CBA suggests the smallpox campaign to have been economically worthwhile. At the same time, however, targeted smallpox spending may have displaced other investments in health on the part of the WHO and participating countries, including basic infrastructure and sanitation.

Cost–benefit analyses suffer from several drawbacks that limit their usefulness as a guide to decisions on health policy. Many published studies are retrospective, perhaps justifying past programs in the defense of health planners. More significantly, it is not easy to quantify costs and benefits, and the same data can be used to skew arguments one way or the other. Many procedures also depend on the prior existence of facilities, trained personnel, and the total related infrastructure, all of which are difficult to account for in cost–benefit calculations.

Although international health institutions heavily promote cost–benefit analyses for health system planning in underdeveloped countries, health services allocation decisions in wealthier nations rarely rely on such cost analyses. Underdeveloped countries are encouraged to promote health services use where the cost is lowest and the health outcomes greatest, while more developed nations often spend exorbitant amounts on health procedures that do not follow these principles. Examples of such expenditures are the high amount of money spent on cosmetic surgery, medication to improve sexual performance, and the amount of money spent on elderly citizens. It is not feasible to enter into a discussion of the enormous literature on costs and benefits of procedures in clinical medicine, including drug therapy and surgery, except to point out that this is an area of active investigation and clashing opinions.

It is important to note that CBA shows impressive results when focused on narrow interventions, such as immunizations, and over short time frames. However, interventions that are much broader in scope, such as education, typically do not provide immediate gains due to large startup costs and diffused effects. Over the long term, social investments yield far greater benefits, but they are undervalued by CBA which favors current savings over future savings.

Ethical Considerations

Although cost analyses are usually presented as value-neutral, the use of any evaluation method has ideological implications. The first assumption is that, according to standard economic thinking, tradeoffs must be made when setting policies regarding health because there are only finite resources available for investment. The limited resources argument has been accused of serving as a rationale for restricting spending on the broader, interlocking determinants of health, which may see gains over a longer period of time, and therefore need to be assessed at a lower net present value than short-term, discrete interventions.

A second crucial ethical concern regarding CBA is the need to put a monetary value on human life and well-being in order to quantify the benefits and the costs of a particular activity or intervention. Any reductions (or increases) in death or disability must be converted into monetary terms in order to be included in the CBA equation.

Valuations of life typically take into account an individual's earning potential at the time of death or disability, placing the highest value on the life of a middle-aged man (assumed most likely to be productively employed). Dorothy Rice, a U.S. health economist, proposed in the 1970s that the monetary value of human life increases until the age of 60, at which point it begins to decline. By these calculations (based on earning potential and contributions to household activity), men at their "most valuable" are worth almost 70% more than women at their "most valuable" (Max et al. 2004).

Although Rice's ideas have been influential (e.g., in the calculation of DALYs, as discussed in Chapter 5), they are based on problematic suppositions regarding who is worth what. For example, in the United States and other settings, women and racial/ethnic minority populations earn less on average than men of European descent and are typically evaluated as having less "value" or monetary worth than white men. Given the lower earning power of working class and marginalized populations and underdeveloped country populations, CBAs sometimes include lower values of life for these groups. Such a calculation is implicit in many settings regarding housing policies for homeless populations, whose ill health or premature death from living on the streets may be insufficient to motivate public investment.

As well, following Rice's methodology, or putting any monetary value on life, may be unacceptable to various cultural and religious groups. For example, in many societies, the elderly are more highly valued, and the declining valuation of life after 60—regardless of productivity or life expectancy—may be considered offensive.

There are other ways of calculating the monetary value of life. For example, "opportunity costs" assess what investment possibility is lost because money is spent on a particular intervention. Once again, the opportunity lost varies by who is making the judgment. Cost utility analysis is a variant of CBA, which uses outcome measures based on people's preferences (gauged through surveys, focus groups, etc.) rather than monetary amounts.

Asking people what is their "willingness to pay" through surveys (or, in litigious societies, through lawsuit outcomes) immediately faces basic questions such as: whose willingness? And paying for what? Not only are these questions challenging to measure, they rarely follow "market logic" because information is imperfect and because healthy people may undervalue relatively low cost, life-extending preventive care in contrast to people in ill health, who value expensive, curative care, even if to less effect. Further, individual choices may not coincide with societal choices, and are mediated by social class, experience, and age (Evans 1984, pp. 255–257).

The inherent problems of placing concrete monetary values on life, health, and suffering has led CBA to be replaced by cost-effectiveness analysis (CEA), which does not require such explicit valuations.

Cost-Effectiveness Analysis

Once health-planning goals are determined, policy-makers must find the best means to reach them. In CEA, the desired health outcome is already decided and the attainment of the outcome is measured in two ways: (1) a comparison of two or more interventions of the same cost and their respective health outcomes; or (2) a comparison of several interventions with the same outcome to determine the variation in the cost of the interventions (also known as cost minimization). In other words, CEA overcomes the problem of monetizing outcomes by evaluating interventions or activities against one another (see Table 11–4). Either spending or the desired effects remain constant, and different routes to achieving these ends are compared.

Cost-effectiveness analyses are also used for screening programs. Here the purpose is not primary prevention of disease but the identification of undetected, early, or asymptomatic cases so that further pathology can be reduced and a costly clinical illness avoided (secondary prevention). Early screening for tuberculosis and trachoma are in this category, as are Pap smears and mammograms. For HIV infections or other conditions for which no cure is currently available, early detection

Table 11–4 Economic Evaluation Techniques for Health

Evaluation Technique	Nature of Benefits	Measurement of Benefits
Cost–benefit analysis	Multiple effects	Monetary units (e.g., dollars or pesos)
Cost-effectiveness analysis	Single effect	Natural units (e.g., lives saved or cases of disease detected)

Source: Adapted from Peacock et al. (2001).

is still economically beneficial if the infected person can be treated and avoid transmission to others who would incur illness, loss of productivity, and medical expenses. The epidemiological information generated from screening programs provides an additional benefit for public health planning.

The WHO promotes CEA as an important tool as it "indicates which interventions provide the highest 'value for money' and helps policymakers choose the interventions and programmes which maximize health for the available resources" (WHO 2006).

An example of CEA is outlined in Table 11–5, in which different health services are compared in terms of cost per DALY (ironically DALYs incorporate a valuation of disability and illness, thus partially defeating one of the purposes of CEA).

Some interventions, such as expanding immunization coverage with standard child vaccines, have a very low cost per DALY; while others, for example coronary-artery bypass grafting, have a very high cost. Following from these calculations, policy makers would be advised that it is more effective to focus scarce resources on childhood immunization, given the relatively greater benefit to be accrued. A general cut-off point for CEA designated by the World Bank is US$100 per DALY averted, although this level is arbitrary and likely to depend on a country's epidemiological profile, income, local desires, and public health infrastructure. We must also recall that DALYs calculate childhood illness and death at a lower level than for adults, so the results are skewed by this and other assumptions built into the DALYs (see Chapter 5 for details). As such, childhood interventions are likely to be undervalued when DALYs are employed.

A deeper problem stems from the way costs are conceptualized. Improved water infrastructure and management/regulation exceeds the $100 per DALY cut-off by a factor of four, whereas improved water management and regulation *without infrastructure investment* is assessed as cost-effective. Yet the valuation of water infrastructure does not include the time, energy, and physical strain of carrying water over long distances or the lost opportunities to attend school by children charged with this responsibility. Further, because these CEA calculations are based on an annual evaluation, they overemphasize initial infrastructure costs rather than appropriately spreading costs and effectiveness over a longer time period.

Table 11–5 Using CEA to Determine Health Priorities

Service or Intervention	Annual Cost Per DALY (US$)
Annual drug therapy treatment of helminthic (parasitic) infections	3
Expanding immunization coverage with standard child vaccines	2–20
Taxing tobacco products	3–50
Provision of insecticide-treated bednets to protect against malaria (sub-Saharan Africa)	5–17
Treating acute myocardial infarction (heart attacks) with an inexpensive set of drugs	10–25
Detecting and treating cervical cancer	15–50
Treating STIs to interrupt HIV transmission	10–100
Improving care of children under 28 days old (including resuscitation of newborns)	10–400
Improved water and sanitation management and regulation	44
Adding vaccines against additional diseases to the standard child immunization program (particularly Hib and HepB)	40–250
Preventing mother-to-child transmission (antiretroviral-nevirapine prophylaxis of the mother; breast-feeding substitutes)	50–200
Improved water and sanitation management and regulation combined with physical infrastructure	413
Performing coronary-artery bypass grafting (bypass surgery) in specific identifiable "high-risk" cases, e.g., disease of the left main coronary artery (incremental to treatment with medications)	>25,000

Sources: Adapted from (Jamison 2006; Varley, Tarvid, and Chao 1998; WHO 2007d; Jamison et al. 2006).

Moreover, CEA, like CBA, almost never addresses the societal determinants of health, such as primary education and increased wages, although these factors have a far larger impact on health outcomes than do specific health care interventions. Some policy analysts assume that if the costs or benefits of a particular course of action are diffuse, it will not be politically acceptable (Stone 1997). Yet social security (a key health determinant) and other diffuse benefits of welfare states enjoyed wide mobilization historically and remain among the most popular public programs across societies.

Other limitations of CEA include the following:

- Since outcomes must be measured in "natural" health units, there are limits to the types of programs that can be evaluated, because CEA cannot be used to compare widely dissimilar programs.
- "Natural health units" reflect only one aspect of program outcomes (e.g., measurement of life years gained does not say anything about the quality of life).

- Even if a program is assessed to be cost-effective, it is not necessarily affordable (Peacock et al. 2001).
- The business model of discounting future savings disadvantages long-term infrastructural efforts.
- "Externalities" are not included, that is, only the direct costs of the service or intervention are evaluated. The time or cost to the recipient relating to one intervention or another is excluded.
- Evaluations are carried out for individual interventions related to individual ailments, but not for activities that have effects in many arenas or for joint efforts that may have synergistic effects (i.e., housing and educational improvements). For example, the multiple benefits of environmental cleanup for numerous cancers and respiratory infections, exercise possibilities, and overall well-being are left out of CEA calculations.
- Cost analyses are depoliticized—it is assumed that if the results are "positive," the activity should be undertaken without taking into account historical trajectory or political context.

In sum, "using simple technical criteria to plan solutions to complex public health problems" (Berman 1982, p. 1054), while a seemingly logical approach to health planning, is marred by numerous shortcomings.

Equity versus Efficiency: Trade-off or False Dichotomy?

Most economic analyses focus on costs in relation to effectiveness and efficiency and either neglect or negate the importance of equity. Indeed, there is believed to be an equity-efficiency trade-off that occurs in economics in general, and in health system financing and delivery in particular (Okun 1975; Hsiao and Heller 2007). As alluded to previously, proponents of this notion hold that since resources are scarce, it is not possible to distribute all goods and services both efficiently and equitably at all times, and therefore decision makers must decide whether they wish to favor equity or efficiency.

Economic evaluations of health implicitly favor efficiency over equity because market mechanisms are notoriously poor at equitably distributing resources. Yet many analysts agree that because of the problems of market failure in health and other social sectors, equity should be favored over efficiency whenever marginalized populations have little access to welfare-enhancing activities (Greenwald and Stiglitz 1986; Collier and Dercon 2006).

As discussed in Chapter 7, a focus on equity implies that any (re)distribution of resources must target the populations with the worst health status, and that health goods and services must be distributed primarily according to need. However, cost analyses and the main health system financing strategies do not have an a priori equity focus, and follow instead from the values of technocrats, elites, and the political and economic trajectories of dominant countries. Especially in the case of highly indebted countries, health system structuring and financing is heavily influenced by IFIs and their accompanying policies, such as SAPs and PRSPs (see Chapters 3 and 9), which pay little more than rhetorical attention to issues of equity. Of course, eliminating inequities in health necessitates a distribution of resources well beyond health care, as most health inequities stem from social, economic, and political factors. Ironically, health economics approaches that only emphasize efficiency are bad for profits as well as for people: the best-run businesses understand that equity and efficiency work hand in hand—educated, healthy, and well-paid workers are more productive than their poorly treated counterparts. Ironically, equity-oriented approaches are typically overlooked as too costly for low-income countries.

Health Market Approaches to Underdeveloped Countries: The 1993 World Development Report

Starting in the 1980s, the World Bank became an increasingly important funder and policy advisor for health care services in underdeveloped countries. Reflecting neoliberal beliefs regarding the superiority of the private marketplace (see Chapter 9), World Bank loans aimed at improving health spending efficiency through decentralization reforms, reduction of covered interventions, and privatization of services. In many settings, these policies accompanied structural adjustment loan conditionalities that stipulated overall social sector budget cuts.

In 1993, the World Bank issued its first health-oriented World Development Report (WDR) entitled *Investing in Health* (World Bank 1993). The report argued that in underdeveloped countries, private practitioners and service providers for sanitation, housing, and garbage collection are "often more technically efficient than the public sector and offer a service that is perceived to be of higher quality" and more accountable (ibid, p. 4). Moreover, it asserted: "The main problem with universal government financing is that it subsidizes the wealthy, who could afford to pay for their own services, and thus leaves fewer government resources for the poor" (ibid, p. 11). Yet the Report's recommendations resulted in even fewer resources for the poor.

The WDR 1993 recommended that underdeveloped countries adopt a "basket" of cost-effective interventions—valued at US$12 and US$21.50 per capita per year for low- and middle-income countries, respectively—as a top public health priority. Only if governments had additional available resources were they advised to fund nonpriority interventions. The basic basket covered immunization, sick-child care, family planning, prenatal and delivery care, treatment for TB, sexually transmitted infections (STIs), and HIV prevention (World Bank 1993). Not included in the recommended basket were treatments for chronic illnesses, such as diabetes and mental illness, emergency medical treatment for moderately severe injuries, or broader public health measures such as housing improvement and sanitation, many of which, the report argued, ought to be provided by the private sector (World Bank 1993).

In conjunction with the report, the World Bank also supported the *Disease Control Priorities in Developing Countries* project (Jamison et al. 1993), which evaluated the burden of disease due to death and disability (see Chapter 5) and helped entrench cost-effectiveness analysis in global health policy making for underdeveloped countries (see ahead for details).

"Investing in Health" became a manifesto for neoliberal health finance reforms, simultaneously highlighting the importance of human health as a key societal investment and the potential of health services in terms of private-sector investment. Numerous underdeveloped countries implemented the strategies proposed in the report, as part of World Bank loans, bilateral aid programs, and new national policies. From Bolivia to Pakistan, these reforms began to dismantle already fragile public coverage of health services.

Almost immediately, activists, advocates, and policy makers denounced the WDR 1993 for its narrow assessment of health and health interventions based almost exclusively on in-house studies; for defining health as a private responsibility and health care as a private good; for failing to recognize the ongoing deleterious effects of World Bank structural adjustment policies on health care systems; and for disregarding the preeminent role of government in protecting health as a human right (Costello and Woodward 1993; Laurell and López Arellano 1996; Global Health Watch 2005). These critiques proved prescient.

The WDR's support for health services privatization, based on the assertion that a private market for health care could manage health services more efficiently, effectively, and equitably than the public sector, was accompanied by promises to address public health system problems, ranging from underfunding (due to debt crises and loan conditionalities) to slow-moving bureaucracies, and in some cases corrupt officials. However, the 1990s privatization reforms did little to resolve these problems, instead increasing health system inequities. In spite of overwhelming evidence that private health services delivery reduces access to care, especially among the marginalized (Rao 1999; Turshen 1999; Waitzkin, Jasso-Aguilar, and Iriart 2007), the World Bank continues to encourage privatization through its policies and publications, most recently a business manual entitled, *Establishing Private Health Care Facilities in Developing Countries: A Guide for Medical Entrepreneurs.*

Health as Productivity: The WHO Commission on Macroeconomics and Health

Since the early 1990s, international health agencies have focused growing attention on health sector financing in underdeveloped countries based on the notion of health as a necessary ingredient for economic growth and poverty reduction. In 2000, the director-general of the WHO joined the fray, establishing the Commission on

Macroeconomics and Health (CMH), chaired by economist Jeffrey Sachs, to "assess the place of health in global economic development." The commission's report, *Macroeconomics and Health: Investing in Health for Economic Development*, proposed that industrialized countries partner with low- and middle-income countries to invest in health as a means of increasing global economic development, productivity, and investment prospects (WHO 2001). The report echoed the WDR 1993, conveying "a double meaning—investing to improve health, economic productivity, and poverty; and investing capital, especially private capital, as a route to private profit in the health sector" (Waitzkin 2003, p. 523).

The Commission justified health investment based on the following findings: (a) countries with lower infant mortality rates experienced higher economic growth; (b) improved health resulted in higher per capita income; (c) countries with a long life expectancy invested more in education and had higher personal savings rates; and (d) personal spending on health was disproportionately shouldered by the most economically marginalized groups, resulting in further impoverishment. Health care spending was estimated to impoverish approximately 100 million people every year, with an additional 150 million pushed into significant financial hardship (WHO 2001).

The CMH found that economic losses associated with excess or preventable disease led to reductions in market income, labor productivity, longevity, and psychological well-being. For example, the total cost of malaria for sub-Saharan Africa in 1999 was estimated at 5.8% of the GDP of the region, and HIV/AIDS at 11.7% of GDP. Recalculated to take into account the age of illness and death from AIDS—typically young adulthood, when people are at their most productive—the cost of AIDS came to over 35% of GDP (WHO 2001, p. 32).

A summary of the report argued that "Increased investments in health…would translate into hundreds of billions of dollars per year of increased income in the low-income countries" (WHO 2001, p. 16), preventing some 8 million deaths annually from HIV/AIDS, malaria, TB, childhood infections, maternal and perinatal conditions, tobacco-related illnesses, and micronutrient deficiencies, as well as reducing fertility.

To achieve these objectives the report proposed huge increases in health sector spending—from an average of US$13 per person in the least-developed countries to a minimum of US$30–40 per person per year—for specific cost-effective interventions combined with a restructured health delivery system. According to the Commission, these increases would come from both underdeveloped countries and a worldwide scaling up of donor financing for "essential interventions" from US$6 billion per year to US$27 billion per year in the space of 5 years. Notwithstanding its ambitious mandate, the CMH had almost nothing to say about the factors influencing health outside of health services per se, including income redistribution and living and working conditions, which together comprise the most fundamental "macroeconomics and health" issues.

Instead, it built upon the focused health services reform approaches laid out in the WDR 1993, such as public sector management improvement, a publicly financed basket of technical health interventions for the poor (but private financing for others), and combined public–private provision of services, including encouragement for consumer prepayment of services and provider competition. The report also stipulated new approaches to donor/recipient relations, with reforms and financing to transpire simultaneously, and funding based upon "performance" (WHO 2001).

The Commission's report has been hailed as a "groundbreaking" blueprint for global health policy that brings together efficiency and generosity, yet it largely continues along previous cost-effective, pro-private market paths for health improvement established by leading donors over the past decades (Katz 2004). While attention to the intertwining of economic conditions and health is welcomed by a wide swath of civil society, occupational and environmental health activists, political parties, social justice movements, NGOs, union members, public health specialists, and others, the Commission's tight "focus on economic productivity diminishes the importance of health as a fundamental human right" (Waitzkin 2003, p. 523). Moreover, the absence of almost all of these key international health stakeholders from the CMH (most commissioners came from the private sector or international financial agencies) raises disturbing questions regarding its (lack of) representativeness.

Due to the CMH report's narrow focus on ill health as the primary cause of poverty—and because of its "stated aim...to legitimize globalization" (Katz 2005, p. 173)—a host of vital macroeconomic and political issues are removed from discussion, including unfair terms of trade, extreme concentration of power and resources, protectionism, debt burden, foreign direct investment, tax havens, free trade zones, intellectual property restrictions, deregulation, and so on. Instead, donor aid, which reinforces foreign influence and pressure and continued dependency of recipient countries, is presented as the sole solution to the health problems of underdeveloped countries. Of course, as discussed in Chapters 3 and 4, donor aid, most of which returns to the donor country through contracts and procurement (Sogge 2002, in Katz 2004), is dwarfed by debt repayment obligations (of late more than five times greater than aid commitments).

Indeed, despite its grand name, the Commission's understanding of the macroeconomic context is limited to health as a motor of productivity and economic growth. The consequences of economic conditions on health are largely overlooked. Moreover, improvements in health are understood to derive almost exclusively from health services, with major determinants of health—education, income, water and sanitation, and agricultural improvement—"disposed of" as "complementary and additional" rather than central to the Commission's recommendations (Katz 2004, p. 762).

As Alison Katz proposes, "in order to assess the usefulness and cost-effectiveness of the strategies proposed by the CMH, policymakers need to compare the benefits accrued to a country in, for example, food and water or public service infrastructure, with investments of the same order in health interventions" (Katz 2004, p. 753). This ambitious and vitally important exercise has yet to be carried out. Instead, the World Bank, the WHO, the U.S. National Institutes of Health, and the Gates Foundation joined forces to sponsor a second edition (2006) of the Disease Control Priorities Project (DCP2)—a bible of cost-effective interventions to "reduce the burden" of dozens of diseases and health problems. Produced by hundreds of researchers from many countries, the DCP2 justifies its disease-control approach in almost identical terms as the CMH: health is a key precursor of productivity, education, and investment, which together generate economic growth. Ill health, by contrast, impedes these factors, thereby preventing growth (Jamison 2006). Largely thanks to the DCP2, CEA is now entrenched as the favored priority-setting mechanism for health aid and domestic health care spending in underdeveloped countries.

In sum, although public health advocates have long argued that: (a) health should be conceptualized as a right in and of itself (and a reflection of social, economic, and political conditions), not just as a potential drain or boost to the economy; and (b) that CEA should only be used after the most pressing needs have been met (Global Health Watch 2005), controlling diseases (particularly those that jeopardize economic growth) through cost-effective measures has become the conventional mantra of the major international health donors.

The Role of International Agencies in Health Financing

In underdeveloped countries, some US$500 billion is spent annually on health care from all sources. This accounts for just one-eighth of global spending on health for more than two-thirds of the world's population. Since up to 80% of health spending in low-income countries is in the private sector (World Bank 2007b) and skewed toward elites, the majority of people in low-income countries have extremely limited (public) financial coverage for health services. As discussed in Chapter 3, international agencies play an important direct or indirect role in policy making in many developing countries. IFIs and other agencies also participate in the financing of health care, significantly so in countries that rely heavily on donor aid (see Table 11–6).

This financial involvement has grown considerably over the past two decades, with development assistance for health going from US$2.5 billion in 1990 to over US$13 billion in 2005. Just four agencies—the World Bank, the Bill and Melinda Gates Foundation, the U.S. government, and the Global Fund to Fight AIDS, Tuberculosis and Malaria—accounted for about one-third of global health financing in 2005, and two agencies, the GAVI Alliance and the Global Fund, accounted for 9% of development assistance for health (WHO 2007a). This attention has shifted over time. For example, the World Bank's health, population, and nutrition activities began only gradually in the early 1970s. By the mid-1990s, the World Bank had become the largest outside financier of health activities in underdeveloped countries. Between 1997 and 2006, its Health, Nutrition and Population division funded new loans to over 500 projects—totaling US$15 billion (World Bank 2007a). Its direct influence is higher in highly indebted and extremely impoverished countries,

Table 11–6 GNI, Debt, Health Expenditures, and Donor Funding in Selected Countries (2006–2007)

	Nicaragua	Ghana	Bolivia	Kenya	Cambodia	P. New Guinea	Zambia
Population (millions)[a]	5.7	23	9.5	37.5	14.4	6.3	11.9
GNI per capita (current US$)[a]	930	590	1,260	680	540	850	800
% GDP spent on health[b]	8.3	6.2	6.9	4.5	6.4	4.2	5.6
External resources for health as % of total health expenditure[b]	9.2	26	6.8	18.1	25.7	37	40.5
External debt as % of GNI[a]	84.8	24.9	49	28.6	50.6	33	23.9

[a] 2007 data (World Bank 2008).
[b] 2006 data (WHOSIS 2008).

where heavy health sector reliance on donor funding is accompanied by quid pro quo policy directives.

Paradoxically, the increased attention to global health has come at a time when international donors play a smaller proportionate role. Between 1972 and 1990, 2.9% of health expenditures in underdeveloped countries was funded through international aid mechanisms. The majority (82%) of these funds originated from tax payments in industrialized countries (i.e., bilateral aid or ODA) and only 1.5% of external aid to health sector finance originated from private foundations (Michaud and Murray 1994). Today, external aid has dropped to less than 1% of health expenditures in underdeveloped countries. (This decline is partially attributable to rising private and national health sector spending in large countries such as China, India, and Brazil.) Yet policies regarding health financing are increasingly made on a global scale. Indeed, as discussed elsewhere in this book, most of the funding is targeted by donors to priority programs of their choice.

Despite this larger trend, countries with limited resources are usually heavily reliant on aid from international donor agencies in order to finance health services. For example, in 1994, international aid made up 84% of the Gambia's total health expenditures (Cassels and Janovsky 1998), and more recently in Surinam 49% of all expenditure on health has come from external financing (Poullier et al. 2002). Overall, in 40 low-income countries more than one-fourth of health spending comes from external aid, and in 20 countries aid covers more than half of health spending (Lane and Glassman 2007).

While external aid makes up a large percentage of national health care budgets in a number of developing countries, health aid is not a substantial foreign aid priority for most donor nations. A 2006 OECD report found that aid for health made up only 4.5% of all of Overseas Development Assistance in 2004 (OECD 2006).

The largest donor agencies have significant influence on national and international health priorities due to their global reach, matching grant strategies that require recipient countries to cofinance many activities through personnel allocations, direct financing and other resources, and agenda-setting capacity. As well, funding criteria may require that discrete targets—typically set by donors—be met within a specified period, and therefore donors tend to favor cost-effective interventions that can meet targets more readily. This pervasive technical targeting approach is under mounting fire for disregarding the underlying determinants of health and the need for infrastructure strengthening (Birn 2005; Cohen 2006; Garrett 2007).

Moreover, health development assistance is currently focused on HIV, malaria, and TB, all but overlooking other health needs. More than a dozen neglected tropical diseases[3] that affect 1 billion people, virtually all of whom are extremely poor, are left out of most aid efforts (Chan 2007), as are environmentally and occupationally related ailments, chronic disease, child health needs, and basic health and sanitary infrastructure.

The importance of better aligning development assistance with the needs of countries was acknowledged by donor countries in the 2003 "Rome Declaration on Harmonization." Donors committed themselves to working closely with recipient countries to ensure greater harmonization, including strengthening government participation, targeting donor assistance to the priorities of the recipient country, streamlining donor missions, and improving reporting (World Bank 2003). In the 2005 Paris Declaration on aid effectiveness, donors adopted a set of targets to guide their activities, with 75% of aid disbursed according to agreed schedules and at least 25% of aid promised to long-term programs as opposed to projects. These declarations have yet to bear fruit (Joint Progress Toward Enhanced Aid Effectiveness 2005).

A similar agreement has been reached by UNAIDS, the Global Fund, and others in the context of HIV/AIDS, called the "three ones:" one HIV/AIDS framework to coordinate the actions of all partners; one national coordinating authority, with intersectoral representation; and one system for monitoring and evaluation. The 2005 Global Task Team (GTT) on Improving AIDS Coordination among Multilateral Institutions and International Donors recommended the development of a scorecard to assess adherence to the three ones. However, the GTT report a year later found many deficiencies in adherence on the part of both donor and recipient countries (WHO 2007a).

Box 11–4 Lack of Harmonization of Development Assistance, Vietnam

"In 2003, Vietnam received approximately 400 separate missions from donors, of which just 2% were undertaken jointly. Donors' use of country systems in Vietnam is extremely low: the share of donor projects using national monitoring and evaluation systems is just 13%; national procurement systems, 18%; and national auditing systems, 9%" (WHO 2005a, p. 68).

A number of other donor initiatives have been established under the rubric of "innovative financing mechanisms." These include: the International Finance Facility for Immunization, which aims to increase funding available for immunization programs, including vaccines and health system strengthening through GAVI's Health Systems Window; Advanced Market Commitments (AMCs) to subsidize the purchasing of vaccines not yet available but which could be funded should such vaccines become available; and UNITAD (the former International Drug Purchase Facility), which aims to finance drugs and diagnostic kits for malaria, TB, and HIV/AIDS, through a tax on airline tickets (WHO 2007a).

Notwithstanding these potentially promising developments, most international health donors admit that without basic health system strengthening, vaccines and medicines have little hope of reaching populations in need, yet few donors have interest in such long-term investments. Indeed, only 12% of aid in 2005 went to overall health sector budgets, and the sector-wide approaches aimed at reducing fragmentation of donor efforts have garnered little participation (Lane and Glassman 2007).

Box 11-5 Corruption in the Health Sector

Corruption in health systems occurs when suppliers, public officials, providers, insurers, or patients take health care resources for personal or private institutional gain. This may take place via embezzlement, bribes, kickbacks, extortion, fraudulent billing, or claims; procurement or sale of counterfeit or knowingly substandard drugs and supplies; conflicts of interest among researchers, purchasers, suppliers, and providers; unnecessary treatment; or refusal to provide services. It may entail outright theft and misrepresentation, or involve profiteering from denial of needed care (particularly in the private insurance sector) or the transfer of patients between private and public practice (Savedoff 2007a).

Corruption is facilitated by the complex nature of health systems, including large imbalances of information, inherent uncertainty, the large number and diversity of actors, the involvement—in many countries—of the public, private, and nonprofit sectors, and the multiple directions of resource flows (Transparency International 2006). The problem of corruption increases greatly as health systems become more privatized and rely more on private providers and suppliers, and out-of-pocket expenditures and user fees.

International agencies cite corruption in low-income nations as a health systems problem, arguing that close monitoring of ODA can circumvent corrupt practices and ensure that health aid reaches target populations. However, various industrialized countries are also marked by extensive corruption in the health sector. Although the scale of corruption is often much greater in industrialized than in underdeveloped countries, these cases are rarely mentioned in international corruption reports.

In 1993, the U.S. Attorney General declared corruption in the health care sector to be the country's "number two crime problem," after violent crime (Sparrow 2006). Since then, the U.S. Department of Justice has fined numerous health-related companies that have defrauded the U.S. government. In 2006 alone, 2,400 cases of health fraud—estimated to involve more than US$60 billion—were investigated (Johnson 2007). The fraud cases included: HCA Inc. (kickbacks to physicians and overbilling Medicare—fined US$1.7 billion in 2003 (Government of the USA 2007); Abbott Laboratories (kickbacks, etc.)—fined US$382 million in 2003; AstraZeneca Pharmaceuticals (for charging for free samples and inflating the prices of drugs—fined US$280 million in 2003);

(continued)

Box 11–5 Continued

Bayer Corporation (for relabeling products sold to HMOs and concealing discounts to avoid paying rebates—fined $143 million in 2003); SmithKline Beecham Corporation (similar to Bayer case—fined US$47 million in 2003) (Government of the USA 2003); and Tenet Healthcare (performed unnecessary cardiac procedures billed to Medicare and Medicaid, paid bounty hunters to track down and kidnap patients) (Tenet Shareholder Committee 2005). Tenet was ordered to pay US$900 million to the U.S. government in 2006 (Johnson 2007).

   Health system corruption removes money from health systems, reduces the effectiveness of public health activities and health care services, jeopardizes population health (especially evident in infant and child health indicators, the most sensitive to health care services), and diminishes the level of societal trust (Savedoff 2007a). Wherever it occurs, corruption in the health sector hurts the poorest and most marginalized populations most, as they may be forced to pay additional "fees" in order to obtain services, or barred from care altogether when services are unjustly denied or eliminated due to insufficient resources (Transparency International 2006).

THE POLITICS OF HEALTH ECONOMICS

Health Economics and Underdeveloped Countries

Most of the concepts of health economics were developed in industrialized countries over the past half-century, after these societies had already undergone major improvements in living and working conditions and established greater or lesser variants of the welfare state (Briggs and Gray 1999; Walker and Fox-Rushby 2000). But in countries where many basic needs remain unmet, these principles may not fit. Money spent for promotive, protective, and primary care services can result in relatively large and rapid improvements in health indicators and have significant benefits to the community at large. Universal coverage of certain cost-effective interventions can be an economically efficient means of improving health and may increase equity if the interventions are focused on the populations with the poorest health indicators (Jamison 2006). However, in many underdeveloped countries, CBA and CEA often lead to short-term responses to larger problems: a band-aid approach to disease control that does not address the underlying conditions that foster illness. In this context, targeted interventions may not provide the lasting outcomes desired, particularly when other issues that affect health are left unaddressed.

   Although initial capital investments in broader determinants of health—such as clean water systems—may be initially costly, their long service life and broad utility can make them very (cost-)beneficial from a health standpoint. As such investments increase, many health problems, particularly those attributable to poverty, will decline. Many underdeveloped countries have high rates of acute infectious diseases that, over the long term, are relatively inexpensive to prevent (through addressing the determinants of health) but over the short term, are far cheaper to continue to treat after the fact (through low-cost interventions). As countries undergo urbanization and modernization, acute infections usually decline, and health dollars (or pesos or rupees) may turn to improving the quality, rather than the length, of life. The problem is that long-term investments are usually underrated by CBA/ CEA and their adherents, who are looking for fast returns on investment.

Health financing agencies frequently expect or require underdeveloped countries to use CEA in order to prioritize the allotment of (scarce) health resources. Much of this guidance and pressure comes from bilateral or multilateral institutions, such as the World Bank and the Global Fund, in the form of loan or grant conditions and particular recommendations aimed at low- and middle-income countries. Yet many of the countries that have attained a high health status themselves reject CEA when planning for and allocating health resources. As well, much of the evidence used for CEA is derived from indicators and research carried out in OECD countries and is unlikely to be relevant to nations with distinct histories, societal pressures, political systems, values and ideologies, and economic conditions. When research is carried out in some developing countries, the validity of the evidence may be weak, yet it still may be used for decision making due to a lack of alternative data sources.

Global Public Goods for Health

The alternative to the conception of health (care) as a private good that can and should be distributed through the marketplace is that of health (care) as a public good, which requires public intervention to ensure effective distribution. In a market for private goods, individuals buy and consume items from a limited pool. (Following from our earlier example, when a person buys a schoolbag, there is one less bag in the market. Unless the buyer decides to share her purchase with others, which may not be feasible, she alone will enjoy the benefits of that bag. Market principles assume that increased demand for bags will lead to a new supply of them.) The inability of the market to adequately supply and distribute goods is known as market failure. Market failure in health occurs because private markets by themselves provide too little of the public goods necessary for health, and therefore government involvement and global cooperation is needed to increase the supply of these goods.

In economic terms, public goods are considered: (a) nonrivalrous, (b) nonexclusive, and (c) nonrejectable. Nonrivalrous means that consumption of a good by one individual does not reduce the availability of the good to others, nonexclusive means that the goods or services are available to all, and nonrejectable means that individuals cannot choose *not* to consume that good (Preker, Harding, and Travis 2000; Woodward and Smith 2003). If an area is provided with routine public garbage collection, the benefit is identical for all residents of the area. Likewise, the air quality improvements due to emissions controls enjoyed by one person do not take away these benefits from others, and nobody can elect *not* to reap the benefits of improved air quality. Environmental cleanup, road safety, fluoridation, clean water, and public education are other examples of public goods.

At a global level, public goods for health have been defined to include: (a) knowledge from research (although private interests insist that profit-making through, for example, patents and exclusive licenses, is a necessary incentive for knowledge generation); (b) policies and regulations, which affect an array of institutions, businesses, and large groups of people; and (c) health systems in general, and infectious disease control in particular, to protect the wider population (Woodward and Smith 2003). Health is also considered by some to be a global public good in terms of its role in human security and development (Kaul, Grunberg, and Stern 1999).

Some health-related goods have an effect on people who do not consume them directly. Economists call these effects externalities. Herd immunity is an example of a positive health externality: as more people are vaccinated against measles and are therefore immune to infection, the amount of circulating measles virus diminishes in the population as a whole, and the likelihood of infection for any nonimmunized person is reduced. As more people become immune and are removed as a potential source of virus, others are more protected. Just as immunization programs carry large positive externalities, inadequate social protection creates negative health externalities.

Paradoxically, although the improvement of health is generally good for economic productivity and consumption, there is little immediate economic incentive for private parties to invest in health. Global public goods are also undersupplied because some governments may not wish to invest in an activity, for example malaria control, that benefits other nations (which may not be making equivalent investments). In light of this, donor agencies sponsor global disease campaigns and set up incentives for the provision of scientific public goods, such as partnership grants for training and research (WHO 2002).

While discussion of the notion of global public goods has raised attention to international health, as yet the global public goods approach has not enabled the extensive needs in global health to be better addressed. First, priorities tend to be set, as in international health generally, through donor agendas. For example, while AIDS, TB, and malaria are global concerns, one or all of these ailments may not be important local problems, yet attention to them squeezes out other priorities. Second, the global public goods approach does not adequately address the underlying determinants of ill health—living and working conditions and the distribution of resources, for instance, would need to be deemed global public goods for this to happen. Third, unlike in national contexts, where taxation systems underpin the provision of public goods (including health), there is currently no ongoing financing mechanism for global health goods. The provision of these goods relies on particular allocations of funds by IFIs, bilaterals, and other donors, or by the collective allocation decisions made by the World Health Assembly. A more stable system of funding for international health as a global public good would need guaranteed streams of resources, such as taxes on international financial transactions and on multinational corporate earnings (Kickbusch and de Leeuw 1999).

Investing in Health through Social and Redistributive Approaches

As discussed in Chapters 4 and 13, donor-led investment in technical interventions (a typical neoliberal approach) is not the only path to health. Indeed, societies that embrace social justice approaches and address (and invest in) the broad determinants of health and well-being have achieved far more than the gains projected by the Commission on Macroeconomics and Health, typically with little or no donor involvement. These two approaches to health are compared in Table 11–7.

This is not to say that the financing of health services is irrelevant. Indeed the reforms advocated by the WDR 1993 have diverted resources away from publicly funded health care in favor of private health services, with dire consequences, including:

- a deterioration of health equipment and services;
- shortages of essential medications and equipment;
- a worsening quality of care; and
- greater difficulty finding and retaining skilled health personnel in the public sector due to low salaries and stressful working conditions.

Table 11–7 Neoliberal and Social Justice Approaches to Health Compared

Neoliberal Approach to Health	Social Justice/Human Rights Approach to Health
Assumptions	
Principal aim is economic growth	Principal aim is fair and sustainable use and distribution of resources
Health results from health services and individual behavior changes	Health results from meeting broad social needs, including health services
Key Features	
Addresses symptoms of health problems	Addresses root causes of health problems
Short-term focus	Long-term focus
Promotes interventions delivered through health services and "magic bullets"	Promotes public works and collective social policies and regulations to meet basic needs, improve living conditions, and decrease inequities
Emphasizes the role of private and out-of-pocket financing for health (where needed, with loans, advice, and conditionalities enforced by international agencies)	Identifies redistribution and economic justice as sources of funds for health, together with fair terms of trade
Maintains the status quo of concentrated wealth and power	Calls for an equitable international economic order
Focuses on individual behavior and tends to blame victims	Focuses on structural poverty, inequality, and violence, and tends to blame systemic imbalances of power and resources

Source: Adapted from Katz (2004, p. 756).

Moreover, as quality of care in the public sector declines, people are less inclined to access care or continue necessary treatment, leading to worsened health conditions and the rise of drug-resistant strains of diseases. As the quality and coverage of health systems have deteriorated due to spending cuts—often carried out under pressure from IFIs—international institutions have become even more influential in setting policy and dictating health funding (Gershman and Irwin 2000).

Good health is clearly in the interest of individuals, but it is also in the best interest of society to minimize the costs of ill health, disability, and premature death. Not only does this offer a major justification for publicly funded preventive, curative, and rehabilitative health care, but also for spending on the social determinants of health.

Consider investments in health in comparison to those in education. Both forms of investment increase an individual's productivity and future earnings and enhance the individual's spending ability. Better health improves the investment in education not only by reducing absences from school, and perhaps improving learning ability, but also by increasing the life span, thus providing a greater long-term return from schooling. It has been shown many times over that education, especially for girls, leads to better family health. The positive effect of maternal education on child survival has also been well-established (Desai and Alva 1998; WHO 2005b; Hatt and Waters 2006). Investments in health and education also have significant external benefits to the community at large.

Social and redistributive approaches to health do not negate the potential health gains from targeted cost-effective interventions but show that for long-term health improvements—such as those achieved in strong welfare states—more is needed. Specific health interventions have had a circumscribed impact in comparison to systematic and comprehensive investment in social and living conditions, meeting basic needs, economic redistribution, and other fundamental determinants of health.

CONCLUSION: HEALTH ECONOMICS VERSUS POLITICAL ECONOMY

Learning Points:

- Health economics has gained increased prominence as the basis for international and national health policy making.
- The principal tools of health economics—cost analyses—are guided by a set of values that prioritize short-term, narrowly focused, technical priority setting.
- Health care spending is not always positively correlated with health outcomes.

When all is said and done, do countries that spend more on health care obtain better health outcomes? Not necessarily!

Plotting annual health care expenditures per capita against life expectancy shows that there is a general correlation between health care spending and health outcomes. However, as Figure 11–1 shows, above annual health care expenditures of approximately US$75/capita, there is no predictable relationship between additional resources devoted to health services and improved health status (Wilkinson and Pickett 2006). For example, Germany spends over 12 times as much on health care/capita as Costa Rica, with virtually no difference in life expectancy.

Likewise, Preston curves, which plot GDP/capita against life expectancy, find a strong positive relationship between the two variables for low-income countries (Bloom and Canning 2007): that the 2.5 billion people living in poverty (40% of the world's population lives on less than US$2/day) have poor health is no surprise. Yet above approximately US$5000 (once basic public health needs are satisfied), the correlation between GDP/capita and life expectancy disappears (Marmot 2006).

Indeed, growth in GDP/capita may even be negatively correlated with progress (Tapia Granados 2005), as seen in the Genuine Progress Indicator (GPI), a compound measure of income distribution, unpaid labor, environmental degradation, leisure time, and other factors (Fig. 11–2). When plotted against GDP, the GPI/capita stagnates, or even declines, as GDP/capita grows.

This discrepancy begs the question of whether health problems in some countries are more expensive to address than in others (which is possible), whether in some countries money is being spent unproductively (which is likely), or whether

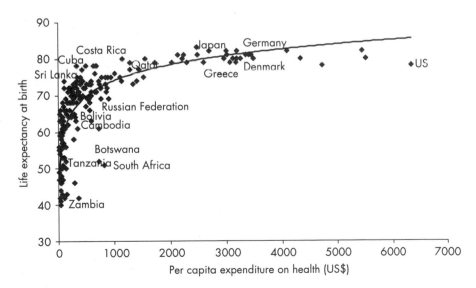

Figure 11–1 The Preston Curve applied to health spending: Life expectancy at birth (2006) and annual per capita expenditure on health (2005) (for 193 countries).
Data Source: WHOSIS (2008).

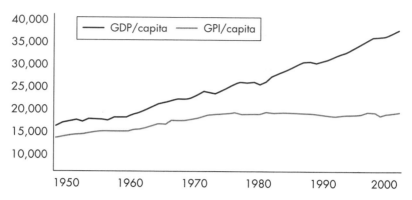

Figure 11–2 Real GDP and genuine progress indicator (GPI) per capita, 1950–2004 for the United States in US$ (2000). The GPI was developed in 1995 in an effort to portray a far more complete picture of social and economic progress than the standard measure of GDP. The GPI begins with GDP data, but then makes adjustments for a variety of factors, starting with income distribution. The value of education, volunteering, and unpaid housework (e.g., childcare) are added to the GPI, while the costs of crime, pollution, environmental damage, and resource depletion are subtracted. The GPI is also adjusted for the durability of consumer goods and infrastructure, "defensive" expenditures to prevent the erosion of quality of life (i.e., water filters and accident compensation), foreign borrowing to cover consumption, and the gain or loss of leisure time. The GPI is used by governmental and nongovernmental policy makers as a scientifically vetted alternative to the GDP for purposes of sustainable development and planning and the measurement of human well-being.
Source: Talberth, Cobb, and Slattery (2007, p. 19). Reproduced with permission from Redefining Progress.

increased health care expenditures play a limited role in reducing mortality and morbidity (which is probable).

It is not known precisely how much of the past increases in life expectancy (or reductions in mortality) are due to general socioeconomic advances, to changes in behavior patterns and ways of life, to the effects of health services, or to other factors. Even those working within the health services sector may not know the relative benefits of public health, prevention, or medical care. Still, as evidenced in Table 11–8, overall economic, political, and social development in multiple sectors—not just the economy, and not only focused on health—are undoubtedly necessary to improve health status in an equitable and sustainable manner.

Much has been written about the impressive health gains—given low levels of GDP/capita—of Cuba, Sri Lanka, Kerala, and Costa Rica (Panikar and Soman 1984; Halstead, Walsh, and Warren 1985; Ghai 2000; Kawachi and Kennedy 2002; Spiegel and Yassi 2004; Withanachchi and Uchida 2006). Mainstream health economists have been particularly puzzled by this seeming paradox, leading them to ask: do these settings enjoy good health outcomes because of particularly effective expenditure on health care (including cost-analysis-based allocation of technical resources) (Savedoff 2007b; O'Donnell et al. 2007)?

Table 11-8 International Comparisons of Health Measures, Health Expenditures, and Inequalities

	Tanzania	Sri Lanka	Bangladesh	Greece	Germany	Egypt	Costa Rica	Chile	Cambodia
Infant mortality rate/1,000 live births (2006)[b]	74	11	52	4	4	29	11	8	65
Life expectancy at birth (2006)[b]	50	72	63	80	80	68	78	78	62
Gini Index[a] (2007)[c]	34.6	40.2	33.4	34.3	28.3	34.4	49.8	54.9	41.7
Net female primary school enrollment ratio (2005)[d]	91	98	96	99	96	91	n/a	89	98
Adult literacy rate (2000–2005)[d]	69.4	90.7	47.5	96	100	71.4	94.9	95.7	73.6
Net migration (1,000s) (2000–2005)[e]	−69	−88	−100	31	200	−105	17	6	2
Energy use (Kg oil equivalent) per US$1,000 (PPP) GDP (2004)[f]	828	124	93	137	163	209	100	171	n/a
Access to potable water (% of population) (2006)[b]	55	82	80	100	100	98	98	95	65
Expenditure on health/ capita (US$) (2006)[b]	18	60	13	2732	3669	93	353	473	30

(continued)

Table 11-8 Continued

	Tanzania	Sri Lanka	Bangladesh	Greece	Germany	Egypt	Costa Rica	Chile	Cambodia
Arable land (% of land area) (2005)[g]	10	14	61	20	34	3	4	3	21
Undernutrition (% of population) (2004)[f]	44	22	30	<2.5	<2.5	4	5	4	33
% of population living below US$1/day (2005)[d]	57.8	5.6	41.3	0	0	3.1	3.3	<2	34.1
Births attended by a skilled health professional (%) (1997–2005)[b]	43	96	13	n/a	100	74	99	100	32

[a]The GINI index measures income inequality within a country on a scale from 0 to 100 (or on a scale from 0 to 1). Countries with GINIs closer to 100 have a greater degree of income inequality. A GINI measurement of 0 would mean that national income is equally distributed among all members of society while a measurement of 100 would mean that 1 person held all the income in that society.

Sources: [b]WHOSIS (2008); [c]World Bank (2008); [d]UNDP (2007); [e]UN Population Division of Economic and Social Affairs of the UN Secretariat (2008); [f]UN (2008); [g]FAO (2008).

While each of these settings has made concerted investments in broad public health efforts, including sanitation, living conditions, and maternal and child health, the reply to the health economics question regarding maximizing health intervention effectiveness is negative: health interventions and economic growth do not offer sufficient explanations for these examples of health success. Instead, we return to the political economy framework (Chapter 4) and to societal determinants of health explanations (Chapter 7), in which equitable social and economic redistribution, undergirded by sustained political support, are central to understanding health outcomes.

As we have seen, health care policy making has become increasingly dominated by economic perspectives, to the point that some health ministries are run by economists rather than public health specialists! Despite the implication of this trend, that public health is a purely technocratic domain, health systems organization—as we shall see in the next chapter—is far more defined by historical and political developments.

Box 11–6 Kerala

Kerala is a Southern Indian state with high health status indicators despite relatively poor economic indicators, including GNI/capita. With Kerala's expenditure on health care of roughly US$10/capita per year, it achieved a life expectancy of 74.6 years in 2000 (Government of Kerala 2005; Jose 2006) just a couple of years shy of life expectancy in the United States, which spends more than 600 times more per capita on health care (WHOSIS 2008). Since the health status of Kerala's population cannot be attributed to health system spending or economic performance—either at the state or national level—analysts have sought alternate explanations (Ekbal 2005):

• A high female literacy rate, which has an inverse relationship with infant mortality.
• A political climate of social justice, emphasizing education and empowerment.
• Governmental priorities of sanitation, drinking water, education, and housing.
• Equitable land distribution.
• A "fair price" food distribution system, providing access to nutritious food at low cost.

While each of the factors above is undoubtedly important in explaining Kerala's health conditions, it is the confluence of these determinants under a redistributive social welfare system, implemented by successively elected Communist governments—beginning in 1957—that best explains the state's long-term success. Given the broad support for such redistributive measures, even non-Communist governments have pursued them, albeit with less vigor. Of course, Kerala, like virtually any setting, is not isolated from global economic forces, and in recent years lack of employment opportunities has led to high levels of out-migration among educated youth, and high economic dependency on remittances (Prakesh 2006). Still, the long experience of social distribution of resources and political distribution of power has enabled Kerala to partially withstand economic pressures to adopt market forces and maintain relatively high wages and social protections.

In sum, the example of Kerala demonstrates that neither efficient health care interventions nor economic growth can fully explain or predict health outcomes. The political economy approach, while offering little guidance on which health care measures are most cost-effective over the short term, is an indispensable tool for understanding what societal investments lead to better health.

NOTES

1. To this day nonunionized workers, whether in developed or underdeveloped countries have few, if any, such protections. Even unionized workers have seen job security and safety eroded unless these rights are protected under strong welfare states (see Chapter 9 for further discussion).

2. Only insofar as expenditures on health serve to eliminate inconsequential symptoms or to enhance social status (e.g., through cosmetic surgery) may they be considered as a form of consumption equivalent to the purchase of any other commodity.

3. The WHO "Neglected Tropical Diseases" category includes onchocerciasis, trypanosomiasis, lymphatic filariasis, schistosomiasis, helminthiasis, and blinding trachoma, among others. See Chapter 6 for details.

REFERENCES

Barrett S. 2004. Eradication versus control: The economics of global infectious disease policies. *Bulletin of the World Health Organization* 82(9):683–688.

Berman PA. 1982. Selective primary health care: Is efficient sufficient? *Social Science and Medicine* 16(10):1054–1059.

Birn A-E. 2005. Gates's grandest challenge: Transcending technology as public health ideology. *Lancet* 366(9484):514–519.

Bloom DE and Canning D. 2007. Commentary. The Preston Curve 30 years on: Still sparking fires. *International Journal of Epidemiology* 36(3):498–499.

Brand D. 1998. A review of important cases and international developments relating to economic and social rights. *ESR Review* 1(1). http://www.communitylawcentre.org.za/Socio-Economic-Rights/esr-review/esr-previous-editions/esr-review-vol-1-no-1-march-1998.pdf. Accessed June 30, 2007.

Briggs AH and Gray AM. 1999. Handling uncertainty when performing economic evaluation of healthcare interventions. *Health Technology Assessment* 3(2):1–134.

Carrin G, Waelkens M-P, and Criel B. 2005. Community-based health insurance in developing countries: A study of its contribution to the performance of health financing systems. *Tropical Medicine and International Health* 10(8):799–811.

Cassels A and Janovsky K. 1998. Better health in developing countries: Are sector-wide approaches the way of the future? *Lancet* 352(9142):1777–1779.

Chan M. 2007. Reaching the people left behind: A neglected success. Keynote speech presented at the Prince Mahidol Award Conference, Bangkok. February 1.

Chernomas R. 1999. *The Social and Economic Causes of Disease*. Ottawa: Canadian Centre for Policy Alternatives.

———. 2005. *The Canadian Health Care System and the Structural Advantages of a Single-Payer System*. Winnipeg: University of Manitoba.

Chernomas R and Sepehri A, Editors. 1998. *How to Choose? A Comparison of the U.S. and Canadian Health Care Systems*. Amityville, NY: Baywood Publishing Company.

Cohen J. 2006. Global health: The new world of global health. *Science* 311(5758):162–167.

Coll AM. 1990. Santé et ajustement structurel. *Vie Santé* 2:13–15.

Collier P and Dercon S. 2006. Review article: The complementarities of poverty reduction, equity and growth: A perspective on the *World Development Report 2006*. *Economic Development and Cultural Change* 55(1):223–236.

Collins T. 2006. The Georgian healthcare system: Is it reaching the WHO health system goals? *International Journal of Health Planning and Management* 21(4):297–312.

Costello A and Woodward D. 1993. The World Bank's *World Development Report. Lancet* 342(8868):440–441.

Desai S and Alva S. 1998. Maternal education and child health: Is there a strong causal relationship? *Demography* 35(1):71–81.

Ekbal B. 2005. People's campaign for decentralised planning and the health sector in Kerala. Issue Paper. People's Health Assembly. http://www.phmovement.org/pdf/pubs/ phm-pubs-ekbal.pdf. Accessed January 3, 2008.

Ekman B. 2004. Community-based health insurance in low-income countries: A systematic review of the evidence. *Health Policy and Planning* 19(5):249–270.

Evans RG. 1984. *Strained Mercy: The Economics of Canadian Health Care.* Toronto, ON: Butterworths.

———. 2003. *Political Wolves and Economic Sheep: The Sustainability of Public Health Insurance in Canada.* Vancouver, BC: Centre for Health Services and Policy Research.

FAO. 2008. Statistics Division 2008. Faostat.fao.org. Accessed September 15, 2008.

Fenner F, Henderson DA, Arita I, Jezek Z, and Danilovich Ladnyi I. 1988. *Smallpox and its Eradication.* Geneva: WHO.

Fuchs VR. 1998. *Who Shall Live? Health, Economics, and Social Choice.* Expanded Edition. Singapore: World Scientific Publications.

Gamkrelidze A, Atun R, Gotsadze G, and MacLehose L. 2002. In MacLehose L and McKee M, Editors. *Health Care Systems in Transition: Georgia. European Observatory on Health Care Systems* 4 (2).

Garrett L. 2007. The challenge of global health. *Foreign Affairs* 86(1):14–38.

Gershman J and Irwin A. 2000. Getting a grip on the global economy. In Kim JY, Millen J, Irwin A and Gershman J, Editors. *Dying for Growth: Global Inequality and the Health of the Poor.* Monroe, Maine: Common Courage Press.

Gertler P and van der Gaag J. 1990. *The Willingness to Pay for Medical Care: Evidence from Two Developing Countries.* Baltimore, MD: Published for the World Bank by Johns Hopkins University Press.

Ghai DP, Editors. 2000. *Social Development And Public Policy: A Study of Some Successful Experiences*: New York: St. Martin's Press; Basingstoke: Macmillan Press in association with United Nations Research Institute for Social Development.

Gilson L and McIntyre D. 2005. Removing user fees for primary care in Africa: The need for careful action. *British Medical Journal* 331(7519):762–765.

Gilson L, Kalyalya D, Kuchler F, Lake S, Oranga H, and Ouendo M. 2001. Strategies for promoting equity: Experience with community financing in three African countries. *Health Policy* 58(1):37–67.

Global Health Watch. 2005. *Global Health Watch 2005–2006: An Alternative World Health Report.* London: Zed Books.

Government of Kerala. 2005. *Human Development Report 2005: Kerala.* Thiruvananthapuram, India: Government of Kerala State Planning Board.

Government of the USA, Department of Justice. 2003. Justice department civil fraud recoveries total $2.1 billion for FY 2003. http://www.usdoj.gov/opa/pr/2003/ November/03_civ_613.htm. Accessed September 9, 2007.

———. 2007. Largest health care fraud case in US settled: HCA investigation nets record total of $1.7 billion. http://www.usdoj.gov/opa/pr/2003/June/03_civ_386.htm. Accessed September 9, 2007.

Greenwald BC and Stiglitz JE. 1986. Externalities in economies with imperfect information and incomplete markets. *Quarterly Journal of Economics* 101(2):229–264.

Gwatkin DR. 2005. Are free government health services the best way to reach the poor? In Preker AS and Langenbrunner JC, Editors. *Spending Wisely: Buying Health Services for the Poor*. Washington, DC: The World Bank.

Halstead SB, Walsh JA, and Warren KS, Editors. 1985. *Good Health at Low Cost*. A Rockefeller Foundation Conference Report. New York: Rockefeller Foundation.

Hatt LE and Waters HR. 2006. Determinants of child morbidity in Latin America: A pooled analysis of interactions between parental education and economic status. *Social Science and Medicine* 62(2):375–386.

Himmelstein DU, Warren E, Thorne D, and Woolhandler S. 2005. Illness and injury as contributors to bankruptcy. *Health Affairs* Jan–June Suppl:W5-63–W5-73.

Hsiao W and Heller PS. 2007. *What Should Macroeconomists Know about Health Care Policy?* Washington, DC: International Monetary Fund.

James CD, Hanson K, McPake B, Balabanova D, Gwatkin D, Hopwood I, et al. 2006. To retain or remove user fees? Reflections on the current debate in low- and middle-income countries. *Applied Health Economics and Health Policy* 5(3):137–153.

Jamison DT. 2006. Investing in health. In Jamison DT, Breman JG, Measham AR, Alleyne G, Claeson M, Evans DB, Jha P, Mills A and Musgrove P, Editors. *Disease Control Priorities in Developing Countries, Second Edition*. Washington, DC: The World Bank; New York: Oxford University Press.

Jamison DT, Breman JG, Measham AR, Alleyne G, Claeson M, Evans DB, Jha P, Mills A, and Musgrove P, Editors. 2006. *Disease Control Priorities in Developing Countries, Second Edition*. Washington, DC: The World Bank; New York: Oxford University Press.

Jamison DT, Henry Mosley W, Measham AR, and Bobadilla JL, Editors. 1993. *Disease Control Priorities in Developing Countries*. New York: Oxford University Press for the World Bank.

Jan S, Dommers E, and Mooney G. 2003. A politico-economic analysis of decision making in funding health service organisations. *Social Science and Medicine* 57(3):427–435.

Johnson C. 2007. US targets health-care fraud, abuse. *Washington Post*, July 19, D01.

Joint Progress Toward Enhanced Aid Effectiveness. 2005. Paris declaration on aid effectiveness: Ownership, harmonisation, alignment, results and mutual accountability. http://www.oecd.org/dataoecd/11/41/34428351.pdf. Accessed September 9, 2007.

Jose VC. 2006. Population: An unbridled horse. Kerala Calling. http://www.kerala.gov.in/kercalsptmbr06/pg44-45.pdf. Accessed September 29, 2007.

Katz A. 2004. The Sachs report: Investing in health for economic development—or increasing the size of the crumbs from the rich man's table? Part I. *International Journal of Health Services* 34(4):751–773.

———. 2005. The Sachs report: Investing in health for economic development—or increasing the size of the crumbs from the rich man's table? Part II. *International Journal of Health Services* 35(1):171–188.

Kaul I, Grunberg I, and Stern MA, Editors. 1999. *Global Public Goods: International Cooperation in the 21st Century*. New York: Oxford University Press.

Kawachi I and Kennedy BP. 2002. *The Health of Nations: Why Inequality is Harmful to Your Health*. New York: The New York Press.

Kickbusch I and de Leeuw E. 1999. Global public health: Revisiting healthy public policy at the global level. *Health Promotion International* 14(4):285–288.

Kim JY, Shakow A, and Bayona J. 2000. Market failures and moral failures: The privatization of health in Peru. In Bambas A, Casas JA, Drayton HA and Valdes A, Editors. *Health and Human Development in the New Global Economy: The Contributions and Perspectives of Civil Society in the Americas*. Washington, DC: PAHO.

Kim JY, Shakow A, Mate K, Vanderwarker C, Gupta R, and Farmer P. 2005. Limited good and limited vision: Multidrug-resistant tuberculosis and global health policy. *Social Science and Medicine* 61 (4):847–859.

Knippenberg R, Traore Nafo F, Osseni R, Boye Camara Y, El Abassi A, and Soucat A. 2003. Increasing clients' power to scale up health services for the poor. Background Paper to the World Development Report. The Bamako Initiative in West Africa. Washington, DC: The World Bank.

Lane C and Glassman A. 2007. Bigger and better? Scaling up and innovation in health aid. *Health Affairs* 26 (4):935–948.

Laurell AC and López Arellano O. 1996. Market commodities and poor relief: The World Bank proposal for health. *International Journal of Health Services* 26(1):1–18.

Marmot M. 2006. Health in an unequal world. *Lancet* 368(9552):2081–2094.

Max W, Rice DP, Sung H-Y, and Michel M. 2004. Valuing human life: Estimating the present value of lifetime earnings, 2000. http://repositories.cdlib.org/ctcre/esarm/ PVLE2000/. Accessed October 9, 2007.

McPake B, Hanson K, and Mills A. 1993. Community financing of health care in Africa: An evaluation of the Bamako Initiative. *Social Science and Medicine* 36(11):1383–1395.

Michaud C and Murray CJL. 1994. External assistance to the health sector in developing countries: A detailed analysis, 1972–1990. *Bulletin of the World Health Organization* 72(4):639–651.

Mills A. 1997. Leopard or chameleon? The changing character of international health economics. *Tropical Medicine and International Health* 2(10):963–977.

Mitton C and Donaldson C. 2002. Setting priorities in Canadian regional health authorities: A survey of key decision makers. *Health Policy* 60(1):39–58.

Murray CJL, Knaul F, Musgrove P, Xu K, and Kawabata K. 2003. *Defining and Measuring Fairness in Financial Contribution to the Health System*. Geneva: WHO.

O'Donnell O, van Doorslaer E, Rannan-Eliya RP, Somanathan A, Raj Adhikari S, Harbianto D, et al. 2007. The incidence of public spending on healthcare: Comparative evidence from Asia. *World Bank Economic Review* 21(1):93–123.

OECD. 2006. Development aid at a glance: Statistics by region. http://www.oecd.org/ dataoecd/59/5/37781218.pdf. Accessed December 3, 2007.

Okun AM. 1975. *Equality and Efficiency: The Big Tradeoff*. Washington, DC: Brookings Institution.

Palmer N, Mueller DH, Gilson L, Mills A, and Haines A. 2004. Health financing to promote access in low income settings—How much do we know? *Lancet* 364(9442):1365–1370.

Panikar PGK and Soman CR. 1984. *Health Status of Kerala: The Paradox of Economic Backwardness and Health Development*. Trivandrum, India: Centre for Development Studies.

Peacock S, Chan C, Mangolini M, and Johansen D. 2001. Techniques for measuring efficiency in health services. Productivity Commission Staff Working Paper. *Commonwealth of Australia*. http://www.pc.gov.au/__data/assets/pdf_file/0018/60471/tmeihs.pdf. Accessed January 9, 2007.

Pettenkofer MJ von. 1941. *The Value of Health to a City: Two Lectures Delivered in 1873*. Translated by HE Sigerist. Baltimore, MD: Johns Hopkins University Press.

Prakesh BA. 2006. Economic policies and performances. Kerala Calling. http://www. kerala.gov.in/kercalnovmbr06/pg15-17.pdf. Accessed August 8, 2007.

Poullier J-P, Hernandez P, Kawabata K, and Savedoff WD. 2002. *Patterns of Global Health Expenditure: Results for 191 Countries*. Geneva: WHO.

Preker AS, Harding A, and Travis P. 2000. "Make or buy" decisions in the production of health care goods and services: New insights from institutional economics and organizational theory. *Bulletin of the World Health Organization* 78(6):779–790.

Rao M, Editor. 1999. *Disinvesting in Health: The World Bank's Prescription for Health.* New Delhi: Sage Publications.

Reichenbach L. 2002. The politics of priority setting for reproductive health: Breast and cervical cancer in Ghana. *Reproductive Health Matters* 10(20):47–58.

Russell S and Gilson L. 1997. User fee policies to promote health service access for the poor: A wolf in sheep's clothing? *International Journal of Health Services* 27(2):359–379.

Save the Children. 2005. *An Unnecessary Evil? User Fees for Healthcare in Low-Income Countries.* London: Save the Children.

Savedoff WD. 2007a. *Transparency and Corruption in the Health Sector: A Conceptual Framework and Ideas For action in Latin America and the Caribbean.* Washington, DC: Inter-American Development Bank: Social Programs Division.

———. 2007b. What should a country spend on health care? *Health Affairs* 26(4): 962–970.

Sepehri A and Chernomas R. 2004. Is the Canadian health care system fiscally sustainable? *International Journal of Health Services* 34(2):229–243.

Sogge D. 2002. *Give and Take: What's the Matter with Foreign Aid?* London: Zed Books Ltd.

Soucat A, Gandaho T, Levy-Bruhl D, De Bethune X, Alihonou E, Ortiz C, et al. 1997. Health seeking behaviour and household health expenditures in Benin and Guinea: The equity implications of the Bamako Initiative. *International Journal of Health Planning and Management* 12 (suppl. 1):S137–S163.

Sparrow MK. 2006. Corruption in health care systems: The US experience. In *Global Corruption Report 2006, Transparency International.* London: Pluto Press in association with Transparency International.

Spiegel JM and Yassi A. 2004. Lessons from the margins of globalization: appreciating the Cuban health paradox. *Journal of Public Health Policy* 25(1):85–110.

Stone D. 1997. *Policy Paradox: The Art of Political Decision Making, Revised Edition.* New York: W.W. Norton and Company.

Talberth J, Cobb C, and Slattery N. 2007. *The Genuine Progress Indicator 2006: A Tool for Sustainable Development.* Oakland: Redefining Progress.

Tapia Granados JA. 2005. Response: On economic growth, business fluctuations, and health progress *International Journal of Epidemiology* 34(6):1226–1233.

Tenet Shareholder Committee. 2005. Greed, scandal & wrongful deaths at Tenet Healthcare Corp. http://www.tenetshareholdercommittee.org/images/Articles/pdf/part_two.pdf. Accessed June 22, 2007.

Transparency International. 2006. *Global Corruption Report 2006.* London: Pluto Press in association with Transparency International.

Tu JV, David Naylor C, Pashos CL, Chen E, Normand S-L, Newhouse JP, and McNeil BJ. 1997. Use of cardiac procedures and outcomes in elderly patients with myocardial infarction in the United States and Canada. *New England Journal of Medicine* 336(21):1500–1505.

Turshen M. 1999. *Privatizing Health Services in Africa.* New Brunswick, NJ: Rutgers University Press.

UN. 2008. UNdata. http://data.un.org. Accessed September 16, 2008.

UNDP. 2000. *Human Development Report 2000.* New York: Oxford University Press for the United Nations Development Programme.

———. 2007. *Human Development Report 2007/2008. Fighting Climate Change: Human Solidarity in a Divided World.* New York: Palgrave Macmillan.

UN Population Division of Economic and Social Affairs of the UN Secretariat. 2008. *World Population Prospects: The 2006 Revision.* Esa.un.org/unpp/index.asp. Accessed September 15, 2008.

Uzochukwu B, Onwujekwe O, and Eriksson B. 2004. Inequity in the Bamako Initiative programme—implications for the treatment of malaria in south-east Nigeria. *International Journal of Health Planning and Management* 19 (Suppl. 1):S107–S116.

Varley RCG, Tarvid J, and Chao DNW. 1998. A reassessment of the cost-effectiveness of water and sanitation interventions in programmes for controlling childhood diarrhoea. *Bulletin of the World Health Organization* 76(6):617–631.

Wagstaff A and van Doorslaer E. 1998. Equity in the finance and delivery of health care: An introduction to the Equity project. In Barer ML, Getzen TE and Stoddart GL, Editors. *Health, Health Care and Health Economics: Perspectives on Distribution.* Chichester, NY: Wiley.

Waitzkin H. 2003. Report of the WHO Commission on Macroeconomics and Health: A summary and critique. *Lancet* 361(9356):523–526.

Waitzkin H, Jasso-Aguilar R, and Iriart C. 2007. Privatization of health services in less developed countries: An empirical response to the proposals of the World Bank and Wharton School. *International Journal of Health Services* 37(2):205–227.

Walker D and Fox-Rushby JA. 2000. Economic evaluation of communicable disease interventions in developing countries: A critical review of the published literature. *Health Economics* 9(8):681–698.

WHO. 2001. *Macroeconomics and Health: Investing in Health for Economic Development. Report of the Commission on Macroeconomics and Health.* Geneva: WHO.

———. 2002. *Global Public Goods for Health. The Report of Working Group 2 of the Commission on Macroeconomics and Health.* Geneva: WHO.

———. 2005a. Improving the effectiveness of aid for health. In *Health and the Millennium Development Goals.* Geneva: WHO.

———. 2005b. *World Health Report 2005: Make Every Mother and Child Count.* Geneva WHO.

———. 2006. An overview of the rationale, activities and goals of WHO-CHOICE. http://www.who.int/choice/description/importance/en/index.html. Accessed December 12, 2006.

———. 2007a. Aid effectiveness and health: Making health systems work. Working Paper No. 9. Geneva: WHO.

———. 2007b. Spending on health: A global overview. Fact sheet No. 319. http://www.who.int/mediacentre/factsheets/fs319/en/. Accessed July 19, 2007.

———. 2007c. TB country profile: Georgia. http://www.who.int/globalatlas/predefinedReports/TB/PDF_Files/geo.pdf. Accessed November 18, 2007.

———. 2007d. WHO-Choice interventions. www.who.int/choice. Accessed February 2007.

WHO AFRO. 1994. *Implementation of the Global Strategy of Health for all by the Year 2000: Second Evaluation. Eighth Report on the World Health Situation.* Vol. 2, African Region, Brazzaville: WHO Regional Office for Africa.

———. 1997. Health policies reviewed by the majority of member states. http://www.afro.who.int/press/1997/regionalcommittee/rc1997090306.html. Accessed May 30, 2007.

WHO EURO. 2007. Life expectancy at birth: European Health for All database. http://data.euro.who.int/hfadb/. Accessed November 18, 2007.

WHOSIS. 2008. Core health indicators. http://www.who.int/whosis/database/core/core_select.cfm. Accessed September 15, 2008.

Wilkinson RG and Pickett KE. 2006. Income inequality and population health: A review and explanation of the evidence. *Social Science and Medicine* 62(7):1768–1784.

Withanachchi N and Uchida Y. 2006. Healthcare rationing: A guide to policy directions in Sri Lanka. *Health Policy* 78(1):17–25.

Woodward D and Smith RD. 2003. Global public goods and health: Concepts and issues. In Smith R, Beaglehole R, Woodward D and Drager N, Editors. *Global Public Goods for Health: Health Economic and Public Health Perspectives.* New York: Oxford University Press.

World Bank. 1987. *Financing Health Services in Developing Countries: An Agenda for Reform.* Washington, DC: World Bank.

———. 1993. *World Development Report 1993: Investing in Health.* New York: Oxford University Press for the World Bank.

———. 2003. Rome declaration on harmonization. February 25, 2003. http://siteresources.worldbank.org/NEWS/Resources/Harm-RomeDeclaration2_25.pdf. Accessed July 25, 2007.

———. 2004. *World Development Report: Making services work for poor people.* New York: Oxford University Press for the World Bank.

———. 2005. Improve maternal health. http://siteresources.worldbank.org/INTECA/Resources/MDG-MaternalHealth.pdf. Accessed November 17, 2007.

———. 2007a. Healthy development: The World Bank strategy for health nutrition and population results. http://siteresources.worldbank.org/HEALTHNUTRITIONANDPOPULATION/Resources/281627-1154048816360/HNPStrategyFINALApril302007.pdf. Accessed November 12, 2008.

———. 2007b. *World Development Indicators 2007.* Washington, DC: The World Bank.

———. 2008. *World Development Indicators 2008.* Washington, DC: The World Bank Group.

Understanding and Organizing Health Care Systems

WHAT IS A HEALTH CARE SYSTEM?

Key Question:

• How do a society's values shape its health care system?

As discussed throughout this text, health derives not just from a society's health care system, but from an array of interlocking political, social, economic, medical, and cultural factors that operate at personal, community, national, and international levels. Moreover, the principal influences on population health, including income, education, production, social welfare programs, tax policy, transportation, and housing, are not a direct part of the health care sector at all. Within the health sector, the elements that most affect health are public health activities such as water supply and sanitation, food inspection, vector insect control, disease surveillance, reduction of industrial pollution, and regulation of pharmaceuticals. Yet most people do not take these societal and public health factors into account when they think about health policy. Instead, they are likely to consider health policy as concerned with the health care system, particularly in terms of clinical or medical care services. Health care policy, then, must be distinguished from a society's broader health policy: health care services, particularly primary health care, form an important—but far from the sole—component of health policy.

The organization of the health care system in each country is a reflection of its political trajectory and societal ideals or values. As such, countries that celebrate individualism, and in which free market economics is the dominant ideology, have largely privately funded and provided health care systems, whereas countries with a strong social democratic ideology and where social solidarity is deeply valued, have primarily publicly funded and organized health systems.

National health care policy is also influenced by the international political and economic order. The proliferation of bilateral, regional, and global trade agreements, which stipulate the opening of domestic markets and the removal of constraints on competition (defined to include the public provision of health and other social services), has diminished the capacity of national governments to shape physical, work, and social policy environments, including the provision of health care services. This chapter briefly addresses the impact of market ideology on recent health reforms, while Chapter 9 analyzes the role of trade agreements and globalization on health.

A health care system is "the combination of resources, organization, financing, and management that culminate in the delivery of health services to the population" (Roemer 1991, p. 31). Health care systems come in a great variety of sizes, forms, and levels of comprehensiveness and effectiveness. Within the structure of every sovereign government there is some entity, usually a ministry of health, which is the official agency charged with responsibilities relating to the health of the population. The ministry of health may be the dominant provider of medical care, or its main function may be to supervise and regulate the work of other organizations.

Most countries have a formal health care policy, which may be enshrined in the national constitution together with the right to health. This policy typically specifies the responsibilities assumed by the state for the health care system. Health ministries may also have mission statements with guiding principles, for example,

> To improve health status through the prevention of illnesses and the promotion of healthy lifestyles and to consistently improve the health care delivery system by focusing on access, equity, efficiency, quality and sustainability (Government of South Africa 2004, p. 4).

and

> Health Canada is committed to improving the lives of all of Canada's people and to making this country's population amongst the healthiest in the world as measured by longevity, lifestyle and effective use of the public health care system (Government of Canada 2006).

These mission statements suggest that health system goals transcend the provision of health care services, but the reality is that health policy is usually focused on curative, medicalized care and underemphasizes community, preventive, and integrated services. In most settings, national health ministries privilege biomedical and behavioral models over a political economy of health approach. Following from Chapter 7, a bona fide health policy—as opposed to a health care policy—would focus on a range of societal determinants of health, many of which are outside of the direct influence of ministries of health (Navarro 2007).

Although health ministry mission statements often resemble one another, the way in which different countries structure their health systems varies considerably. One common misconception is that most European countries have monolithic systems of "socialized medicine" under which a person need only appear on a clinic doorstep to be showered with free services. Perhaps equally widespread is the erroneous idea that most developing countries have no health care systems at all. As with most stereotypes, neither of these images is accurate.

An important characteristic of health care systems is their relation to a society's cultural and political values. According to Donald Light (1997) these fall under four main categories:

1. *Mutual aid values*: the underlying aim of the health system is to help fellow members of society and their families when they are ill.
2. *Societal/state values*: the main goal of the health system is to strengthen the nation through a vigorous, healthy population.
3. *Professional values*: the purpose of the health system is to provide the best possible care to every sick patient (who meets the criteria of the health care system).
4. *Corporatist values*: the role of the health care system is to join buyers and sellers, providers and patients, who then decide on the range and cost of services to be provided.

Health care systems are further shaped by the extent to which health is viewed as a public good and human right as opposed to a commodity or privilege. Although such values may not be explicitly stated in national health care policy, the practices and principles of a health care system typically signal its underlying values and thus help explain its organization.

The organization of health care systems is also the fruition of historical processes and political and economic structures. The roles played by class-based political parties, civil society organizations, trade unions, big business, economic elites, and social movements; how the economy is regulated; the extent to which states redistribute resources; historical legacies of colonialism; and the state's power vis-à-vis international business interests and global economic policy all have bearing on the structure of health care systems.

This chapter begins with a presentation of health system typologies, followed by a historical analysis of various health systems around the world, and a discussion of more recent health system reforms. It then turns to the building blocks and principles of health care systems, with an examination of primary health care as the most important component of any health care system. In many countries "Western" (allopathic), homeopathic, and traditional medicine operate simultaneously; this chapter will focus primarily on allopathic medicine.

HEALTH SYSTEM TYPOLOGIES

Key Question:

• What are the major ways of classifying health care systems?

There are many different ways of interpreting and understanding national health care systems. Not only do various typologies overlap but many countries have multiple health care systems (for different occupational or population groups), and have both public and private delivery and financing mechanisms, making categorization difficult.

Political Economy of Health Systems

The simplest means of classifying health systems is according to two variables: (1) the financing and delivery of health care services, and (2) whether each of these occurs in the public or private sector. Financing is the means by which funds are collected to pay for health care services. This may be mostly through public revenues (taxes, social insurance funds, income from state-owned enterprises) or predominantly through private insurance and/or user fees at the source of delivery. Delivery is the means by which health care is provided. Under a system of public delivery, hospitals and clinics are usually owned and operated by the state, with medical practitioners employed, contracted, or subsidized by the government. In a system of private delivery, health care professionals, and the clinics, offices, and hospitals in which they work, operate as private sector entrepreneurs or businesses (usually not-for-profit in systems that have public financing). Health care delivery and financing may involve a mix of private and public funds (usually dominated by one approach), or just one or the other.

Table 12–1 highlights the fact that private and public systems of financing and delivery are found in both highly industrialized and underdeveloped countries. At the same time, few countries fit purely into a single category. For example, the health care system in the United Kingdom—which is largely publicly financed and delivered—includes a private sector, while the system in the United States—which is mainly private—includes publicly financed services for members of the military, senior citizens, the disabled, and certain extremely low-income groups.

Although this typology offers a useful starting point for understanding the main organizational differences between health systems, it does not offer an explanation of how these differences materialized. In writing about the United States, Vicente Navarro has argued, "we cannot understand...our health care system by looking [solely] at the actors and agents of its delivery...The economic and political order—capitalism—governs the financing and delivery of our health services"

Table 12-1 Public versus Private Financing and Delivery of Health Care Services

Health Care Financing	Health Care Delivery	
	Public	*Private*
Public	(National Health Service) United Kingdom[a] Cuba Spain[a]	(National Health Insurance) Korea[b] Canada[b] New Zealand[b] Thailand[b]
Private	NA[c]	(Pluralistic–private with some public) Ghana U.S.[d]

[a]Also has a small private health sector.
[b]Universal coverage, largely publicly financed, but mix of public/private delivery.
[c]There are no health systems that are privately financed and publicly delivered.
[d]Mostly private but with public financing for senior citizens, the disabled, military and veterans, and certain indigent groups.

Source: Adapted from Roemer (1991).

(Navarro 1993, p. 11). This political economy approach to health systems analysis seeks to take into account:

- the political system and distribution of political power;
- the ownership and social structure of production;
- distribution of income and resources; and
- historical attributes (e.g., the role of labor movements, the legacy of colonialism, the imposition of structural adjustment policies).

Only when we understand these larger factors shaping the context of health care policy can we consider financing mechanisms, coverage and protection, and methods of health care delivery.

Roemer's Typology: Economic Level and Health Care Policy

Perhaps the best known and most widely replicated typology is Milton Roemer's classification of health care systems which includes two key parameters: (1) the level of economic development of a country (measured in GNP/capita), and (2) the degree to which the market and/or the state influence the distribution of health care goods and services. In 1991, Roemer revised his typology (see Table 12–2) in order to differentiate between underdeveloped, resource-rich countries with relatively high GNP/capita from those with a similar GNP/capita but a more developed industrial sector. Roemer's typology distinguishes among four different types of health care policies, based on the level of state protection against market forces (e.g., from entrepreneurial and permissive to socialist and centrally planned), with policies becoming increasingly protective as one moves to the right across the columns.

Table 12-2 Roemer's Health System Typology

Economic Level	Health Care Policy			
	Entrepreneurial and Permissive	Welfare Oriented	Universal and Comprehensive	Socialist and Centrally Planned
Affluent and industrialized	United States	Canada Germany Netherlands Japan	Norway United Kingdom	Former Soviet Union Former Czechoslovakia
Developing and transitional	Thailand Philippines South Africa	Brazil Egypt Malaysia Mexico	Costa Rica	Cuba
Very poor	Bangladesh Nepal Honduras	Botswana Tajikistan	Sri Lanka	China Vietnam
Resource rich	Nigeria	Libya Gabon Venezuela	Kuwait (except "guest" workers)	

Note: In a previous period, Nigeria, China, South Africa, and Vietnam fell into different categories.

Source: Updated (with arrows) from Roemer (1991).

Clearly much has happened to the economies and politics of countries cited by Roemer. This is an important lesson as it illustrates the changing nature of the world's economic, political, and social systems. For example, neither the Soviet Union nor Czechoslovakia exist as countries today, and China is neither strictly socialist nor very poor. However, the classification system remains a useful starting point for discussion.

Roemer's typology also does not take into account the fact that many countries have a mixture of public and private financing and delivery systems, or that privately delivered systems may be for-profit, nonprofit, or a mixture of both. Moreover, the financing and delivery of health services are not always equitably distributed within a country. In Brazil and South Africa, for example, the private sector accounts for two-thirds of total national health expenditures but only a small portion of the population can afford to use private services. In many countries, persons already covered by compulsory public health insurance can buy additional private policies to obtain better coverage or amenities such as private hospital rooms that are not included in the public insurance plan. These trends also skew health spending.

Of course if the peculiarities of each health system were included, we would be left without a typology at all. Still, Roemer's typology might be enhanced by distinguishing further among the various arrangements of state, market, and family or household in capitalist countries, including (Esping-Andersen 1990; Chung and Muntaner 2007):

- *liberal welfare states*, which provide only a minimum safety-net (e.g., the United States, which offers basic health and social services for the elderly and some indigent groups);
- *wage earner welfare states*, which are more generous than liberal states and provide largely employment-based (rather than citizenship-based) benefits (e.g., Australia);
- *conservative-corporatist welfare states*, which are more generous than wage earner states and provide health and social services based on religious affiliation, union membership, or residence (e.g., Italy); and
- *social democratic welfare states*, which are the most redistributive, providing universal benefits to all residents (e.g., Nordic states).

Comparisons without a Typology: Resources Spent on Health

Many international comparisons of health systems—such as those made by the OECD—do not employ a typology at all, but rather list measurable health care system attributes. Nations are commonly compared based on how much they spend on health care services in terms of the percentage of GDP (or GNP). While dramatic differences may be found, it does not follow that the higher the percentage of GDP spent on health care the better the health status of the nation as seen in Figure 11–1. This results from several factors:

1. The distribution of health resources may not relate to need. According to the inverse care law, as proposed by Julian Tudor Hart in 1971, "The availability of good medical care tends to vary inversely with the need for it in the population served. This...operates more completely where medical care is most exposed to market forces, and less so where such exposure is reduced" (Hart 1971, p. 405). In most countries the rich spend more on health care—or the state spends more on health care for the rich—than the populations most in need. In highly redistributive welfare states, this problem is corrected through systems of targeting within universal programs, as per Marx's dictum, "to each according to need, from each according to ability."
2. Access to resources such as clean water, housing, sanitation, maternal education, wages, and many other societal factors also affect health (see Chapter 7).
3. Medical care (spending) is unable to correct for overall inequalities in wealth (which correlate with health status).

The proportion of GDP spent on health care continues to spiral upward in industrialized countries. In the United States, over 15% of GDP went to health care spending—about US$6,700 per capita in 2006. That year, OECD member countries spent on average 8.9% of their GDP on health care, up from 7.1% in 1990 and 5% in 1970 (Kaiser Family Foundation 2007; OECD 2008). In these countries, annual health care spending per capita ranges from approximately US$1,000 to $4,500 (except the United States, the high expenditure outlier, and more recent OECD members Mexico and Turkey with US$600 to $800 per capita annual health care expenditures). By contrast, per capita health care spending in lower-income countries ranges from US$2 to $550/year, generally accounting for 1% to 7% of GDP. For example, Madagascar spends 2.7% of GDP on health, which equates to US$24 per capita per year (WHO 2006d).

In some low-income countries, the percentage of GDP spent on health care may appear to be relatively high, but the actual per capita monetary expenditure is often extremely low, as seen in Figure 12–1. As well, the high cost of purchasing drugs and medical equipment can squeeze out spending on primary health care (PHC). This problem has worsened in recent years due to WTO-enforced patent regimes and the high cost of drugs for AIDS, multidrug resistant tuberculosis, and other ailments (see Chapter 9). The majority of underdeveloped countries must import all or most of their drugs (with the notable exceptions of India, Argentina, Brazil, South Africa, Thailand, and Mexico, which have significant pharmaceutical production capacity).

As discussed in Chapter 11, greater health care spending does not systematically lead to improved health outcomes. Moreover, numerous countries have achieved *Good Health at Low Cost* (Halstead, Walsh, and Warren 1985). The most widely cited examples of resource-poor areas with favorable population health outcomes are Sri Lanka, Cuba, and the state of Kerala in India (see Chapter 13 for more details).

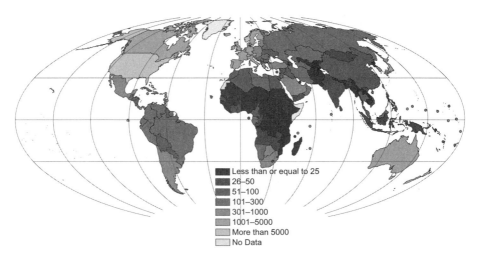

Figure 12–1 Total expenditure on health per capita, 2004 (in US$). *Source*: Courtesy of the WHO (WHO 2007a).

Table 12–3 Comparison of Health Indicators: Cuba, the United States, and Sweden, 2006 (unless otherwise indicated)

Health Indicator	Cuba	U.S.	Sweden
GNI per capita (PPP Int$)[a]	$1,170[b]	$44,070	$34,310
Health expenditure as % of GDP	7.6	15.2	9.2
Health expenditure per capita (PPP Int$)[a] (2005)	$333	$6,347	$3,012
Life expectancy (years)	78	78	81
Infant mortality rate (deaths/1,000 live births)	5	7	3
Physicians per 10,000 people (2000–2004)	59	26	33
Nurses and midwives per 10,000 people (2000–2002)	74	94	109

Note: Aggregate numbers can hide discrepancies between population groups. For example, for 2002–2004 infant mortality among the white population in the United States was 5.7 deaths/1,000 live births but more than twice as high—13.7 deaths/1,000 live births—among African-Americans (Centers for Disease Control and Prevention 2007). Such health differences by social group are discussed in detail in Chapter 7.

[a]Purchasing Power Parity in international dollars. See http://www.who.int/choice/costs/ppp/en/index.html.
[b]Estimate that may not correspond to the same year.

Source: WHOSIS (2008).

For example, as shown in Table 12–3, even though Cuba's GNI and health expenditure per capita are much lower than that of the United States, the two countries have similar health indicators. According to spending comparisons alone, it is hard to understand what makes Cuba's health outcomes so good (surely it is not just the sun and sea!). But by now readers are sufficiently versed in a political economy of health explanation to understand that these examples of success derive from societal determinants of health that are far more extensive than health care services alone.

Not only does increased health sector spending not necessarily lead to better health, but at the extreme, excessive spending on health services may prevent societies from marshalling resources to other key determinants of health, such as adequate housing and occupational health measures.

Examining the proportion of total health expenditures paid privately versus publicly constitutes another means of comparing health systems. Private payments as a percentage of total expenditure on health care in OECD countries are comparatively lower than public expenditures. This is because most industrialized countries have publicly financed health insurance systems. Indeed, the public sector accounts for the majority of total health spending in all *high-income* OECD countries *except* the United States.

Even in universal health care systems, not all services (e.g., pharmaceuticals, dental care, private hospital rooms) or residents (e.g., foreign "guest" workers) are publicly covered. However, universal public coverage generally reduces private expenditure on health care services. As seen in Table 12–4, the five countries with the lowest private health expenditures as a percent of total expenditures all have universal health systems.

Private health expenditures include both out-of-pocket payments and private health insurance. While developing country private health insurance premiums currently comprise less than 10% of the worldwide market, this trend has been accelerating, especially in Asia and Eastern Europe (Drechsler and Jutting 2007). In many countries, out-of-pocket expenditures dwarf private health insurance spending.

Table 12–4 Private Expenditures as % of Total Health Spending in Selected Countries, 2006 (unless otherwise indicated)

Country	Private Expenditures as % of Total Health Spending
Guinea	87.7
India	80.4
Burundi	75.4
Cambodia	73.9
South Africa	58.1
China	58.0
Jordan	58.0
Greece	57.5
Mexico	56.7
United States	54.2
Haiti	51.4 (2005)
Venezuela	50.5
Republic of Korea	47.0
Iran	44.4
The Gambia	41.7
Russia	36.8
Canada	29.6
Botswana	23.3
Saudi Arabia	22.8
New Zealand	22.2
Sweden	18.8
United Kingdom	12.6
Cuba	9.3

Source for data: World Health Organization (2008). National Health Accounts by country, http://www.who.int/nha/country/en/index.html Accessed September 5, 2008.

As total private expenditures increase, those with the fewest disposable resources suffer disproportionately. An increasing dominance of private health care expenditures usually exacerbates social inequalities in health, and may provoke increases in preventable illnesses as people are forced to postpone needed healthcare. Private expenditure as a percent of total spending on health may change quickly, depending on a country's economic conditions and government policies, especially in countries without universal health systems.

Ranking Health Systems: *The World Health Report 2000*

In its 2000 *World Health Report*, the WHO developed a new typology based on measurable performance indicators of health care systems. Countries were ranked according to the following five variables (WHO 2000):

1. overall level of health;
2. distribution of health in the population;
3. overall level of responsiveness;
4. distribution of responsiveness; and
5. distribution of financial contributions.

France ranked the highest, followed by Italy and several small European states (Andorra, San Marino, and Malta).

The report sparked great controversy. Some argued that the WHO ranking did not take into account levels of citizen satisfaction with each country's health system (Blendon, Kim, and Benson 2001). For example, the United States ranked highest in the world in terms of responsiveness to citizen's needs, despite having 15% of its population uninsured and another 15% underinsured. Numerous analysts, focusing on methodological flaws, found that the indices (many extrapolated indirectly) were unclear, of questionable validity, not useful to decision makers, and did not take into account the values and histories of the countries in question (Nord 2002; Deber 2004). Nonsensically, Colombia ranked higher than Canada on fairness in financing, despite Canada's more equitable system of taxpayer contributions, more comprehensive coverage, and greater overall efficiency (Walt and Mills 2001).

Other analysts accused the report of being more ideological than scientific. According to Navarro, the report was influenced by a political environment in which the technocratic and market-based priorities of the WHO's major donors dominated. The report assumed that "...the most prominent health problems our societies face can be resolved by technological-scientific medical bullets or interventions, without reference to changes in the social, political, and economic environments in which these problems are produced" (Navarro 2000, p. 1601). This critique was echoed in an assessment by Brazil's Oswaldo-Cruz Foundation, which questioned why the WHO had discarded its previous principles and strategies for improving health, such as the primary health care approach, and why it failed to recognize the universal right to health and publicly delivered health care as a basic element of health systems comparisons (Oswaldo Cruz Foundation 2000).

In sum, while quantitative comparisons of health systems may be useful for certain planning exercises, they remain problematic. They may be driven by ideological motives or rest on the false assumption that health is solely the product of health services spending. Certainly, the quality and range of quantitative data could be improved, and its limits for analytic and policy-making purposes could be addressed through the use of appropriate qualitative data. An example of the kind of qualitative evidence that might be used to compare health systems is presented in Table 12–5. The next section explores the historical and political context of health systems evolution, taking into account a complex array of qualitative and quantitative evidence.

Table 12–5 Evolution of Health Systems

Health System	Type 1: Private	Type 2: Pluralistic	Type 3: National Health Insurance	Type 4: National Health Service	Type 5: Socialized Health Service
Political and ideological values	Health care as an item of personal consumption	Health care as primarily a consumer good	Health care as an insured, guaranteed service	Health care as a state-supported service	Health care as a right and state-provided public service
Position of the physician	Solo entrepreneur	Solo entrepreneur and member of practitioner group	Private solo or group practice and/ or employed by hospitals	Private solo or group practice and/ or employed by hospitals	State employee
Ownership of facilities	Private	Private, not-for-profit, and public	Not-for-profit and public	Mostly public	Entirely public
Source of financing	Private out-of-pocket payments	Mix of private, out-of-pocket, and public	Primarily public single-payer	Public monopsony	Public monopsony
Administration and regulation	Market	Market, some government	Government	Government	Government
Prototype	Most countries until the 19th or 20th century	United States Peru	France Canada Japan Korea	Great Britain Sweden (de facto)	Former Soviet Union Cuba

Sources: Adapted from Rodwin (1984); Field (1978).

THE ORIGINS OF HEALTH CARE SYSTEMS

Key Question:

• What historical and political factors have led to different trajectories of health care system development?

Family members and local healers have always cared for the sick, and religious institutions have a long tradition of providing charitable care. But, an organized system to oversee the health of a large population is a relatively recent development linked to the rise of the modern state, beginning in the 18th century. In particular, industrial development, the rapid growth of cities, and the demands of imperial powers highlighted the need for a healthy labor force and military. By the 19th century, increasingly organized workers and city dwellers made claims on their governments to provide health care alongside other social services. Notwithstanding these common pressures, a diversity of organizational arrangements emerged based upon the particular historical trajectories, political forces, economic interests, and social values of each setting. Around the world, necessity, controversy, and ingenuity have generated many different strategies but none is perfect. As we cannot possibly describe the health care systems of all countries, here we present several important patterns, as archetypes, and compare the circumstances of their development.

National Health Insurance: Germany

Germany's system of social insurance originated in the 1880s and provides one of the earliest examples of state-guaranteed health care coverage. The working class that developed during the late 18th and 19th century industrial revolution—when small tenant farmers were uprooted and forcibly transformed into factory workers across much of Europe—sought protection against the vagaries of wage employment under capitalism. They began to form voluntary mutual-help groups, whose members agreed to make regular contributions to a common fund that would provide cash benefits in the event of sickness or unemployment.

These semi-autonomous health funds were organized along occupational, ethnic, religious, political, or geographic lines. Over time, tens of thousands of voluntary funds were organized. The Prussian Parliament formalized the system into law in 1854, requiring regular contributions from workers to be matched by their employers. Three decades later, after orchestrating the unification of Germany, Chancellor Otto von Bismarck—faced with the increasingly militant demands of organized labor and city dwellers—introduced a series of social insurance programs to protect vulnerable urban workers from the hazards of dangerous factories and life in unsanitary environments. The 1883 Sickness Insurance Act made sickness fund coverage mandatory for low-wage workers and established

596 Textbook of International Health

guidelines for regulation. The following year Bismarck introduced a law covering
workers in case of industrial accidents, with all contributions made by employers. While the industrial sector decried these programs as unfair burdens, they
effectively boosted worker productivity and profits. Bismarck's political strategy
was motivated by the need to suppress social unrest and preempt the growing
success of socialist parties through emphasis on "carrots" over repressive "sticks"
(Sigerist 1943).

This was the dawn of the concept of social security, which spread to other countries in Europe, Japan, South America, and beyond. By 1985, 70 countries had
adopted Germany's form of health care insurance along with wage-loss compensation for sickness and medical treatment (Roemer 1991). In Germany and elsewhere,
social security protection was soon extended to "old age" pensions, disability,
unemployment, maternity, death, and widows' benefits, children's allowances, and
other measures.

Despite the disruption of two world wars and Hitler's fascist Third Reich,
Germany's highly decentralized system has proven extremely durable. Today the
majority of Germans—about 88%—participate in the mandatory sickness insurance
schemes, with 7% covered by private health insurance and 5% by insurance for
civil servants (funded partly by government and partly by private insurance). About
10% of those covered under the public plan (the "sickness funds") purchase supple-
mentary insurance for additional benefits such as private hospital rooms (Busse and
Reisberg 2004, Busse 2008). In 2006, public sources accounted for approximately
77% of total health financing (WHOSIS 2008).

The sickness funds provide a comprehensive package of benefits to members
and their families, including disease prevention, health promotion, and ambulatory,
hospital, and dental care. Other benefits include maternity and nursing care, drugs
and appliances, cash payments for loss of income during illness, funeral benefits,
and even visits to health spas. Long-term care needs are covered through a separate
insurance system, which is mandatory for the whole population.

Box 12–1 Basic Features of Germany's Social Insurance System (WHO 2006d)

- Publicly funded social health insurance compulsory for employees earning up to €48,000 (2007) and their dependents.
- Health insurance is provided via more than 200 competing nonprofit, autonomous, nongovernmental health insurance funds—"sickness funds"—publicly financed through payroll (employer and employee) and income taxes.
- Public, private nonprofit, and a small but growing number of private hospitals are reimbursed for patient care by sickness funds through a prospective system of diagnosis-related fees.
- Ambulatory care physicians, mostly in solo private practice, are paid by capitation or fee-for-service, under regulated rates.
- Patients are free to select any provider though they are offered incentives to use gatekeepers.

The sickness schemes are nonprofit organizations. They do not provide medical care directly but function as financial intermediaries. Physicians in Germany are not employed by the funds. They work as private practitioners and can be separated into two classes: those who provide ambulatory care (medical services that do not require hospitalization) and those who work in hospitals. Hospital-based physicians are salaried by their hospitals, which receive operating income by billing the sickness funds. Ambulatory care doctors in the national health insurance system charge for services provided and are paid according to predetermined rates set by the regional physician's association. Payment is made on a capitation basis (i.e., a set amount for each patient, independent of the number of visits) (Altenstetter 2003, Busse and Reisberg 2004) or as a fee for each medical procedure, as negotiated between sickness funds and doctors' associations. A patient (fund member) may select any ambulatory care physician.

Due to the fragmented historical development of the funds in Germany and other settings, a great number of actors, often with competing interests unions, employers, providers, government—have become involved in negotiations of health care system structuring. As a result, countries with national health insurance may have separate plans for government employees, postal, railroad, and communications workers, miners, sailors, and others. Many countries also maintain independent social security funds for agricultural workers and the self-employed, for whom membership may be voluntary. It is mainly because of these diverse interests that few countries, at least in Western Europe, have been able to fully consolidate all of these plans, although some have been able to merge existing insurance schemes into comprehensive national programs (e.g., Israel). Others have close to 100% population coverage under one social security plan (e.g., Austria).

Fragmented funding systems can lead to inequities among groups of beneficiaries, if not regulated by government agencies, and can further entrench competing plans. Nevertheless, a general consensus in Europe holds that health care is a community responsibility, not a private one. Health care financing remains predominantly public, with delivery of services split between private and public arrangements.

National Health Service: United Kingdom

The United Kingdom has a long tradition of mutual aid societies and of government regulation of medical practice and the welfare of the poor. In 1804 there were 1 million members of "friendly societies" in England (which, like Germany's sickness funds, provided health coverage and other assistance to members in need), growing to 7 million by the turn of the 20th century. By the 1840s, some employers supported these societies because they were good for business. Meanwhile the Poor Law Reform of 1834 authorized, but did not guarantee, medical relief for the indigent. In Britain, "where provision for the acute sick by charitable effort was inadequate to provide for all who needed care, the acute sector of hospital care was, from 1870 onward, gradually supplemented by public authorities" (Abel-Smith 1965, p. 33). As elsewhere, until circa 1900, those who could afford to stayed away from hospitals, preferring to be cared for at home where the risk of death was lower.

By 1911, the British government was determined to make medical care more generally available to the poorest sectors of the population and passed the Health Insurance Act. A national health insurance scheme came into effect in 1912, mandating basic medical benefits for workers earning, at that time, under £160/year. Doctors were paid through local insurance committees made up of insured workers, doctors, and government officials. Reimbursement was usually on a capitation basis. Approved mutual aid societies were also permitted to sell additional insurance to workers (e.g., for dental coverage), and to the general public on a voluntary basis.

World War I, the Depression, and World War II left large numbers of people unemployed. In 1942, the government-commissioned Beveridge Report recommended the provision of state insurance to cover unemployment, ill health, old age, and widowhood as well as allowances to meet family needs. The report famously called for: "A comprehensive national health service [which would] ensure that for every citizen there is available whatever medical treatment he requires, in whatever form he requires it" (Beveridge 1942, p. 158). In its subsequent proposal for a postwar national health service, the Ministry of Health reiterated William Beveridge's recommendation, emphasizing the need to "divorce the care of health from questions of personal means" (Ministry of Health of Great Britain 1944, p. 47).

The report's biggest contribution was to unify social policy across classes by proposing a single social insurance scheme for the whole nation, financed through income taxes. Basic protection—through a public and universal health service—against the hazards of illness and mortality and the vagaries of the economy was, like the vote, to be every citizen's birthright.

Plans for the national health service (NHS) were opposed by the British Medical Association, which feared loss of physician autonomy and insisted on the right to remain in private practice. For almost 2 years Socialist Minister of Health Aneurin Bevan waged an uphill battle against doctors and the Conservative Party. He shepherded the NHS's launch in 1948 (Webster 1998). In short order, health insurance coverage was extended to the whole of the population, benefits were expanded, and hospitals were nationalized (in order to control their size, location, and operations). Central councils and committees were also established, but by no means was the NHS fully centralized. Regional hospital boards were created, each centered in a university medical school, and hospital management committees oversaw nonteaching hospitals. County and borough councils were charged with community and environmental health services. Various other countries such as Sweden, Spain, and Chile adopted similar models (though Chile underwent a major privatization reform in the 1980s, creating a highly inequitable health care system [Unger et al. 2008]).

After Bevan's battle, the NHS emerged with three categories of doctors: general practitioners (GPs), specialists, and public health physicians. As in the German system, community and hospital-based specialists are clearly distinguished. Primary medical care is provided by GPs, with whom individuals must register for general medical services. Although GPs contract with the NHS as self-employed professionals, they receive subsidies for their staff and for the cost of maintaining their premises, and they participate in NHS pension programs. Other health professionals, such as dentists, optometrists, and pharmacists, practice on a more independent commercial basis with few subsidies.

Box 12–2 Basic Features of the NHS

- Comprehensive coverage for all residents.
- One system funded mostly through taxation (with structural differences under the devolved local administrations in Northern Ireland, Scotland, and Wales).
- Mostly free at the point of service, although cost sharing is growing.
- The national government oversees primary care and delivery of most specialty and hospital care services through trusts, contracting to the private sector for some elective surgery.
- Hospital physician consultants (specialists) are generally employed in public hospitals.
- Independent GPs act as gatekeepers to specialized care and are paid via primary care trusts through a mix of capitation, salary, and fee-for-service methods.

The NHS has undergone a series of reforms but none as significant as those launched in the 1980s, when a conservative political shift led to tightening budgets and growing incentives for private health insurance. Conservative Prime Minister Margaret Thatcher was zealous in reducing the role of government in Britain, infusing market forces in a 1982 NHS reorganization. But she was forced to defend the principle of universal access to health care regardless of ability to pay, due to the U.K. population's collective support for health care as a right (Maynard and Bloor 1995). Reforms in the 1990s created "internal markets," whereby, in a highly unpopular program, GPs were encouraged to compete against one another as fundholders responsible for purchasing care for their patients (Light 2003).

In the late 1990s, Britain's New Labour government reversed some reforms of previous decades and increased focus on primary care. Since 2000, however, emphasis on the internal market has increased inequities in access. Although the Labour government has injected large amounts of new funding into the NHS and reduced waiting times, the maze of reforms and often insidious competitive mechanisms have prevented regional cooperation (Toynbee 2007). Out-of-pocket payments grew to almost 12% of total health expenditures in the United Kingdom in 2005. Still, thus far, the NHS has managed to retain one of its key characteristics—a tax based system. In recent years government health spending accounted for close to 90% of the total, mostly funded by general taxes (OECD 2004;WHOSIS 2008). In 2005, approximately 12% of the population held some form of private health insurance

(Foubister, Thomson, and Mossialos 2006), accounting for less than 1% of total health expenditures.

A Centrally Planned Health Care System: The Former Soviet Union

In contrast to the stepwise creation of health care systems in Germany and Britain, the Soviet system was born of radical change. The Bolshevik Revolution of 1917 defeated the monarchy and created a new government that was almost immediately faced with economic crisis and civil war. Soon after the Bolsheviks seized power, the scattered medical activities of individual departments were unified by the Council of Medical Boards. Local councils took charge of health affairs including the rural medical system (the Zemstvo), and all private hospitals, clinics, and pharmacies were nationalized. In July 1918, the People's Commissariat of Health Protection was established as the central body in charge of the entire health system of the new nation.

Initially, the major issue in the Soviet Union was not the health of factory workers, for there were few in the predominantly rural country, but the control of epidemic diseases. Typhus infected tens of millions, and millions died. In 1919, the Russian Communist Party (the Bolsheviks) emphasized the importance of broad measures of health and sanitation aimed at the prevention of diseases. As Lenin famously declared in 1919, "Either socialism will defeat the louse, or the louse will defeat socialism." Accordingly, the Russian Communist Party set as its immediate tasks (Roemer 1991):

1. the implementation of broad sanitary measures such as the improvement of health conditions in residential areas (protection of soil, water, and air); the establishment of communal feeding on scientific-hygienic principles; the organization of measures to prevent the outbreak and spread of contagious disease; and the enactment of sanitation legislation;
2. the control of social diseases (e.g., tuberculosis, venereal diseases, alcoholism); and
3. the provision of accessible, free, and efficient medical and pharmaceutical services.

Due to the vastness of the territory and the diversity of conditions, health commissariats were set up in a decentralized manner in each constituent republic. Under the new Constitution of 1923, and reaffirmed in 1936, the federal government established general rules for the protection of health, with uniform principles of Soviet medicine applied in all republics:

> The Soviet state acknowledges the right of every citizen of the USSR to obtain not only full medical attention, but also material assistance during illness, in old age

or in invalidism at the expense of the state. Soviet mothers have the right to obtain the material assistance of the state during pregnancy, childbirth, and the rearing of their children. These rights are guaranteed by the Constitution of the USSR (1936 Constitution, Article 120).

The health commissar, Nikolai Semashko, planned for government control of all aspects of Soviet public health. All medical establishments were interlinked and designed to achieve the same objectives: a reduction in the death rate of the population, continuous improvement of health, and an increase in the average life span through amelioraton of working and living conditions.

In the 1930s, the Soviet government set up special medical institutes that produced tens of thousands of new doctors to meet the country's ambitious health agenda. In a matter of just a few years, the Soviet Union had one of the world's highest doctor–population ratios based on a highly trained medical workforce. Around the same time, occupational health and community clinics were prioritized so that the needs of industrial workers and city dwellers could be addressed (Sigerist 1937).

A distinctive feature of Soviet public health was strong central planning. The national government projected the numbers of health workers needed and placed personnel accordingly. Local facilities also made requests for equipment and personnel, which were combined at each level and forwarded up through the system; allocations of resources came from the top down. Still, as in most countries, the health system was marked by unequal quality across regions and remained underfunded as it was often the last item planned for in the budget.

From the users' point of view, the system began at the local polyclinic, a multifunction health center located primarily in urban areas and industrial settings. Adults, pregnant women, children, and workers attended distinct, specially staffed and equipped institutions. Rural areas had health posts staffed by paramedical personnel, initially *feldshers* (assistant doctors), and then mostly midwives and nurses. Patients with complex conditions could be referred up the system to district-level or larger hospitals.

All personnel in the Soviet system were full-time government employees. Although private practice was strictly banned, persistent complaints about inefficiency and lack of service led to unofficial "moonlighting" or paid private practice by physicians during their off hours. With *glasnost* (openness) and *perestroika* (restructuring) in the late 1980s, a small amount of private practice was tolerated, and a few private clinics and fee-for-service practices operated openly in the larger cities.

The polyclinic-based system was adopted by other socialist countries including Cuba, North Korea, Vietnam, Poland, Czechoslovakia, and other Eastern European countries with greater or lesser fidelity depending on prevailing economic and social conditions.

Box 12–3 Basic Features of the Former Soviet Model

- Centrally planned and operated facilities and service provision.
- Strong focus on prevention, occupational health, and community health.
- Doctors employed by the state; medical training centrally planned.
- Full coverage—free of charge—for all citizens through networks of facilities starting in the local neighborhood or workplace.
- Funded through general revenues (from state-owned enterprises).

The dissolution of the USSR and the creation of the Russian Federation in 1991 provoked the de-modernization of Russia's economy, large-scale privatization, and one of the world's most rapid and remarkable declines in GDP. This dramatic economic dismantling (which occurred to an equal or lesser extent in the former Soviet republics) resulted in major changes in the organization of the health system, including the opening of the private health care market. In line with political decentralization, Russia's health system was also decentralized. It is currently divided into federal, regional, and municipal levels of administration, with geographic location, as under the Soviet system, determining the site of care (Tragakes and Lessof 2003).

The new Russian Constitution retained the right to free medical care, and subsequent government administrations have operated according to the principle of care based on need rather than ability to pay. However, the public health care system has met with severe budgetary constraints, even as oil revenues have filled government coffers. A mandatory health insurance system based on payroll taxes was introduced in 1993, but severe shortages, long waiting times, and quality of care problems remain. The health care system has also suffered a significant loss of personnel, drug supplies, and equipment, especially outside Moscow and St. Petersburg, while facing burgeoning rates of both chronic (e.g., heart disease, cancer) and new and reemerging infectious diseases (e.g., AIDS, tuberculosis, diphtheria, whooping cough). Most health services continue to be provided by the severely underfunded public sector, with the private sector remaining small, mostly covering the new elites and the middle class in major cities. Still, private spending makes up over 35% of all health expenditures, 78% of which is paid out of pocket (WHO EURO 2003a; WHO 2006c).

From Communist Barefoot Doctors to Market Socialist Hodgepodge: The People's Republic of China

With approximately one-fifth of the world's population, China has become one of the world's most rapidly growing economic powers, following a history of turbulence and violent swings of policy. The millennia-long Imperial period, marked in various degrees by semi-feudal agrarianism and a centralizing bureaucratic state, ended in 1911. During the ensuing nationalist period under the Kuomintang government, public health authorities sought to control epidemic diseases, and

China opened up to Western medicine brought by Christian missionaries, Chinese immigrants, and the Rockefeller Foundation (which invested colossal sums to found and operate the Peking Union Medical College starting in 1915). However, these efforts reached only a small portion of the population. Internal strife and the trauma of Japanese occupation left much of China sick and impoverished at the end of World War II.

The successful revolution of Mao Zedong's forces and the establishment of the People's Republic of China in 1949 resulted in a period of cooperation with, and influence by, the Soviet Union lasting until 1960. Prior to the 1950s, China's vast rural areas were served almost exclusively by practitioners of traditional medicine. In towns and cities, there were also private physicians and some missionary clinics and hospitals. In 1949, all private capital and property, including hospitals, were nationalized by the state, and rural land was taken from landlords and distributed to collectives of peasants. These rural communes, which operated from the 1950s to 1970s, maintained a three-tier system of health facilities, with county hospitals, commune (township level) clinics, and brigade (village level) health centers.

During the Cultural Revolution from 1965 to 1975, formal medical education was halted, and physicians and professors were sent to do active labor in the countryside. Physicians could no longer practice in the private sector. Shanghai, for example, had 10,885 private physicians in 1950; this was reduced to 1,514 in 1965 and to zero in 1966. Cooperative medical schemes developed in rural areas based on grassroots insurance plans in which commune members decided what benefits to provide, the amount of copayments needed for various services, and so on. Most of the primary medical care was provided by "barefoot doctors"—local workers selected by their comrades to be given several months of medical training, usually at the county level. These part-time, low-level medical workers then returned to their brigades and were awarded work points, donated by their comrades, for doing medical work in lieu of labor in the fields. In this way, accessible, low cost, basic medical services were extended to 90% of villages. The state also conducted patriotic health campaigns to educate and motivate the peasantry. Enormous health gains were experienced in this period thanks to vast improvements in living and social conditions, including the new primary health care system. China's barefoot doctors were seen as a model for health care delivery across the world and an exemplar for the approach promoted by the Alma-Ata International Conference on Primary Health Care held in 1978.

After Chairman Mao's death in 1975, Chinese society changed radically, and the policies of the Cultural Revolution were criticized and repudiated. China officially adopted a "socialist market economy," medical schools reopened, the private practice of medicine was sanctioned, and the commune system was dismantled in favor of individual production. Village health workers were no longer paid collectively and many barefoot doctors either stopped practicing or upgraded their skills and opened private practices as rural doctors. Health stations were privatized. A new household responsibility system replaced the communes, leading to private production of crops and private payment for medical services.

By the early 1990s, cooperative medical schemes remained for roughly 5% of rural residents, while all others had to pay for medical services out of pocket. In the mid-1990s the Chinese government acknowledged that in poor rural areas medical expenses could be ruinous to peasants with low incomes, and it began to renew rural medical schemes based on the principle of decentralized, geographically based social insurance. Some of these health programs are supported by profits from new nonagricultural enterprises. Generally termed "cooperative health care schemes," they are based on insurance principles with risk sharing, strict budgets, and negotiation with providers and third-party payers. Funds are generated from households, collectives, and local governments, and are used to reimburse defined health care expenses. Run on a not-for-profit basis and aimed at ensuring services at a low cost, the schemes are administered by management committees representing various interested parties (Feng et al. 1995). Although growing, rural health insurance plans cover only 42% of rural residents (Meng 2007).

Urban residents are served by two main programs. One is the publicly funded Government Insurance System (*gongfei yiliao*) for civil servants, college students, and disabled military officers, which serves about 30 million people. The other is the Labor Insurance System (LIS or *laobao yiliao*) for workers in state-owned and collective enterprises. The LIS is financed by employer contributions and serves about 200 million people. Those who are not eligible for coverage under these systems, such as persons employed in the private sector, pay privately for their medical care. Prepaid employment-based health plans are used in cities, but 70% of urban residents remain without health insurance (Ho 1995; Zhengzhong 2005; Meng 2007).

Health services in China today are in fact far less "socialized" than in many Western countries and are plagued by numerous problems (Blumenthal and Hsiao 2005). Many health professionals and hospitals have to generate their own income because medical fees are kept low by government regulation. This has led to the overprescription of drugs, as this is one of the only ways a practitioner can turn a profit. As a result, people who are well-off are often overmedicated, while the poor are unable to afford medicines. Because there are few regulatory controls, privatization has also led to soaring rates of unnecessary procedures, including caesarean-sections and surgery. Despite rapid economic growth, public spending on health has decreased and disparities in health status have worsened (Eggleston, Rao, and Wang 2005; Huong et al. 2007).

Box 12–4 Basic Features of Health Care under China's "Market Socialism"

- Formerly acclaimed "barefoot doctor" system abandoned.
- Two separate systems: better-resourced and organized urban system, poorly resourced and organized rural system.
- Hodgepodge of public and private funding and provision schemes.
- High levels of private health expenditure with inadequate budgets in the public sector.

In sum, health sector reforms in China over the past 30 years have resulted in the creation of two public health care systems—an urban system which has some resources and is better organized, and a rural system with few resources and poor organization leaving 80% of the country's 700 million rural residents without health insurance coverage (Liu and Rao 2006). China's system is also highly fragmented: the Ministry of Labor and Social Security is responsible for urban health insurance, the Ministry of Civic Affairs for poor urban and rural households, and the Ministry of Health for rural areas of the country (Hu 2004). Commercialization of the health sector, as well as a weakened state, have had a particularly deleterious effect on rural communities (Liu 2004; Huong et al. 2007). Moreover, China's growing health inequalities show that economic growth—especially growth that is not equity-based—does not necessarily generate health improvements. (Liu, Hsiao, and Eggleston 1999; Gong, Walker, and Shi 2007).

Unsystemic Health Care: The United States

It is difficult to speak of a health care system in the United States—it is one of the world's most fragmented, chaotic, and irrational examples of health services organization. Strikingly, the United States has the world's most technologically advanced medicine, contributes hugely to medical research, and spends by far the largest total and per capita amount on health care—over US\$6,700/person in 2006, or more than 15% of its GDP. Yet 47 million people (almost one-sixth of the population in 2006) have no health insurance at all, and millions more are underinsured (WHO 2006d; DeNavas-Walt, Proctor, and Smith 2007). In total, 42% of adults are either uninsured or underinsured (Schoen et al. 2008). This appalling irony has led U.S. health care to be characterized as a "paradox of excess and deprivation" (Enthoven and Kronick 1989, p. 29).

Despite a series of social and political struggles, the United States is the only industrialized nation that does not provide universal health insurance to its citizens. Various analysts have studied why this is the case, ascribing the problem, variously, to deep-seated individualist values, special interest groups and stakeholders (Quadagno 2004), and the absence of a labor party that mobilizes around working class needs (Navarro 1989; Hoffman 2003). Even amidst the misery of the 1930s Great Depression, national health insurance was blocked from inclusion in the country's social security package by a powerful alliance of insurance companies, business interests, physician groups, and hospital associations (Birn et al. 2003).

The private employer-based health insurance system that is in place today was entrenched during World War II, when the mobilization of millions of soldiers left a shortage of workers, and companies sought to attract laborers to their factories with health insurance benefits. Unions later included these benefits as part of their bargaining rights. Meanwhile, insurance companies proliferated and became highly profitable.

Notwithstanding wide popular support for national health insurance, legislative efforts aimed at passing a universal plan in the 1940s and 1970s were again defeated by coalitions of insurance companies, health care providers, and business and economic elites. Fragmented gains were made in the 1960s with health plans established for two population groups not covered by workplace-based insurance: one for senior citizens (Medicare), and another scaled-down, state-based plan for certain categories of indigent persons such as pregnant women and children (Medicaid).

By this time, decades of political pressure from physician and hospital lobbies had led to a wasteful oversupply of personnel and facilities. This was based on the pervasive assumption that more is almost always better: more hospitals offering more intense services, more professionals with more training, and more researchers devising expensive new treatments. By the 1980s, many acute care hospitals were operating at just 60% capacity, and medical specialists outnumbered generalists by three to one. Innumerable politicians, unions, advocates, workers, and employers were frustrated and alarmed by the excessive costs and gross inefficiency of the health sector. However, efforts in the early 1990s to control the health care behemoth, including a major initiative by then President William Clinton to provide universal coverage—funded by employers and taxpayers and delivered by competing managed care organizations—failed, largely due to the opposition of highly profitable insurance corporations.

Some form of managed care—the integration of health care financing and delivery via contracts in which providers assume certain financial risk and move from being patient advocates to allocators of health care spending—has existed in the United States for more than a century. Early forms of such prepaid health services were provided by employers for immigrant workers, and group practice in various forms emerged to fill the demand for services. In the early 20th century, health maintenance organizations (HMOs)—which cover all health care for workers in designated clinics and hospitals based on a prepaid fee—were organized for hydro-industrial workers in the western United States and for municipal workers in New York City and elsewhere. By the late 1990s there were over 600 HMOs in the United States, plus many other types of managed care plans with a bewildering variety of structures. Some are for-profit companies, and others, such as Kaiser-Permanente, are nonprofit organizations.

The distinctions among prepaid health plans, traditional indemnity insurance, and other arrangements have broken down in a maze of mergers, acquisitions, and joint ventures. The drive to control explosive growth in health care costs has propelled managed care from a novel alternative to the cornerstone of the U.S. health care delivery system. The term managed care organization (MCO) has become a wastebasket expression used to describe organizations that have overall accountability for the health of an enrolled population, and that integrate financing or insurance functions with management of health care delivery. MCOs exert control over patients, who are permitted to utilize only a limited range of contracted providers and are penalized for going to other providers (whose charges are not—or not fully—covered by the plan); MCOs exercise control over providers through "utilization management" (approval/rejection of medical decisions) to contain medical expenditures and through penalties and incentives.

The United States remains dominated by private health insurance coverage and has the largest for-profit health care sector in the world, accounting for 54.2% of health care spending in 2006. Services are organized through a variety of employer-based, individual, occupational, or geographically based insurance plans, and a complicated mix of public insurance programs for the military, war veterans, senior citizens, children, and the "categorically poor." Last-resort municipal hospitals and clinics are also available in some cities. There are currently over 1,300 health insurance companies operating in the United States (AHIP 2007), with the dominant form of insurance coverage provided through employment contracts. Even for the approximately 170 million people with employment-based insurance, there are varying levels of coverage, with copayments (or coinsurance), premiums, deductibles, and spending ceilings regulated by arcane contracts governing which of the country's 819,000 physicians and surgeons, and 7,500 hospitals can be accessed (U.S. Census Bureau 2005).

All U.S. states have a public insurance system (of varying quality) for low-income individuals, covering 59 million people at some point during the year (Medicaid). Approximately 44 million people over the age of 65 and long-term disabled persons under 65 are covered by a near-universal (for the elderly) social security and premium-funded national medical and hospital insurance plan (Medicare) Although three-fourths of Medicaid beneficiaries are poor children and (primarily) working parents, most Medicaid spending is concentrated on the acute and long-term care needs of persons with disabilities and low-income senior citizens. (U.S. Census Bureau 2008; www.kff.org).

Those not covered by employment-based or public insurance plans may apply for insurance with a private company, but premiums for individuals or small groups are usually set at exorbitant rates. Moreover, people with preexisting medical conditions or who are at risk of developing a condition are often denied coverage. Insurance companies may also select which counties/regions to operate in, thereby "cherry picking" not only the healthiest individuals, but also the healthiest and/or most profitable geographic areas (Hellander 2002).

Limits to public and private health insurance leave over 18% of the under 65 population without coverage. In 2006 the number of uninsured grew to 47 million people (16% of the total population, with almost half of adults either uninsured or underinsured), over 70% of whom were employed. Almost 12% of children and more than one-third of people of Hispanic descent were uninsured (DeNavas-Walt, Proctor, and Smith 2007). The lack of universal insurance in the United States contributes to worse health outcomes, an inability to access care (Kennedy and Morgan 2006), and personal bankruptcy. Indeed, one-half of all bankruptcies in the United States are caused by medical debts (Himmelstein et al. 2005). The U.S. health system is also characterized by an inordinate amount of funding spent on administration rather than on health care. Twenty-seven percent of all health system employees work in administration, and of every dollar spent on health in the United States, 31 cents goes toward administrative costs (Woolhandler, Campbell, and Himmelstein 2003). Health in the United States is a highly profitable, multibillion dollar industry. In 2001, 23 CEOs of the top insurance companies received a total of US$172.5 million in salaries and stock options (Hellander 2002). The profits of many of these companies come from price-fixing, fraud, and monopolistic control over the market (Hellander 2002).

Box 12–5 Basic Features of Health Care Delivery in the United States

- Public coverage for persons who are elderly, people living with a long-term disability, and certain indigent groups.
- Large uninsured population.
- Proliferation of for-profit, market-driven health care plans with a maze of incentives (discounts and bonuses) and disincentives (penalties, high coinsurance, noncoverage) for providers and patients.
- Mix of public and private financing and delivery.

The United States spends the most on health care of any country in the world—over US$2 trillion in 2006, with public (government) spending amounting to over US$900 billion (WHO 2008). Yet the proportion of health expenditures publicly funded—approximately 46%—is far lower than the OECD average of 73% (OECD 2008). Moreover, the United States has fewer physicians and nurses per capita, fewer hospital beds, and a shorter average length of hospital stay than most OECD nations (OECD 2005; 2007). Partly due to poor access to care, the United States also has lower life expectancy and a higher infant mortality rate than the OECD average. In spite of enormous spending levels, and notwithstanding provision of high quality care for a small minority able to afford the best coverage, health care provision in the United States falls far short of meeting population needs.

HEALTH CARE SYSTEM REFORM

Key Questions:

- What are the different forces driving health care reforms?
- What are the features of health care reform?

The WHO's *World Health Report 2000* noted that during the last century there were three generations of health system reforms (WHO 2000):

1. The founding of social insurance and national health care systems.
2. The promotion of primary health care and a drive for affordable coverage.
3. Diverging reform aims, including, simultaneously, greater access to care for poorer populations, cost controls, and increased private provision of health care services.

Table 12–6 Characteristics of Health Sector Reform

Regulation

  • policy changes (e.g., liberalization)

  • changes in regulatory structures

Financing

  • user fees, insurance schemes, external financing mechanisms

Resource Allocation

  • defining which services will be covered

  • management and supervisory contracts

  • reforms in payment systems

Provision

  • commercialization, privatization, competition

  • quality improvement activities

  • primary health care, decentralization

Source: Adapted from Gilson and Mills (1995).

In recent decades, many countries have undergone significant health care system reforms with four main characteristics, listed in Table 12–6. Some have been driven by rising expenditures, others by concerns over quality of care, and still others by pressures from international financial agencies. Two main (contradictory) trends have emerged in patterns of reform: one toward public administration and universality, and another toward privatization and market incentives.

Here we review five patterns of reform processes.

Reform in Stratified Systems: Latin America and the Caribbean

In many Latin American countries, the health sector is characterized by stratified health care arrangements. In countries such as Brazil, Peru, and Colombia, separate health insurance and social security schemes were founded in the early 20th century to cover particular occupational groups (e.g., civil servants, miners, railway workers, oil workers, industrial workers). Strong labor movements in the region have ensured that formally employed workers, including civil servants, receive publicly financed health coverage. Most of these schemes operate publicly, with health workers—themselves government employees—working in public facilities. Wealthy elites who do not want to be part of a public insurance scheme pay for health services out of pocket or buy private insurance. Those working outside the formal sector (including agricultural workers, informal vendors, and day laborers) are typically served by a resource-strapped set of public clinics and hospitals, almost always overcrowded, and often inaccessible to rural residents.

As such, the region has developed multitiered, fragmented health systems with employment sector and level of wealth determining medical coverage: elites obtain services in the private sector, formal workers are covered under separate social insurance schemes, and the large informal workforce and indigent populations receive services in underfunded public facilities or pay out of pocket for private health care. In Mexico, for example, the armed forces obtained health care coverage in 1926, petroleum workers in 1935, railroad workers in 1938, private sector workers in 1943, federal civil servants in 1960, and so on (Hernández Llamas 1982). In 2000 over 50% of the population had no health insurance coverage and relied on public clinics of uneven quality, supplies, and staffing. Poor, indigenous, and rural populations were overrepresented in this group (Knaul et al. 2005). Meanwhile over half of health care expenditures occurred in the private sector, mostly covering a small elite.

Beginning in the 1980s, most Latin American countries implemented extensive health sector reforms, many of which entailed privatization of both health and social security systems, as advised by the World Bank and other international financial agencies (Armada, Muntaner, and Navarro 2001). At the same time, the region has experienced increased penetration of private health insurance, especially the lucrative managed care sector (Iriart, Merhy, and Waitzkin 2001)

Brazil's 1988 reform, though not able to withstand privatization altogether, attempted to rectify disparities in health care access and financing, while retaining the primacy of public funding (Elias and Cohn 2003). Based on the notion of health care as a universal right, it created a Unified Health System for all those who were not included in previous health insurance schemes. The plan sought to increase equity of federal health funding among regions, and created local decision-making councils to ensure that health system planning met regional needs. Brazil's 1988 reform entrenched three forms of service provision and financing (Almeida et al. 2000):

1. a publicly funded and delivered system, responsible for high-cost, high-volume care (and now providing extensive PHC through over 29,000 family health teams across the country);
2. a system of private service providers contracted by the government; and
3. a "free choice" private sector system based on either out-of-pocket payments or corporate insurance plans specializing in more profitable services.

The most recent round of reforms undertaken in Mexico is the 2004 *Popular Health Insurance Program*, aiming to cover the country's 50 million uninsured through voluntary health insurance coverage for a defined package of interventions (Knaul and Frenk 2005; Frenk et al. 2006). However, instead of merging coverage for the uninsured population with the social security system, the legislation created a new separate system, financed by premiums from the state and federal governments and participating families (with the poorest 20% exempt). Although phased in only gradually, the reform has already been touted by its crafters for having increased insurance coverage and decreased rates of impoverishment due to out-of-pocket medical expenditures (Gakidou et al. 2006). But private health care expenditures (over 53% of the total), remain at the prereform level, indicating that the reform falls far short of its early self-evaluation. Moreover, because many of the previous barriers to access persist (including inadequate facilities)—and because inequitable and fragmented financing and coverage systems remain entrenched—the populations who have historically benefited from, or been disadvantaged by, a segmented system remain the same as before the reform (Lloyd-Sherlock 2006; Laurell 2007).

For the most part, recent health care reforms in Latin America have yielded limited gains, focusing more on equity in access than on equity in resource allocation, quality, and utilization. While coverage for previously excluded groups has been extended, it remains patchy and fragmented. Moreover, the introduction of user fees, competition among providers, and the privatization of facilities have caused health care access to deteriorate throughout the region, from Guatemala to Argentina. Services for poor and marginalized populations are mostly provided by the underresourced public sector with the private sector covering the rich. The continuation of multiple and exclusive systems reinforces inequities, particularly in access to quality care (Flores 2006).

Post-Socialist Reform: Countries of the Former Soviet Bloc

With the breakup of the Soviet Union and the Soviet bloc in the early 1990s, Poland, Hungary, and other Eastern European countries, the newly independent republics of Eastern Europe and Central Asia, as well as Russia itself, were faced with depleted government resources. Health systems had already begun to deteriorate in prior decades due to underinvestment, poor quality of care, corruption, and an overall shortage of resources (Barr and Field 1996). By the mid-1990s, virtually all formerly socialist countries undertook reforms in health and other social sectors.

Advised by economists at the World Bank that privatization would help attract additional funds, and therefore provide a larger financial base from which to deliver care (World Bank 1993), most formerly socialist countries opened the health sector to private insurance and reinstituted private medical practice. While the socialist principle of universality remained intact at a rhetorical level, market incentives generated parallel public–private systems of health care delivery, further weakening the public system (Balabanova et al. 2004).

As outlined earlier, Soviet (and Soviet bloc) health systems were characterized by centralized, universal access to health services, which contributed—as part of economic redistribution and vast improvements in literacy, nutrition, housing, and other social conditions—to a steep decline in communicable diseases and increased life expectancy (Tulchinsky and Varavikova 1996). Since the 1980s, many of the former Soviet bloc countries have experienced a reversal of these trends, with worsening infant mortality rates, a drastic increase in infectious diseases, particularly

TB, and mounting stress-related ailments such as cardiovascular disease. Patterns of access to and use of health care services are marked by widening inequalities, with pensioners and large numbers of low-income workers facing the biggest barriers (Balabanova et al. 2004). As discussed in Chapter 4, this deterioration in health is largely attributable to the social and economic shift to a capitalist economy, the loss of employment security, and the dismantling of the social welfare state, including health care systems.

Reform in Emerging Economies: South Korea, South Africa, and India

The contradictory nature of health reforms is exemplified by countries with fast-growing, emerging economies, which have pursued both publicly financed universal health systems and market-based reforms.

South Korea's health system was implemented in steps, in conjunction with rapid economic growth beginning in the 1970s. A targeted basket of interventions steadily expanded until full implementation of national health insurance was reached in 1989. More recent reforms have subsumed the multiple insurance schemes that were in existence into a single-payer system. These health reforms were possible not only due to increased economic resources, but also to an increase in democratic participation of many key stakeholder groups and to a political environment conducive to change.

Private hospitals and practitioners deliver over 90% of services in South Korea, with the public sector primarily responsible for public health campaigns. This has created some geographical disparities, as proportionately more services are provided in urban than rural areas. In the most recent health care reform in 2000, the South Korean government increased public health financing, and as a result out-of-pocket spending has declined sharply (Jeong 2005). Over a short time frame, the Korean polis and populace have demonstrated an impressive commitment to national health insurance.

South Africa has undergone even faster implementation of universal health coverage than South Korea, but through a mixed public–private financing system. The post-apartheid government, elected in 1994, made health care a universal right for the first time, starting with coverage for pregnant and breast-feeding women and children under 6. Within 2 years, primary health care services were provided free at the point of delivery to the entire population (Health Systems Trust 1999; Pillay 2001). Currently, the public sector is responsible for about 85% of the population, accounting for 44% of total health care expenditure. The private sector accounts for 56% of health care expenditure serving just 15% of the population. As in the United States, South Africa's private health sector is dominated by a large number of health insurance plans, which have experienced significant cost escalations in the past few years. For example, private hospital care expenditures doubled between 1997 and 2005 (Blecher and Harrison 2006).

Health sector reform in South Africa has involved decentralization of services from the national government to provincial governments and within provinces to health districts. The national government remains responsible for developing legislation and policies, while provincial governments are charged with providing primary health care and hospital care, and municipalities carry out environmental health measures (Government of South Africa 2004). Despite the advances made by the public sector—including the removal of user fees, an expansion in the number of primary health care facilities, the introduction of community service requirements for a wide range of health professionals, and increased spending in the public sector (an annual average increase of 5.6% in real terms since 2002)—there remain considerable inequities by region and social group. Per capita health funding in 2006/2007 was as much as twice as high in some provinces as in others (Blecher and Harrison 2006), and poor and rural populations continue to have significantly less access to health care than people living in urban areas or who are privately insured. South Africa's health system continues to face great challenges, including enormous social inequalities, the HIV/AIDS epidemic, and marginal living conditions for the majority of the population.

Postindependence India sought to create a Soviet-style state health system, geographically organized and with heavy investments in facilities construction and training of health personnel. However, the system fell short of providing accessible care to the majority of the population, particularly outside the major cities, and it came apart in the early 1990s. India was then pressured by the IMF and World Bank to cut health sector spending and follow market reforms, including institution of user fees and health facility privatization.

Currently two publicly financed health insurance schemes offer mixed public/private delivery for a tiny proportion of India's nearly 1 billion citizens. The central government health scheme covers over 4 million government workers and their families, while some 30 million state government workers, private industry employees and their families are covered by the employee state insurance scheme. While these schemes have been shielded from reform, the vast majority of health spending in India (87%) now takes place in the private sector. Approximately 135 million people in the middle and upper economic strata (some 13% of the population) spend the vast majority of health rupees (though few have insurance coverage). The remaining 800 million people—India's marginalized and working class—are forced to pay out of pocket for most of their health care needs.

Cost Management Reforms in Industrialized Countries

In recent years, Western European countries, as well as Canada, New Zealand, Japan, and Australia—constituting the majority of OECD nations, where universal, publicly financed coverage is standard—have faced different concerns. Rising health expenditures have motivated market-based reforms (reflecting the dominant trend toward private sector involvement in social services), with various countries turning to cost management as a means of reducing spending and improving efficiency.

Although all OECD countries have experienced increases in health spending, single-payer systems (monopsonies) have been much more successful at containing costs than their multiple-payer counterparts. For example, in 1970, health care expenditure as a percentage of GDP was 7% for both the United States (a multi-payer system) and Canada (which was just shifting from a multipayer to a single-payer system), whereas in 2004 health expenditures comprised 15.3% of GDP in the United States, compared to 9.9% in Canada (OECD 2007). Indeed, per capita health care spending in Canada is now approximately half that of the United States (i.e., US$3,430 per capita in Canada, as compared to US$6,401 per capita in the United States in 2005) (OECD 2007). This is largely because private health sector spending is harder to regulate, has higher administrative costs, and directs significant sums to marketing and profits.

Health care spending has grown faster than GDP in many industrialized countries largely due to unregulated spending, including increased use of technology and pharmaceuticals, and provider incentives. Although such cost increases are often attributed to the health care problems of aging populations, careful studies show that *healthy* seniors generate far more expenditures than the sick. This points to changing patterns in the intensity of health care utilization on the provider side (more diagnostic tests, more interventions), and does not necessarily reflect the greater needs of the elderly (Barer, Evans, and Hertzman 1995; Zweifel, Felder, and Meiers 1999).

Most OECD nations continue to operate under the principle that need must determine access to care, but inequitable access to care persists due to (Docteur and Oxley 2003):

1. practitioner shortages and poor distribution of health care services across geographic regions;
2. delays in receiving treatment; and
3. sociocultural barriers due to differences in language, cultural norms, and economic status, particularly in the context of recent waves of immigration to Europe from Africa and Asia.

Some European reforms have focused on improving the supply of health care practitioners through recruitment of foreign-trained workers targeting services to underserved regions, and providing financial incentives to practitioners for performing high volume services and reducing waiting times.

Further reforms have focused on regulating prices, instituting budget caps, and implementing cost-sharing measures with the private sector. Because spending cuts have been met with public resistance, more recent reforms emphasize efficiency measures, including reduced length of hospital stays, increased competition among providers, and decentralized decision making. These have had mixed results. Lessons from cost containment reforms thus far suggest the following:

- Publicly funded, single-payer systems result in lower overall spending due to better regulation, less duplication, greater access, higher quality care, and improved efficiency (Sepehri and Chernomas 2004).
- Efforts to control the volume of services delivered have been successful, particularly in the hospital sector; however, these may not be sustainable in the long run.
- Budget caps in various forms have successfully contained expenditures, but have had limited effects on efficiency.

Reform in Underresourced Systems: Sub-Saharan Africa

In many of the least developed countries, already fragile health sectors have been further eroded since the 1980s due to significant cutbacks in public sector spending under structural adjustment programs. As discussed in Chapter 11, these programs have forced health systems to scale down the number of publicly funded health services and to start charging fees.

In much of sub-Saharan Africa, health sector reform has included (Murthy et al. 2004):

- reductions in public coverage and an increase in private insurance;
- the introduction of user fees; and
- changes in priority-setting and organizational mechanisms as a result of external aid.

Almost all of the reforms have resulted in greater reliance on the private sector, with a smaller role for the state, and a reduction in local participation and accountability mechanisms.

Reforms in underresourced systems have been particularly influenced by the advice and loan conditionalities of the World Bank and the IMF, as well as by the WHO and bilateral aid programs. Most international players have emphasized market efficiency and cost-effectiveness over equity, needs, and rights-based approaches. The proliferation of donors and programs has also resulted in bureaucratic confusion and duplication of recipient government activities, with further harmful effects on vast marginalized populations. In recent years, the World Bank and other agencies have sought to redress some of these problems by coordinating health reforms through "sector wide approaches" (SWAps; see Chapter 3) and targeting the poorest populations through special programs (Gwatkin, Wagstaff, and Yazbeck 2005). Both efforts are constrained by donor exigencies, including short time frames, outside priority-setting, and conditionalities, which can undermine domestic planning processes and overall health system development (Welch 2000; Pettifor, Thomas, and Telatin 2001; WHO 2004; Oxfam International 2004).

In sum, apart from settings that have developed public health insurance systems such as Costa Rica, Kerala, and Cuba, there are few examples of successful health sector reforms in underdeveloped countries (Berman and Bossert 2000). Indeed, the deleterious consequences of pursuing privatization reforms were made more acute by the simultaneous increase or reemergence of infectious diseases such as TB, malaria, and HIV/AIDS, which are far better addressed through universal and comprehensive health systems that are free at the point of care.

PRINCIPLES AND BUILDING BLOCKS OF A HEALTH CARE SYSTEM

Key Questions:

- What are the components of a health care system?
- How do these components interrelate?

How would you design a health system? This section examines the various principles and building blocks of health care systems and the interactions among them (see Table 12–7) in order to understand their role in the delivery of health services. Maternal and child health vignettes will be used throughout as illustrations.

Principles of Health Care Systems

There are a few basic principles that underpin health care systems and different degrees to which these inform health care system design.

Universality

The extent to which a health care system is universal indicates the proportion of residents who have a legal right to obtain benefits and care. Canada is viewed as a model of a universal health care system, as all legal residents have access to benefits wherever they are in the country. However, some groups remain excluded such as new immigrants in their first few months after arrival, undocumented persons, and migrant and other temporary laborers.

Some governments assume full responsibility for providing health care to their citizenry, and medical care is made universally available at no or little charge. More commonly, full medical care supported directly by the central government is provided only for specific segments of the population. Almost everywhere, members of the military are in this category, usually with their immediate families. Other groups often covered by government-supported medical services include

Table 12–7 Health System Principles and Building Blocks

Principles	Building Blocks	Interface Between Principles and Building Blocks
Universality	*Facilities*	*Health insurance plans*
Accessibility	• hospitals	*Financing*
• geographic	• clinics	• public sector: taxation, loans,
• economic	• offices	direct foreign support
• cultural	• long-term care homes	• benefactors: philanthropists,
Portability	*Personnel*	NGOs, religious/ethnic groups
Equity	• doctors	• household/individuals: per-
• access	• nurses	sonal assets, medical savings
• utilization	• traditional healers	accounts, informal/in-kind
• resource allocation	• technicians	donations
• delivery quality	• pharmacists	• mixed: employment, compul-
• delivery effectiveness	• dentists	sory, voluntary
• health status	• midwives	*Regulation*
Comprehensiveness	• support staff	• legislative
Affordability and	• administrative staff	• unofficial, traditional
sustainability	*Equipment and technology*	• external
Quality	• e-health and	*Training, recruitment, and retention*
Participation	telemedicine	*of personnel*
• patient decision making	• pharmaceuticals	*Remuneration*
and choice	• physical infrastructure	• capitation
• community/policy	•	• contract
making		• fee-for-service
Organizational coherence,		• none (voluntary)
health promotion, and		• salary
intersectoral cooperation		*Policy and planning*
		• resource allocation
		• programs
		Management
		• information systems
		• capacity building
		• decentralization and district
		health systems

pensioners, inmates of prisons, and members of aboriginal or tribal populations. Along with general public health services, the health of pregnant women, mothers, and young children may also be considered a government responsibility and may exist independently of other programs.

In many countries, public health services such as immunizations or the control of epidemics, are provided for all citizens. As well, certain diseases may be the subjects of specified services (sometimes called vertical or categorical) in which preventive, diagnostic, and curative care is offered universally, typically free of charge. Tuberculosis, leprosy, and sexually transmitted diseases usually fall into this category. Ambulance and emergency services are also commonly provided to all by local governments (although patients are sometimes billed for these services).

Accessibility

Accessibility is key to the utilization of health care services. In a highly accessible health care system, all members who fit the eligibility criteria are equally able to obtain care, without barriers. Accessibility may be influenced by geography, resource availability (e.g., the number of clinics or health professionals per capita), financing mechanisms, as well as cultural or social factors. Most countries have a greater concentration of physicians relative to the population in urban areas, particularly in the national capital, compared to rural areas. Health professionals may also congregate in high-income areas. Other health system components such as laboratories and medical equipment demonstrate an even more skewed distribution than that of doctors, with accessibility limited for those who live in rural areas or impoverished peri-urban zones.

People may not use health services even when they seem to be reasonably accessible. Subtle barriers to access include illness or impairment, transportation costs and limited availability, distance to the provider, the facility's hours of operation, attitudes of health professionals, cost in terms of payment for health care services or time lost from work, and family care responsibilities. There are also more complex sociocultural barriers such as differences in language and healing beliefs, and discrimination based on race, class, sex, religion, and other factors.

Box 12–6 Maternal and Child Health Example: Bureaucratic and Resource Barriers

"Dashnyam...[from Mongolia]...manifested symptoms of pre-eclampsia...[and] the doctor urged her to go to the provincial hospital's maternity waiting home. However, her admission was delayed for over a week to solve bureaucratic issues, initially because she had no proof of having health insurance, and then because there were no beds available. Eventually Dashnyam delivered via caesarian section, but suffered severe haemorrhage. After a delay in finding the anaesthetist, the bleeding was eventually stopped by emergency surgery but the hospital had no blood for transfusion. She died from haemorrhagic shock" (WHO 2005, p. 22).

Portability

Portability is a health care system principle in many countries with universal plans. Under this principle, citizens may obtain care throughout the country and are not confined to one geographic location or medical practitioner.

Equity

According to the International Society for Equity in Health, equity in health is "the absence of systematic and potentially remediable differences in one or more aspects of health across populations or population groups defined socially, economically, demographically, or geographically." Equity in health care services relates closely to other principles and may be defined in the following terms (Flores 2006):

1. Equity in access to health care services—physical, organizational, or cultural accessibility.
2. Equity in the utilization of health care services—tied to costs of care and modes of financing.
3. Equity in resource allocation—demonstrated through absence of disparities in allocation of services and infrastructure between, for example, urban and rural populations or formally and informally employed workers.
4. Equity in the quality of services.
5. Equity in the delivery of effective services.
6. Equity in health outcomes.

Inequities in health systems further exacerbate social and political inequities, as the poorest and most vulnerable populations have higher absolute and disease-specific rates of morbidity and mortality than the most privileged, yet less access to care. Ill health that is a result of health care system inequities may also lead to further impoverishment and vulnerability and thus to greater inequities in health. This has been termed "the medical poverty trap" (Whitehead, Dahlgren, and Evans 2001).

Comprehensiveness

The extent to which a health care system is comprehensive depends on what ser vices are provided and/or covered either through insurance mechanisms or direct public provision. While comprehensiveness is a foundational principle for many OECD countries, it has typically been undermined in underdeveloped nations lacking universal health systems. As discussed elsewhere, international agencies have in recent decades emphasized coverage of a limited "basket" of services rather than a comprehensive range of services (as reflected in the World Bank's 1993 *World Development Report*). Of course, what is considered comprehensive changes as medical research and practice develop. Priority-setting efforts seek to determine how to measure comprehensive care in different political and cultural contexts.

Affordability and Sustainability

A stable health care system must be affordable for both health system users and society as a whole. Affordability describes the extent to which the system can be financed through agreed upon means (taxes, out-of-pocket payment, etc.), and also how well it "fits" with social values. A system that is financially accessible, uses resources appropriately, and is societally acceptable is more likely to be sustainable in the long term.

Quality

Box 12–7 Maternal and Child Health Example: Poor Quality Care

Rosa is a pregnant indigenous woman living in rural Mexico, where she has access to both a public clinic and a private practitioner. She believes that private care is superior to that in the public clinic, as she knows many women who have endured long waits to receive public care. Although the private practitioner will charge her for prenatal visits, she chooses to access care there. She does not know that there are fewer standards for private practitioners, and that the quality of care she will receive is likely to be of lower quality than if she had visited the public clinic.

Quality is difficult to measure, but it is a key determinant of health service utilization, system productivity, and health outcomes. Persons who lack access to care cannot obtain services, but those who are dissatisfied with quality may refuse to use them. When provision of even minimal services is a struggle, the quality of health care may not be foremost in the minds of health planners and providers. However, accessibility and quality go hand in hand in ensuring good care for all.

Methods of measuring quality include asking patients to report on their experience of care (gauging their level of satisfaction), measuring differences in type of care received by income, ethnic, and geographic group, examining the availability and use of certain technologies and resources, and documenting the care received and tests performed (Das and Gertler 2007). Of course, health status and health outcomes are critical measures of health system quality.

Participation

The participation of citizens in the design of health care systems may lead to increased equity and responsiveness to needs, as system users are likely to know what kind of health system will work best for them. As well, community participation can help determine whether health care is of acceptable quality. Community/citizen participation in health care planning and implementation may also be of value in decision making regarding resource allocation and system design, ultimately enhancing satisfaction and utilization of services.

Participation also occurs at the patient level: decisions must be made regarding whether to access care, where to go, how much to spend (if applicable), and what course of treatment to follow. As we have seen, membership in some national health plans is compulsory and only one medical care system exists for many health interventions. This may limit the choice that citizens have in selecting health care providers or deciding what level of care they need. Other systems offer a wide array of choice in terms of service providers, though typically only the well-off have the knowledge and financial resources to select—or challenge the decisions made by—providers.

Organizational Coherence, Health Promotion, and Intersectoral Cooperation

A well-integrated system limits duplication and waste in administrative functions, enhances efficiency, and minimizes confusion on the part of providers and the public. A crucial component of a coherent health system is health promotion to address determinants of health that extend well beyond health care. Enhancing health and well-being at a population level limits the occurrence of preventable ailments and curbs the use of unnecessary curative care. The ability of a health care system to adequately address public health concerns also depends on the level of cooperation between various sectors. Sectors such as urban planning, agriculture, labor, manufacturing, education, public safety, and trade all influence health outcomes, and can work effectively in tandem with the health sector to enhance public health.

Building Blocks

The basic building blocks or infrastructure of a health care system include its facilities, health care professionals, and equipment. Health care delivery may also be distinguished by its level of specialization and relationship to the social context:

- *Primary care*: services offered to the population at the point of entry into the health system (e.g., at a clinic or with a nonspecialized health care professional), ideally combining preventive and curative, personal and community, individual and environmental aspects.
- *Secondary care*: standard inpatient services and specialist consultations, often on referral from primary care providers.
- *Tertiary care*: highly specialized services such as neurosurgery or neonatal intensive care, available in hospitals equipped with advanced technology.

In countries where social insurance mechanisms are highly developed, benefits are generally divided into ambulatory or general physician care (i.e., primary care) and specialist and hospital care (i.e., secondary care). In low-income settings, tertiary care services, if available, may be limited to university teaching hospitals or national-level institutions.

Box 12–8 Maternal and Child Health Example: Infrastructural and Economic Barriers

"Bounlid, from the Lao People's Democratic Republic, is seven months pregnant and feeling tired. She is finding it much harder to work and her family's income has slipped. Because of this [she says], 'I've had no antenatal care and I don't expect to have any for the rest of my pregnancy. I plan to give birth at home, as I did with my other four children. It is too expensive for most people in my village to give birth with a skilled attendant at the clinic, which in any case has very basic facilities and no telephone or ambulance if there were complications'" (WHO 2005, p. 43).

Facilities

Facilities refer to clinics, hospitals, nursing homes, health centers, pharmacies, medical schools, etc. Each health system differs in its management of facilities and the private/public mix of financing. Hospitals and apothecaries have histories that go back centuries, but clinics and health centers developed mostly in the 20th century as part of health system planning efforts aimed at offering well-organized, community-based services. In recent years, with the growth of private health markets and the adoption of ambulatory hospital care as a cost-cutting measure, free-standing specialized clinics have also proliferated. Scandinavian countries have made particular efforts to rationalize their hospital systems through reducing the number of hospital beds by 40% (WHO EURO 2003b).

Box 12–9 Long-Term Care Facilities and Hospices

Long-term care (LTC) facilities and hospices are rarely considered a mainstay of health systems, but as populations age, the need for these facilities is increasing. By 2050, 2 billion people will be over the age of 65, with 85% of this number projected to be living in underdeveloped countries. In many nations, a cultural shift has occurred simultaneous to this demographic shift, whereby women are increasingly employed outside the home and can no longer care for older family members as they have traditionally done (WHO 2002). This has generated a greater need for LTC facilities and hospices for older populations, who may require complex, continuous health care.

Few industrialized countries have planned for these changing needs, and many underdeveloped countries face even greater challenges in providing adequate care to the elderly due to the increased migration of young people (WHO 2002). While some countries have developed publicly funded and/or delivered LTC facilities and payment plans to replace informal caregivers, most do not yet have policies or plans in place to meet the needs of aging populations. As a result, LTC facilities and/or hospices may not be available, the regulation of these facilities may be lax, or there may be fragmented quality, accessibility, and affordability of long-term care.

Sweden has a strong institutionally-based medical care system with a hierarchy of municipal health centers (which each provide primary ambulatory care for about 15,000 people), secondary care district and county hospitals, as well as regional hospitals for tertiary subspecialty care. There are few family practitioners and the public has direct access to specialists via hospital outpatient departments (WHO EURO 2003b).

In Japan, where all hospitals must be nonprofit, 15% are operated by local governments, 5% by the national government, and the remainder are privately operated. Since there are few nursing homes, hospitals have taken on this role, with over 45% of inpatients over the age of 65 hospitalized for more than 6 months (Ikegami and Campbell 1997; Ikegami 2004). Thus, long stays averaging more than 3 weeks are the norm in Japan, more than double the length of hospital stay in most developed countries (WHO 2006b).

Religious health care facilities are present in many parts of the world. In Latin America, from the earliest days of colonial settlement, such institutions were operated by local charitable welfare boards made up of leading citizens, with heavy involvement of the Catholic Church. As time passed, government subsidies assisted with the high cost of running them. In many countries, religious facilities are an important source of medical care for the poor. Hospitals and clinics (and even health care systems as a whole) often operate according to religious principles, which may include segregating patients by sex, prohibiting certain practices (e.g., abortion), and specializing in particular types of care. The staff and patients of faith-based institutions do not necessarily practice the faith of the hospital or clinic.

Box 12–10 Maternal and Child Health Example: Inequalities in Health Care Facilities

Mary lives in a mid-sized city and is married to the owner of a large factory. She does not have health insurance, but her husband's salary makes it possible for her to attend private prenatal clinics, where she receives a full range of tests, services, and advice at every visit. Although she must pay out of pocket for the private care, she likes the cleanliness and tranquility of the clinic. Clara works for Mary's husband and has no health insurance. When she becomes pregnant, she does not want to take time off work because she needs money to pay for clinical visits. At the after-hours clinic that she attends, she has to wait for long periods only to see staff who are too tired and busy to address her questions about prenatal nutrition.

Personnel

For many people, the responsiveness, effectiveness, and quality of a health system is gauged by how they are treated by an individual health professional. Health professionals personify the values and underlying goals of any health system and act as the "gatekeepers" into the system.

PHYSICIANS   Physicians are typically categorized as "generalists" or "specialists." Generalists (e.g., family doctors, internists, pediatricians) attend to a wide variety of problems and preventive needs ideally through the continuous care of a stable set of patients in primary care settings. Specialists (e.g., thoracic surgeons, gastroenterologists, cardiologists) practice in tertiary care hospitals and private offices, concentrating on a narrower set of ailments which require specialized knowledge and technical expertise. Both types of physicians may also practice within secondary care settings. Human resource experts recommend that health systems maintain parity between specialists and generalists. However, the lure of specialization coupled with inadequate planning means that many countries produce far too many specialists, causing shortages of generalists. For example, in the United States only 35% of medical graduates in 2001 became generalists (Sheldon 2003).

In developing countries government medical services and social security hospitals and clinics usually employ salaried physicians. In many countries all new physicians must undertake a period of full-time government service (Blumenthal 1994), generally in rural areas. Because of low wages across Latin America, Africa, and Asia, many physicians devote part of the day to government service and maintain a private practice. In some European countries, a system of split practice finds many physicians dividing their time between government service, service under a private medical insurance plan, and their own personal practice.

NURSES   At both the primary care and hospital care levels, nurses play a crucial role. Yet in a great many countries in the developing world there are fewer nurses than physicians. In Latin America and in the Middle East, where nursing is sometimes looked down upon as a low-prestige occupation (suitable only for women), the number of nurses is very low. In the United States the majority of physicians are male, while the majority of nurses are female (WHO 2006d), whereas in the former Soviet Union most doctors and nurses were women. There is a relatively high ratio of nurses in the United States (7.9/1,000 persons), but thousands of foreign nurses are recruited each year, particularly from the Philippines, where there is only one nurse for approximately 2,500 people.

Considering the variety of forms medical practice can take, it may be difficult to distinguish the role of a nurse from that of a physician. Certainly some nurses are better trained and assume more responsibility for patient care than some doctors, particularly in medically underserved areas. Although there is no set physician to nurse ratio, where there are very few nurses and support staff relative to physicians, health delivery is more inefficient and costly.

TECHNICIANS AND OTHER HEALTH PROFESSIONALS   Nurses and doctors—while essential—are not the only health professionals who work within a health care system. In order for health care systems to run smoothly, there is also a great need for technicians, pharmacists, support staff, and medical auxiliaries. Technicians operate and maintain valuable health equipment (e.g., x-ray machines and chemotherapy pumps), and they conduct and analyze the results of tests on human specimens. Pharmacists dispense, and sometimes prescribe, appropriate and safe pharmaceuticals. Health system support staff such as maintenance and cleaning staff, administrative personnel, and paramedics ensure that doctors and nurses are able to perform their duties with minimal delay or difficulty, and also provide valuable services in their own right. Medical auxiliaries, including physician assistants and nurse practitioners, are trained to provide an array of primary care services. They are well established in some places but underused in most industrialized countries.

TRADITIONAL HEALERS   Notwithstanding the many systems described above, much of the world's population has little access to modern medical care, and vast numbers get no care at all. Among those receiving some modern medical care, many also consult traditional healers. Globally, the use of traditional healing exceeds that of scientific or Western medicine by a factor of at least two to one.

Only a few countries, most notably India and China, have made concerted efforts to integrate indigenous medical practice with modern medicine. In India, public insurance schemes cover both allopathic doctors and practitioners of Ayurvedic, homeopathic, Unani, and Siddha medicine. In China, persons may elect to receive traditional (herbal, acupuncture, moxibustion, etc.) or modern medical treatment or a blend of both. Following the Alma-Ata conference in 1978, a number of countries integrated traditional birth attendants into their maternal and child health programs.

Acknowledging the importance of traditional healing, heads of state of the African Union (AU) declared 2001–2010 as the Decade of African Traditional Medicine. Member states of the AU have sought to "mainstream" traditional medicine by integrating African traditional healers into their health care systems.

Box 12–11 Maternal and Child Health Example: Health Human Resources Shortages

The maternal mortality ratio in Malawi increased from 752/100,000 live births in 1992 to 1,120 in 2000. Confidential inquiries into the maternal deaths found three reasons for the increase: (1) the impact of HIV/AIDS; (2) a drop from 55% in 2000 to 43% in 2001 in the percentage of women delivering in health facilities; and (3) deterioration in the quality of care provided by health facilities, with only one in four mothers receiving standard care in 2001. It was also noted that in rural areas a single midwife rendered care on a 24 hour/7 days a week basis and that 10% of maternity units were not functional due to lack of staff. The WHO suggests that a ratio of 2.28 doctors, nurses, and midwives per 1,000 population is necessary to ensure skilled attendance at birth; Malawi had only 0.02/1,000 doctors and 0.59/1,000 nurses in 2004 (WHO 2005).

Equipment and Technology

The equipment used in health care delivery is also of vital importance to how well a health system functions. Proper equipment and supplies help ensure that health practitioners are able to provide necessary care. Basic supplies, including clean syringes, latex gloves, and disinfectant can prevent many communicable diseases. Surgical items, namely sutures and IV drips, turn potentially fatal procedures into lifesaving ones. Technologically advanced imaging equipment such as MRI machines can provide health care practitioners with a clearer picture of how best to proceed with treatment.

Unfortunately, properly functioning and appropriate equipment is very inequitably distributed at a global level. The WHO estimates that in many developing countries, up to 50% of medical equipment is not in use due to malfunction, lack of training on correct use, or inadequate spare parts and supplies. More than 85% of the health care equipment that is used in underdeveloped countries is purchased outside the country (WHO 2007b). The prices for this equipment are set on the international market, making it prohibitively expensive. Other barriers to obtaining needed equipment include patents, licensing, and trade laws (see Chapter 9) (WHO 2000). These barriers have led to a growing gap in access to, and use of, medical equipment and other technologies between developed and underdeveloped countries and, within many countries, between elites able to pay for using them and the majority of the population who are not.

Key issues in the equitable dissemination of technology are: relevance according to local and regional health needs, affordability, and absorbability of equipment (i.e., ability to integrate particular technologies into health systems and provide skilled human resources to employ them). The concept of "appropriate technology" has been coined to address these concerns in terms of appropriateness to the level of care (primary vs. tertiary care) and to the particular context (which includes need, affordability, having human resources in sufficient quantities and with the requisite skills to use it, etc.). Additional dimensions of appropriateness include ability to manufacture, maintain, and replace parts locally and energy consumption (Gibbons 2003).

The designation of "appropriateness" raises a number of questions. Who decides on what is appropriate? Appropriate for whom? Does it imply, in practice, simple technologies for the poor and high-end expensive technologies for the rich?

Many people think that technology is transferred exclusively from developed countries to the developing world. However, this is not always so. As discussed elsewhere, many important drugs, such as quinine, artemisinin, and emetine, were derived from knowledge and practices in developing countries. Methods developed in Brazil in the 1930s helped to make mass miniature radiographic screening practical. The first successful heart transplant took place in South Africa in the 1960s. And so on. Developing countries also have much to share regarding the provision of public health and the ingenuity necessary for the equitable application of technologies.

There are a number of ways in which technology transfer can take place. Countries may import the technology using their own resources and request assistance in training personnel or they may follow trial and error processes (Grieve 2004). Countries may also develop their own "hardware" or production capacity by copying (either legally or illegally) from other countries. Or there may be collaboration between high- and low-income countries in developing a product to lower costs and improve diffusion (e.g., the software industry in India). A critical element in technology transfer is its sustainability without long-term dependence on the donor. This may require investments by both the donor (training, long distance support, etc.) and the recipient (investment in and commitment to the new technology). Most importantly, under conditions of deprivation and inequality, the greatest research and technology needs relate to schooling and literacy, water and sanitation, housing, and income stability, few of which are currently addressed by technology transfer activities.

New technologies, despite their contribution to prevention, treatment, and rehabilitation, have their limitations. Because special equipment is often concentrated in urban areas, there may be large turnaround times between, say, collecting a patient specimen and the diagnosis and communication of results to treat that patient. For instance, the benchmark 48-hour turnaround time for TB sputa results remains a challenge in many African countries—it may take as long as 7 days to get results from laboratories. Such delays mean patients are often lost to treatment and may spread infection to others in their families and communities.

E-HEALTH AND TELEMEDICINE   A potentially important vehicle to increase access to health care in rural areas and even bridge the technology and equipment gap between developed and developing countries is e-health—that is, medical communication and treatment using the internet and other communications technologies. Telemedicine refers to the use of telecommunications (such as telephone or videoconferencing) for the provision of health services at a distance. For example, the Indian Space Research Organization has connected 22 specialist hospitals with 78 rural hospitals using geostationary satellites, leading to tele-consultations for more than 25,000 patients in 2004 and 2005 (Bagchi 2006). Benefits of e-health and telemedicine include: improving the knowledge base of health professionals, continuing professional development, and consultations with senior colleagues; improved access to specialist care for patients in peripheral areas and for nonambulant patients; empowerment of patients and their families who have access to the internet to look up symptoms of diseases and simple self-care techniques (with certain downsides); and improved efficiency in the use of scarce resources, including specialists and expensive medical equipment.

Most developed countries also use e-health and telemedicine to provide a range of services to remote areas (such as in Canada's north or Australia's outback) or to enhance diffusion for specialized services in general (as in the United Kingdom and Sweden). Middle-income countries, including South Africa, have established e-health facilities at tertiary and regional hospitals so that generalists at district hospitals can seek medical opinions from specialists.

In addition to linking rural and urban areas within countries, e-health and telemedicine can also connect health professionals in developing countries with counterparts in developed countries. The Swinfen Charitable Trust provides email facilities and digital cameras to health professionals in developing countries and links them with specialists in developed countries. To date 120 hospitals in 34 countries have been linked (Wootton et al. 2004). Recognizing the potential of e-health and telemedicine to improve access to health information, the WHO established a global e-health observatory in 2005. As an example, the WHO's Evidence-Informed Policy Network (EVIPnet), using e-health approaches, promotes the use of health research in policy making in low- and middle-income countries.

These developments notwithstanding, it is important not to overplay the advantages of e-health and telemedicine. While useful for a certain number of patients, these technologies do not address the underlying health system and infrastructure inadequacies and inequities—not to mention the billions of people who lack even basic health services coverage—that make e-health and telemedicine necessary in the first place.

PHARMACEUTICALS   Access to and affordability of medicines—as well as the development of drugs for diseases of the marginalized—constitute a pressing international health concern, as discussed in Chapters 3 and 9.

Box 12–12 The Political Economy of Big Pharma

The ethical problems and human injustices posed by profit-making in the health sector are most vividly played out in the pharmaceutical industry. This US$400 billion global business is market-driven to the extreme, with companies determining what drugs to research and develop, where to distribute them, and how to set prices. Big Pharma (the ten largest drug companies) has enjoyed unparalleled profits in the last 30 years—between 14% and 25% of sales, at least three times the median profits of Fortune 500 companies (the 500 largest companies in the United States). Pharmaceutical executives earn staggering eight figure salaries (nine figures when stock options are included) (Angell 2004). Some years ago, the combined profits of the world's top five pharmaceutical corporations were found to be twice the total GDP of all nations in sub-Saharan Africa (WHO 1996).

The industry claims that it prices drugs in order to be able to invest in research and development (R&D) and bring drugs from the laboratory to clinical trials and then to market. Yet not only are these costs heavily subsidized by public sector funding (with government grants subsidizing much of the university-based research that underpins new drug development), but in 2001 (consistent with other years) Big Pharma's marketing and administration costs (approximately 35% of sales) were almost three times as high as its R&D costs (13%). Moreover, pharmaceutical companies themselves carry out little research on original drugs. In recent years most newly approved drugs have been "copycat" or "me-too" drugs, which have slight molecular variations from existing drugs and only marginal differences in efficacy. Nonetheless, they have earned patent protection because the U.S. Food and Drug Administration's approval process only judges "new" drugs against placebos, not against other drugs already on the market (Angell 2004). Another tactic is "evergreening"—obtaining separate patents for multiple attributes of a single drug—thereby extending patent protection periods by many years.

Despite Big Pharma's claims of high R&D spending, over half of drug earnings go straight to profit and marketing (including direct-to-consumer advertising, medical journal article advertisements, and physician gifts and incentives). Further, there is no evidence to support pharmaceutical company claims that drug prices are high in the United States because it must subsidize R&D for the rest of the world (Light and Lexchin 2005). Pharmaceutical profit-making is also ensured by national governments through the patenting system, which since 1994 has been extended internationally through the WTO's TRIPS Agreement (see Chapter 9). As such, for a period of 20 years, pharmaceutical manufacturers have an exclusive government-guaranteed monopoly over marketing and sales, and often increase prices in order to squeeze out the maximum profit before the patent expires.

Because profits, not human health, are what drives the pharmaceutical industry, it engages in all sorts of unethical tactics, including biased research studies, suppression of unfavorable results and information on negative side effects, questionable marketing practices, and safety violations. In sum, drug companies, like other corporations are necessarily amoral: their main obligation is to make profits for shareholders, and they are only required to obey the law, not pursue ethical or socially responsible ends (Lexchin 2006), such as making drugs available to those who need them.

Amidst this profiteering, hundreds of millions of people across the underdeveloped world—and millions of North Americans—cannot afford prescription drugs. Often they must decide between essential needs such as food or household heating, and medications. Although the WHO has declared that essential medicines must be available in adequate amounts, at all times, of good quality, and at affordable prices, 30% of the world's population (80% of whom live in developing countries) still lacks access to these basic supplies (Global Health Watch 2005).

For many households in both industrialized and lower-income countries, expenditures on medicines are a growing share of out-of-pocket expenses. In most developing countries, over 50% of household health expenditures go toward medicines. In OECD member states, pharmaceutical expenditures are fueling a rapid increase in health spending (WHO 2000; OECD 2008) due to increased use and raised prices, even of essential medicines. As we saw in Chapters 6 and 9, this has posed a particular problem for HIV/AIDS drugs (ARVs), which remain unaffordable to millions who need them despite several initiatives aimed at lowering prices and distributing ARVs free of charge.

(continued)

Box 12-12 Continued

The profit-making imperative and the patent protection system have led to a gap in funding for drug research and development for many of the ailments prevalent in underdeveloped countries. For example, for over 40 years, there was no research into new drugs for the treatment of TB (see Table 12–8). Drug companies prioritize blockbuster drugs—antibaldness and virility pills, multiple versions of antidepressants, and antiallergy, arthritis, cholesterol, and blood-pressure lowering medications—that generate high sales in industrialized countries. Meanwhile drugs for neglected diseases that disproportionately affect the most marginalized (some 350 million people) have been "all but forgotten by drug developers" (Orbinski and Burciul 2006, p. 117).

In addition to problems stemming directly from the pharmaceutical industry's exorbitant prices, patent protection regime, and inadequate drug development for ailments of the poor (see Box 12–12), is the issue of counterfeit and substandard medicines. These include everything from mixtures of chalk and water (found in Kenya in 2005); expired medicines that are still being sold (as in Peru in 2005); donations of inappropriate (expired, dumped, or useless) medicines (as in Bosnia and Herzegovina in the mid-1990s) (Berckmans et al. 1997); and medicines containing no active ingredient, as in the case of the malaria treatment artesunate sold in Southeast Asia. Another practice is to package and sell medicines that have been rejected for inferior quality by a legitimate manufacturer. An estimated 1% of medicines in developed countries and 10% in developing countries are either counterfeit or substandard (WHO 2006a). The sale of counterfeit and substandard medicines is big business especially in developing countries with annual earnings estimated to be US$32 billion (Wertheimer, Santella, and Chaney 2004).

Counterfeit and substandard medicines can cause serious harm, including death. Effects include: deterioration in clinical condition due to administration of a non-therapeutic product or one of lower than expected dosage; death resulting from toxic preparations; and the development of resistance to a particular drug or class of drugs. Artesunate, manufactured in China, is a case in point. Since 2000, between

Table 12-8 Drug Pipeline for TB as Compared to Cancer and Cardiovascular Diseases

	TB	Cancer	Cardiovascular Diseases
Number of compounds under development (including existing drugs being retested)	6	399	146
Number of pharmaceutical companies	12	178	82
Compounds/1,000 DALYS	0.17	5.16	0.98

Source: Adapted from Doctors Without Borders/Médecins Sans Frontières (MSF) (2006). Development of new drugs for TB Chemotherapy: Analysis of the current drug pipeline. www.doctorswithoutborders.org/news/tuberculosis/tb_xdr_report_10–2006.pdf.

33% and 53% of artesunate sold in Southeast Asia was counterfeit. This has led to unnecessary deaths and drug resistance in countries with high malaria rates (Newton et al. 2008).

To combat this problem, regulatory and inspection mechanisms should be strengthened within countries and between countries. Enhanced public awareness of the dangers of counterfeit and substandard medicines is key, but unless high quality medicines are made affordable, the attractiveness of cheaper counterfeit drugs will remain.

In recent years a set of strategies have been proposed to address the inadequacies of the private sector domination of pharmaceutical development and distribution. These include:

- Dual policy whereby governments pay for research and development innovations and ask the private sector to manufacture the product or drug. As a result, companies would not need to hike the cost of medicines to recoup their R&D investment (Weisbrod 2004). But, as discussed in Box 12–12, this is already how considerable pharmaceutical research is funded in the United States, and it has had virtually no impact on drug prices or profiteering.
- "Open source" research not covered by patents—modeled on open source software development and "no license" products such as Linux (Huang and Weber 2006). This idea has potential to lower prices, if adopted.
- Advance price and purchase commitments, as under the U.S. Orphan Drug Act and the production of meningitis C vaccine in the United Kingdom. These approaches use incentives to encourage pharmaceutical companies to invest in R&D for otherwise "unprofitable" ailments, with quid pro quo guarantees of preset prices or volume/level of promised purchase. Other incentives include tax credits, expedition of regulatory processes, and periods of exclusive sales (Towse and Kettler 2005).

The Center for Global Development has similarly spearheaded the idea of advance purchasing commitments to pharmaceutical companies to incentivize them to bring late stage or existing vaccines for ailments afflicting the "global poor" to market. In a quid pro quo that would eliminate the business risk of developing vaccines for low-profit markets, governments, large foundations, or multilateral agencies would promise to purchase the vaccines, and pharmaceutical companies would promise to sell them on a cost-plus basis with minimal profits (Center for Global Development 2005). Yet critics argue that not only is this approach of questionable value and little sustainability—providing windfalls to companies that have already carried out research and development rather than fostering new research (Light 2005)—but that this "pull mechanism" amounts to a subsidy for super-rich pharmaceutical companies without any assurances. Instead these companies should be made accountable for existing research subsidies received through public funding.

On another front, the Institute for OneWorld Health is a private nonprofit pharmaceutical firm (likely the only) launched in 2000, which aims to develop "safe, effective, and affordable new medicines for people with infectious diseases in the developing world" (http://www.oneworldhealth.org/). Its current focus is on therapies for diarrhea, leishmaniasis, and other "neglected diseases." While its mission is honorable, One World Health's sustainability and accountability remain questionable: it currently operates as a product development PPP with a private board.

To date, the only pharmaceutical agencies that have successfully separated business interests from the scientific research and development of medicines are those that are publicly operated and accountable, such as Brazil's Butantan Institute and Biomanguinhos and Cuba's biotechnology sector (Thorsteinsdóttir et al. 2004).

This existing public pharma strategy may be the most promising idea of all.

Interface Between Principles and Building Blocks

The way in which a health care system is administered and managed can ensure that delivery of care is in line with its principles.

Health Insurance Plans

The underlying philosophy of private insurance schemes is different from that of national health plans. Insurance schemes spell out predetermined levels of compensation or responsibility in specific circumstances, while national health plans typically assume responsibility for all risks and health needs.

In many national health care programs, short-term sickness benefits are provided directly as services, or they may be provided as cash benefits through a variety of reimbursement schemes. In countries with sickness funds, benefits differ depending on the political strength and negotiating skill of the various parties involved. In some countries, patients from higher-income families pay higher contributions. Where private health insurance is sold, policyholders may be required to purchase separate coverage for ambulatory, hospital, surgical, indemnity, or other types of benefits.

Benefits such as pharmaceuticals are also managed differently in different health care systems. In many countries, drugs given in hospital are paid for through a hospital coverage plan, while those for use at home are bought by the patient. The common practice in resource-poor countries of issuing very small amounts of drugs free or at minimal cost, prevents wastage, minimizes the risk of overdose, and may discourage patients from reselling drugs. However, repeated visits are inconvenient and expensive for patients, and wasteful of staff time. Insufficient dosages of drugs may also lead to resistance by microorganisms.

Financing

Health care financing is a universal lightning rod for comment and criticism (see Chapter 11). It is a crucial element of health care systems. All financing systems are subject to continual flux in response to changes in world and local economies, social and political thinking, programmatic needs, technological advances, and the demographic and epidemiological picture. There are five main means through which health care systems are financed:

1. *General tax revenues*: mainly used in high- and some middle-income countries where personal income is relatively high. (N.B. In socialist countries where there are no income taxes, revenues from state industries fund health care and other social services.)
2. *Social security/social insurance*: payroll or other contributory taxes funding mandatory schemes for particular population groups or an entire population.
3. *Voluntary insurance*: privately purchased, through or by employers or purchased by individuals from private companies.
4. *Donations*: including charity or philanthropic gifts and bi-/multilateral grants or loans, particularly to low-income countries.
5. *Household/out-of-pocket payments*: may be a small amount (e.g., copayment with an insurance company), a sliding fee based on household income, or the full cost of health services provided.

Private financing—whether through insurance, out-of-pocket spending, or donations—is usually highly inequitable. It is therefore essential to analyze how financing differs by population group and how this affects accessibility, quality, and comprehensiveness of care.

Box 12–13 Maternal and Child Health Example: Lack of Insurance Coverage

Anna works full time in a restaurant in a U.S. city. She and her employer used to share the cost of the insurance premiums, which covered most of the expenses of her first pregnancy and delivery. However, the insurance company then raised its rates, which her employer passed on to the workers. Anna could no longer afford the premiums and lost her insurance coverage. She is pregnant again and has not qualified for personal insurance, as pregnancy is considered a "preexisting condition," which most insurance plans will not cover. Although there is a public insurance plan for low-income pregnant women, she is not eligible, as she earns more than the income cut-off for the program. Anna worries about not being able to cover the costs of pregnancy and delivery, as she knows that childbirth without complications can cost upward of US$6,000, and she has heard stories of deliveries that cost much more. She has searched for affordable prenatal care clinics, but has found them overcrowded and bureaucratic. She has estimated that each prenatal care visit will cost US$200–$300. As a result, she delays seeking prenatal care, and does not go regularly—with potentially dangerous effects on her health and that of her unborn child.

Regulation

The issue of oversight and responsibility for health and medical services is vital, complex, and dependent on the particular political and economic context of each country. The state typically has the largest role to play in health system regulation, regardless of the extent to which it is publicly delivered and financed. Health care is not effectively regulated through the private sector, as market systems are notoriously poor at self-monitoring. Regulatory purposes and practices may include the following (Mills, Rasheed, and Tollman 2006):

- *Protecting public safety and improving health*: legislating quality standards, planning training curricula, and regulating training and accreditation facilities.
- *Creating transaction standards*: designing reimbursement mechanisms.
- *Improving efficiency*: monitoring practice patterns and allocating new equipment and facilities.
- *Improving quality*: licensing facilities, insurance companies, and health practitioners.
- *Enhancing equity*: implementing incentives to provide care in remote areas or to specific populations.
- *Correcting market failures*: planning where and by whom various services should be offered and controlling prices of medical care and medication.

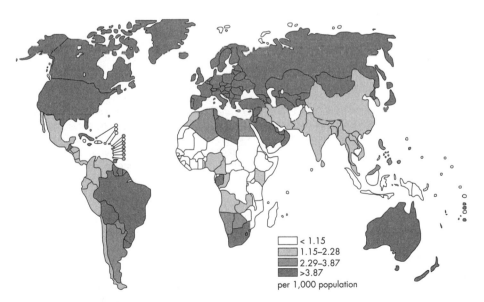

Figure 12–2 Global health worker density. The Joint Learning Initiative has estimated that at minimum there must be 2.5 health workers per 1,000 people in order to carry out essential health interventions (e.g., immunizations). However, this number is insufficient for most complex health interventions (e.g., ARV therapy for HIV) (Joint Learning Initiative 2004). *Source*: Courtesy of the WHO (WHO 2006d).

Not all regulatory practices may be implemented at all times depending on political will and the relative power of the parties involved, the availability of resources, and historical factors that may privilege certain practices over others.

Training, Recruitment, and Retention of Personnel

Training and recruitment of medical personnel can ensure appropriate supply and skills composition for a health system and can set quality standards, particularly for the public sector. Enrollment in medical schools in Asia, Africa, and Latin America has increased greatly in recent years. Despite the shortage of medical doctors in most regions (see Fig. 12–2), there are also arguments against training more physicians in developing countries:

- It is economically impossible to produce enough physicians. The actual cost of training a doctor may be higher in poor countries than in wealthier ones, due to the fact that faculties, libraries, and physical facilities are extremely expensive to maintain.
- The conventional medical school curriculum may not be relevant to local needs in developing countries.
- After physicians are trained it may be difficult to retain them in their home countries—large numbers join the "brain drain" and migrate to more developed countries.

Box 12–14 The "Brain Drain," the Shortage of Health Workers, and Cuba's Solution

Health workers form an essential component of any health system, yet there is a severe global shortage—estimated at more than 4 million workers. Health workers are often underpaid (sometimes limited by public sector wage ceilings imposed by the IMF), poorly distributed among population groups and regions, inaccessible to the poorest populations, lack continuing professional training, and work in high-stress environments. Even in countries without overall shortages, marginalized populations remain underserved, particularly in rural or remote regions, urban slums, and areas with high prevalence of certain ailments such as HIV/AIDS. For example, in Bangladesh, 35% of health workers are urban-based, although 85% of the population lives in rural areas. In countries that do have health worker shortages, many trained workers are unemployed due to problems in health system administration and the downsizing that occurred in the 1980s and 1990s as a result of structural adjustment programs (Joint Learning Initiative 2004). Although 15% of all doctors in Mexico are unemployed, for example, many health posts remain unstaffed in rural regions. In part, this stems from inequitable pay rates between regions.

In recent years, there has been increased attention to the problem of the "brain drain" (the emigration of skilled workers from their country of origin to another country). Some analysts have long viewed the migration of health workers from developing to industrialized nations as yet another way in which resources—such as capital and natural resources—flow from "south to north," with poorer countries essentially subsidizing wealthier nations and maintaining conditions of underdevelopment (Navarro 1981). As such, developing countries are in fact "donors" of aid rather than recipients. Unlike direct investment flows, most "donor" health systems do not benefit from the arrangement. Instead, they are left struggling to maintain a national health workforce.

(continued)

Box 12-14 Continued

In 2000, over 20% of all practicing physicians in the United States, Canada, Britain, New Zealand, and Australia, were foreign-trained, mostly from developing countries. By 2005 this proportion climbed to 25% to 33% (OECD 2005, 2007), with India, Pakistan, and the Philippines as the leading sources of these physicians. Over half of all doctors in the Canadian province of Saskatchewan, for example, trained abroad, primarily in South Africa (Labonte et al. 2006), and 10% of all doctors in Britain are from India (Mullan 2005). Developed countries aggressively recruit internationally trained nurses, too, with the proportion of foreign-trained nurses working in the United States, for example, rising from 8.8 % of the total in 1990 to 15.2 % in 2000, over one-fifth of whom were from low-income countries (Polsky et al. 2007). The Philippines, alone, has lost more than 100,000 nurses to migration since 1990 (Joint Learning Initiative 2004), and 50% of Ghana's nurses have emigrated to Canada.

While in absolute terms, far more doctors emigrate from the Indian subcontinent than elsewhere (almost 80,000 [Mullan 2005]), the relative loss of health workers is greatest in sub-Saharan Africa. In 2000, some 65,000 African-born doctors and 70,000 nurses were working in developed countries. Health worker migration rates range from 1% of nurses from Egypt to 70% of physicians from Angola (Clemens and Pettersson 2007). Caribbean countries are also increasingly affected by health workforce migration, and many rural and underserved areas are now reliant on visiting physicians from Cuba.

Relatives of health professional migrants from some countries, such as the Philippines, benefit from remittances sent home by nurses practicing overseas, though migrant doctors rarely leave any savings behind. Moreover, many Filipino hospitals and clinics have been left without any staff as whole cohorts migrate, effectively shutting down services and denying care to local populations. In countries with an unequal health worker distribution and/or shortage, such as Thailand, training nurses and technicians for work in rural and underserved areas has mitigated some of these problems (Joint Learning Initiative 2004).

In other settings, such as Tanzania, training capacity has been severely undermined as a result of structural adjustment policies which capped public university enrollment and public employment positions, even as the soaring number of people with HIV/AIDS necessitates more health workers. These circumstances have combined to create a shortage of over 17,000 health workers in Tanzania, and 700,000 doctors in Africa as a whole. Even if Tanzania were to stop out-migration of health workers, personnel shortages would increase by 1,000 people every year (Joint Learning Initiative 2004). Indeed, in 36 African countries, even if all migrant health workers were to be repatriated, only 12% of workforce shortages would be alleviated (Dumont and Zurn 2007).

The HIV/AIDS pandemic poses a triple threat to the health workforce—increased workloads in terms of numbers of patients seen, emotional strain as a result of providing long-term palliative care, and increased infection rates (in part occupationally acquired) and mortality among workers themselves. In Malawi, for example, 45% of mortality in health workers in 2002 was due to AIDS (Joint Learning Initiative 2004).

The migration of health professionals is influenced by both push and pull factors. Many countries in the developed world recruit health professionals from developing regions through direct campaigns or indirectly by providing easy access to visas. This is also exacerbated by working conditions in the workers' country of origin, where there may be low wages and stressful conditions due to staff shortages and an underresourced health system (Hicks 2004). Many workers note that there is a lack of opportunity for professional advancement and postgraduate training and may sense that their work is inadequately recognized, appreciated or supported in their home country. Finally, it has been suggested that the "export" of physicians is encouraged by some governments to increase remittances of hard currencies (Joint Learning Initiative 2004).

In response to growing recognition of a "brain drain," some countries have turned to direct training of health workers for shortage areas. The WHO, the former Soviet Union, and some Western countries

(continued)

635

Box 12-14 Continued

have a long tradition of training professionals from underdeveloped countries, but these fellowships have declined in recent decades. Ironically, several underdeveloped countries are themselves currently addressing the shortage of doctors not only in developing countries, but also in developed countries such as the United States. In 2000, the Cuban government founded the Latin American School of Medicine (ELAM) dedicated to training doctors to treat underserved populations in their home countries (ELAM 2006). Particularly intent on training students from minority and impoverished backgrounds, ELAM provides full scholarships to accepted applicants, who are required as a condition of their acceptance to return to their communities and serve marginalized communities (Mullan 2004). In 2008, over 10,000 students from 27 different countries, including the United States, were enrolled at ELAM (Remen and Holloway 2008). Over the past decades Cuba has also sent tens of thousands of its own doctors to work in underdeveloped settings, including South Africa, Angola, Venezuela, and Nicaragua—a form of health cooperation enabled by its large investment in physician training since the 1959 revolution (Beldarraín Chaple 2006). (Cuba currently has twice as many physicians per capita as the United States.)

Box 12-15 Medical Tourism

The flip side of the brain drain is "medical tourism," whereby patients (mostly from industrialized countries) travel to developing countries expressly to receive health care services, ranging from surgery to dental work. A relatively new phenomenon, medical tourism attracts foreign currency to developing countries and saves money (between 75% and 90% of costs) to patients in countries where substantial numbers of people lack health insurance and out-of-pocket costs for privately delivered or elective services are high (especially the United States). Private insurance companies may even encourage medical tourism to cut costs, and some governments implicitly favor—or even subsidize—care-seeking abroad as a savings measure and a strategy to reduce waiting lists.

A burgeoning number of countries, including Lithuania, Argentina, South Africa, Turkey, Israel, and Jordan, participate in this multibillion dollar business. The Malaysian government promotes health tourism as a fast-growing sector; and Thailand has hospitals just for foreigners, accredited by U.S. boards. The largest medical tourism market is India: health-tourism-india.com advertises orthopedic and cardiac surgery, treatment of eye diseases, among other services, with options to visit tourist sites! Some countries offer unique services, such as Cuba's treatment for retinitis pigmentosa (night blindness). Hungary and Costa Rica are top cosmetic surgery destinations. Mexico, too, has thriving pharmaceutical, medical, and dental services for North Americans. A related practice is the outsourcing from developed to developing countries of diagnostic tests, which are transmitted electronically and read by doctors who charge lower fees and are located in different time zones (e.g., an after-hours emergency room in the eastern United States may send x-rays to pathologists in India, rather than hiring its own overtime staff).

Although beneficial to some, medical tourism distorts already fragile developing country health systems, with particular damage to primary care and services for the poor. In expanding the private sector, medical tourism draws resources (such as expensive technologies) and health professionals (through higher remuneration) away from the public health sector, already evident in India and Thailand (Ramírez de Arellano 2007). Even when the public sector benefits from medical tourism revenues, two-tiered systems are usually created, with foreign patients treated in separate (better) wards with dedicated facilities, equipment, and health professionals.

Medical tourism is a paradoxically perfect example of how health care policies in high-income countries (especially lack of universal health insurance in the United States) jeopardize health services resources in poorer countries.

Remuneration

Physicians function under a variety of payment mechanisms (see Table 12–9). They may operate on a fee-for-service basis in which they directly bill a patient (who then claims reimbursement from their health insurance plan, if they have one) or they may bill the government. Fee-for-service is popular with physicians in many countries such as Belgium, France, Sweden, Switzerland, and Japan.

Capitation is another form of remuneration which is used in the United Kingdom, Spain, the Netherlands, in HMOs in the United States, and to some extent in Italy and Denmark. Under this system, a physician is paid according to the number of patients in their practice, not by the number of services performed. Under capitation, there is a clear incentive to minimize return visits and unneeded patient contact.

Table 12–9 Provider Remuneration Mechanisms

Remuneration Mechanism	Description	Benefits	Limitations
Fee-for-service	Physician/facility is reimbursed by the government, patient, or insurance plan for each service performed (for each patient)	Remuneration closely linked to provider output	Inflationary, with incentives for unnecessary treatment
Capitation	Provider is paid (by the government, insurance plan, etc.) a set fee per patient over a set period of time, regardless of actual volume of services provided	Administratively simple; predictable expenditures	Encourages selection of young, healthy patients; incentive to enroll excessive numbers of patients and underserve them; may include a "gag clause" (doctors barred from discussing treatment options not covered by the insurance plan); precarious balance of neglect and prevention
Per case	A flat fee is charged per illness episode (e.g., for a hospital stay)	Encourages minimal use of resources	May lead to misrepresentation of diagnosis in order to generate higher payment
Salary/global budget	Annual wages or budget for total work performed	Simplest to administer and budget; no perverse incentives	Potential loss of productivity
Mixed	Combination of the above mechanisms	Mixed, depending on system	Mixed, depending on system

Source: Adapted from Glaser (1993).

There is also the complex system of sickness funds used in Germany and elsewhere, in which regional physicians' associations contract with funds on a quarterly basis to provide care for members. Sickness insurance funds pay a negotiated lump sum to physicians' associations, which pass a share on to each participating doctor, depending on the services provided, and weighted according to standard fee schedules. Other fee-for-service systems do not have a "lump-sum" budget and patients may make a copayment. Capitation and negotiated-sum systems retain a measure of selection by both practitioner and patient, and they preserve the private entrepreneurial status of the doctor who may not wish to be regarded as anyone's employee.

Health facilities may be financed in a number of ways including:

- global budgets for the year;
- retrospective fee-for-service reimbursement;
- all-payer (the same retrospective fee-for-service negotiated for all facilities);
- per diem (prospective payments, set in advance, adjusted for severity of case);
- per case/stay (prospective payments, set in advance, adjusted for severity of case);
- private fund raising and donations; and
- mixed payment systems.

Remuneration mechanisms may have a large influence on the incentives to provide care and also affect overall system costs, quality, access, and equity.

Box 12–16 Maternal and Child Health Example: Provider Reimbursement Incentives

Julie lives in a small town in Canada and her provincial health insurance plan covers all prenatal care visits. The OB/GYN physician living in her area is not accepting new patients, so she remains with her family physician and books monthly appointments. Her doctor will be reimbursed for each visit, although the fee-for-service model has meant that s/he must keep each visit to a few minutes. Julie has many questions for her doctor, but she is told to limit herself to only the most pressing issue at each visit, and she always feels rushed out of the office.

Box 12–17 Encouraging Publication of Health Research by Developing Country Researchers

According to the editor of the *Lancet*, "The invisibility to which mainstream science publishing condemns most Third World research thwarts efforts of poor countries to strengthen their indigenous science journals—and with them the quality of research in regions that need it most. It may also deprive the industrial world of critical knowledge" (Richard Horton as cited in Gibbs 1995, p. 92). Regardless of the research area, publications by scientists from developing countries, in particular by African researchers, are significantly underrepresented in mainstream journals (Paraje, Sadana, and Karam 2005).

(continued)

Box 12-17 Continued

Why is it important that researchers from developing countries conduct research and share their findings internationally? Local researchers may better understand the context—and therefore the issues—that need to be addressed through research; the best methods to conduct research; the most appropriate ways to obtain informed consent; and so on. As well, local researchers are often able to interpret the results of their research more appropriately—for use in policy making, for example. Local researchers may also be able, under certain circumstances, to convince policy makers to base decisions on research findings.

The publication of the work of developing country researchers in international journals has further benefits: it lends credence to their work and enables professional advancement; it allows greater sharing among countries; and it increases the profile of challenges faced in developing countries.

There are also selfish reasons for industrialized countries to ensure that research and medical information from the developing world is shared. Diseases do not respect international boundaries, as demonstrated by SARS and avian influenza. Research in developing countries may thus prove beneficial to the national interests of developed countries (Goehl 2007).

Many reasons have been advanced for the low publication rates by Africans in particular, and by developing country scientists and physicians in general. These include: lack of funding for research in developing countries (as illustrated by the 10/90 gap; see Chapter 3); poor research facilities; limited technical support; inadequate training; lack of expertise to write in English and other languages; fear of rejection; little culture of publishing; insufficient time to commit to research given competing priorities (e.g., clinical work or teaching); preference to publish in local or regional rather than international journals; limited access to information, for example inability to conduct wide literature searches given the lack of access to journals; and brain drain—skilled researchers are often attracted to work in developed countries (Sumathipala, Siribaddana, and Pate 2004; Mason 2007).

In 2004, the WHO convened a meeting of editors of scientific journals to address these challenges, and the editors of its own journal, the *Bulletin of the World Health Organization*, have put in place a number of strategies to assist developing country authors: articles are not rejected on the basis of problems with English but rather for not being original, scientific, or important in the international context (Momen 2004). Some journals actively solicit submissions from developing country scientists. The *Journal of Public Health Policy* does so. Its editors also developed "AuthorAID"—a system to match authors from the developing world wishing assistance with senior scientist mentors and professional editors (Freeman and Robbins 2006).

Another initiative is the International Network for the Availability of Scientific Publications (INASP), an NGO formed in 1992 under the auspices of the International Council for Science. The INASP provides advisory and referral services as well as access to university and research libraries and hosts meetings of scientists and health professionals to help enhance the diffusion of research findings (Pakenham-Walsh and Priestley 2002). As well, the China Medical Board's Program in Biomedical Editing in Beijing has, since 1996, run courses and trained a corps of editors in Southeast Asia.

An encouraging development in recent years has been the establishment of open access journals, such as the Public Library of Science (*PLoS*) journals, and the growth of online full-text databases such as PubMed, Bioline, and Scielo, based in Brazil. The WHO's Health InterNetwork Access to Research Initiative, among others, aims to provide internet access to the journals of major publishers to scientists in developing countries (www.who.int/hinari/en/).

The creation of strong national and regional journals also assists in building the capacity of researchers from developing countries to publish internationally. The WHO has assisted regional associations of medical editors in Africa and in the Eastern Mediterranean in this effort (Momen 2004). The African Journal Partnership provides mentorship between editors in developed countries and those in Africa. Two African journals, *Mali Medical* and *African Health Sciences*, have been assisted through this partnership to become indexed in PubMed (Goehl 2007).

Notwithstanding these promising efforts, there remains much to be done in challenging "publication imperialism."

Policy and Planning

Determining a national health care policy is a complex undertaking as resources are often scarce and there are multiple competing interests. The WHO has defined a national health policy as "an expression of goals for improving the health situation, the priorities among those goals, and the main directions for attaining them" (WHO 1979, p. 14). There are multiple levels of policy planning (Frenk 1995):

- *Systemic level planning*: related to the structure and function of the system, by specifying the institutional arrangements for regulation, financing, and delivery of services.
- *Programmatic level planning*: related to the substantive content of the system, by specifying its priorities, for example through a universal package of health care interventions.
- *Organizational level planning*: concerned with the actual production of services, by focusing on issues of quality assurance and technical efficiency.
- *Instrumental level planning*: generates the institutional intelligence for improving system performance through information, research, technological innovation, and human resource development.

Policies may be imposed on a country by various intergovernmental entities and agreements, such as the European Union, NAFTA, and others. As members of these organizations and as signatories of treaties, governments may therefore be bound to accept a range of policies. However, most of the pressures that determine fundamental policies exist internally. Major players in health policy formation include the state, through its leaders and bureaucracy, political parties, the medical profession, employers and other commercial interests, unions, and the citizenry or beneficiaries of the system. Advocacy groups of all kinds also play a role.

Planning is the process by which a society envisions a better future and charts a way to get there. The purpose of planning is to determine how, when, and where to employ resources to achieve policy goals most effectively. Effective planning involves liaison with various parties within or outside the government, or with international agencies that have an interest in what is at stake. Resources that are planned for are primarily financial, although human (e.g., physicians, nurses, administrators) and capital (e.g., MRIs, clinics) resources must also be considered. Both the private and public sectors are involved in resource allocation. Determining how resources are allocated has equity implications, as marginalized or vulnerable populations may or may not receive resources proportionate or relevant to their needs. As the private sector is unlikely to equitably distribute resources without regulation, this responsibility typically falls to government.

Policy, planning, and resource allocation all lead to program development, which is what is visible to the users of the health care system (e.g., immunization and health promotion campaigns). Because health programs cannot function in a vacuum, a high degree of intersectoral cooperation is needed. However, in countries with a decentralized political structure, where decision making is spread among overlapping and competing authorities, perceived threats to power bases may hamper collaboration. Ultimately, planning is a political process, which has profound implications for workers, marginalized groups, the health sector, corporate interests, and the population at large.

Box 12–18 Maternal and Child Health Example: Health Planning within Larger Societal Reforms

Sri Lanka has shown dramatic improvements in maternal health and currently has the lowest maternal mortality ratio (MMR) in South Asia. From 1,500 maternal deaths/100,000 live births in the early 20th century, the MMR fell to 42/100,000 in 1992 and further to 27/100,000 in 2002. These dramatic improvements were enabled by extensive coverage by skilled midwives, increased access to primary care, and improvements in the quality of maternal care received. Simultaneously—and distinct from other countries in the region—improvements in health care were accompanied by increases in overall standards of living, significant investments in education and social services, and the improved status of women (WHO 2005).

Management

Good health system management is necessary in all countries and at every level—from national budget-setting and policy making to individual facility and health worker supervision and evaluation. Managers and management systems are critical to a large number of activities including: determining priorities and projecting future needs; allocating and monitoring resources; establishing needs in terms of human and physical resources, including health workers, infrastructure, transport, maintenance, technology, and equipment; developing and implementing policy and programmatic strategies; and evaluating system performance (Reinke 1988).

The effective functioning and operation of health facilities is also largely determined by management capacity and structure. Outlining a facility's goals and objectives, determining budgetary and other resource allocations, supervising staff, and overseeing and evaluating policies and programs are all the purview of management. Health systems management also plays an important role in health worker recruitment, retention, and training (usually at the regional or national level). At national, district, and facility levels, management is central to the creation of supportive work environments that favor health worker recruitment and retention, well beyond salary levels per se, such as (Segall 2003):

- providing adequate physical resources (infrastructure, medicines, equipment);
- undertaking continuing education and training activities with staff;
- ensuring support and feedback from supervisors;

- engaging health workers in managerial decision making;
- maintaining sufficient recognition and incentives (financial and otherwise) for good job performance; and
- hiring adequate numbers of staff.

Finally, integrating health information systems (which focus on discrete health indicators such as infant mortality rates) with management information systems (which focus on tracking funds, staff, equipment, activities, achievement of goals, etc.) is essential for effective health systems management. Data collection and information systems are discussed in greater detail in Chapter 5.

Despite its importance, management remains one of the most problematic aspects of health care delivery. In many settings, management is compromised by insufficient resources and a lack of clear direction from regional or national authorities. In resource-constrained health systems, providing adequate training and funds for administrative purposes may not be seen as high a priority compared to ensuring sufficient numbers of frontline health care workers and other resources. As a result, both management and service delivery may suffer. Some countries—particularly those with universal single-payer systems such as Costa Rica and Norway—have health systems that allocate resources efficiently among these various needs.

Countries with significant private sector spending tend to face greater management problems, due to duplication of functions and inequitable resource distribution. For example, in South Africa, although 80% of the population uses public health services, 60% of all generalists operate in the private sector (Breier 2006). While such discrepancies may be addressed through improved management, major policy questions regarding health systems organization and budgetary allocations are political rather than managerial decisions. As such, whether government and private sector managers are public-spirited and responsive to the needs of the people, or motivated by self-serving interests, their ability to maneuver is limited by the political and bureaucratic context.

In other places, management may be overemphasized. Settings with multiple social security and health insurance arrangements tend to spend excessively on management and administration. In Latin America, for example, management and support workers make up an average of 43% of the total health workforce (WHO 2006d). Duplication of roles and unnecessary and inflated management expenditures often occur at the expense of health care delivery in rural areas and in public facilities. Nowhere is wasteful management spending more apparent than in the United States where administrative costs have grown over 2,500% since 1970 (over 10 times greater than the increase in number of physicians) and now account for 31% of health spending, despite the fact that 47 million people have no health insurance at all.

Various countries, for example Italy and Brazil, have strong unions of health workers who negotiate with management over these issues, leading to higher rates of retention and greater stability.

Management and administrative support workers make up one-third of all health workers globally and themselves are in need of support and training (WHO 2006d). Unfortunately, managerial capacity can be overwhelmed by competing needs for planning, supervision, and evaluation, particularly when there is inadequate staff and unclear roles and responsibilities between levels of government. In many under-developed settings, this may be exacerbated by the presence of multiple donor-run programs, which rarely fall within national health system management control yet demand significant, often duplicative administrative support due to requirements for compiling data, evaluating programs, seconding staff, and submitting reports.

Box 12-19 Decentralization and District Health Systems

Since the 1980s, many countries have introduced public sector decentralization reforms, including the decentralization of health services. Decentralization entails the transfer of authority and respon-sibility for health services delivery, including planning, resource allocation, and procurement, to subnational levels of government—namely municipalities, districts, and provinces—or to parastatal agencies and private contractors. Under decentralization, the national government typically retains broad policy making and financing responsibilities, although the latter may also be devolved to the local level. Because centralized systems can be overly bureaucratic, rigid, and unresponsive to local population needs, decentralization has been promoted as a strategy to achieve greater equity, effi-ciency, participation, intersectoral collaboration, and accountability (Mills 1994).

A normative model of decentralized health organization known as District Health Systems (DHS)—the regional building blocks of national health systems—was developed by the WHO and its regional offices following the 1978 Alma-Ata primary health care conference. The conference declaration called for integrated preventive and curative services at the local level, community par-ticipation in decision making, and attention to the social and political determinants of health (Segall 2003). Guidelines for DHS have offered a useful model for numerous countries seeking to develop, manage, and strengthen health care provision at the district level (usually encompassing 100,000–300,000 people) in terms of integrating primary and community health care centers and district hospitals at the secondary level, implementing referral and cross-referral systems, and managing health teams and community health workers (Walley, Wright, and Hubley 2001).

Much of the recent pressure to decentralize has come from bilateral and multilateral financial and development agencies. Although decentralization has been hailed as efficient and democratic, it has faced numerous problems and has yet to demonstrate improvements in health system performance (Bossert and Beauvais 2002). Some governments have been unwilling to delegate real decision mak-ing or spending powers to lower level authorities. As well, in various settings there has been little preparation or training for decentralization, and local management capacity and expertise are lacking. Perhaps most importantly, decentralization has often taken place simultaneous to considerable budget cuts and health care privatization. This has meant placing more responsibility on the shoulders of local authorities without giving them sufficient resources or the policy-making abilities to carry out these functions (Collins and Green 1994; Araújo 1997; Birn, Zimmerman, and Garfield 2000).

PRIMARY HEALTH CARE

Key Question:

- What are the implications of a primary health care approach for health systems organization?

The *Alma-Ata Declaration on Primary Health Care*, issued in 1978 and signed by 175 countries, represented a milestone in international agreements on priorities for health. It stimulated, and was stimulated by, lively international debates and discussion (Werner and Sanders 1997).

The Alma-Ata conference and declaration sought to reorient the narrow, increasingly medicalized approach that characterized much international health activity into an integrated political and technical health endeavor. While such ideas had been expressed previously through social medicine movements (see Chapter 4) and other efforts around the world, the Alma-Ata conference provided a world stage for promotion of this health philosophy.

At the conference, WHO's then Director-General, Halfdan Mahler, threw down the gauntlet to attending governments in the form of challenges including (Mahler 1978):

- Are you ready to address yourselves seriously to the existing gap between the health "haves" and the health "have nots" and to adopt concrete measures to reduce it?
- Are you ready to ensure the proper planning and implementation of primary health care in coordinated effort with other relevant sectors, in order to promote health as an indispensible contribution to the improvement of the quality of life of every individual, family, and community as part of overall economic development?
- Are you ready to make preferential allocation of health resources to the social periphery as an absolute priority?
- Are you ready to introduce, if necessary, radical changes in the existing health delivery system so that it properly supports primary health care as the overriding health priority?
- Are you ready to fight the political and technical battles required to overcome any social and economic obstacles and professional resistance to the universal introduction of primary health care?
- Are you ready to make unequivocal political commitments to adopt primary health care and to mobilize international solidarity to attain the objectives of health for all by the year 2000?

Box 12–20 Selections from the *Declaration of Alma-Ata*

I   Health, which is a state of complete physical, mental, and social well-being, and not merely the absence of disease or infirmity, is a fundamental human right...the attainment of the highest possible level of health is a most important worldwide social goal whose realization requires the action of many other social and economic sectors in addition to the health sector.

V   Governments have a responsibility for the health of their people, which can be fulfilled only by the provision of adequate health and social measures.

VI   Primary health care is essential health care based on practical, scientifically sound, and socially acceptable methods and technology made universally accessible to individuals and

(continued)

Box 12–20 Continued

families in the community through their full participation and at a cost that the community and country can afford to maintain at every stage of their development in the spirit of self-reliance and self-determination.

VII Primary health care:

1. reflects and evolves from the economic conditions and sociocultural and political charac-teristics of the country and its communities, and is based on the application of the relevant results of social, biomedical, and health services research and public health experience;

2. addresses the main health problems in the community, providing promotive, preventive, curative, and rehabilitative services accordingly;

3. includes at least...promotion of food supply and proper nutrition; an adequate supply of safe water and basic sanitation; maternal and child health care, including family plan-ning; immunization against the major infectious diseases; prevention and control of locally endemic diseases; appropriate treatment of common diseases and injuries; and provision of essential drugs;

4. involves...all related sectors and aspects of national and community development;

5. requires and promotes maximum community and individual self-reliance and participation in the planning, organization, operation, and control of primary health care, making fullest use of local, national, and other available resources;

6. should be sustained by integrated, functional, and mutually supportive referral systems, leading to the progressive improvement of comprehensive health care for all, and giving priority to those most in need; and

7. relies, at local and referral levels, on health workers, including physicians, nurses, mid-wives, auxiliaries, and community workers as applicable, as well as traditional practitioners as needed, suitably trained socially and technically to work as a health team and to respond to the expressed health needs of the community.

Source: WHO (1978).

The consensus reached at Alma-Ata was confirmed in a resolution at the next (32nd) World Health Assembly held in May 1979, and over the following years a defined strategy was developed according to which PHC was honed as the instrument by which to achieve the goal of "health for all by the year 2000." From the begin-ning, PHC programs were visualized as an integral, permanent, and pervasive part of the formal health care system in any country and not as separate add-on programs. However, as discussed in Chapter 3, PHC soon faced political and ideological chal-lenges, and broadly-defined PHC was selectively dismantled into a technical shadow of its former comprehensive approach. Still, the principles of primary care endure.

The PHC approach emphasizes:

- equity and the right to health;
- comprehensiveness, with an emphasis on prevention and protection of health through addressing the "underlying social, economic and environmental determinants of health" (Global Health Watch 2005, p. 209) (see Chapter 7);
- the integration of many levels of health care;
- the use of culturally and socially appropriate health technology and care; and
- community involvement in the health sector.

In a comprehensive review of PHC in industrialized countries, Barbara Starfield and her colleagues found it to be associated with better health outcomes, improved equity, and lower health care costs in the private and public sector. Six explanatory mechanisms were identified:

1. PHC increases access to a variety of health services for relatively deprived population groups;
2. Common health issues are best treated by a primary care physician;
3. PHC is associated with improved disease and illness prevention;
4. PHC manages health issues at an early stage, before they can progress to more serious conditions requiring more complex care;
5. PHC focuses on the individual rather than on a specific disease or ailment; and
6. PHC leads to avoidance of inappropriate or unnecessary care.

These findings were consistent across countries and population groups, showing that health care systems anchored in primary care are considerably more effective and equitable—and less costly—than systems based upon targeted interventions and high levels of medical specialization (Starfield, Shi, and Macinko 2005).

The *Alma-Ata Declaration* went well beyond the medical aspects of health care—it emphasized that all members of society should be treated fairly and humanely and that they should have equal access to the same basic rights, including the right to health. Unfortunately, aside from countries with well-developed welfare states, the Alma-Ata approach has not been widely followed by most signatories. Still, in 2008, the WHO reiterated its commitment to PHC and affirmed that the principles of PHC are just as valid today as they were 30 years ago.

Box 12–21 Maternal and Child Health Example: Primary Health Care

Ester lives in a Cuban town with a maternal health clinic nearby. She is encouraged to visit the clinic as frequently as she wishes. There she receives nutrition and health education free of charge, and she is given the opportunity to pose any questions she has. The doctors and nurses take the time to speak with her about her pregnancy, delivery, and raising the child. She knows the practitioner team that is responsible for the health care of her neighborhood, and she trusts that they will provide her with advice and care as needed.

CONCLUSION

Learning Points:

- Health care systems are a crucial but are not the sole determinant of health.
- Understanding the values underlying health care systems enhances comparative analyses.

- Health care systems are shaped by a variety of historical trajectories and political factors.
- The primary health care approach is central to the development of equitable health systems.

> "Of all the forms of inequality, injustice in health care is the most shocking and inhumane."
> —Martin Luther King, Jr

As we have seen, many factors must be taken into account when analyzing health care systems. The main features of a health care system (delivery, financing, management, organization) cannot be considered in purely technocratic terms: values, principles, the interests of particular parties, historical precedent, and political struggles are all fundamental influences on health care systems. The United States shows a disturbing example of how undemocratic political processes act against the interests and demands of the majority of the population who favor a national health insurance system, while countries such as Denmark or Cuba demonstrate how political processes enhance health services coverage.

Due to the pervasiveness of neoliberal ideologies in recent years, many countries, both developed and underdeveloped, have turned to the private sector to provide health care services. As discussed here and in Chapter 11, such shifts can lead to growing inequities in access to services and health outcomes. At the same time, a growing number of countries recognize the role of publicly funded systems with a PHC emphasis in the efficient and equitable distribution of health care services and defend existing social insurance programs or are developing them anew.

REFERENCES

Abel-Smith B. 1965. The major patterns of financing and organisation of medical services that have emerged in other countries. *Medical Care* 3(1):33–40.

AHIP. 2007. America's health insurance plans. http://www.ahip.org/. Accessed June 20, 2007.

Almeida C, Travassos C, Porto S, and Elena Labra M. 2000. Health sector reform in Brazil: A case study of inequity. *International Journal of Health Services* 30(1):129–162.

Altenstetter C. 2003. Insights from health care in Germany. *American Journal of Public Health* 93(1):38–44.

Angell M. 2004. *The Truth about the Drug Companies. How They Deceive Us and What to Do About It.* New York: Random House.

Araújo Jr JL. 1997. Attempts to decentralize in recent Brazilian health policy: Issues and problems, 1988–1994. *International Journal of Health Services* 27(1):109–124.

Armada F, Muntaner C, and Navarro V. 2001. Health and social security reforms in Latin America: The convergence of the World Health Organization, the World Bank, and transnational corporations. *International Journal of Health Services* 31(4):729–768.

Bagchi S. 2006. Telemedicine in India. *PLoS Medicine* 3(3):e82.

Balabanova D, McKee M, Pomerleau J, Rose R, and Haerpfer C. 2004. Health service utilization in the Former Soviet Union: Evidence from eight countries. *Health Services Research* 39(6 Pt 2):1927–1950.

Barer ML, Evans RG, and Hertzman C. 1995. Avalanche or glacier? Health care and the demographic rhetoric. *Canadian Journal on Aging* 14(2):193–224.

Barr DA and Field MG. 1996. The current state of health care in the Former Soviet Union: Implications for health care policy and reform. *American Journal of Public Health* 86(3):307–312.

Beldarraín Chaple E. 2006. La salud pública en Cuba y su experiencia internacional (1959–2005). *História, Ciencias, Saúde—Manguinhos* 13(3):709–716.

Berckmans P, Dawans V, Schmets G, Vandenbergh D, and Autier P. 1997. Inappropriate drug-donation practices in Bosnia and Herzegovina, 1992 to 1996. *New England Journal of Medicine* 337(25):1842–1845.

Berman PA and Bossert TJ. 2000. A decade of health sector reform in developing countries: What have we learned? In *DDM Symposium: "Appraising a Decade of Health Sector Reform in Developing Countries."* Washington, DC: Data for Decision-Making Project.

Beveridge W. 1942. *Social Insurance and Allied Services: American Edition.* New York: The Macmillan Company, Inter-departmental Committee on Social Insurance and Allied Services.

Birn A-E, Zimmerman S, and Garfield R. 2000. To decentralize or not to decentralize, is that the question? Nicaraguan health policy under structural adjustment in the 1990s. *International Journal of Health Services* 30(1):111–128.

Birn A-E, Brown T, Fee E, and Lear W. 2003. Struggles for national health reform in the United States. *American Journal of Public Health* 93(1):86–91.

Blecher M and Harrison S. 2006. Health care financing. In *South African Health Review.* Durban: Health Systems Trust.

Blendon R, Kim M, and Benson J. 2001. The public versus the World Health Organization on health system performance. *Health Affairs* 20(3):233–243.

Blumenthal DS and Hsiao W. 2005. Privatization and its discontents-the evolving Chinese health care system. *New England Journal of Medicine* 353(11):1165–1170.

Blumenthal DS. 1994. Geographic imbalances in physician supply: An international comparison. *Journal of Rural Health* 10(2):109–118.

Bossert TJ and Beauvais JC. 2002. Decentralization of health systems in Ghana, Zambia, Uganda and the Philippines: A comparative analysis of decision space. *Health Policy and Planning* 17(1):14–31.

Breier M. 2006. New human resource plan foresees fewer foreign doctors. *Human Sciences Research Council Review* 4(2).

Busse R. 2008. The health system in Germany. *Eurohealth* 14(1):5–6.

Busse R and Reisberg A. 2004. Germany. In *Health Systems in Transition.* Copenhagen: WHO EURO.

Center for Global Development. 2005. *Making Markets for Vaccines: Ideas into Action.* Washington, DC: Center for Global Development.

Centers for Disease Control and Prevention. 2007. Infant, neonatal, and postneonatal mortality rates, by detailed race and Hispanic origin of mother: United States, selected years 1983–2004. In *Health, United States, 2007.* Hyattsville, MD: Centers for Disease Control and Prevention, National Center for Health Statistics.

Chung HJ and Muntaner C. 2007. Welfare state matters: A typological multilevel analysis of wealthy countries. *Health Policy* 80(2):328–339.

Clemens M and Pettersson G. 2007. New Data on African Health Professionals Abroad. Working Paper 95. Washington, DC: Center for Global Development.

Collins C and Green A. 1994. Decentralization and primary health care: Some negative implications in developing countries. *International Journal of Health Services* 24(3):459–475.

Das J and Gertler PJ. 2007. Variations in practice quality in five low-income countries: A conceptual overview. *Health Affairs* 26 (3):w296–w309.

Deber R. 2004. Why did the World Health Organization rate Canada's health system as 30th? Some thoughts on league tables. *Longwoods Review* 2(1):2–7.

DeNavas-Walt C, Proctor BD, and Smith J. 2007. Income, poverty and health insurance coverage in the United States. U.S. Census Bureau.

Docteur E and Oxley H. 2003. *Health Care Systems: Lessons from the Reform Experience.* Paris: OECD.

Drechsler D and Jutting J. 2007. Different countries, different needs: The role of private health insurance in developing countries. *Journal of Health Politics Policy and Law* 32(3):497–534.

Dumont J-C and Zurn P. 2007. *Immigrant Health Workers in OECD Countries: An Assessment of the Situation in the Broader Context of Highly Skilled Migration.* Paris: OECD.

Eggleston K, Rao K, and Wang J. 2005. *From Plan to Market in the Health Sector? China's Experience.* Tufts University: Department of Economics.

ELAM. 2006. *Historia.* http://www.elacm.sld.cu/historia.html. Accessed June 20, 2007.

Elias PEM and Cohn A. 2003. Health reform in Brazil: Lessons to consider. *American Journal of Public Health* 93(1):44–48.

Enthoven A and Kronick R. 1989. A consumer-choice health plan for the 1990s. Universal health insurance in a system designed to promote quality and economy. *New England Journal of Medicine* 320(1):29–37.

Esping-Andersen G. 1990. *The Three Worlds of Welfare Capitalism*: Princeton, NJ: Princeton University Press.

Feng X, Tang S, Bloom G, Segall M, and Gu X. 1995. Cooperative medical schemes in contemporary rural China. *Social Science and Medicine* 41(8):1111–1118.

Field MG. 1978. *Comparative Health Systems: Differentiation and Convergence.* Rockville: National Center for Health Services Research.

Flores W. 2006. Equity and health sector reform in Latin America and the Carribbean: From 1995 to 2005. International Society for Equity in Health—Chapter of the Americas. Report commissioned by the International Society for Equity in Health—Chapter of the Americas. http://www.iseqh.org/docs/HSR_equity_report2006_en.pdf. Accessed May 10, 2007.

Foubister T, Thomson S, and Mossialos E. 2006. Private medical insurance in the United Kingdom. Brussels: WHO, on behalf of the European Observatory on Health Systems and Policies.

Freeman P and Robbins A. 2006. The publishing gap between rich and poor: The focus of AuthorAID. *Journal of Public Health Policy* 27:196–203.

Frenk J. 1995. Comprehensive policy analysis for health system reform. *Health Policy* 32(1):257–277.

Frenk J, González-Pier E, Gómez-Dantés O, Lezana MA, and Knaul FM. 2006. Comprehensive reform to improve health system performance in Mexico. *Lancet* 368(9546):1524–1534.

Gakidou E, Lozano R, González-Pier E, Abbott-Klafter J, Barofsky JT, Bryson-Cahn C, et al. 2006. Assessing the effect of the 2001–2006 Mexican health reform: An interim report card. *Lancet* 368(9550):1920–1935.

Gibbons D. 2003. Appropriate technology in Tanzania. *Wide World* 15(1):12–14.

Gibbs W. 1995. Lost science in the third world. *Scientific American* 273(2):92–99.

Gilson L and Mills A. 1995. Health sector reforms in sub-Saharan Africa: Lessons from the last ten years. In Berman PA, Editor. *Health Sector Reform in Developing Countries: Making Health Development Sustainable.* Boston, MA: Harvard University Press.

Glaser WA 1993. How expenditure caps and expenditure targets really work. *The Milbank Quarterly* 71(1):97–127.

Global Health Watch. 2005. *Global Health Watch 2005–2006.* London: Zed Books.

Goehl TJ 2007. Access denied. *Environmental Health Perspectives* 115(10):A482–A483.

Gong S, Walker A, and Shi G. 2007. From Chinese model to U.S. symptoms: The paradox of China's health system. *International Journal of Health Services* 37(4):651–672.

Government of Canada. 2006. Health Canada, Mission and Vision. http://www.hc-sc.gc.ca/ahc-asc/activit/about-apropos/index-eng.php#mission. Accessed April 23, 2007.

Government of South Africa. 2004. *Strategic Priorities for the National Health System: 2004–2009.* Pretoria: Department of Health.

Grieve RH. 2004. Appropriate technology in a globalizing world. *International Journal of Technology Management and Sustainable Development* 3(3):173–187.

Gwatkin DR, Wagstaff A, and Yazbeck AS, Editors. 2005. *Reaching the Poor with Health, Nutrition, and Population Services: What Works, What Doesn't, and Why.* Washington, DC: The World Bank.

Halstead SB, Walsh JA, and Warren KS, Editors. 1985. *Good Health at Low Cost, A Rockefeller Foundation Conference Report.* New York: The Rockefeller Foundation.

Hart JT. 1971. The inverse care law. *Lancet* 297(7696):405–412.

Health Systems Trust. 1999. Health and related indicators. *South African Health Review 1999.* Durban South Africa: Health Systems Trust.

Hellander I. 2002. A review of data on the health sector of the United States. *International Journal of Health Services* 32(3):579–599.

Hernández Llamas H. 1982. Historia de la participación del estado en las instituciones de atención médica en México: 1935–1980. In Ortiz Quesada F, Editor. *Vida y muerte del Mexicano.* México, DF: Folios Ediciones.

Hicks V. 2004. Strategies to confront crisis. In Wibulpolprasert S and Hempisut P, Editors. *Health Human Resources Demand and Management.* Nonthaburi, Thailand: Joint Learning Initiative.

Himmelstein DU, Warren E, Thorne D, and Woolhandler S. 2005. MarketWatch: Illness and injury as contributors to bankruptcy. *Health Affairs* W5:63–73.

Ho L-S. 1995. Market reforms and China's health care system. *Social Science and Medicine* 41(8):1065–1072.

Hoffman B. 2003. Health care reform and social movements in the United States. *American Journal of Public Health* 93(1):75–86.

Hu T-w. 2004. Financing and organization of China's health care. *Bulletin of the World Health Organization* 82(7):480.

Huang A and Weber A. 2006. The Health of Nations: 'Open source' research and the economics of life and death in the developing world. *Berkeley Science Review* 45–50.

Huong DB, Phuong NK, Bales S, Chen J, Lucas H, and Segall M. 2007. Rural health care in Vietnam and China: Conflict between market reforms and social need. *International Journal of Health Services* 37(3):555–572.

Ikegami N. 2004. Japan's health care system: Containing costs and attempting reform. *Health Affairs* 23(3):26–35.

Ikegami N and Campbell JC. 1997. *Containing Health Care Costs in Japan.* Ann Arbor, MI: University of Michigan Press.

Iriart C, Merhy EE, and Waitzkin H. 2001. Managed care in Latin America: The new common sense in health policy reform. *Social Science and Medicine* 52(8):1243–1253.

Jeong H-S. 2005. Health care reform and change in public–private mix of financing: A Korean case. *Health Policy* 74(2):133–145.

Joint Learning Initiative. 2004. *Human Resources for Health: Overcoming the Crisis.* Cambridge, MA: Harvard University Press.

Kaiser Family Foundation. 2007. Health care spending in the United States and OECD countries. http://www.kff.org/insurance/snapshot/chcm010307oth.cfm. Accessed June 2007.

Kennedy J and Morgan S. 2006. Health care access in three nations: Canada, insured America and uninsured America. *International Journal of Health Services* 36(4):697–717.

Knaul FM, Arreola H, Mendez O, and Miranda M. 2005. *Preventing Impoverishment, Promoting Equity and Preventing Households from Financial Crisis: Health Insurance through Institutional Reform in Mexico.* México: DF: Fundación Mexicana para la Salud.

Knaul FM and Frenk J. 2005. Health insurance in Mexico: Achieving universal coverage through structural reform. *Health Affairs* 24(6):1467–1476.

Labonte R, Packer C, Klassen N, Kazanjian A, Apland L, Adalikwu J, et al. 2006. The brain drain of health professionals from sub-Saharan Africa to Canada. In *African Migration and Development Series No. 2 (South African Migration Project—SAMP).* Cape Town: Idasa Publishing.

Laurell AC. 2007. Health system reform in Mexico: A critical review. *International Journal of Health Services* 37(3):515–535.

Lexchin J. 2006. The pharmaceutical industry and the pursuit of profit. In Cohen JC, Illingworth P, and Schuklenk U, Editors. *The Power of Pills: Social, Ethical and Legal Issues in Drug Development, Marketing and Pricing.* London: Pluto Press.

Light D. 1997. Comparative models of "health care" systems. In Conrad P, Editor. *The Sociology of Health and Illness.* New York: St. Martin's Press.

———. 2003. Universal health care: Lessons from the British experience. *American Journal of Public Health* 93(1):25–30.

———. 2005. Making practical markets for vaccines. *PLoS Medicine* 2(10):e271.

Light D and Lexchin J. 2005. Foreign free riders and the high price of US medicines. *British Medical Journal* 331(7522):958–960.

Liu Y. 2004. China's public health care system: Facing the challenges. *Bulletin of the World Health Organization* 82(7):532–538.

Liu Y, Hsiao W, and Eggleston K. 1999. Equity in health and health care: The Chinese experience. *Social Science and Medicine* 49(10):1349–1356.

Liu Y and Rao K. 2006. Providing health insurance in rural China: From research to policy. *Journal of Health Politics, Policy and Law* 31(1):71–92.

Lloyd-Sherlock P. 2006. When social health insurance goes wrong: Lessons from Argentina and Mexico. *Social Policy and Administration* 40(4):353–368.

Mahler H. 1978. Speech at the opening ceremony, Alma-Ata, September 6. International Conference on Primary Health Care, 6–12 September 1978, Alma-Ata, Kazkhstan, (USSR former). ID number P21/87/5. Geneva: WHO Archives.

Mason PR. 2007. The need for a journal of infection in developing countries. *Journal of Infection in Developing Countries* 1(1):3–6.

Maynard A and Bloor K. 1995. Health care reform. Informing difficult choices. *International Journal of Health Planning and Management* 10(4):247–264.

Meng Q. 2007. *Developing and Implementing Equity-Promoting Health Care Policies in China. Health Systems Knowledge Network.* Geneva: WHO Commission on Social Determinants of Health.

Mills A. 1994. Decentralization and accountability in the health sector from an international perspective: What are the choices? *Public Administration and Development* 14(3):281–292.

Mills A, Rasheed F, and Tollman S. 2006. Strengthening health systems. In Jamison DT, Breman JG, Measham AR, Alleyne G, Claeson M, Evans DB, Jha P, Mills A, and Musgrove P, Editors. *Disease Control Priorities in Developing Countries.* New York: Oxford University Press.

Ministry of Health of Great Britain, and Department of Health for Scotland. 1944. *A National Health Service.* London, HMSO. Cmnd 6502.

Momen H. 2004. The role of journals in enhancing health research in developing countries. *Bulletin of the World Health Organization* 82(3):163.

Mullan F. 2004. Affirmative action, Cuban style. *New England Journal of Medicine* 351(26):2680–2683.

———. 2005. The metrics of the physician brain drain. *New England Journal of Medicine* 353(17):1810–1818.

Murthy RK, de Pinho H, Ravindran STK, and Romero M. 2004. Health sector reforms and sexual reproductive health services. In *Technical Consultation on Health Sector Reform and Reproductive Health: Developing the Evidence Base.* Geneva: WHO.

Navarro V. 1981. The underdevelopment of health or the health of underdevelopment: An analysis of the distribution of human health resources in Latin America. In Navarro V, Editor. *Imperialism, Health and Medicine.* Farmingdale, NY: Baywood Publishing Company.

———. 1989. Why some countries have national health insurance, others have national health services, and the U.S. has neither. *Social Science and Medicine* 28(9):887–898.

———. 1993. *Dangerous to Your Health: Capitalism in Health Care.* New York: Monthly Review Press.

———. 2000. Assessment of the world health report 2000. *Lancet* 356(9241):1598–1601.

———. 2007. What is a national health policy? *International Journal of Health Services* 37(1):1–14.

Newton PN, Fernández FM, Plançon A, Mildenhall DC, and Green MD, et al. 2008. A collaborative epidemiological investigation into the criminal fake artesunate trade in South East Asia. *PLoS Medicine* 5(2, e32):209–219.

Nord E. 2002. Measures of goal attainment and performance in the World Health Report, 2000: A brief, critical consumer guide. *Health Policy* 59(3):183–191.

OECD. 2004. *The OECD Health Project: Private Health Insurance in OECD Countries.* Paris: OECD.

———. 2005. *Health at a Glance 2005: OECD Indicators.* Paris: OECD.

———. 2007. *OECD Health Data 2007 Statistics and Indicators for 30 Countries-CD-ROM Version.* Paris: OECD.

———. 2008. OECD Health data 2008: How does the United States compare. Paris: OECD. http://www.oecd.org/dataoecd/46/2/38980580.pdf. Accessed September 2008.

Orbinski J and Burciul B. 2006. Moving beyond charity for R&D for neglected diseases. In Cohen JC, Illingworth P, and Schuklenk U, Editors. *The Power of Pills: Social, Ethical and Legal Issues in Drug Development, Marketing and Pricing.* London: Pluto Press.

Oswaldo Cruz Foundation. 2000. Report of the workshop Health systems performance: The World Health Report 2000, December 14–15, Rio de Janeiro, Brazil.

Oxfam International. 2004. From Donorship to Ownership: Moving toward PRSP Round Two. Oxfam Briefing Paper. Oxford, UK: Oxfam International.

Pakenham-Walsh N and Priestley C. 2002. Towards equity in global health knowledge. *QJM* 95(7):469–473.

Paraje G, Sadana R, and Karam G. 2005. Public health: Increasing international gaps in health-related publications. *Science* 308(5724):959–960.

Pettifor A, Thomas B, and Telatin M. 2001. *HIPC: Flogging a Dead Process*. London: Jubilee Plus.

Pillay Y. 2001. The impact of South Africa's new constitution on the organization of health services in the post-apartheid era. *Journal of Health Politics, Policy and Law* 26(4):747–766.

Polsky D, Ross SJ, Brush BL, and Sochalski J. 2007. Trends in characteristics and country of origin among foreign-trained nurses in the United States, 1990 and 2000. *American Journal of Public Health* 97(5):895–899.

Quadagno J. 2004. Why the United States has no national health insurance: Stakeholder mobilization against the welfare state, 1945–1996. *Journal of Health and Social Behavior* 45(extra issue):25–44.

Ramírcz de Arellano AB. 2007. Patients without borders: The emergence of medical tourism. *International Journal of Health Services* 37(1):193–198.

Reinke WA. 1988. *Health Planning for Effective Management*. New York: Oxford University Press.

Remen R and Holloway L. 2008. A student perspective on ELAM and its educational program. *Social Medicine* 3(2):158–164.

Rodwin VG. 1984. *The Health Planning Predicament: France, Quebec, England, and the United States*. Berkeley, CA: University of California Press.

Roemer MI. 1991. *National Health Systems of the World. Vol. 1: The Countries*. Oxford: Oxford University Press.

Schocn C, Collins SR, Kriss JL, and Duly MM. 2008. How many arc undcrinsurcd? Trends among U.S. adults, 2003 and 2007. *Health Affairs* 27(4):w298–w309.

Segall M. 2003. District health systems in a neoliberal world: A review of five key policy areas. *International Journal of Health Planning and Management* 18(S1):S5–S26.

Sepehri A and Chernomas R. 2004. Is the Canadian health care system fiscally sustainable? *International Journal of Health Services* 34(2):229–243.

Sheldon G. 2003. Great expectations: The 21st century health workforce. *The American Journal of Surgery* 185(1):35–41.

Sigerist HE. 1937. *Socialized Medicine in the Soviet Union*. New York: W. W. Norton & Co.
———. 1943. From Bismarck to Beveridge: developments and trends in social security legislation. *Bulletin of the History of Medicine* 13(4):365–388.

Starfield B, Shi L, and Macinko J. 2005. Contribution of primary care to health systems and health. *Milbank Quarterly* 83(3):457–502.

Sumathipala A, Siribaddana S, and Pate V. 2004. Under-representation of developing countries in the research literature: Ethical issues arising from a survey of five leading medical journals. *BMC Medical Ethics* 5:5.

Thorsteinsdóttir H, Sáenz TW, Quach U, Daar AS, and Singer PA. 2004. Cuba—Innovation through synergy. *Nature Biotechnology* 22 (Supplement):DC19–DC24.

Towse A and Kettler H. 2005. Advance price or purchase commitments to create markets for treatments for diseases of poverty: Lessons from three policies. *Bulletin of the World Health Organization* 83(4):301–307.

Toynbee P. 2007. NHS: The Blair years. *British Medical Journal* 334(7602):1030–1031.

Tragakes E and Lessof S. 2003. Russian Federation. In Tragakes E, Editor. *Health Systems in Transition*. Copenhagen: WHO EURO.

Tulchinsky TH and Varavikova EA. 1996. Addressing the epidemiologic transition in the Former Soviet Union: Strategies for health system and public health reform in Russia. *American Journal of Public Health* 86(3):313–320.

Unger J-P, De Paepe P, Cantuarias GS, and Herrera OA. 2008. Chile's neoliberal health reform: An assessment and a critique. *PLoS Medicine* 5(4):e79.

U.S. Census Bureau. 2005. *National Nurses Week (May 6–12) and National Hospital Week (May 8–14)*. Washington, DC: U.S. Census Bureau.

————. 2008. *Income, Poverty, and Health Insurance Coverage in the United States: 2007*. Washington, DC: U.S. Census Bureau.

Walley J, Wright J, and Hubley J. 2001. *Public Health: An Action Guide to Improving Health in Developing Countries*. New York: Oxford University Press.

Walt G and Mills A. 2001. Commentary. *Lancet* 357(9269):1702–1703.

Webster C. 1998. *The National Health Service: A Political History*. New York: Oxford University Press.

Weisbrod BA. 2004. Solving the drug dilemma. *Institute for Policy Research News* 26(1).

Welch C. 2000. Structural adjustment programs and poverty reduction strategy. *Foreign Policy in Focus Policy Brief* 5(14) http://www.fpif.org/fpiftxt/2833. Accessed May 12, 2007.

Werner D and Sanders D. 1997. Alma-Ata and the institutionalization of primary health care. In *Questioning the Solution: The Politics of Primary Health Care and Child Survival*. Palo Alto, CA: HealthWrights.

Wertheimer AI, Santella TM, and Chaney NM. 2004. Counterfeit pharmaceuticals—update on current status and future projections. Business briefing. *Pharmagenerics* http://www.touchbriefings.com/cdps/cditem.cfm?NID=955. Accessed May 9, 2007.

Whitehead M, Dahlgren G, and Evans T. 2001. Equity and health sector reforms: Can low-income countries escape the medical poverty trap? *Lancet* 358(9284):833–836.

WHO. 1978. Declaration of Alma-Ata. International Conference on Primary Health Care. Alma-Ata, USSR. http://www.who.int/hpr/NPH/docs/declaration_almaata.pdf. Accessed March 8, 2007.

————. 1979. *Formulating Strategies for Health for All by the Year 2000*. Geneva: WHO.

————. 1996. *Report of the Ad Hoc Committee on Health Research Relating to Future Intervention Options*. Geneva: WHO.

————. 2000. *The World Health Report 2000. Health Systems: Improving Performance*. Geneva: WHO.

————. 2002. *Key Policy Issues in Long-Term Care*. Brodsky J, Habib J, and Hirschfeld MJ, Editors. Geneva: WHO.

————. 2004. *The World Health Report: Changing History*. Geneva: WHO.

————. 2005. *The World Health Report 2005: Make Every Mother and Child Count*. Geneva: WHO.

————. 2006a. *Counterfeit Medicines*. Fact sheet No 275. http://www.who.int/mediacentre/factsheets/fs275/en/. Accessed March 9, 2008.

———— (Regional Office for the Western Pacific). 2006b. *Japan*: Country health profile. http://www.wpro.who.int/countries/05jpn/health_situation.htm. Accessed April 23, 3006.

————. 2006c. *National Health Accounts: Russian Federation*. http://www.who.int/nha/country/rus/en/. Accessed May 2007.

————. 2006d. *World Health Report 2006: Working Together for Health*. Geneva: WHO.

————. 2007a. Health expenditure in the world. http://www.who.int/nha/en/. Accessed September 13, 2007.

————. 2007b. Medical devices and equipment. http://www.who.int/medical_devices/en/. Accessed April 8, 2007.

————. 2008. *National Health Accounts: United States of America.* Geneva: WHO. http://www.who.int/nha/country/usa.xls. Accessed March 2008.

WHO EURO. 2003a. Russian Federation. In *Health Systems in Transition.* Copenhagen: WHO EURO.

————. 2003b. Sweden. In *Health Systems in Transition.* Copenhagen: WHO EURO.

WHOSIS. 2008. WHO statistical information system. http://www.who.int/whosis/en/. Accessed September 2008.

Woolhandler S, Campbell T, and Himmelstein DU. 2003. Costs of health care administration in the U.S. and Canada. *New England Journal of Medicine* 349(8):768–775.

Wootton R, Youngberry K, Swinfen P, and Swinfen R. 2004. Prospective case review of a global e-health system for doctors in developing countries. *Journal of Telemedicine and Telecare* 10(1):94–96.

World Bank. 1993. *World Development Report 1993: Investing in Health.* Washington, DC: World Bank.

Zhengzhong M. 2005. *Health System of China: Overview of Challenges and Reforms.* Bangkok: United Nations Economic and Social Commission for Asia and the Pacific..

Zweifel P, Felder S, and Meiers M. 1999. Aging of population and health care expenditure: A red herring? *Health Economics* 8(6):485–496.

13

Toward Healthy Societies: From Ideas to Action

Key Questions:

- What makes for a healthy society?
- How do international health policies and activities aid or impede the making of healthy societies?

In 1968 Julius Nyerere, the first president of postcolonial Tanzania, poignantly laid out his aims:

> to build a society in which all members have equal rights and equal opportunities; in which all can live in peace with their neighbours without suffering or imposing injustice, being exploited, or exploiting; and in which all have a gradually increasing basic level of material welfare before any individual lives in luxury (Nyerere 1968, p. 340).

Up to this point in the text, we have critically examined the history of international health, the key contemporary actors, the global epidemiology of morbidity and mortality, and the structural forces that shape differences in health patterns both within and between countries. In contrast to Nyerere's aspirations, the dominant international health donors (also called global health initiatives and global health partnerships) prioritize technical silver bullets—such as vaccines (e.g., through the GAVI Alliance) and provision of antiretrovirals (ARVs) for HIV/AIDS—usually at the expense of integrated and comprehensive approaches. What Nyerere proposed in 1968 was to achieve healthy societies by building peaceful communities: providing social and economic security in ways that protect the vulnerable; allowing freedom of expression and opportunities for full participation in civic life; and providing universal and equitably distributed services, including water, sanitation, education, shelter, and health care. The sum total of individual quick fixes to these problems does not add up to such a comprehensive strategy.

This chapter explores how, and under what conditions, Nyerere's goals can be realized, building on some of the key issues that were raised in Chapter 7. We contrast orthodox, selective, and disease-control approaches to international health with broad-reaching societal efforts aimed at addressing the underlying causes of ill health. This chapter highlights a range of these successful endeavors. We focus on the makings of healthy societies not only in theory but in practice—efforts that have made a difference in municipalities, regions, countries, and globally. Many of the case studies that we use in this chapter (as elsewhere in the book) are from underdeveloped settings, illustrating that under the right conditions, developing countries can generate lessons for us all. By focusing on societal change through the lens of political economy, these approaches provide a counterbalance to mainstream efforts in global health.

THE "DISEASE CONTROL" CONCEPTION OF INTERNATIONAL HEALTH: ITS SUCCESSES AND LIMITATIONS

As outlined in Chapters 2 and 3, the first generation of international campaigns that focused on particular diseases were launched a century ago by the Rockefeller Foundation and various colonial authorities. These were later followed by disease campaigns championed by the WHO. Based on a defined target of eliminating a single disease, a number of these efforts achieved their aims. The problem of anemia-inducing hookworm was addressed in some areas through latrine-building, promotion of shoe-wearing, and, especially, antihelminthic treatment; yellow fever was controlled through extensive antilarval efforts, and, later, a vaccine. Most notably, the global eradication of smallpox in 1980, based on an aggressive immunization campaign, has been called one of the single greatest feats of international public health.

Attempts to eliminate malaria, however, were more problematic. Early 20th century efforts focused on reducing larval breeding sites of the mosquito vector (*Anopheles*) through swamp drainage, use of larvicidal fish, and the spraying of larvicidal oils. Before DDT (insecticide) spraying was introduced in the mid-1940s, housing and sanitation improvements, such as screened windows (to keep mosquitoes out) and piped water and sewage (to diminish the use of water receptacles, thereby eliminating breeding sites), enabled malaria's disappearance from North America and Europe. When the WHO launched its Global Malaria Eradication Campaign in 1955, such multipronged methods were ignored in favor of an almost exclusive focus on DDT. Within a few years, an estimated 1 billion people were no longer threatened by malaria. However, in the late 1960s, when the technology (DDT) faltered due to mosquito resistance and political opposition to the campaign's vertical (top-down) structure, together with concerns over DDT's environmental effects, the campaign was abandoned. With little further attention to other malaria control methods, malaria reemerged in many settings as a more severe problem than before the eradication campaign began (see Chapter 6). In the wake of this fiasco, the technical approach to international health was not buried, however, but rather resurrected through a new effort—smallpox eradication—aimed at transcending the flaws of the global malaria campaign.

Smallpox Eradication

Smallpox had several advantages over malaria as a target for eradication. First, there were millennia of experience with its control. Smallpox inoculation was practiced in ancient India and China, where the idea of preventive medicine was well entrenched (Needham 1980). The lack of an animal host and the availability of an effective vaccine—able to be delivered, by the 1960s, via easily administered bifurcated needles and rapid jet vaccinators—were also important factors in its control.

The eradication of smallpox was facilitated by still other ingredients. The WHO's global campaign, launched in 1967, was divided into defined phases reminiscent of, but even more totalizing than, the global malaria campaign:

- *Attack phase*: Where smallpox was endemic with a substantial number of unvaccinated persons, a mass vaccination program was instituted, aiming for 100% coverage. When documented coverage reached 80% and the incidence of smallpox fell below five cases per 100,000 inhabitants, the program was considered ready to move into the next phase.
- *Consolidation phase*: At this point mass vaccination was terminated, and it was considered necessary to vaccinate only new arrivals and newborns. Surveillance activities were augmented, case detection improved, and an effort was made at concentrated local vaccination of case contacts. Where no new cases occurred for over 2 years, yet another phase was entered.
- *Maintenance phase*: Surveillance and reporting were normally shifted to the national or regional health service, and any cases detected received intensive investigation.

Moreover, although there was limited financial support allocated to the campaign by WHO and large donors (originally US$440,000 to vaccinate 1.2 billion people in some 33 countries—using Soviet vaccines), numerous experts and laboratories collaborated to prepare handbooks and offer advice.

Yet the heroic account of single-minded global cooperation is vastly oversimplified. Most expenses were met by the affected countries themselves (see Table 13–1), many of which faced severe hardship in setting aside these funds. Nor was there consensus over the approach or the vaccines to be used. In India in particular, there was enormous division among national, state, and local officials; one key issue

Table 13-1 Cost of the Smallpox Eradication Program

Source of Funds	Amount (constant US$)
WHO regular budget	37,930,000
WHO voluntary fund for health promotion	43,168,946
Bilateral aid	32,246,898
Estimated national expenditures	200,000,000
Total (approximate)	**313,000,000**

Sources: WHO (1980). Based on Basch (1999, Table 14–2).

was whether to use an Indian-produced oral smallpox vaccine to demonstrate self-sufficiency (Bhattacharya 2004).

As outlined in Chapter 11, smallpox campaign chief D.A. Henderson has argued that the total US$313 million expenditure over 10 years of the campaign (more than US$1 billion today) was the best global health investment ever made (Fenner et al. 1988). But other than in South Asia, smallpox was not a leading global health problem on the eve of the campaign. Most importantly, the activities *not* carried out because of smallpox spending—sanitation, housing, and primary care improvements—were not included in this calculation.

The Child Survival Campaigns

As mentioned in Chapter 3, UNICEF launched its "child survival revolution" in 1982, shortly after the Alma-Ata conference. UNICEF described this initiative as a "throw-back to the great disease campaigns of the 1950s [in which] UNICEF now proposed to vanquish common infections of early childhood using simple medical technologies" (UNICEF 1996b).

Four main techniques were employed: growth monitoring (G), oral rehydration therapy (O), breast feeding (B), and immunization (I) against the six vaccine-preventable childhood killers (tuberculosis, diphtheria, whooping cough, tetanus, polio, and measles). Collectively, this approach was known as "GOBI." Later, family planning, female education, and food supplementation were added to the original GOBI, resulting in the acronym GOBI-FFF.

Not withstanding its ambitions, the child survival initiative was narrowly conceived and met with numerous implementation problems. These included: ritualistic growth monitoring without addressing the reasons for poor nutrition; oral rehydration therapy without addressing the underlying causes of diarrhea (i.e., the need to provide clean water and proper sanitation); breast-feeding programs that lacked social support; and centrally controlled, top-down immunization programs that ran contrary to the philosophy of community-based primary health care. The technical orientation of the child survival initiative was also accompanied by a focus on individual behavior change:

> The poor are charged with ignorance and inappropriate behavior, and are asked to change their life-styles to better adjust to the circumstances in which they are embedded. For example, they are asked to adjust to the realities of contaminated water by treating diarrhea, rather than being coached in methods for demanding improved waterworks from their local governments...We should be fully aware of the implications of doing band-aid work where major surgery is needed (Kent 1991, p. 53).

Despite these criticisms, UNICEF has claimed that the child survival strategy contributed to a significant reduction in infant and child mortality in many developing countries (UNICEF 1996b). Yet child mortality declines started in the 1960s and were steepest before 1980—well before the start of UNICEF's child survival campaign (Black, Morris, and Bryce 2003).

Moreover, an estimated 10.6 million children under 5 continue to die annually—most in sub-Saharan Africa and South Asia—from preventable causes such as pneumonia, low birth weight, diarrhea, and, in some regions, malaria and AIDS. Children are more susceptible to illness due to their immature immune systems. This biological fragility is greatly exacerbated by conditions of poverty, which include lack of safe water and sanitation, malnourishment, exposure to indoor air pollution, overcrowding, low quality housing, and inadequate access to primary health care (Victora et al. 2003). Indeed, poverty, poor nutrition, and lack of access to basic services continue to be the major underlying cause of death among children, even as immunization coverage has increased to 79% (UNICEF 2008; GlobalNutritionSeries.org 2008). UNICEF's belated call for a more integrated approach to improving child health (UNICEF 2007a)—while widening the focus of child survival programs—remains overly centered on the delivery of health services and the management of global health programs, rather than on addressing social conditions broadly.

Which Selective Interventions Work and What Is the Evidence?

In the mid 2000s, a highly publicized review titled *Millions Saved: Proven Successes in Global Health*, conducted by the Washington, DC-based Center for Global Development, based its selection of exemplary global health efforts on five criteria (Levine, Group, and Kinder 2004):

1. scale (national, regional, and global);
2. importance (measured by disease burden);
3. impact (measurable impact on population health);
4. duration (programs that functioned for at least 5 years); and
5. cost-effectiveness (using a threshold of US$100 per disability adjusted life year (DALY) saved; see Chapter 5 for an explanation of DALYs).

The authors of the report stated that:

> While some of the improvement in health is the result of overall social and economic gains, about half of it is due to specific efforts to address major causes of disease and disability—such as providing better and more accessible health services, introducing new medicines and other health technologies, and fostering healthier behaviors (Center for Global Development 2004, p. 1).

Of the dozens of cases submitted for consideration by several hundred global health experts, seventeen success stories were identified (with three more added subsequently). These include the eradication of smallpox, HIV prevention in Thailand, TB control in China, reduction of tobacco use in Poland, and measles elimination in southern Africa. In their review, the authors noted six key ingredients of success for global health programs:

1. predictable and adequate funding from both local and international sources;
2. political leadership and champions;
3. affordable technological innovation within an effective delivery system;
4. technical consensus about the appropriate biomedical or public health approach;
5. effective management of health delivery systems; and
6. effective use of information.

These elements of success are hardly a surprise and have been documented previously (Halstead, Walsh, and Warren 1985; Chatora and Tumusiime 2004; MIHR 2005). The question stands: if these ingredients are (self-)evident, why are they not incorporated on a wider scale? Other aspects of the report are also problematic.

On one level, the reliability of the evidence used by *Millions Saved* may be questioned. For example, the claim of successful national TB control in China is inaccurate, even with recent increases in case detection. This is because the Chinese TB program has not extended to poor populations living in rural areas of the country (Jackson et al. 2006). One key issue is that TB treatment costs up to 55% of the annual income of poor households. Another indication that TB control is not reaching marginalized populations is China's high multidrug-resistant TB rate.

Similarly, while the *Millions Saved* report noted that by 2000 there were just 117 measles cases in southern Africa, the WHO *Weekly Epidemiological Record* reported 3,626 clinical cases and 667 confirmed cases in 2005. Although this increase may be the result of a number of factors, such as migration and deteriorating health systems, it demonstrates that even when effective vaccine technology is available, diseases remain subject to social factors.

On another level, *Millions Saved* recounted only part of the highlighted stories of success. For example, it cited the saving of mothers' lives in Sri Lanka—the reduction of maternal mortality by 90% since the 1950s—as attributable to a universal, free health care system with extensive rural coverage, trained midwives, good data for decision making, and targeted efforts to marginalized groups. These are all undoubtedly important factors. What's missing is the *context* of these policies—what enabled them, what sustained them, and what other measures accompanied them. Most of the cited Sri Lankan success in improving maternal mortality took place in an era of redistributive policies under socialist governments, from the country's independence in 1948 until the late 1970s (see ahead). These policies included not just midwife training and free and universal health care services, but also universal education (with one of the highest literacy rates in the world), land reform, economic security measures, concerted efforts at gender equality, universal suffrage since 1931, and much more. (Some of these advances were jeopardized by civil war and privatization starting in the 1980s.)

This dissenting evidence suggests that there is a need to look far more carefully at the mythical success stories of international health and the criteria employed in defining success. Differential effects (e.g., rural–urban, female–male, elites-workers-peasants) must be assessed. Long-term effects (far beyond 5-year success rates) and opportunity costs of targeted programs in the absence of societal approaches also warrant further scrutiny. Most importantly, as we shall explore ahead, the decontextualization of international health successes leads to a biased understanding of what measures work and under what conditions. It is both short-sighted and unscientific to separate narrowly evaluated policy and technical successes from the larger societal and political successes that redistribute power and resources (including access to technical resources) and enable health improvement.

Box 13–1 Scaling Up Versus Building Stairs, Bridges, and Foundations

In recent years the notion of "scaling up"—that is, taking a project from pilot to broad application—has become a popular concept among international health donors. A program is tested out in a local district—for example, directly observed therapy (DOTS) for TB—and when the obstacles are ironed out, it is applied to an entire province or country. This concept suggests a bottom-up model, rather than the widely criticized top-down approach of vertical campaigns. Scaling up is often supported by donors who are ultimately interested in seeing technically-based campaigns (such as DOTS-plus) applied to large regions. A prime concern in scaling up efforts is "absorptive capacity," that is, whether authorities in other regions and at other levels (beyond the pilot program) are able to effectively utilize programs and resources according to donor criteria and rules (de Renzio 2005). For example, the 3 by 5 effort to distribute ARV treatment to millions of people was hamstrung in many countries by limited management capacity, lack of health workers, insufficient diagnostic capacity, and so on, making it very difficult to scale up AIDS treatment (Kim 2004).

In focusing on particular programs, however, the concept of scaling up fails to take into account the larger societal environment in which programs are operating. For example, are local governments broadly representative or do they serve the interests of elites? Are there permanent, comprehensive social services offered to the population or do programs come and go? Are the staff so focused on meeting the evaluation criteria of funders that local needs are secondary? The very metaphor of scaling up—a single being climbing a vertical structure—implies a narrow and

(continued)

Box 13–1 Continued

precarious form of social service delivery. A more politically contextualized metaphor might be "building stairs, bridges, and foundations," which implies that programs are protected, solid, and connected to the larger community. A national, public social welfare system would be the embodiment of such a metaphor.

In a related vein, the upstream/downstream (or distal/proximal) dichotomy has taken on added salience among international public health advocates in recent years, based on the argument that upstream (presumably underlying) factors should be addressed so that problems do not then emerge downstream. While the preventive sentiment in this idea is palpable, the dichotomy is ultimately false. Social conditions are not far away (distal or upstream) for the billions of people who live in precarious housing without plumbing or steady access to water. At the same time, downstream efforts, such as clean stoves and ventilated homes, are vital and inevitably reflect the upstream political context in their design, implementation, dissemination, and reception. As such, explicit discussion of the pathways and distribution of power and resources that affect health at all levels is a more useful guide to designing public health endeavors than choosing between the stark alternatives of upstream/downstream or distal/proximal approaches (Krieger 2008).

Limitations of the Single Disease Campaigns

A number of researchers and international organizations have recognized the limitations of the selective, single disease approach and related vertical programs (i.e., programs that are carried out or supervised, largely or wholly, by a specialized service with its own personnel), as opposed to an integrated, comprehensive approach (Gonzalez 1965; Mills 2005). For example, a UNICEF recount of WHO's malaria campaign stated that it:

> failed because its chief architects misjudged the willingness of humans and malarial mosquitoes to live, eat, sleep and generally behave according to technical assumptions…The most important lesson to be learned from the programs of the 1950s was that the people of Africa, Asia and Latin America were not a blank sheet of paper on which experts from the industrialized world could write their own version of progress (UNICEF 1996a).

In the case of Mexico, the decline of malaria predated the DDT campaign of the late 1950s; moreover, the campaign undermined more comprehensive national public health measures that were already in place, including land reform, education system improvements, strengthened public services, rural development, sanitary measures, and health education, as well as malaria-specific efforts focusing on irrigation, ditch draining, and medical treatment (Gómez-Dantés and Birn 2000).

Regardless of the deficiencies of DDT-based malaria campaigns in different settings, smallpox eradication resurrected the legitimacy of vertical, technically based campaigns. Yet notwithstanding the hailing of the smallpox campaign, the disease-specific approach to international health does little to address overall health or well-being. As soon as one disease is addressed, other problems emerge to replace it. By focusing on one disease at a time, it appears that the population as a whole is getting healthier, even when mortality rates and life expectancy remain unaffected. Attacking diseases one by one—rather than improving the underlying determinants of most ailments—thus becomes an end in itself.

For example, in Box 13–2 health administrators describe the challenges of implementing a vertical TB program in Assam province, India, where the primary health care system is nonfunctional. This case suggests that vertical programming that is successful in the short term may be disruptive in the long-term. Moreover, single disease programs can address one problem, all the while exacerbating another. India's vertical polio eradication program, for example, has led overall immunization coverage to decrease, resulting in an increase in diphtheria cases. Sometimes vertical programs are so narrowly focused that they overlook, or fail to treat, people who present with problems not directly related to the campaign in question (Piller and Smith 2007), missing key opportunities to provide services to populations who otherwise have little access to health care.

Box 13–2 Why Vertical Programs Do Not Work: The Case of TB in Assam

An official in the Revised National TB Control Programme, Assam province, India noted,

> The lack of integration between the TB programme and the general healthcare system is the main reason why the programme has not attained its goals. The PHC health staff do not support the TB programme because it does not offer cash incentives. These vertical programmes are creating distortions, and there is no collaboration in the implementation of programmes (Chinai 2006).

Similarly, a TB program manager reported,

> Our cure rate here is 76%, when it should be 85%. The defaulter rate should not exceed 5%; here it is 11%. The death rate should not exceed 4%; here it is around 7%. The cure rate cannot come down because of the high defaulter and death rates. Our programme largely deals with old cases where erratic treatment under the earlier government programme, or factors such as frequent default rates or irrational treatment through a private practitioner have made a cure difficult to achieve. We are failing to reach out to new cases because of lack of convergence between vertical programs and de-motivated staff within the general healthcare system (ibid).

Another limitation of vertical programs is their focus on "biological transmission control concepts, rather than by the entitlements of citizens to health care" (Devadasan et al. 2007, p. 638). That is, vertical campaigns are based more on biological than infrastructural or social concerns. Vertical programs can also cause distortions in health systems as health care workers are drawn away from primary care to receive training for and staff new disease-specific programs. Meanwhile, their former positions delivering primary care remain unfilled.

Some argue that vertical programming does not necessarily weaken health systems, but instead has a strengthening effect. The polio eradication program in Latin America, according to *Millions Saved*, bolstered infrastructure and surveillance systems. Similarly, the river blindness program in central and east Africa increased access to primary health care, and the volunteers in Nepal who distributed vitamin A were later involved in a number of other programs such as deworming (Center for Global Development 2004).

Despite these instances of successful vertical programs, *Millions Saved* acknowledged that several important causes of morbidity and mortality remain significant challenges. These include: the impact of inequality on health outcomes (99% of childhood deaths are in developing countries, concentrated among the poorest population sectors); the high rates of HIV/AIDS, particularly in sub-Saharan Africa; the decrease in the rate of improvement in child health during the past 20 years, largely due to deaths that are preventable and treatable; and the rapid increase of cardiovascular and chronic diseases in all countries, but especially in developing countries (Levine 2007).

In sum, "the longer we isolate public health's technical aspects from its political and social aspects, the longer technical interventions will squeeze out one side of the mortality balloon only to find it inflated elsewhere" (Birn 2005, p. 519). Ultimately "No health system in the world is actually built on 'vertical' programs" (Maciocco and Italian Global Health Watch 2008, p. 47). Yet international health

---

Box 13-3 Limits to Technical Approaches to International Health

The Bill and Melinda Gates Foundation's "Grand Challenges in Global Health" initiative illustrates the limits of reductionist technical approaches. The initiative was launched in 2003 to stimulate scientific researchers to develop "solutions to critical scientific and technological problems that, if solved, could lead to important advances against diseases of the developing world" (http://www.gcgh.org/channels/gcgh). Notwithstanding the need for scientific solutions to be integrated with the societal determinants of health, the Gates Foundation "turned to a narrowly conceived understanding of health as the product of technical interventions divorced from economic, social, and political contexts" (Birn 2005, p. 515). The Grand Challenges deliberately excluded integrated social-scientific approaches to target major public health problems, instead focusing on technical efforts such as vector control, vaccine innovation, and drug treatment.

Analysis of one of the 14 Grand Challenges, "improv[ing] nutrition to improve public health," shows why decontextualized technical approaches are misguided. This Grand Challenge entails:

creat[ing] a full range of optimal, bioavailable nutrients in a single staple plant species" (http://www.gcgh.org/channels/gcgh). According to such an approach, "the malnutrition problem in the developing world could disappear with no need to produce and distribute more than a single crop in any particular region. The glitch: reliance on a single crop is a recipe for disaster. Such reliance on potato production to improve caloric intake and agricultural efficiency—and reserve large tracks of arable land for export-oriented agriculture—resulted in the devastating 1840s Irish potato famine, which either killed or forced emigration on a quarter of the population (Birn 2005, p. 516).

(continued)

Box 13–3 Continued

Few in the world would choose a single fortified staple for every meal or feed their children micronutrients instead of fruits, vegetables, and protein. Moreover, there is consensus on the part of nutritionists that a well-balanced diet should draw from all food groups. If this is the global standard, why should it not apply to all people? Yet the Grand Challenges approach to nutrition is promoted as a promising breakthrough for the world's poor. It also overlooks:

> key distributional questions. Many of the regions with the worst malnutrition problems—such as Central America, the Andes, East Africa, and India—have extremely fertile growing conditions and produce some of the world's most nutritious fruits and crops. As Nobel-winning economist Amartya Sen has demonstrated, malnutrition and famine are not caused by technical roadblocks but rather by political and economic ones: local populations are priced out of their food entitlement due to poor income distribution and market shifts, such as production for export, that have little to do with food supply or nutritional content (Birn 2005, p. 516).

Individually and as a whole, the Grand Challenges—like most of the Gates Foundation's initiatives—share an assumption that scientific and technical aspects of health improvement can be separated from political, social, and economic aspects. Ultimately, goals such as new vaccine development or connecting schools to the internet—in the absence of better living and working conditions and democratic decision-making processes—remain technological quick fixes, yielding no permanent or broadly shared improvements in human well-being. Without taking social and political realities into account, the Gates Foundation's patronage of even the most powerful technologies cannot meet its stated goal of reducing inequalities in health.

efforts, such as the Global Fund and those cited by *Millions Saved*, continue to operate on this premise.

The limitations of vertical programming point to the need for more comprehensive strategies. The next section focuses on "healthy societies," demonstrating how holistic and integrated approaches, grounded in political economy understandings, can achieve significant and sustainable health gains.

HEALTHY SOCIETIES: CASE STUDIES

As discussed in Chapters 4 and 7, the determinants of health are complex. They cannot be addressed adequately through unidimensional interventions, even when medicines and vaccines are available, nor through a sole focus on the behavior of individuals. The largest set of healthy societies are high-income, industrialized nations. However, these countries do not provide uniform levels of protection and health; they vary based on the structures of power and distribution of resources. And, strikingly, a number of developing countries have achieved welfare states, and health levels, comparable to those of much wealthier settings.

Developed Welfare States

Industrialized countries with egalitarian and redistributive welfare states based on universal social rights have better health outcomes than those with more liberal welfare states, where protections are based on particular, often tightly targeted, policies that may come and go with different administrations. The solidity of social welfare structures established in social democratic states means that even occasional conservative governments continue to provide broad protection to their populations (see Table 13–2). What accounts for good health in these countries?

Navarro and his colleagues found that political parties in power in OECD countries subscribing to social democratic principles—for the study period between 1950 and 1998—had greater success in reducing infant mortality rates than did other political parties in power (Navarro et al. 2003). Chung and Muntaner similarly compared four types of welfare states by two health indicators—infant mortality and low birth weight—between 1960 and 1994 (Chung and Muntaner 2007) and determined that countries with social democratic traditions had significantly better health outcomes than liberal-corporatist, wage-earner, and Christian democratic welfare states (see Chapter 12 for clarification of these terms). These indicators reflect social, economic, and cultural factors, including redistributive social benefits, such as family cash benefits and family services (Tanaka 2005). Additional studies have found that women and adolescents in strong social welfare states (especially in Scandinavia) have better health levels than their counterparts in states that have higher dependence on the market and individual contributions to social welfare (Raphael and Bryant 2004; Zambon et al. 2006).

Sweden, in particular, has a long history of addressing the societal determinants of health, yielding positive results in its health indicators (see Table 13–2) and its Human Development Index of 0.956 in 2005 (sixth in the world ranking) (UNDP 2005). The Swedish welfare state has explicitly tackled the socioeconomic gradient, discrimination, and living conditions and promoted meaningful and equitable citizen participation at all levels of public life (Vallgårda 2007). Despite having achieved one of the lowest levels of health inequities in the world, Sweden remains highly concerned about persistent social inequalities in health. The most recent public health strategy focuses on the health of the most vulnerable groups in Swedish society, with the overall aim of "creat[ing] social conditions that will ensure good health for the entire population" (Government of Sweden 2007, p. 1),

Table 13–2 Mortality Rates for Selected Welfare States

Country	Infant Mortality Rate/1,000 Live Births (2006)	Under-5 Mortality/1,000 Live Births (2006)	Maternal Mortality/100,000 Live Births (2005)
Denmark and Sweden	3	4	3
Norway	3	4	7
United Kingdom	5	6	8
Uruguay	13	15	20

Source: WHO (2008b).

including universal social security, healthier and safer working conditions and environments, extensive public transport, the fostering of good nutrition, and reduced use of tobacco, alcohol, and illicit drugs (through regulation and restrictions), as well as the provision of medical care and protection from communicable diseases.

What sets some welfare states apart from others? Key features of welfare states are redistribution of resources and social safety nets—social assistance for the vulnerable, including paid maternity leave for all pregnant women, "old age" security, health services, housing or income support, unemployment subsidies, and other benefits provided universally or as necessary. Resources are pooled and provided for all based on need—rather than ability to pay—with significant cross-subsidization deriving from the principles of universalism and solidarity. Such comprehensive approaches, rather than single technical interventions applied in isolation, have a broad impact.

Developing Welfare States: Costa Rica, Cuba, Sri Lanka, Uruguay, and Kerala State, India

Unlike the countries referred to in the section above, Costa Rica, Cuba, Sri Lanka, Uruguay, and Kerala State, India are underdeveloped settings. While there are many differences among them, they all share one feature: significantly better health outcomes than one would expect given their level of development (i.e., GDP/capita) (see Table 13–3). The importance of these cases lies precisely in their ability to

Table 13–3 Data on Selected Determinants of Health and Mortality Rates for Three Developing Countries and the United States

	Costa Rica	Cuba	Sri Lanka	United States
% population using improved drinking water sources (2006)	98	91	82	99
% population using adequate sanitation facilities (2006)	96	98	86	100
Net primary school enrollment/ attendance (2006)	92	97	97	92
Total adult literacy rate (2000–2005)	95	100	91	99
Infant mortality rate/1,000 live births (2006)	11	5	11	6
Under-5 mortality/1,000 live births (2006)	12	7	13	8
Adjusted maternal mortality ratio (deaths/100,000 live births) (2005)	30	45	58	11
Total health services expenditure per capita, per year (2006) (U.S. international dollar rate)	742	363	213	6,714
GNI per capita (2006) (US$)	4,980	1,170	1,300	44,970

Sources: UNICEF (2007a); WHO (2008b); WHO and UNICEF (2008).

show sustained declines in mortality and other health indicators. Not fitting neatly into the welfare state categories developed for industrialized countries, they may be considered, in the case of Costa Rica, Uruguay, and Sri Lanka, state protectionist (Martínez Franzoni 2008) and in the case of Cuba and Kerala, socialist and communist. Together they provide bona fide models for the level of social protection that can be achieved in low-income settings.

Costa Rica

Costa Rica, with a population of 4.13 million people, is perhaps best known for its lack of armed forces, burgeoning ecotourism industry, and universal health care system. With no significant expenditure on arms or the military since the late 1940s, resources have been freed up for other functions of government, especially the provision of basic social services. Costa Rica's economy was traditionally based on the export of primary products, mostly bananas and coffee. Like other developing economies, it was dependent on fluctuating commodity prices set by international markets. Unlike most others, however, Costa Rica developed a comprehensive welfare state in the 1940s and now has the highest universal coverage and scope of services of all Latin America (Martínez Franzoni 2007).

In the 1960s, Costa Rica began to develop its manufacturing capacity and to export goods to the Central American Common Market. Although the economic crisis of the 1980s led to severe recession in Costa Rica, the country (with considerable foreign assistance) continued to invest in social services and the public health sector—particularly primary health care—thus maintaining gains made in infant mortality and health status (Mesa-Lago 1985; Morgan 1987). Also notable is that high health indicators have been achieved with modest health spending—US$305 per capita (WHO 2006)—the latter stabilized by the central role of payroll taxes (rather than other income taxes and revenue sources) in funding health care services. Today, Costa Ricans enjoy the longest life expectancy in the Americas, after Canadians.

To what can one ascribe these health gains in Costa Rica? At the level of organization of health services, several features of the system stand out including: publicly provided services (rather than services contracted out to the private sector); a single public insurer; no purchaser-provider split or autonomy for hospital managers; and the fact that users of health services are involved in the management of services (Unger et al. 2007).

Other factors are also key, such as Costa Rica's ability to partially resist neoliberal reforms when its economy faltered (i.e., fending off privatization of social service provision), although the quality and funding for some services deteriorated markedly at this time (Seligson and Martínez Franzoni 2009). Still, Costa Rica's emphasis on the principles of collectivism and worker solidarity, and the state's prioritization of human development (with high levels of literacy and gender-empowerment)—all part of Costa Rica's long tradition of social protection—have helped cushion it against the worst hardships of recent economic crises (Martínez Franzoni 2008).

Cuba

Cuba is a socialist country whose commitment to redistributive policies was forged following its 1959 revolution, at the height of the Cold War. The revolution spurred nationalization of productive assets and extended broad social welfare protections to all Cubans. Under Fidel Castro's almost half-century watch, the government prioritized the provision of social services—water, sanitation, housing, health, and education—to all. This safety net remained intact even after the USSR's demise in 1991 plunged the country into an economic crisis, adding to the burden of trade sanctions imposed by the United States. The impact of Cuba's investment in education, health, and other social services are palpable in its positive health outcomes. As seen in Table 13–3, Cuba's infant and under-5 mortality rates are better than those of the United States, which spends significantly more per capita on health and has a GDP/capita almost 40 times that of Cuba (WHO 2006). Box 13–4 suggests a range of factors that help explain the health status of Cubans, including the role of citizen participation.

The "special period in peacetime"—the term used for the period of severe oil shortages and economic crisis in the 1990s—heralded various health-enhancing policies, such as local food production. Prior to the early 1990s, most Cuban cities

---

Box 13–4 Factors Contributing to the Success of Cuba's Social Services

Even a World Bank review admitted that Cuba's success derived at least partially from the following (with points 1 and 3 almost the exact *opposite* of standard World Bank advice):

1. The public sector is dominant and health is a government priority.
2. Cuba's social policy objectives have remained unchanged since 1960.
3. Government spends a relatively large part of the GDP on health, and this spending remained high, even during the mid-1990s crisis, at the expense of defense.
4. Cuba has demonstrated a remarkable capacity to mobilize the population, and community participation is rather well ensured.
5. Policies are based on comprehensive monitoring and evaluation, backed up with quality data.

Source: Adapted from Erikson, Lord, and Wolf (2002), cited in de Vos, de Ceukelaire, and van der Stuyft (2006, p. 1609).

---

were heavily dependent on the rural sector and foreign imports for food security. However, after Cuba's favored trade relationship with the USSR ended, the island lost over half of its oil, fertilizer, and pesticide imports. Many families had difficulty meeting their immediate food needs and the average daily caloric intake per person dropped to 1,863 calories and 46g of protein—74% and 61% of recognized basic needs (Cruz and Medina 2003).

To combat food shortages, Cuba's Ministry of Agriculture created the world's first public urban agriculture program, coordinating: access to land; technical support services to farmers; research and development; new supply stores with tools and agricultural inputs for small farmers and urban residents; sale points for growers; and new marketing schemes (Murphy 1999; Perez Rojas and Vila 1998). Laws banning the use of chemical pesticides within city limits were also passed, leading gardeners to rely almost exclusively on organic fertilizers, including chicken or cow manure, compost from household food waste, and, occasionally, worms. By 1995, thanks to civic and governmental efforts, the food shortage was largely overcome, and Cuba is now seen as a global leader in urban and sustainable agriculture (Warwick 1999; Rosset 2000; Food First 2003; Alleson 2005). Urban gardens, which occupy more than 1,000 hectares in Havana, produce 60% of all the vegetables that are consumed in Cuba (Cruz 2001) and have created approximately 100,000 jobs in the city (Cruz and Medina 2003). Additionally, Havana residents now have access to a more nutritious and diverse diet than before the "special period." Even with the resignation of Castro and signs of Cuba's opening to the global market, its population enjoys the health legacy of the country's broad social investments.

If Cuba has been so successful in improving the health of its people, why was it not included as a case study in *Millions Saved* and why have other developing and middle-income countries not followed suit? Politics, to be sure! The ability of Cuba to maintain its health gains in the face of harsh economic conditions and in spite of a longstanding U.S. trade embargo, indicates that it is Cuba's socialist redistributive and collective policies that have enabled the health gains made since the Cuban Revolution and ensured their sustainability (Spiegel and Yassi 2004).

Sri Lanka

Sri Lanka is another underdeveloped country that has achieved significant improvements in the health of its population (see Table 13–3), having adopted collective social policies over the past seven decades. This is despite a meager US$31 per capita spent on health care services (WHO 2006). Infant and child mortality are low, and the country has a relatively high life expectancy of 74 years at birth (UNICEF 2007b). Though the UNDP attributes these achievements to district-level health care services (UNDP 2005), the explanatory factors are far more comprehensive. They include: high levels of autonomy for women and gender equality; universal right to vote; free education; high levels of female literacy; provision of subsidized rice; well-developed water and sanitation systems; and a publicly funded health system based on the principles of equity and efficiency with no user fees, which protects against illness-induced impoverishment (McNay, Keith, and Penrose 2006; Russell and Gilson 2006).

Maternal mortality—while higher than in Cuba and Costa Rica—is also lower than in most developing countries, as a result of free health care, commitment to female education, increased use of antenatal and natal services provided by publicly trained midwives, integration of family planning into the maternal health program, and a well-functioning health information system. All of these factors, in turn, are reflective of the broader claims made on the state (outlined above) beginning with universal suffrage in the 1930s (Fernando, Jayatilleka, and Karunaratna 2003).

These achievements in health and social policy have largely persisted through more than two decades of civil war, which has resulted in significant loss of life, injuries, displacement, and loss of revenues for social services. Understanding why this is the case may provide lessons for other conflict situations. Certainly public investment in social welfare has historically been supported by the majority of Sri Lanka's population since long before the civil war began in 1983 (Meegama 1986). Moreover, demand for social services remains high—even in northeastern Sri Lanka, where the conflict is concentrated, education, health, and other services continue to be supported by all parties. Still, the war and, especially, two decades of neoliberal cutbacks are taking their toll on Sri Lankan social services, which remain nominally universal but have deteriorated considerably in terms of equity and public funding.

Uruguay

Several other countries have effectively augmented social protection policies in the wake of political and economic crises. In just 16 years (1990–2006), after a brutal dictatorship in the 1970s and 1980s, Uruguay was able to build on its welfare state tradition and reduce the infant mortality rate by half, from 20 deaths/1,000 live births to 11/1,000 (UNICEF 2007a). More recently, following a sustained economic crisis and inadequate resources for social services in the early 2000s, Uruguay's newly elected social democratic government implemented a national Plan de Atención Nacional a la Emergencia Social (PANES—Plan to Address the Social Emergency) in 2005. When PANES took effect, one-third of the population lived in poverty and/or were without stable employment; over half of all children were born into poverty; 10% of Uruguayans had no health coverage; and over 50% of workers lacked social security benefits. PANES sought to address these issues from a human rights perspective with three main objectives:

1. to guarantee access to the basic necessities for the most vulnerable households;
2. to develop an integrated and participatory social plan to lift people out of poverty; and
3. to create structural opportunities for full social inclusion for all families participating in PANES.

Concretely, PANES provided the poorest households (8% of the population, half of whom were categorized as indigent) with a monthly stipend; increased public sector employment; furnished nutritional support, health promotion activities, and sanitation improvements; provided assistance to people living on the streets; and funded the improvement of housing in informal settlements. A year after it was initiated, PANES had reached 80,000 households, created 7,100 jobs, reduced unemployment by 12%, and provided 40,000 pregnant women with nutritional supplementation (Gobierno de Uruguay 2006). Within 2 years, the country's rate of extreme poverty was cut by more than half. By the end of 2007, school attendance had significantly increased and child employment decreased for those aged 6 to 13 years old (Amarante, Burdín, and Vigorito 2007).

While some of these improvements were related to overall economic recovery, Uruguay's dual focus of strengthening welfare protection through family stipends and an increased minimum wage (Arim, Vigorito, and Salas 2006), combined with targeted support for the most vulnerable, has helped the country return to its position as one of the *least unequal* countries in Latin America, with associated benefits for health and well-being. In 2008 Uruguay began implementing a new equity plan that redistributes more income to poor families with children by reforming the current family allowance system (initially implemented in 1943). This transformation of PANES into a family wage has a much wider target, starting with 20% of the population and aiming to cover over half the country's 500,000 children by 2009 (Borgia 2008).

Kerala State, India

Although not a country, the case of Kerala warrants examination in the context of health and social welfare developments. Kerala is a southern Indian state of approximately 32 million people. One of the poorest states in the country, it has a per capita income of less than US$3,000 (Government of Kerala 2005). Despite its relative poverty, Kerala is an anomaly within India and other developing settings because of its good health outcomes relative to its level of economic development (see Table 13–4 and Chapter 11). The reasons for this success are multifactorial, but most agree that the history of organized political struggle for social and economic rights in the country are partly, if not largely, responsible. Voter turnout in Kerala is high, and a large proportion of the population is engaged in civic activity. Kerala is one of the few regions in the world where a communist party has been elected in democratic parliamentary elections. For most of the past 40 years, Kerala has been run by the (Marxist) Communist Party of India. Although it has no health subcommittee, the party perspective is that all societal factors affect health in some way.

UNICEF has found that Kerala, Barbados, Botswana, Costa Rica, Cuba, the Republic of Korea, Malaysia, Mauritius, and Sri Lanka all have better health and education outcomes than neighboring locales with similar levels of income. These countries and regions share several key characteristics: state (rather than market) sponsored social services; education spending in excess of spending in neighboring

Table 13–4 Selected Health Outcomes, Kerala and India

	Kerala	India
Infant mortality rate (2000)	14/1,000	71/1,000
Life expectancy at birth	74.6 (2000)	63.3 (2003)
Human Development Index (2003)	0.773	0.602

Source: Government of Kerala (2005).

countries; high teacher–pupil ratios; free primary schooling; and universal primary school enrollment (UNICEF 1999). Kerala's health outcomes also result from subsidized staple foods, the elimination of absentee farm landlords, the redistribution of land to small farmers and landless laborers, as well as large social investments in health, infrastructure, agricultural credits, and housing (Franke and Chasin 1992; Parayil 1996).

Box 13–5 Creating Healthy Societies through Cooperation: Health Alliance International

On occasion, an international health organization can help contribute to the making of a healthy society, but such an effort requires commitment and adherence to principles of solidarity.

Over the past three decades members of the organization Health Alliance International (HAI), mostly from the United States, have worked to promote public health and social justice in Mozambique, with a shared commitment to strengthening public infrastructure and the national health system.

Following Mozambique's independence in 1975, the Ministry of Health (MOH) developed a comprehensive national plan to rapidly expand health care to its rural population, despite scarce human and financial resources—including only 40 physicians for 11 million people. In the late 1970s numerous foreign physicians and public health advocates moved to Mozambique to support the new socialist government's ambitious primary health care plans. As *cooperantes*, they worked as MOH employees paid at local rates and accountable to local authorities. Though widely supported, the country's social programs were soon undermined by a 14-year proxy war backed by South Africa's apartheid government. Health infrastructure and personnel became military targets.

In 1987, at the request of the Mozambican government, a group of North American *cooperantes* came together to form the Mozambique Health Committee, which would later become HAI. The organization was formed to support the rebuilding of severely damaged health infrastructure. In the 1980s and 1990s, HAI continued to support the MOH to strengthen the provision of primary care in the central provinces of Manica and Sofala through technical assistance and material support. By this time, the country was faced with new threats to the health system including structural adjustment programs and privatization.

Starting in 2003, the Mozambican MOH was one of the first countries in Africa to initiate a national HIV treatment program, and HAI has been a strong advocate for and partner in this effort. Currently, as Mozambique has experienced a huge influx of foreign aid that has further stretched the MOH's management capacity and already inadequate workforce, HAI has moved into the realm of advocacy. One of its key advocacy efforts has been to lead a group of NGOs in the development of an International NGO Code of Conduct for Health System Strengthening to call for organizations to "do no harm" and support ministries of health in their role as leaders of the health sector (see Chapter 14). HAI's involvement in Mozambique's government-purveyed primary health care efforts serves as an important counterexample to the prevailing model of NGOs competing against or displacing publicly provided health services (Fort 2008).

Kerala's accomplishments build upon female empowerment in at least four forms: significant investments in girls' education; high levels of women's political participation; high rates of female employment; and a relatively advanced age of first marriage (similar to Sri Lanka). These factors have led to greater acknowledgement and protection of the rights of women (UNICEF 2001); unlike the rest of India, Kerala has low levels of abortion of female fetuses. Kerala was also the first region in the world to be declared "baby-friendly" by the WHO and UNICEF.

In the political realm, a number of initiatives have increased female participation in civil society, including microenterprise investment, savings clubs, antipoverty programs, and localized decision making and planning. Women's enhanced participation in decentralized planning processes has also taken place through the Campaign for People's Planning initiated in 1996 (Isaac and Franke 2002; Kadiyala 2004; Muraleedharan 2005), which has a major focus on health equity (Elamon and Ekbal 2004).

Despite its historic success, Kerala—and its social solidarity measures—are currently under assault in the context of privatization and deregulation (Thankappan 2001; Varatharajan, Thankappan, and Jayapalan 2004). Analyzing and disseminating the elements of Kerala's long-term achievements can serve as a useful step toward preserving them.

These examples illustrate that even in resource-constrained settings, welfare states with comprehensive social programs can, in a relatively short period of time, bring about large health and social justice gains. At the same time, following the pressures on public social spending of recent decades, the welfare state architecture across the world needs renewal, taking into account concepts of solidarity (Filgueira 2007). Several efforts in Latin America are seeking to face these challenges.

Latin American Social Medicine in Action: Porto Alegre, Brazil; Mexico City, Mexico; and Misión Barrio Adentro, Venezuela

Three recent examples of innovative social interventions that focus on systemic changes have their roots in Latin American Social Medicine (LASM), a movement almost a century old that was founded on the ideas of Rudolf Virchow of Germany and Salvador Allende of Chile and institutionalized by Belgian hygienist René Sand. Sand—who worked for the Rockefeller Foundation's International Health Board and was later appointed Professor of Social Medicine at Brussels University—is credited with creating an academic discipline out of social medicine during the 1920s and 1930s, and with supporting the establishment of social medicine as a field of study at the University of San Marcos in Lima, Peru and at the Oswaldo Cruz Institute in Rio de Janeiro in Brazil (Cueto 1999; Porter 2006).

LASM is based on the "economic, political, subjective, and social determinants of the health-disease-care process of human collectivities" (Tajer 2003, p. 2023). LASM became an important regional movement, as institutionalized in various schools of public health in Chile, Brazil, and elsewhere and especially through the work of committed health professionals who organized nationally and regionally to fight for better health. As Waitzkin and his colleagues show,

Social medicine in Latin America has emerged as a sometimes dangerous but very productive field of work. A focus on the social origins of illness and early death inherently challenges the relationships of economic and political power in Latin America. As a result, participation in social medicine has led to suffering and even death for some of the movement's most talented and productive adherents (Waitzkin et al. 2001, pp. 1599–1600).

Regionwide, the organizational expression of LASM is the *Asociación Latinoamericana de Medicina Social* (ALAMES), established in 1984.

Box 13–6 ALAMES's Guiding Principles and Key Aspects of its Political Agenda

Principles:

- Health is a prized asset of human beings; for health to be a reality requires a radical defense of life and well-being.
- Health is a human and social right and a public good; this places a duty on the state to guarantee it and on society the responsibility to demand it.
- Health, as a public good and human right, must be detached from the logic of the marketplace.
- Addressing health inequities is an ethical imperative; it involves changes in the social, economic, political, environmental, and cultural determinants of health as well as the recognition that the diversity of health needs must be considered in the design of social and institutional responses.

Political Agenda:

- Demand social policies that affect the structural determinants of health.
- Ensure the health of workers, defending and building upon the rights they have already acquired.
- Demand the consolidation and construction of universal and free health systems.
- Defend the right to health in the face of war, militarization, and violence.
- Demand that health inequality be eliminated with urgent and diverse public programs which include prevention, protection, education, curative, and rehabilitative assistance, as well as the organization and management of health services in such a way as to expand organized social participation and the effective control of the state by society.
- Promote alliances for a radical defense of life among movements working for the rights to health, water, food security and land, the environment, and gender equality, and the rights of indigenous and Afro-American populations, among others.

Source: Torres Tovar (2007). Courtesy of *Social Medicine/Medicina Social*.

Mexico City, Mexico

A recent example of how social medicine principles can be put into practice has taken place in Mexico City. Despite the 2000 election of a right-wing federal government that implemented neoliberal policies, the social democratic government of Mexico City, elected at the same time, has implemented comprehensive and redistributive policies to address the inequities among population and geographic groups. The city's Integrated Territorial Social Program is based on four tenets: the right of the municipal population to social benefits; large-scale and universal social programs; progressive income redistribution; and a collective, rather than targeted, focus (Laurell 2003). The program aims for universal coverage, with the poorest sectors of the city reached first.

Box 13–7 Components of Mexico City's Integrated Territorial Social Program

· Housing and neighborhood renewal.
· Scholarships for children of single mothers.
· Free breakfast in public schools.
· Compensation for increased milk prices.
· Economic aid for the disabled.
· Job training scholarships.
· Micro credits for household production.
· Funding to peasants for the protection of remaining rural areas.
· Pensions and health care for senior citizens.

Source: Adapted from Laurell (2007).

In 2001, the city introduced pensioner programs (food support and free health care, including the provision of medicines) as the first step toward universal pensions for the elderly. By the end of 2002, almost all those aged 70 years and older were enrolled in the program. In 2005, the city established a system of health surveillance, including home visits for the elderly.

A second program targeted those without health insurance and provided free health care and pharmaceuticals to families. By mid-2006, 94% of eligible families were enrolled in the free health care and pharmaceuticals program. To fund these programs, the city government implemented a range of measures to eliminate corruption, tax evasion, and inefficiencies, including reduction in salaries of top officials. The municipal government now spends about 10% of total expenditure on health with a budget increase of 59% between 2000 and 2005 (Laurell 2007).

Other policies adopted include resource allocation based on equity and a new model for service delivery based on the primary health care approach. There is also a focus on community participation in planning and supervising program activities. Community concerns have been documented in 137 local plans. Significantly, health personnel have been trained to work with local communities to generate these plans.

Broadly and simultaneously implemented, these measures have, according to preliminary evidence, contributed to lower death rates, including reductions in maternal mortality and mortality from AIDS. Rapid declines in infectious and nutrition-related diseases have also been documented. However, as throughout Mexico, the rate of chronic diseases has increased (Laurell 2007), bringing new challenges for the local government.

Porto Alegre, Brazil

Porto Alegre, Brazil offers another example of collective action based on social medicine principles. In 1989, the city began a participatory budgeting process that allows citizens to set priorities for an important proportion of municipal resources. Participatory budgeting extends the usual form of representative democracy by directly engaging citizens in determining their needs—hence it is called a "new form of citizenship." Participatory budgeting is based on four principles: "redirecting public resources for the benefit of the poorest; creating a new relationship between municipalities and citizens (i.e., a new form of governance); rebuilding social ties and social interest; and inventing a new democratic culture and promoting active citizenship" (Lieberherr 2003, p. 1). In essence, both representative and participatory democracy principles are at work in Porto Alegre. Municipal government is comprised of formally elected representatives and is complemented by elected district delegates who participate in many capacities, including the budgeting process.

Most analysts of the Porto Alegre experiment have praised its inclusiveness of a wide range of citizen groups—in particular, poor segments of the population. The Porto Alegre experience was honored as an exemplary urban innovation at the UN Summit on Human Settlements in 1996. According to Wagle and Shah, it "stood out for demonstrating an efficient practice of democratic resource management" (Wagle and Shah 2003, p. 1).

The participatory budget process has benefited the citizens of Porto Alegre in a number of ways. In the first 10 years (1989–1999) more than US$700 million was invested in public works, largely for the provision of water and sanitation. Spending on social services, including health, education, housing, and welfare, increased from 91.2 million reais in 1989 to 361.6 million in 2000. In addition, school dropout rates decreased from 9% in 1989 to 1.46% in 2000 (Menegat 2002). Between 1989 and 1996, there was an increase from 80% to 98% of households with access to water services; a jump from 46% to 85% of people with access to the sewerage system; a doubling of the number of children enrolled in schools; 30 km of roads paved annually in the poorest neighborhoods; and a 50% increase in tax revenues (Wagle and Shah 2003).

Various observers argue that the participatory process in Porto Alegre is "self-reinforcing... when neighbors discovered that others got their streets paved or a new bus stop they wondered why. The simple answer was that only the beneficiary had gone to budget meetings" (Goldsmith and Vainier 2001, p. 2). This suggests that the concrete outcomes of involvement resulted in dramatic increases in participation. In 2000, the budgeting process involved an extraordinary 30,000 citizens (Menegat 2002).

Misión Barrio Adentro, Venezuela

Arguably the best recent example of LASM as an international health endeavor is Venezuela's "Misión Barrio Adentro," an alternative model to neoliberal health reforms. In the early 2000s President Hugo Chávez initiated a series of reforms, launched by a new 1999 constitution declaring health to be a human right guaranteed by the state; that the health system should be publicly funded with free health care at the point of delivery; and that health promotion and prevention should be prioritized (Muntaner et al. 2006). Misión Barrio Adentro was founded as a community–national–international mechanism to meet these constitutional obligations.

Launched in 2003 at the behest of the mayor and constituents of one of Caracas's poorest neighborhoods (*barrios*) who were fed up with incessantly delayed government promises for health care and Venezuelan doctors' refusal to serve them, Misión Barrio Adentro turns the principles of international health cooperation upside down. Rather than an international agency selecting the activity and setting the terms of cooperation, community-level committees—now throughout the country—host over 14,000 Cuban doctors and dentists to live in their neighborhoods and serve as their practitioners following a principle of solidarity (at a popular level) and exchange (at the level of the state—i.e., Cuban doctors for Venezuelan oil) rather than aid (Jardim 2005). These doctors are not privileged short-term consultants, but rather eat and sleep in the same shantytown dwellings where they practice.

The bona fide "bottom-up" approach of Barrio Adentro emphasizes participatory democracy and management covering a wide range of areas, including housing, education, employment, and neighborhood improvement. Thus far, barrio-dwellers have evaluated the open-ended health program to be a great success by the simplest of measures: before they had no primary care services and now they do. Over 3,200 popular health clinics have been built in the program's first 5 years, with almost 9,000 popular health committees created (Armada et al. 2009). As of 2006, virtually the entire population has access to primary health care and dental care thanks to Barrio Adentro, a more than doubling of access to quality primary care in just 3 years (Pan American Health Organization 2006). Over the long term, the enormously popular Barrio Adentro program aims to strengthen access to primary health care by improving health care infrastructure and increasing training of Venezuelan doctors from poor barrios so dependence on foreign doctors diminishes. A further challenge arises from the need to fully institutionalize Barrio Adentro and integrate it with the existing state public health system. To date, Barrio Adentro has been associated with infant mortality improvements that went from 21.3 deaths/1,000 live births in 1998 to 13 deaths/1,000 births in 2007, simultaneous to a halving of poverty rates and significant increases in preschool and primary school attendance, among other indicators (Alvarado et al. 2008).

As one woman from Catia, a large slum in Caracas, noted:

> I think it is something great, really the best thing that has happened here in Venezuela... I think Barrio Adentro is a good way of doing things because the services are actually in the [neighbor]'hoods supporting people who truly need them...Never before had we seen a doctor come to a barrio to provide care. And we have learned a lot—at least in terms of organizing ourselves as a community. We are helping one another and our neighbors (Catia resident, 2005).

These national, state, and citywide examples reveal a number of common threads. First, grassroots organizing and bottom-up representation in the political process are key to making the voices of poor and marginalized groups heard. Second, collective commitment to social justice and equity and comprehensive approaches are critical to ensuring a healthy population. Finally, a key strategy to achieve such a commitment is social action. Such action is often easier to achieve at the local level, as shown in the next section.

Box 13–8 A Critique of "Pro-Poor" Approaches to Policy Making: Why Not Antipoverty Instead?

So-called pro-poor policies are at the center of development initiatives aimed at poverty reduction. By definition, these policies are targeted to "the poor" and aim at lifting them out of poverty. Examples of pro-poor policies include cash transfers to the poorest households, the provision of free or highly subsidized water and electricity to the poor, free health care for the poor, and so on. At first glance such policies appear to make sense, but if one considers both the contexts in which pro-poor polices are applied as well as their practical implementation, a number of problems become apparent.

Pro-poor programs are typically designed without a clear understanding of why people are poor—that is, what national (e.g., access to land, education, employment opportunities) and international conditions (e.g., trade barriers) create poverty in the first place.

From a methodological perspective, a pro-poor approach assumes that one is able to identify the poor (often the poorest of the poor) in every society. Yet the marginalized poor are by definition hard to reach, living in remote or precarious areas, sometimes moving frequently from place to place, and often not captured in social services registries or surveys. In many countries, the most marginalized groups, including refugees and undocumented workers, may not have proof of identity, nationality, or residence and may fear deportation, discrimination, or punishment (see Chapter 7). Second, from an operational point of view, such a strategy requires significant administrative capacity to implement—capacity which does not always exist and therefore requires new investments.

Even if the poor are identified, social programs may not reach them, as has been shown across the developing world, where health programs targeted to the poor disproportionately benefit those who are better-off (Gwatkin, Wagstaff, and Yazbeck 2005). When they do reach poor populations, health and social programs are often insufficient. For example, 6 L of free water are provided per *household* per day in South Africa, far less than the WHO-recommended 20 L per *person* per day (Dugard 2007). It is also key to recognize that health is not necessarily a local priority, especially in poor villages where roads, employment, housing, and so on can be far more important. As discussed throughout this text, policies outside the health or social services sector have a major impact on poverty and health outcomes but are usually excluded from pro-poor efforts.

Why do so many pro-poor policies not benefit the poor? Perhaps the most important reason is that the poor are rarely given the chance to participate in decisions affecting them, regarding what policies will best meet their needs, and how various interventions should be delivered. Unequal societies create poverty, and people are poor because the societies in which they live are unequal. What is necessary, therefore, are social policies that reduce societal inequalities, which in turn require political struggle to challenge the power of vested interests in the status quo (Johnson and Start 2001).

HEALTHY PUBLIC POLICY: HEALTH PROMOTION, THE HEALTHY CITIES PROGRAM, AND GREEN CITIES

Health Promotion

Health is experienced "by people within the settings of their everyday life; where they learn, work, play, and love" (WHO 1986, p. 3). But the determinants of health exist and are produced and reproduced at macro, meso, and micro levels and must be understood in this complex fashion. In 1986, an international health conference took place in Ottawa, Canada to build on the principles of the *Alma-Ata Declaration* of 1978 (see Chapters 3 and 12). The document produced, entitled *The Ottawa Charter for Health Promotion*, set out a plan of action for achieving "health for all," the stated aim at Alma-Ata. Health promotion was envisioned as "the process of enabling people to increase control over, and to improve, their health" (WHO 1986, p. 1). The Charter outlines eight fundamental prerequisites for health—peace, shelter, education, food, income, a stable ecosystem, sustainable resources, and social justice and equity—with five action areas for reaching the goal of health for all by 2000:

1. *Creating supportive environments*: conserving natural resources and creating working and living conditions that promote health.
2. *Strengthening community action*: ensuring communities are in control of matters affecting their health and are able to voice opinions and concerns.
3. *Developing personal skills*: increasing the opportunities for people to make healthy choices through education and action.
4. *Reorienting health services*: moving health systems beyond curative care toward prevention and overall health promotion, in a culturally sensitive manner.
5. *Building healthy public policy*: ensuring that health is a component of policy development in all government sectors.

Ideally, actions that incorporate the principles of health promotion aim to reduce social inequalities in health as opposed to raising average population health (Ridde 2007). As such, health promotion potentially embraces a broad approach covering numerous societal determinants of health. For example, in Orissa, India an aid program set up in 1999 to help communities rebuild after a cyclone addressed economic needs and lack of employment, physical infrastructure, education, and training programs as well as developing health-specific interventions such as first aid training and maternal and child health programs. All projects were, and continue to be, designed and implemented in partnership with the community (Mukhopadhyay 2007).

Although the health promotion field purports to address personal, local, and global determinants of health together, in practice most health promotion efforts focus on the behavioral level—for example, encouraging people to quit smoking, modify their diet, practice safer sex, improve personal hygiene, and increase their physical activity. This is evidenced by the burgeoning of personal health education workshops, social marketing campaigns, and media and government campaigns in recent decades, which rarely address advocacy or action regarding the social, political, and economic determinants of health. For example, despite the documented negative effects of debt, unfair trade, and international financial agency policies (such as loan conditionalities) on health and well-being in a wide swath of underdeveloped countries (see Chapters 4 and 9), a recent review of peer-reviewed health promotion journals found that virtually no attention was being paid to these issues (Mohindra 2007). Moreover, biomedical and scientific perspectives and products are increasingly shaping health promotion messages (e.g., vaccines, nicotine and other drug-replacement therapies, appetite suppressants) (Buchanan 2000), further ingraining the emphasis on the individual.

Undoubtedly, certain individually focused interventions may affect health in the short term, such as reduced AIDS transmission due to use of condoms. However, viewed from a political economy perspective, behaviorally oriented health promotion efforts have little long-term effect because they do not adequately address the broader structural influences on health (see Chapters 4 and 7). Integrating technical, personal, social, and political approaches is certainly a grand challenge, but as illustrated in the healthy society cases above, it is one that is feasible.

Various countries (e.g., Brazil and Sweden) have sought to infuse the Ottawa Charter's principles of health promotion (specifically equity, community action, and primary care-oriented health systems) into social policies that extend far beyond the health sector. Others have limited their efforts to the articulation of health promotion goals and objectives without adopting clear strategies for realizing them, such as the Healthy People 2010 project of the U.S. government (www.healthypeople.gov/).

The limited scope of mainstream approaches to health promotion also threatens to amplify social inequalities in health (Buchanan 2000), as seen in the case of smoking cessation campaigns in industrialized countries. While these campaigns are widely touted for drastically reducing rates of tobacco use, smoking cessation has occurred unevenly between socioeconomic groups, leading to a marked increase in inequities within countries (Giskes et al. 2007). For example, 50% of Canadians smoked in 1965, dropping to 20% of the overall population in 2004, following increased tobacco control, taxes, and behavioral messages. However, currently approximately 70% of aboriginal and homeless populations smoke (Greaves et al. 2006).

In sum, while the original conception of health promotion represented a promising approach to improving health and its determinants, its mainstream practice is frequently in conflict with its fundamental principles and, as such, its potential impact is limited.

The Healthy Cities Program and Green Cities

The Healthy Cities Program (HCP) is a creative health promotion initiative that uses public policy and institutional incentives to improve "the physical, social, economic and spiritual dimensions of urban development...in the home, the school, the workplace, the city and other places or 'settings' where people live and work" (WHO EURO 2003, p. 11). The HCP movement began in Toronto, Canada in 1984

Box 13–9 Wherefore International Efforts? Promise and Limitations of the Framework Convention on Tobacco Control

Tobacco use accounts for more than 5 million deaths annually—more than the mortality attributed to HIV/AIDS, tuberculosis, and malaria combined (WHO 2008a). To address tobacco-related ill health, the WHO Framework Convention on Tobacco Control (FCTC), was passed by the World Health Assembly in 2003 and to date 160 governments and other parties have signed on. The first global health treaty of its kind, the FCTC sets out price, tax, and regulatory measures to reduce demand for tobacco, such as product packaging, education, and elimination of tobacco advertising, promotion, and sponsorship. Core supply-reduction provisions include measures to halt the illicit trade in tobacco and sales to minors, and economically viable alternatives for tobacco farmers.

There are various challenges to the full implementation of the FCTC, primarily the lack of political boldness on the part of governments to implement it, the limited capacity of states to regulate the tobacco industry, and the sophistication of tobacco advertising. For example, the political leverage of British American Tobacco (BAT) in Kenya has delayed legislation on smoking and led to a bill compelling farmers to sell tobacco leaves to BAT rather than its competitors (Patel, Collin, and Gilmore 2007). Youth are increasingly the target of tobacco advertising, and as globalization homogenizes values and lifestyles, tobacco companies are able to enter developing markets with greater ease (Hafez and Ling 2005). Without incentives for farmers to produce products other than tobacco, and without significant political will on the part of governments, the ultimate success of the FCTC is jeopardized.

Given the power of, and lobbying strategies employed by, the US$500 billion tobacco industry to protect its billions in profits, it is not surprising that the latest WHO report on the implementation of the FCTC revealed that "no government is fully implementing all key effective interventions—monitoring, smoke-free environments, treatment of tobacco dependence, health warnings on packages, bans on advertising, promotion and sponsorship, and tobacco taxation" (WHO 2008a, p. 42). Only 5% of the world's population is protected by comprehensive smoke-free laws, and, incredibly, 74 countries still allow smoking in schools and health facilities. Two countries, Uruguay and New Zealand, are at the forefront of full implementation of the FCTC.

The struggle to stem tobacco use shows that even with significant evidence and consensus at hand, challenging powerful corporate forces and their government allies is no simple task.

---

and HCP initiatives were implemented in many European cities soon thereafter. HCP is also showing promise for enhancing local health planning in various developing countries (Harpham, Burton, and Blue 2001; WHO EURO 2003).

Numerous HCPs are active in Latin America. In the early 1990s in Bogotá, Colombia, a city marred by violence and inequality, municipal authorities worked together on an overarching healthy city plan which included: increased lighting in public areas; increased parking fees to reduce traffic; improved public transit and car-free days; "women only" evenings to encourage women to walk and shop in the city center; improved sanitation and water services; and stricter enforcement of bar hours. In order to increase citizen participation in and acceptance of the proposed changes, street performers and artists were hired to promote a culture of respect, and incentives for positive behavior were instituted. From 1993 to 2003, water consumption dropped dramatically, traffic fatalities declined from 1,300/year to 600/year, homicide rates dropped from 80/100,000 to 22/100,000, and use of public transportation increased (Jackson et al. 2007).

HCPs were also launched in the Eastern Mediterranean region starting in 1990. Iran's HCP has been cited as a role model for the region, building on its long urban planning tradition. Its healthy cities network incorporates the federal ministries of health, information, culture, labor, housing and urban development, education, industry, power, environment, and welfare as well as the mayor of Tehran (National Secretariat for Healthy Cities Program 2005). Some of the outcomes of its healthy cities approach include: increased green space and urban agriculture; screening for numerous health problems; improved drinking water and sanitation; mental health promotion; reduction in traffic mortality and injury; improved solid waste management; increased job opportunities through HCP projects; reduced migration from towns/cities with HCP; skills training for women; and community engagement.

As reviewed in Chapter 10, a variety of local environmental initiatives also show promise for urban health improvement, akin to the healthy cities movement. Portland, Oregon, for example, has been hailed as a premier "green city," with a quality of life consistently ranked amongst the highest in the United States (Stephenson 1999). Portland's growth containment policies—including a growth boundary, strong regional government, major investment in public transit, and minimum density legislation—are considered exemplary in demonstrating that the "compact city" model of growth is possible. As well, there is a regional system of parks, natural areas, greenways, and trails for fish, wildlife, and people, including 57 urban natural areas and 34 trail and greenway corridors.

Public transport can also contribute to a city's health, as seen in Helsinki, Finland, where strong political commitment has resulted in over half of all trips being made through environmentally friendly means (approximately 30% by public transit, 16% on foot, and 9% by bicycle). By contrast in the United States, excepting a few cities, only 5% of trips are made on public transit (Beatley 2000). Few nations encourage bicycle use as much as the Netherlands. In a country of 16 million people, there are 17 million bicycles. The Netherlands has the highest proportion of bike lanes and paths in Europe, some 20,000 km total (compared to 110,000 km of streets and roads). Nationally, about 27% of all trips are made by bicycle and about 40% of these are for trips shorter than 2.5 km (Beatley 2000).

Viewed from a political economy perspective, healthy cities and green cities that develop effective local measures such as alternative transport models, organic food production, and universal social services are nonetheless limited in their ability to address, for example, systems of trade, conflict, and global environmental pressures. Notwithstanding its Toronto roots, the healthy cities movement there was not sustained, mostly due to the larger political context of neoliberalism in the 1990s. Budget cuts to healthy cities projects occurred simultaneous to deregulation, growing inequalities, deteriorating social conditions—such as a rise in homelessness and child poverty—and inaction in the face of worsening pollution and air quality (Raphael 2001, 2003). As well, the movement has been undermined by an increasing emphasis in the health promotion field on individual actions and responsibility. The HCP approach has other limitations: namely, that it is unlikely

Box 13–10 Challenges of National and International Approaches to Combating Female Genital Cutting

The issue of female genital cutting—practiced in an estimated 28 countries in Africa, the Middle East, and Asia, and among immigrants in other countries—illustrates the importance of integrating culturally appropriate health policies with international efforts to protect women's health and well-being.

Genital cutting—also known as female circumcision and female genital mutilation (FGM)—can take different forms: (a) removal of the clitoral hood; (b) removal of the clitoris and labia minora; (c) excision of part or all of the external genitalia and narrowing of the vaginal opening; and (d) cutting, pricking, stretching, or introduction of substances into the female genitalia. The practice dates back more than 5,000 years, as discovered through examination of Egyptian mummies. It is estimated that between 100 and 140 million women worldwide have undergone genital cutting, with an additional 3 million girls undergoing the procedure each year (UNICEF 2005).

A number of reasons have been advanced for this practice, including signification of readiness to marry; a form of anticolonial resistance to rape; religious tradition; a marker of cultural and or ethnic pride; a coming of age ritual for girls; a belief that it preserves virginity and prevents adultery; and a belief that the female genitalia is unclean and its removal is important to maintain hygiene (Boddy 2002). The health consequences of genital cutting are often dire, including short- and long-term problems due to pain, hemorrhage, tetanus, sepsis, urinary incontinence, difficulty with vaginal intercourse, infertility, depression, and even death.

Combating female genital cutting is enormously complex. In countries where it is a cultural norm, girls who do not undergo genital cutting may be precluded from marriage. Critiquing FGM can be tantamount to accusing mothers and grandmothers, who have purview over this practice, of abuse. International movements against FGM have been charged with hypocrisy, particularly where male circumcision is practiced and, especially, where female beauty rituals involve unhealthy cosmetics, painful shoes and clothing, or dangerous plastic surgery (Boddy 1991).

There have been various national and international efforts to eliminate female genital cutting. Fifteen African countries and various others have banned the practice altogether. In 1959, Egypt imposed sanctions (fines and imprisonment) against those who carried out genital cutting. However, given its widespread practice, the government shifted strategies in 1994, allowing the practice of genital cutting at government health facilities 1 day a week. Two years later, this was disallowed. In 1999, the Egyptian government, in partnership with a number of UN agencies, embarked on a project to eradicate FGM by 2010. In some places, a symbolic form of genital cutting is carried out, which retains the ritual component without the damaging health and psychological impact. In Indonesia, mass surgeries are carried out by trained practitioners under sponsorship of the Assalaam Foundation, an Islamic educational and service organization.

Some Western and feminist anti-FGM movements have been accused of religious and racial intolerance. During British colonial rule in Sudan, outside interference was met with resistance, and more women underwent FGM than previously. In Kenya, by contrast, the Norwegian Lutheran Mission worked with local communities to eradicate the practice. Key to their success appears to have been the introduction of alternate rites, which also focus on purity and womanhood (afrol.com 2008).

Notwithstanding these differences, there is growing international consensus that FGM is a human rights and health violation and that the practice must be abandoned (OHCHR et al. 2008).

to be generalizable given the local nature of decisions and developments (Awofeso 2003).

Despite these reservations, the healthy cities movement has considerable potential to galvanize local communities to take action, especially in conjunction with social redistribution efforts at higher political/administrative levels, for example in the state of Kerala or national governments in Sri Lanka and Costa Rica.

CONCLUSION: THE MAKINGS OF SUCCESSFUL POLICIES FOR HEALTH

Learning Points:

- Redistributive welfare state efforts are far more effective than vertical disease campaigns in achieving healthy societies.
- It is important to take a broad approach when evaluating successful health policies and interventions, lest control of diseases overshadow the greater importance of health improvement.
- Various developing countries and regions that have invested broadly in social welfare have made extraordinary gains in health conditions. In several settings, (e.g., Costa Rica and Mexico City) redistributive welfare policies have been implemented *despite* neoliberal pressures.
- Bona fide health promotion efforts require attention to the societal determinants of health at local, national, and global levels.
- Collective commitment to social justice and equity through social action and grassroots organizing—as well as through more formal political channels—is essential to the making of healthy societies.

Even as more and more money is infused into international health aid, many critics, and even insiders, agree that existing global health models are bankrupt: they address international agency criteria rather than local needs, focus more on disease control than on health improvement, and favor technical approaches to the exclusion of living and working conditions. Moments of crisis should not lead us to despair, however. New ideas and worldwide mobilization around health demonstrate that conditions can improve, given concerted political effort.

What then are the ingredients of success? Clearly, while some interventions may work in several settings, a one size fits all strategy applied in a cookie cutter fashion is likely to fail. This chapter has argued that unless social, political, and economic realities are taken into account, prescriptive, vertical disease campaigns can yield little overall health betterment, and may even be more harmful than helpful.

Both developed and developing country settings offer effective examples of how to improve the health of populations (Oxfam International 2006). Such steps include:

- universal provision of key services, especially those empowering women and girls;
- elimination of user fees for education, health, and other social services;
- subsidized clean water, sanitation, and housing;
- enhanced public sector capacity to deliver services;
- expanded services to rural and marginalized urban areas; and
- investment in human resources, especially those that provide social services and education;

in conjunction with:

- living wage laws;
- extended unemployment insurance;
- universal family benefits;
- housing guarantees or subsidies; and
- broad-scale social security.

Such measures are not novel: still, history shows that political struggle for true equity and a highly mobilized society are necessary to ensure that they are implemented.

Government service provision and the role of government in redistributing power and resources are essential to the realization of comprehensive social policies aimed at redressing structural inequities in society. International movements and organizations may also have a role to play in both advocating for and supporting policies that move countries toward greater social justice. Examples of these efforts are provided in Chapter 14.

As this chapter shows, countries, states, and cities with strong histories of social action, collective and redistributive policies, and citizen participation are able to achieve long-term improvements in health outcomes regardless of the level of GDP/capita. Guaranteeing universal access to comprehensive tax-funded social security benefits is the most sustainable approach. This counters the neoliberal claim that governments ought to be left on the sidelines. Indeed, healthy societies require that there be a greater, not a lesser, degree of government involvement in social policy-making and implementation, as long as governments represent broad public interests rather than narrow private interests.

Historical analysis also shows that technical quick fixes that ignore the underlying societal determinants of health are limited in scope, reversible, and inevitably poorly distributed across societies (exacerbating existing inequalities). When integrated, technical and redistributive approaches can lead to permanent health improvement, but technical approaches alone can not resolve the health challenges of the underdeveloped or the developed world.

What then is the role of international health in this arena? How can people and organizations involved in international health positively influence long-term and sustainable actions to improve health and well-being? These issues will be explored in the next, and final, chapter of this textbook.

REFERENCES

afrol.com. 2008. Missionaries successful in curbing female mutilation in Kenya. www. afrol.com/Categories/Women/wom018_fgm_kenya.htm. Accessed February 12, 2008.

Alleson I. 2005. Building and evaluating organizational linkages in food security initiatives: A preliminary analysis of international collaboration in Cuba. Paper read at the Second Annual Conference for Social Research in Organic Agriculture in conjunction with the 24th Annual Organic Agriculture Conference, University of Guelph, Canada.

Alvarado CH, Martínez ME, Vivas-Martínez S, Gutiérrez NJ, and Metzger W. 2008. Social change and health policy in Venezuela. *Social Medicine* 3(2):95–109.

Amarante V, Burdín G, and Vigorito A. 2007. *Evaluación cuantitativa del impacto del PANES*. Primer informe de avance: Instituto de Economía, Facultad de Ciencias Económicas, Universidad de la República, Montevideo, Uruguay.

Arim R, Vigorito A, and Salas G. 2006. Las políticas de transferencias de ingresos y su rol en el Uruguay 2001–2006. Working paper. Report number 41056. Washington, DC: World Bank.

Armada F, Muntaner C, Chung H, Willams-Brennan L, and Benach J. 2009. Barrio Adentro and the reduction of health inequalities in Venezuela: An appraisal of the first years. *International Journal of Health Services* 39(1):161–187.

Awofeso N. 2003. The Healthy Cities approach—reflections on a framework for improving global health. *Bulletin of the World Health Organization* 81(3):222–223.

Basch PF. 1999. *Textbook of International Health, Second Edition*. New York: Oxford University Press.

Beatley T. 2000. *Green Urbanism: Learning from European Cities*. Washington, DC: Inland Press.

Bhattacharya S. 2004. Uncertain victories: A review of the administration of the final phases of the eradication of smallpox in India, 1960–80. *American Journal of Public Health* 94(11):1875–1883.

Birn A-E. 2005. Gates's grandest challenge: Transcending technology as public health ideology. *Lancet* 366(9484):514–519.

Black RE, Morris SS, and Bryce J. 2003. Where and why are 10 million children dying every year? *Lancet* 361(9376):2226–2234.

Boddy J. 1991. Body politics: Continuing the anticircumcision crusade. *Medical Anthropology Quarterly* 5(1):15–17.

———. 2002. The female circumcision controversy: An anthropological perspective. *Journal of the Royal Anthropological Society* 8(1):181.

Borgia F. 2008. Health in Uruguay: Progress and challenges in the right to health care three years after the first progressive government. *Social Medicine/Medicina Social* 3(2):110–125.

Buchanan DR. 2000. *An Ethic for Health Promotion*. New York: Oxford University Press.

Catia resident. 2005. Interviewed by René M. Guerra Salazar in Caracas, Venezuela, August.

Center for Global Development. 2004. Millions saved: Proven successes in global health. *CGD Policy Brief, Global Health Policy Research Network* 3(3):1–8

Chatora R and Tumusiime P. 2004. *Management, Leadership and Partnership for District Health*. Brazzaville: WHO.

Chinai R. 2006. TB in Assam: Why vertical health programmes don't work. http://infochangeindia.org/20061201105/Health/Features/TB-in-Assam-Why-vertical-health-programmes-don-t-work.html. Accessed February 5, 2008.

Chung H and Muntaner C. 2007. Welfare state matters: A typological multilevel analysis of wealthy countries. *Health Policy* 80(2):328–339.

Cruz MC. 2001. Participatory planning in the city of Havana, Cuba. *Urban Agriculture Magazine 5*, December.

Cruz MC and Medina RS. 2003. *Agriculture in the City: A Key to Sustainability in Havana, Cuba*. Kingston: Ian Randle.

Cueto M. 1999. Negotiated health, discourses and practices on social medicine in Peru: 1920–1950. In Esteban Rodríguez Ocaña, Editor. *The Healthy Life: People,*

Perceptions, and Politics. Granada: European Association for the History of Medicine and Health and the International Network for the History of Public Health.

de Renzio P. 2005. Scaling up vs. absorptive capacity: Challenges and opportunities for reaching the MDGs in Africa. ODI Briefing Paper. http://www.cgdev.org/content/calendar/detail/3069/. Accessed February 12, 2008.

Devadasan N, Boelaert M, Criel B, van Damme W, and Gryseels B. 2007. The need for strong general health services in India and elsewhere. *The Lancet* 369(9562):638–639.

de Vos P, de Ceukelaire W, and van der Stuyft P. 2006. Colombia and Cuba, contrasting models in Latin America's health sector reform. *Tropical Medicine and International Health* 11(10):1604–1612.

Dugard J. 2007. A pro-poor critique of prepayment water meters in South Africa: The Phiri story. *Critical Health Perspectives* 2.

Elamon J and Ekbal B. 2004. *Kerala People's Campaign for Decentralized Planning.* http://www.pitt.edu/~super1/lecture/lec3441/index.htm. Accessed February 12, 2008.

Erikson D, Lord A, and Wolf P. 2002. *Cuba's Social Services: A Review of Education, Health and Sanitation.* Washington, DC: World Bank.

Fenner F, Ainslie Henderson D, Arita I, Jezek Z, and Danilovich Ladnyi I. 1988. *Smallpox and its Eradication.* Geneva: WHO.

Fernando D, Jayatilleka A, and Karunaratna V. 2003. Pregnancy-reducing maternal deaths and disability in Sri Lanka: National strategies. *British Medical Bulletin* 67:85–98.

Filgueira F. 2007. Cohesión, riesgo y arquitectura de protección social en América Latina. *Serie politicas sociales* 135.

Food First. 2003. Food First: Institute for food and development policy. http://www.foodfirst.org/. Accessed April 14, 2004.

Fort M. 2008. Personal email communication, February 27.

Franke RW and Chasin BH. 1992. Kerala State, India: Radical reform as development. *International Journal of Health Services* 22(1):139–156.

Giskes K, Kunst AE, Ariza CC, Benach J, Borrell C, Helmert U, et al. 2007. Applying an equity lens to tobacco-control policies and their uptake in six Western-European countries. *Journal of Public Health Policy* 28(2):261–280.

GlobalNutritionSeries.org. 2008. The Lancet Series: Maternal and child undernutrition. http://www.globalnutritionseries.org/. Accessed February 12, 2008.

Gobierno de Uruguay. 2006. Mides-Plan de Emergencia: 16 meses construyendo ciudadanía. http://www.mides.gub.uy/panes/julio_06.html. Accessed May 17, 2007.

Goldsmith WW and Vainier CB. 2001. Participatory budgeting and power politics in Porto Alegre. *Land Lines* 13(1):1–5.

Gómez-Dantés H and Birn A-E. 2000. Malaria and social movements in Mexico: The last 60 years. *Parassitologia* 42(1–2):69–85.

Gonzalez CL. 1965. Mass campaigns and general health services, Public Health Paper No. 29. Geneva: WHO.

Government of Kerala. 2005. *Human Development Report 2005: Kerala.* Thiruvananthapuram, India: Government of Kerala State Planning Board.

Government of Sweden. 2007. *The National Public Health Strategy for Sweden in Brief.* Stockholm: Swedish National Institute of Public Health.

Greaves L, Johnson J, Bottorff J, Kirkland S, Jategaonkar N, McGowan M, McCullough L, and Battersby L. 2006. What are the effects of tobacco policies on vulnerable populations? *Canadian Journal of Public Health* 97(4):310–315.

Gwatkin DR, Wagstaff A, and Yazbeck AS. 2005. *Reaching the Poor with Health, Nutrition and Population Services: What Works, What Doesn't and Why.* Washington, DC: World Bank.

Hafez N and Ling PM. 2005. How Philip Morris built Marlboro into a global brand for young adults: Implications for international tobacco control. *Tobacco Control* 14(4):262–271.

Halstead SB, Walsh JA, and Warren KS, Editors. 1985. *Good Health at Low Cost, Rockefeller Foundation Conference Report.* New York: Rockefeller Foundation.

Harpham T, Burton S, and Blue I. 2001. Healthy city projects in developing countries: The first evaluation. *Health Promotion International* 16(2):111–125.

Isaac TM and Franke RW. 2002. *Local Democracy and Development: The Kerala People's Campaign for Decentralized Planning.* Lanham, MD: Roman & Littlefield Publishers.

Jackson S, Sleigh AC, Wang GJ, and Liu XL. 2006. Poverty and the economic effects of TB in rural China. *International Journal of Lung Disease* 10:1104–1110.

Jackson SF, Perkins F, Khandor E, Cordwell L, Hamann S, and Buasai S. 2007. Integrated health promotion strategies: A contribution to tackling current and future health challenges. *Health Promotion International* 21(Suppl.1):75–83.

Jardim C. 2005. Prevention and solidarity: Democratizing health in Venezuela. *Monthly Review* 56(8).

Johnson C and Start D. 2001. *Rights, Claims and Capture: Understanding the Politics of Pro-Poor Policies* (Working Paper 145). London: Overseas Development Institute.

Kadiyala S. 2004. Scaling up Kudumbashree—collective action for poverty alleviation and women's empowerment. FCND discussion papers 180. Washington, DC: International Food Policy Research Institute (IFPRI).

Kent G. 1991. *The Politics of Children's Survival.* New York: Praeger Publishers.

Kim JY. 2004. Plenary Address: Scaling up access to care in resource constrained settings: What is needed? In *XV International AIDS Conference.* Bangkok.

Krieger N. 2008. Proximal, distal, and the politics of causation: What's level got to do with it? *American Journal of Public Health* 98(2):221–230.

Laurell AC. 2003. What does Latin American social medicine do when it governs? The case of the Mexico City Government. *American Journal of Public Health* 93(12):2028–2031.

———. 2007. Granting universal access to health care: The experience of the Mexico City Government. *Case Study Commissioned by the Health Systems Knowledge Network.* WHO Commission on Social Determinants of Health. www.who.int/entity/social_ determinants/resources/csdh_media/mexico_universal_access_2007_en.pdf. Accessed January 7, 2008.

Levine R, What Works Working Group, and Kinder M. 2004. *Millions Saved: Proven Successes in Global Health.* Washington, DC: Center for Global Development.

Levine R. 2007. *Case Studies in Global Health: Millions Saved.* Boston, MA: Jones and Bartlett.

Lieberherr F. 2003. Participatory budgets: A tool for a participatory democracy. *Urban News* 7. Berne: Swiss Agency for Development and Cooperation.

Maciocco G and Italian Global Health Watch. 2008. From Alma Ata to the global fund: The history of international health policy. *Social Medicine* 3(1):36–48.

Martínez Franzoni J. 2007. Costa Rica's pension reform: A decade of negotiated incremental change. In Kay SJ and Sinha T, Editors. *Lessons from Pension Reform in the Americas.* New York: Oxford University Press.

———. 2008. *Domesticar la incertidumbre en América Latina: Mercado laboral, política social y familias.* San José: Universidad de Costa Rica, Instituto de Investigaciones Sociales.

McNay K, Keith R, and Penrose A. 2006. *Bucking the Trend: How Sri Lanka has Achieved Good Health at Low Cost—Challenges and Policy Lessons for the 21st Century.* London: Save the Children.

Meegama SA. 1986. The Mortality Transition in Sri Lanka. New York: United Nations.

Menegat R. 2002. Participatory democracy and sustainable development: Integrated urban environmental management in Porto Alegre, Brazil. *Environment and Urbanization* 14(2):181–206.

Mesa-Lago C. 1985. Health care in Costa Rica: Boom and crisis. *Social Science and Medicine* 21(1):13–21.

MIHR (The Centre for Management of IP in Health R&D). 2005. *Innovation in Developing Countries to Meet Health Needs.* Geneva: WHO.

Mills A. 2005. Mass campaigns versus general health services: What have we learnt in 40 years about vertical versus horizontal approaches? *Bulletin of the World Health Organization* 83(4):315–316.

Mohindra KS. 2007. Health public policy in poor countries: Tackling macro-economic policies. *Health Promotion International* 22(2):163–169.

Morgan LM. 1987. Health without wealth? Costa Rica's health system under economic crisis. *Journal of Public Health Policy* 8(1):86–105.

Mukhopadhyay A. 2007. Aparajita Orissa. *Promotion and Education* 14(2):74–75.

Muntaner C, Guerra Salazar RM, Benach J, and Armada F. 2006. Venezuela's Barrio Adentro: An alternative to neoliberalism in health care. *International Journal of Health Services* 36(4):803–811.

Muraleedharan K. 2005. Participatory development: Issues and lessons: Gendering governance and empowering women through participatory programs in Kerala. http://www.eldis.org/fulltext/MURALEEDHARAN_participatory_development.pdf. Accessed February 12, 2008.

Murphy C. 1999. Cultivating Havana: Urban agriculture and food security in the years of crisis. Development Report No. 12. Oakland, CA: Food First Institute for Food and Development Policy.

National Secretariat for Healthy Cities Program. 2005. Healthy cities program and healthy villages program with BDN (basic development needs) approach in Islamic Republic of Iran. http://www.emro.who.int/cbi/pdf/healthycities_iran.pdf. Accessed September 18, 2007.

Navarro V, Borrell C, Benach J, Muntaner C, Quiroga A, Rodríguez-Sanz M, et al. 2003. The importance of the political and the social in explaining mortality differentials amongst countries of the OECD, 1950–1998. *International Journal of Health Services* 33(3):419–494.

Needham J. 1980. *China and the Origins of Immunology.* Hong Kong: University of Hong Kong.

Nyerere J. 1968. *Socialism and Rural Development. Freedom and Socialism.* Dar es Salaam: Oxford University Press.

OHCHR, UNAIDS, UNDP, UNECA, UNESCO, UNFPA, UNHCR, UNICEF, UNIFEM, WHO. 2008. *Eliminating Female Genital Mutilation: An Interagency Statement.* Geneva: WHO.

Oxfam International. 2006. *In the Public Interest: Health, Education, Water and Sanitation for all.* Oxford: Oxfam International.

Pan American Health Organization. 2006. *Mission Barrio Adentro: The Right to Health and Social Inclusion in Venezuela.* Caracas: PAHO/Venezuela.

Parayil G. 1996. The "Kerala model" of development: Development and sustainability in the Third World. *Third World Quarterly* 17(5):941–957.

Patel P, Collin J, and Gilmore AB. 2007. "The law was actually drafted by us but the Government is to be congratulated on its wise actions": British American Tobacco and public policy in Kenya. *Tobacco Control* 16:e1; doi:10.1136/tc.2006.016071.

Perez Rojas N and Vila CT. 1998. Las unidades basicas de producion cooperativa (UBPC): Hacia un nuevo proyecto de participacion. In Arango M, Editor. *Cuba Periodo Especial: Perspectives.* Habana: Editorial de Ciencias Sociales.

Piller C and Smith D. 2007. Unintended victims of Gates Foundation generosity. *Los Angeles Times,* December 16.

Porter D. 2006. How did social medicine evolve, and where is it heading. *PLoS Medicine* 3(10):1667–1672.

Raphael D. 2001. Letter from Canada: Paradigms, politics and principles—an end of the millennium update from the birthplace of the healthy cities movement. *Health Promotion International* 16(1):99–101.

————. 2003. Barriers to addressing the societal determinants of health: Public health units and poverty in Ontario, Canada. *Health Promotion International* 18(4):397–405.

Raphael D and Bryant T. 2004. The welfare state as a determinant of women's health: Support for women's quality of life in Canada and four comparison nations. *Health Policy* 68(1):63–79.

Ridde V. 2007. Reducing social inequalities in health: Public health, community health or health promotion. *Promotion and Education* 14(2):63–67.

Rosset PM. 2000. Cuba: A successful case study of sustainable agriculture. In Magdoff F, Foster J and Buttel F, Editors. *Hungry for Profit: The Agribusiness Threat to Farmers, Food and the Environment.* New York: Monthly Review Press.

Russell S and Gilson L. 2006. Are health services protecting the livelihoods of the urban poor in Sri Lanka? Findings from two low-income areas of Colombo. *Social Science and Medicine* 63(7):1732–1744.

Seligson M and Martínez Franzoni J. 2009. Limits to Costa Rican Heterodoxy: What Has Changed in "Paradise"? In Mainwaring S and Scully T, Editors. *The Politics of Democratic Governability in Latin America: Clues and Lessons.* Palo Alto, CA: Stanford University Press.

Spiegel JM and Yassi A. 2004. Lessons from the margins of globalization: Appreciating the Cuban health paradox. *Journal of Public Health Policy* 25(1):85–110.

Stephenson RB. 1999. A vision of green: Lewis Mumford's legacy in Portland, Oregon. *Journal of the American Planning Association* 65(3):259.

Tajer D. 2003. Latin American social medicine: Roots, development during the 1990s, and current challenges. *American Journal of Public Health* 93(12):2023–7.

Tanaka S. 2005. Parental leave and child health across OECD countries. *Economic Journal* 115(501):F7–F28.

Thankappan KR. 2001. Some health implications of globalization in Kerala, India. *Bulletin of the World Health Organization* 79(9):892–893.

Torres Tovar M. 2007. ALAMES: Organizational expression of social medicine in Latin America. *Social Medicine* 2(3):125–130.

UNDP. 2005. Human Development Report 2005. International Development at a Crossroads: Aid, trade and security in an unequal world. New York: UNDP.

Unger J-P, de Paepe P, Buitrón R, and Soors W. 2007. Costa Rica: Achievements of a heterodox health policy. *American Journal of Public Health* 98(4):636–643.

UNICEF. 1996a. The 1950s: Era of the mass disease campaign. In *Fifty Years for Children: The State of the World's Children.* New York: UNICEF. http://www.unicef.org/sowc96/1950s.htm.

————. 1996b. The 1980s: Campaign for child survival. In *Fifty Years for Children: The State of the World's Children.* New York: UNICEF. http://www.unicef.org/sowc96/1980s.htm

———. 1999. The state of the world's children, 1999: Education. www.unicef.org/sowc99/summary4.htm. Accessed February 9, 2008.

———. 2001. *Progress since the World Summit for Children: A Statistical Review.* New York: UNICEF.

———. 2005. *Female Genital Mutilation/Cutting: A Statistical Exploration.* New York: UNICEF.

———. 2007a. The state of the world's children, 2008: Child survival. http://www.unicef.org/sowc08/docs/sowc08.pdf. Accessed February 12, 2008.

———. 2007b. *UNICEF Humanitarian Action: Sri Lanka in 2007.* New York: UNICEF.

———. 2008. Expanding immunization coverage. http://www.unicef.org/immunization/index_coverage.html. Accessed September 11, 2008.

Vallgårda S. 2007. Health inequalities: Political problematizations in Denmark and Sweden. *Critical Public Health* 17(1):45–56.

Varatharajan D, Thankappan KR, and Jayapalan S. 2004. Assessing the performance of primary health centres under decentralized government in Kerala, India. *Health Policy and Planning* 19(1):41–51.

Victora CG, Wagstaff A, Schellenberg JA, Gwatkin D, Claeson M, and Habicht J-P. 2003. Applying an equity lens to child health and mortality: More of the same is not enough. *Lancet* 362(9379):233–241.

Wagle S and Shah P. 2003. Case study 2—Porto Alegre, Brazil: Participatory approaches in budgeting and public expenditure management. *Social Development Notes.* Note no. 71.

Waitzkin H, Iriart C, Estrada A, and Lamadrid S. 2001. Social medicine then and now: Lessons from Latin America. *American Journal of Public Health* 91(10):1592–1601.

Warwick H. 1999. Cuba's organic revolution. *The Ecologist* 29(8):457–460.

WHO. 1980. *The Global Eradication of Smallpox. Final Report of the Global Commission for the Certification of Smallpox Eradication.* Geneva: WHO.

———. 1986. Ottawa charter for health promotion: First International conference on health promotion. Geneva: WHO.

———. 2006. *World Health Report 2006: Working Together for Health.* Geneva: WHO.

———. 2008a. *Report on the Global Tobacco Epidemic.* Geneva: WHO.

———. 2008b. *World Health Statistics.* Geneva: WHO.

WHO EURO. 2003. Healthy Cities Around the World: An Overview of the Healthy Cities Movement in the Six WHO Regions. International Healthy Cities Conference, Belfast, Northern Ireland. Copenhagen: WHO EURO.

WHO and UNICEF. 2008. *World Health Organization and United Nations Children's Fund Joint Monitoring Programme for Water Supply and Sanitation. Progress on Drinking Water and Sanitation: Special Focus on Sanitation.* New York: UNICEF and Geneva: WHO.

Zambon A, Boyce W, Cois E, Currie C, Lemma P, Dalmasso P, Borraccino A, and Cavallo F. 2006. Do welfare regimes mediate the effect of socioeconomic position on health in adolescence? A cross-national comparison in Europe, North America and Israel. *International Journal of Health Services* 36(2):309–329.

14

Doing International Health

Key Questions:

- How does the traditional approach to doing international health compare to the political economy approach?
- What are the connections among personal motivations, institutional aims, and the geopolitical context of international health?
- What alternatives to traditional international health help foster true cooperation?
- How do we measure success in international health?

We hope that taking a course or reading this book on your own will have made you passionate about the importance of international health and sparked your desire to become involved—in small or large measure—in addressing the challenges of international health.

What motivates your interest to work in the field of international health? How will you go about finding where and how your participation is needed given your interests and abilities? What is the appropriate arena for your activism and involvement? Should you obtain international experience before completing your education? What should you learn about local, national, and international needs? From what kinds of sources? How will you ensure the accountability and ethical compliance of your own work and that of your organization? These are all important questions that should be contemplated by anyone considering employment or volunteering in the international health arena (Sarfaty and Arnold 2005).

There are various ways of thinking about work in international health. Some consider it a learning adventure for well-meaning health professionals and students from industrialized countries who travel to underdeveloped settings to help alleviate health problems. Others regard international health in terms of humanitarian and/or technical assistance from developed to underdeveloped countries during times of need or disaster. Still others see international health in terms of mutual cooperation aimed at improving health and social conditions, whether among developing countries, through international agencies and NGOs, or among networks of health workers, organizations, and professionals. A more radical way of viewing international health is as a transformative process, both for people living in conditions of poverty and inequality *and* for students, health professionals, and community actors who wish to be part of an agenda for change, whether in their home country or overseas.

Notwithstanding these idealistic perspectives, most international health work, as we have seen, is marked by pervasive self-interest on the part of donor countries, organizations, and other actors—whether regarding the control of threatening communicable diseases crossing the globe, the forging of strategic political alliances, the acquisition of primary resources, the expansion of production and consumer markets, or the protection of commercial interests. As we have discussed throughout the text, international health activities are not a neutral sphere of action. They are embedded in particular social contexts and intertwined with economic and geopolitical forces. At whatever level you are involved, understanding the political economy underpinnings of international health can make your work more informed and effective and can enable you to challenge the forces that reproduce local, national, and international inequalities.

International health today is marked by the history of past activities. As discussed in Chapter 2, starting circa 1500 leading European powers ventured "overseas" to explore, settle, convert, colonize, profit from, "civilize," and exploit peoples and lands of less powerful societies. Health activities played a central part in the imperial enterprise. (Of course, power imbalances also exist(ed) *within* virtually every country, with one or more groups or classes oppressing others.) After colonies gained independence in the 19th and 20th centuries, these unequal relationships persisted: bona fide cooperation among countries for the most part took a back seat to more exploitative interaction. Those involved in any international health endeavor should be conscious that this legacy has not been forgotten by millions of people living in conditions of poverty and inequality. In the present, we need to continuously bear in mind the troubling possibility that even the most well-intentioned and informed international health endeavor may perpetuate inequalities in power across the world.

Contradictions abound in the field of international health. Much global health activity is premised on a one-way diffusionist model of assistance from high- to low-income nations. Yet past and present, a unidirectional understanding of ideas, resources, and expertise moving from developed to underdeveloped settings is overly simplistic. Not only do far more "southern" health professionals go to work in "northern" settings than vice versa (as part of the "brain drain"—see Chapter 12), there are countless public health lessons from underdeveloped countries that can be applied to industrialized countries. This is, for instance, the way that the community health movement in the United States got its start in the 1960s, based on lessons learned from South Africa and Israel. South–to–South collaboration— that is, developing countries assisting one another—has also existed in previous eras and, though vastly understudied and underreported, is gaining ground today. The deployment of Cuban doctors and engineers to African, Asian, and Central American countries and, more recently, South African aid toward the reconstruction of the Democratic Republic of the Congo are just two examples of this growing trend.

This chapter lays out a hopeful realist—rather than a hopeless idealist or cynical realist—approach to international health work. Returning to the premise that "health problems, issues and concerns...are best addressed by cooperative actions and solutions" (Institute of Medicine 1997, p. 2), we explore how to move beyond traditional approaches to foster a more cooperative form of international health. This chapter is designed to help readers navigate the complex world of international health from an analytic perspective, as well as provide some pointers for the more practical and ethical aspects of engaging in international health work. We review the challenges, possibilities, and limits of international health work from personal and institutional perspectives, while bearing in mind the larger constellation of forces and interests discussed in previous chapters. Then we outline alternative approaches to engaging in international health. The chapter closes with reflections on how success is gauged in the international health field.

TRADITIONAL WAYS OF DOING INTERNATIONAL HEALTH

The traditional approach to international health presumes that those in powerful countries have a monopoly on the necessary knowledge, technical expertise, and resources to ameliorate the problems of people living in underdeveloped countries. This modus operandi has resulted in waves of health professionals descending on a country to sort out its health problems according to donor agency or personal agendas. These efforts often ignore the social and political context and the existing health and welfare infrastructure, or hold them in disregard, and set up parallel health systems that do not build local capacity. Under this approach, health professionals in developing countries (who have likely been seconded from their posts) are overseen by outside "experts" or consultants who impose their own values and tools and negate, or even denigrate, the importance and usefulness of local knowledge and the existing organization of social and medical services. In another variant of this approach, transnational professional elites from low-income countries are trained as "experts" at universities in North America, Europe, Australia, and elsewhere; upon return to their home country, they may impose their knowledge on those working within the ministry of health or other institutions, or serve as interlocutors for, or even representatives of, outside donors.

Medical officers of the British army deployed to India in the 19th century exemplify the "traditional approach" to international public health. While Britain's Army Medical Service prided itself on bringing "sanitary science to India, stopping the ravages of cholera and improving the whole conditions there" (Harrison 1994,

p. 227), the primary mission was to protect the health of British soldiers and colonists; any benefit to the local population was of secondary concern. Moreover, many of India's health problems—ascribed to local cultural deficiencies—were in fact created by the British through conquest and agricultural practices that "disrupted traditional systems of drainage exposing huge tracts of the country to the ravages of malaria and waterborne disease" (ibid.).

While those involved in international health today might (smugly) distance themselves from such attitudes and activities, it is important to bear in mind that much of the renewed interest in global health is based on analogous self-interest: the global transmission of disease has been portrayed as a threat, for example, to "American security, prosperity, and interest in economic development abroad" (Kassalow 2001, p. 5). Moreover, as discussed in Chapter 9, many health problems across the world derive from inequalities generated by local, national, and global patterns of economic and environmental exploitation.

Mainstream approaches to aid—including those that express profound moral sentiments in favor of reducing poverty and improving health in developing countries—often fall into a colonialist mode, whereby solutions emanate from powerful quarters and are imposed on the less powerful. This "white man's burden," as per the phrase coined by British imperial poet and author Rudyard Kipling, supposes that aid stems from generosity and responsibility on the part of powerful donors, while disregarding the past and present pilfering of less powerful economies and peoples.

A slew of recent books by Western economists critical of development aid patterns—and each with a nostrum for change—only reproduces this mentality, whether calling for more aid, less aid, or better aid (Sachs 2005; Easterly 2006; Collier 2007; Ncayiyana 2007). Jeffrey Sachs, for example, argues that aid is a "practical bargain": a set of simple steps realizable "at a cost that would be nearly unnoticeable to the world's wealthiest nations" that would "eas[e] the economic and environmental strains" imposed on impoverished nations (Sachs 2008, p. 36). While the "practical bargain" of aid is appealing to those comfortable with the status quo of power and resource distribution across the world and within countries, this approach—in contrast to negotiated cooperation—offers limited prospects for addressing the underlying determinants of international health problems. Ironically—and tragically—most development aid critiques fail to take into sufficient account the role of colonial exploitation in enabling Western industrial development in the first place and in creating vast inequalities between and within countries (Shiva 2005).

In a related vein, missionary doctors in early 20th century China proselytized both Christianity and hospital-based medicine, with little regard for local needs or beliefs (Cheung and New 1985). The part played by Protestant and Catholic medical missionaries in disseminating Western medicine to European colonies in Latin America, Asia, and Africa has been hailed by some: to this day, across Africa many hospitals are run by missionaries, providing care that might not otherwise be available.

Yet missionary work historically facilitated imperialist exploitation. Exploitation's continuance—by both internal and external interests—is arguably the most important determinant of poor and unequal health in Africa today. Some missionaries have vocally decried human rights violations, and various large religious charities emphasize social justice rather than proselytization in their health aid (see Chapter 3). In other respects, modern day "medical missionary" work has not changed much from past patterns, with medicine employed as a conduit to religious conversion.

Box 14–1 Trypanosomiasis in East Africa

The exacerbation of African sleeping sickness (trypanosomiasis) after the colonization of East Africa is a testament to the myopic and prejudicial nature of the traditional approach to "doing international health." African sleeping sickness spreads via the tsetse fly vector, resulting in a parasitic infection that first attacks the immune system, then other organ systems, and finally the central nervous system, eventually killing infected humans and cattle.

Various African societies have long known that trypanosomiasis (known as *nagana*) attacked cattle, but the local populations were able to contain the disease through herding practices in the unclaimed wilderness areas between neighboring territories (Ford 1971). With the imposition of international boundaries by European colonists, frontier zones were destroyed and the locally maintained ecological equilibrium disappeared, causing an increase in tsetse fly populations and in the spread of trypanosomiasis. As poor farmers were forced to combine their cattle into larger herds, sleeping sickness became epidemic, increasing human infections. In the late 19th century, during the tumultuous period of German occupation and local resistance movements in East Africa, trypanosomiasis "depopulated" large parts of Tanzania and neighboring Uganda, killing an estimated one-tenth of the population.

Colonial medical authorities attributed the high death rates from trypanosomiasis—as well as tuberculosis, malaria, and other ailments—to the poor hygiene and diet of Africans and to the lack of immunity to diseases to which they had no prior exposure. This paradigm located sickness in the individual's body rather than in the body politic (Turshen 1984). Political and medical authorities alike failed to consider that the "civilizing" process—wars of conquest, the slave trade, the imperial division of Africa, and the increased exploitation of land and resources—was driving these epidemics (Hoppe 2003). Today trypanosomiasis continues to be epidemic, infecting an average of 100,000 people per year in Uganda alone and threatening 60 million more across sub-Saharan Africa (Fèvre, Picozzi, and Fyfe 2005). In 2003 the humanitarian NGO Médecins Sans Frontières (MSF), together with the UNDP/UNICEF/World Bank/WHO's Special Programme for Research and Training in Tropical Diseases (TDR), and the health research institutes of Brazil, France, India, Kenya, and Malaysia, helped form the Drugs for Neglected Diseases initiative (DNDi) to stimulate collaboration and provide support for drug development for human African trypanosomiasis and other "neglected diseases."

PRACTICING INTERNATIONAL HEALTH: PEOPLE, ORGANIZATIONS, AND THE WORLD ORDER

As you contemplate your potential or actual role in international health, it is essential to recognize the possibilities and limits of your own participation. We can conceive of international health as operating at three levels:

1. motivations and actions of individuals;

2. missions and interventions of organizations; and
3. logic and structures of the world order.

The three levels operate simultaneously, but each is constrained by the next higher level. Individual motives or institutional missions may conflict with the logic of global capitalism, and the impact of individuals and institutions is limited by the world order. At the same time, they can help transform free market capitalism into, for example, a world order made up of welfare states that share a commitment to protecting human well-being and reducing inequality under a system of democratic governance. Though individual actions by themselves cannot transcend the world order, they can contribute to changing it, in part through the formation of organizations and movements.

Individual Level: Motivations and Training and Work Experience

Motivations

There are numerous reasons for wanting to engage in international health work. While the desire to be of service may seem laudable, justifying overseas engagement—for those in a position to travel abroad—based on generosity and "helping" people is illusory, especially when "help" has not been sought. Indeed, most people who undertake a health-related work or volunteer experience in another country find that the greatest benefit is to themselves. Countless medical relief trips run every year by well-meaning nonprofit and for-profit organizations are nothing more than "global health tourism." Such trips are typically financed by the participants themselves, who pay large sums of money for the chance to sew up wounds in the Amazon (complete with rainforest river cruises on the weekend), treat exotic diseases in the jungles of Rwanda (with side tours to see silver back gorillas), or distribute eyeglasses to Tibetan refugees in the foothills of the Himalayas (with the possibility of an audience with the Dalai Lama). Such expeditions often do more harm than good, leaving behind no capacity for follow-up and applying "band-aids" to deep problems (Bezruchka 2000).

In reality, the bulk of international health work—that is, work involving some connection to an organization, issue, or policy from another country or to a regional, bilateral, or multilateral entity—is carried out by local health workers, community organizers and leaders, mothers, traditional birth attendants, and others, often with very limited resources and little payment for their work. We may not typically consider people working in their home country, year after year, as taking part in international health: clearly the perspective and relative contribution of those engaged in a lifetime of work differs greatly from those of outsiders flying in and out. As such, it is important for foreigners and for highly trained developing country (trans)nationals who decide to engage in health work to recognize that they are in

---

Box 14–2 Personal Motivations for Working in International Health

1. Desire for a broader perspective on public health.
2. Scientific research and/or teaching interests.
3. Desire to improve clinical skills.
4. Genuine humanitarianism—desire to serve those in need.
5. Desire to change local or national health policy in one's own country, drawing from international experience.
6. Desire to improve conditions or ensure access to care for friends, siblings, children, and neighbors.
7. Idealism—the wish to counter mainstream efforts and change the world.
8. National pride or chauvinism expressed, for example, through commitment to foreign policy goals.
9. Employment and professional opportunities.
10. Religious conviction or "sense of mission."
11. Desire for adventure and travel to exotic locales.
12. Challenge of a different setting in which new skills can be mastered.
13. Curiosity—desire to encounter interesting cultures and customs.
14. Provide charitable service.

Source: Based in part on Krogh and Pust (1990).

---

a position of power and that they need to be very careful not to abuse this power. Foreigners and transnationals enjoy relative wealth, advanced education, the power to leave (the country or community), and the luxury to challenge decisions without jeopardizing their livelihood, as well as organizational access to resources and influence over policymaking. All of these factors shape the interactions of transnational and foreign health professionals with ministries of health, communities, local health workers, leaders, and educators.

It is still commonplace for citizens of high-income nations to display ethnocentrism, paternalism, or condescension toward people from developing countries. Students may assume that they can provide some benefit to a community without understanding the political or social dynamics, the language, or the role of outside organizations. Child Family Health International, an NGO that organizes international placements for students, recently published excerpts of how some participants described their experiences overseas: "The local coordinator was a buffoon [who] talked too much about nothing useful"; "Although one of the doctors explained a few medical things to us, she was generally very bitter towards us because of the wealth of our country versus the almost primitive nature of the medicine in these small villages" (Shaw 2007, p. 3). The arrogance and lack of even a basic understanding of the social context suggests that these students should never have been sent on an international placement.

Other aspects of ethnocentrism include the failure to appreciate the importance of local understandings of disease and ill health, such as the belief that diarrhea in children is caused by supernatural forces (Kauchali, Rollins, and Solarsh 2002),

> **Box 14–3** Voices from the Ground
>
> "I graduated as a medical doctor from Calcutta twenty-three years ago. Since then I have worked as a: resident in Obstetrics/Gynecology and Paediatrics; community practitioner; manager of a community health project and hospital; community trainer; trainer of health providers and managers; consultant to government, international NGOs, and UN bodies; public health researcher; and health and human rights advocate. I now direct a national health policy resource centre. My core concern has always remained the health of poor and marginalized women. This motivation to 'do good' was later sharpened to a political–economic understanding of health through experience and reading.
>
> There have been remarkable changes in the arena of public health in India in the twenty odd years of my work. I was alone in a class of 150 to choose to work in a village, and was considered an oddity. Today the number of doctors opting for rural postings has increased, with very lucrative jobs offered by international programs. Numerous international organizations have come into the country offering salaries which seem inflated, especially since the sector is what I would call a 'misery' sector and the economic difference between the professional and the villager is so vast as to mitigate against empathy.
>
> International organizations have their own missions and agendas which can vary from the explicit political and social agenda of USAID to the more operational mission of international NGOs. Since these organizations are well-financed, they have the potential to skew local priorities. I have found this to happen especially with the global polio eradication initiative, or in the way institutional delivery is promoted at the behest of WHO and other UN bodies. The other issue of concern is the lack of space provided to local experience and insight because of the importance accorded to 'evidence.' My current endeavour is to find ways and opportunities for lived experiences to become 'evidence' so that policies are informed by ground reality and not information analysed out of context through professional sophistication."
> Abhijit Das, Centre for Health and Social Justice, Delhi, India 2008.

and the imposition of "best practice" biomedicine on communities that employ traditional medicine (Krumeich et al. 2001). This goes well beyond issues of cultural sensitivity. As discussed in Chapters 4 and 7, the Western biomedical model has conceptual and practical limitations and biases—it is individualistic, mechanistic, invasive, generally ignores holistic understandings and the societal context of health, can do little for many chronic conditions—and is not always the best option for addressing health problems. People working in international health should not only be open to traditional healers, different conceptions of health and healing, and so on, but should also recognize that these approaches may be more appropriate than the biomedical model. Understanding and discussing the weaknesses of the biomedical model is very important in dispelling the assumption that it is the only appropriate means of tackling health problems. Moreover, attempting the integration of traditional healing and biomedicine is not simply a matter of healers being tolerated by official health systems but requires that healers be respected and taken seriously for their knowledge and abilities.

As you embark on or redirect your career in international health, be reminded that excessive idealism, overconfidence (in your tools, role, abilities, or approach), and ignorance about the realities of international health can pose insurmountable impediments and grave damage on local populations.

Training and Work Experience

A laboratory researcher investigating drug resistance in local populations, an entomologist working in a vector control program, a computer expert setting up a health information system, an administrator of a maternal and child health program, an economist, a social worker, an accountant, an office manager or project manager, an activist, or a teacher can all make a significant contribution to international health. Each will have acquired a level of training and expertise to contribute in their field. For example, competence as a trained health care provider (physician, nurse practitioner, etc.) is necessary for those doing clinical work, and an advanced degree, such as a DrPH (for applied research in public health) or PhD is important for researchers. As health is shaped by multiple factors, policy analysts, community organizers, engineers, and a host of other professions also play key roles.

A common question for young professionals is when or whether to invest time in formal training in international health. This could include a Master of Public Health (or a Master's degree in Global Health), a diploma in tropical medicine and hygiene, a summer course in tropical medicine (e.g., offered by Tulane and Johns Hopkins universities, both in the U.S., and by the Gorgas Institute in Peru), or a doctorate in public health to deepen research abilities. Some international health workers undergo training after medical/nursing/graduate school, others before, and some skip it altogether. Since there is no single "right path," it is useful to seek the advice of mentors.

Given the breadth of international health, it is impossible to develop all necessary skills a priori. Job descriptions may call for expertise in vital statistics, health economics, social mobilization, program administration, sanitation, multiple languages, or any of the topics covered in this book. Twenty years of experience can lead to great proficiency in, say, organizing region-wide immunization programs or developing healthy housing standards, but will not necessarily impart knowledge about reducing air pollution or monitoring social inequalities in health. Skills in budget and program development and monitoring and evaluation, whether learned on the job or in training courses, have become increasingly relevant to any position.

Moreover, even for those with training, dogged effort is needed to stay abreast of developments in the broader field. The job is made both easier and more challenging by online medical, health, and social science databases, listserves, and a profusion of Web sites. Care should be applied in evaluating the credibility of all sources, and findings should be considered in social and political context. Relevant knowledge is not only disseminated through leading medical journals but also in many kinds of sources emanating from multiple locales. Bioline International and Scielo offer open access to a range of health-related journals from Asia, Africa, and Latin America (www.bioline.org.br/). Numerous activist organizations, such as Focus on the Global South, People's Health Movement, Navdanya, ALAMES, and others, have useful Web sites (see the Appendix: List of Web sites).

One of the most important aspects of being an effective international public health practitioner is communication: speaking local languages is key. You may start by learning one or more important regional languages such as French, Spanish, Arabic, Russian, Swahili, Hindi-Urdu, or Mandarin. In most developing countries, however, this still limits communication to dominant social and cultural groups. While mastering local languages is not always feasible, at the very least, it is important to acknowledge that a great deal will be missed without speaking the language. Many English speakers are accustomed to speaking in their native tongue wherever they go, yet over half the world's population is bilingual. For those whose work takes place internationally, language skills are imperative.

Formal training in international health, usually obtained from a school or program of public health, is common though not obligatory: many people who consider themselves international health professionals entered the field circuitously. International health training in medical and nursing schools is limited though growing: generally a few hours per year are devoted to international issues as part of classes in nutrition, epidemiology, travel medicine, or tropical diseases. The Alma-Ata Global Health Network has found increasing interest in international health but reluctance on the part of universities to fund such programs (Nicholson, Lewis, and Martineau 2007). The Global Health Education Consortium, bringing together faculty from more than 70 health professions schools in Canada, the Caribbean, Central America, and the United States, prepares training materials and organizes conferences with the aim of raising the number of global health educators (Global Health Education Consortium 2008). Some schools, such as the University of Toronto, the London School of Hygiene, New York University, and the University of Washington have responded to student coalitions, conferences, and initiatives by setting up formal global health training programs.

There are also organizations that provide courses for individuals interested in either a career or volunteer work in international health. For example RedR-IHE, an NGO with offices in the United Kingdom and Australia, offers courses in relief work focusing on such issues as international humanitarian law, understanding gender and cross-cultural issues, and personal health and safety (RedR Australia 2008). International health volunteers and workers, especially those providing humanitarian aid in disaster or conflict situations, may find that they are not prepared to work under highly stressful conditions (Bjerneld et al. 2004). Formal training in how to survive while working abroad is increasingly common. Professionals working abroad for the U.S. government or the WHO are mandated to take a week-long training course in security, housing, mental health coping techniques, and communication skills.

It is important to note that most international health training programs focus on traditional and technical approaches, often paying only minor attention to the political economy and social perspectives presented in this book. We encourage students to push their own or prospective institutions to cover the political economy of international health in greater depth so that they do not finish their academic careers thinking that health aid provided through donor organizations is the solution to global and local social inequalities in health.

Rajesh Gupta and Paul Farmer (2005, pp. 3–4) provide three "admonitions" to students and course directors:

1. Know the setting: students should learn about the "political, sociocultural, and economic history" of the country and recognize that "in no settings does treatment end with a simple prescription or procedure; effective therapy needs invariably reflect the social conditions of patients."
2. Expand the notion of treatment: "Civil strife, war, health sector reform, or even the lack of consistent electricity may profoundly affect (treatment) goals ... the combination of prevention and treatment is more synergistically powerful than either alone."
3. Continue involvement upon returning home: international placements should not be voyeuristic episodes to see "how the majority lives" but bestow a continuing responsibility on the intern to address the problems experienced long after leaving—that is, they should address health and disease at global as well as local levels through advocacy, activism, education, and other solidarity measures. Recognizing how home country/imperialist policies affect the health of populations internationally and taking part in efforts to address them is much less glamorous yet urgently needed.

Many health professionals obtain their first international health experiences through a student placement or internship. The WHO, PAHO, and other UN and bilateral agencies including the Canadian International Development Agency (CIDA), and technical agencies such as the CDC, offer an array of international health internships (see www.who.int/employment/internship/en/). The United Nations Volunteer Program (www.unv.org) provides international health opportunities for people early in their professional careers. The program is especially useful for individuals from countries with few other funding sources.

Various university and foundation grants (e.g., the Barry Freeman Fellowship at the University of Iowa and the Rotary Foundation) fund international placements and fellowships. The U.S. Fulbright program and the National Institutes of Health's (NIH) Fogarty International Center also support research, clinical, and teaching opportunities in international public health. The NIH's Web site hosts a directory of grants and fellowships for international health (www.fic.nih.gov/funding/graddir06.htm), including funding from the Aga Khan Foundation and the Wellcome Trust. The Canadian Society for International Health has similar listings (www.csih.org/en/opportunities/fundopps.asp). Other useful Web sites for finding international health placements include: the American Medical Student Association Web site (www.amsa.org/global/ih/travelfunding.cfm), the University of Arizona (www.globalhealth.arizona.edu/Funding_Links.htm), idealist.org, and the University of Washington's International Health Group which mostly funds medical students (depts.washington.edu/ihg/funding.htm).

Many humanitarian organizations and international NGOs also offer internships, for example the Asia Foundation, CARE-USA, Save the Children-USA, and Winrock International. Individuals interested in health and human rights activities (described below) can pursue internships with Physicians for Human Rights, Amnesty International, and Human Rights Watch.

It is regrettable but understandable that few developing countries provide fellowships or grants to study international health. Notable exceptions to this are programs sponsoring South-to-North training and South-to-South training, such as the GK Fellowships at Gonoshasthaya Kendra in Bangladesh (part of the International People's Health University, www.phmovement.org/iphu/en/fellprog), and Canada's International Development Research Centre (IDRC)-supported Teasdale-Corti Global Health Research Partnership Program (www.idrc.ca).

Electives in developing countries have also become an essential part of surgery residencies (Ozgediz et al. 2005) to train surgeons how to operate in resource-constrained environments. Certain internal medicine residency programs—for example, at Case Western Reserve, Harvard, and Yale universities—are organized around global health education and work hard to place their residents overseas (Gupta et al. 1999).

Some developed countries regard the international work experience of health specialists as a form of training that serves their own institutional purposes, such as reducing turnover, increasing motivation, and improving delivery of care. The U.K. Department of Health, for example, encourages its employees to take "career breaks" to carry out international humanitarian and health work (Department of Health 2003). In its *Toolkit to Support Good Practice*, the Department outlines various concrete skills it expects from employees who obtain overseas experience: better prioritization and allocation of scarce resources; improved planning, monitoring, and auditing; ability to assess health needs of local communities; and enhanced leadership, teamwork, and intersectoral collaboration. While this is undoubtedly a self-serving agenda, it also has the potential to implement multidirectional learning efforts that are central to international health cooperation.

Exciting as these opportunities may be, it is important to recognize that international placements can put an enormous burden on settings with already stretched resources. Health workers in developing country programs and institutions are often given little or no compensation for acting as supervisors or trainers for those from overseas. As in the case of "global health tourism," students and other visitors usually walk away with lots of knowledge and new skills, but leave little behind in the community. In addition, outsiders may disrupt social services that are in place by bringing in short-term treatments/solutions that are not available once they leave.

Every country has laws and regulations governing the practice of different types of health professionals. Students still in training who find themselves in clinical settings must not expect to examine patients, prescribe medicines, or engage in any other clinical activity that they would not legally be allowed to do at home. This dictum, however, is often defied by students who see the underdeveloped world as a training ground to hone their skills. Trained health professionals also frequently break this rule and practice medicine in countries in which they are not licensed, assuming that their training (typically in developed countries) is equivalent or superior to that required by local health professionals. Not only is this illegal, it may be dangerous: different treatment standards in each country mean that outsiders cannot presume that what they have been trained to do is appropriate for a different setting (e.g., bringing in new antibiotics where penicillin is the standard treatment).

Those trained or acculturated in Western biomedicine often overlook the many indigenous practices, including acupuncture, yoga, and t'ai chi, that have been adopted and "validated" by modern science and accepted as better than biomedicine for various health problems. One-fourth of modern medicines are made from plants first used traditionally (WHO 2003b). For example, quinine (from cinchona tree bark) was used by indigenous peoples in what is now South America long before it was adopted by Western physicians for the treatment of malaria. Similarly, the herbal remedy *Artemisia annua*, used in China for almost 2,000 years, has become a breakthrough malaria preventive (formulated as artemisinin).

Furthermore, various health systems include diagnosis and treatment protocols and local licensing procedures for Ayurveda, Tibetan medicine and psychiatry, homeopathy, Chinese medicine, and Islamic medicine, among others. Indeed, local healing systems and traditional healers are being increasingly incorporated into national and international public health activities. A growing number of programs allow allopathically (Western-) trained professionals to study Tibetan medicine and psychiatry in Nepal and India (www.himalayanhealth.com), for example. Similar programs exist for Ayurveda, Chinese medicine, and traditional herbal medicine.

In addition to understanding local traditions and needs, any person interested in international health engagement needs to be tolerant, self-critical and reflective, a good listener, patient, able to work with people in diverse fields and with varied backgrounds, open minded, humble, and have or be able to develop expertise that is relevant within the work context. As discussed above, it is also necessary to be cautious of power differentials and make a concerted effort not to disrupt local systems. Finally, it is essential to become historically, culturally, and politically aware—that is, to appreciate the relationship among local conditions and national and international policies and forces, as well as the profoundly political underpinnings of most international health aid.

Ultimately, the effectiveness of international health workers and, by extension, the programs that they support, depends as much on understanding language, culture, and broad sociopolitical issues as on possessing particular technical skills.

Apart from authors writing about research ethics (Bhutta 2002), little advice on "doing international health" has been written from a developing country vantage point. This is unfortunate, as much perspective and balance would be gained if, for example, developing country policymakers, advocates, and health workers (who work alongside donor country workers), as well as the "recipients" of assistance also shared their experiences.

International Health Research: Challenges and Ethical Dimensions (Individual and Institutional Levels)

In addition to expertise, experience, and political economy knowledge, a strong foundation in the ethics of international health and research is indispensable. Ethics resides at the intersection of individual and organizational roles and responsibilities.

Scientific research can play a vital role in international health, especially when health technologies are integrated with public health services (and systems) *and* with efforts to address the societal determinants of health examined in Chapter 7, including neighborhood and living conditions, social security and worker protections, and inequalities of power and resources within and between countries. Alas, this goal is rarely met. Indeed, the conduct of international health research, particularly in underdeveloped countries, faces a series of challenges.

In 1990 the Commission on Health Research for Development estimated that less than 10% of global funding for health research was used to address the health problems of developing countries, which at the time accounted for 90% of preventable causes of premature death and disability (Matlin 2005). This finding—and the companion term "10/90 gap"—still holds today. Moreover, only a minute portion of international health research spending focuses on combined social and technical approaches to health improvement.

In conjunction with the 10/90 gap is a parallel problem: the research agenda of underdeveloped countries is mostly set by "development partners" rather than according to locally defined priorities (COHRED 2007). This means, for example, that "neglected diseases" (see Chapter 6) prevalent in certain developing countries receive little attention. Even well-recognized diseases, such as tuberculosis, may benefit little from research on new medications as compared to other diseases (see Table 12–8). Moreover, virtually no research addresses how disease processes and poor social conditions interact. These deficiencies result partly from the influence of the private sector, particularly pharmaceutical companies, on public policies: research spending by the private, for-profit sector—approximately half of the $US126 billion in global health research and development expenditure in 2003 (Intergovernmental working group on public health 2007)—has resulted in greater inequities rather than fewer.

As such, attention to international health research—and expanding health research in underdeveloped countries—can be justified on a number of grounds. Clearly, conducting research on diseases including schistosomiasis, trachoma, and malaria requires knowledge of and applicability to endemic areas. Similarly, research on the organization of programs such as rural primary health care may be appropriately conducted only in places where they operate. The challenge of addressing ill health and marginalization simultaneously—while relevant to both developing and developed countries—requires particular research attention in settings with limited resources and extreme inequalities.

Despite these vast needs, much international health research has not benefited the majority of developing country populations. As discussed in Chapter 2, there has been long experience with unilateral, opportunistic research endeavors: colonial health research was historically aimed at resolving imperial needs, whether safeguarding soldiers and settlers, protecting trade, or improving the productivity of workers in profitable industries. Today, well-funded foreign experts from industrialized countries or international agencies may travel to developing countries on short stints to gather material or collect data for their own publications—gaining personal advancement, perhaps with little acknowledgment of the efforts of local colleagues. In extreme cases, developing country research may be appropriated, local scientists denied rightful authorship, and study populations mistreated. Wherever it takes place, collaboration, not exploitation, is the key to scientific work. Interestingly, although each year thousands of health researchers from developed countries receive grants to carry out studies in developing countries, it is virtually unheard of for a team of researchers from, for example, India or Senegal to receive funding to investigate health problems in, say, Canada or France.

But "research imperialism" is only part of the story. Rising costs and restrictions on research and development in industrialized countries have made it increasingly attractive to conduct drug trials in locales where expenses are low and administrative oversight may be relatively lax. Rates of particular diseases may be higher in developing countries, making it easier to reach required study sample sizes. Undoubtedly, more stringent justification is needed for conducting pharmaceutical trials in developing countries, especially when only a fraction of the local population might benefit from the results, and the study sponsors leave little or nothing behind in terms of health systems infrastructure.

Of course, resident scientists in developing countries are often as well trained as foreigners, and they are certainly more knowledgeable about the local situation. Scientific contributions from developing countries include, to name just a few: the identification of American trypanosomiasis by Brazilian Carlos Chagas in 1909; Chinese researchers' isolation of the traditional plant extract artemisinin for the treatment of malaria; Cuba's combined social and biotechnology achievements (including universal primary health care and education, food and housing security, and the first meningitis B vaccine), leading to one of the world's best child health records; and Botswana's solar-rechargeable hearing aid. Much of this work, including the budding biotechnology industry in various countries, has been spurred by national scientific research and funding councils (such as Mexico's CONACYT).

Informed Consent and Research Ethics Guidelines

Notwithstanding their potential benefits, the means used to produce new knowledge and products may themselves cause harm, a concern that was only systematically addressed as of the mid-20th century. In the years just after World War II, the Nuremberg War Crimes trials demonstrated the importance of defining standards for judging the physicians and scientists who had conducted heinous medical experiments on concentration camp prisoners in Nazi Germany and for preventing future violations. The Nuremberg Code of 1947 established the requirement for voluntary consent of all human medical research subjects. Following this prototype, many codes of research ethics have been promoted by various professional groups, all based on the principle of informed consent and the notion of individuals as autonomous (free-acting) agents.

Yet even after these codes were developed, harmful research continued. Perhaps the most infamous case was the Tuskegee Syphilis Study in the United States, conducted by the U.S. Public Health Service between 1932 and 1972 on over 400 poor African-American men in the U.S. state of Alabama. The recruited men believed that they were being treated for syphilis—with which they had been diagnosed—but in fact were never treated or were inadequately treated, resulting in at least 40 deaths (Gamble 1997; Reverby 2000). Similarly, in the mid-1950s, an almost 20-year study of viral hepatitis in more than 700 mentally retarded children, many infected with the disease, was launched at the Willowbrook State School in Staten Island, United States, without obtaining consent (for a list of similar cases see www.clarion.edu/academic/adeptt/bpcluster/cases.htm).

Revelation of these ethical violations led to more stringent regulation and control over research involving human subjects. In the United States, the basic document is found in the 1974 Code of Federal Regulations (Title 45, Part 46, Public Law 93–348). This act also established a National Commission for the Protection of Human Subjects of Biomedical and Behavioral Research, which stated the basic ethical principles and guidelines for research involving human subjects as follows (Belmont Report 1979):

- *Respect for persons*: Individuals should be treated as autonomous agents. Persons with diminished capacity are entitled to protection.
- *Beneficence*: Persons are treated in an ethical manner, not only by respecting their decisions and protecting them from harm, but also by making efforts to secure their well-being.
- *Justice*: Decisions on who ought to receive the benefits of research and bear its burdens should be made on the basis of "fairness in distribution" or "what is deserved."

According to U.S. law and practice, each research subject must be provided with the following information:

- A statement indicating that the study involves research and describing whether and how confidentiality will be maintained; an explanation of the purposes of the research and the expected duration of the subject's participation; a description of the procedures to be followed; and identification of any procedures which are experimental.
- A description of any reasonably foreseeable benefits and risks or discomforts to the subject and disclosure of appropriate alternative procedures or courses of treatment, if any, that might be advantageous to the subject.
- For research involving more than minimal risk, an explanation as to whether any compensation or treatments are available.
- An explanation of whom to contact for answers to pertinent questions about the research and research subjects' rights and how to report a research-related injury.
- A statement that participation is voluntary, that refusal to participate or desire to discontinue participation (at any time) will involve no penalty or loss of benefits to which the subject is otherwise entitled.

Normally, informed consent is documented in writing and signed by the subject or their representative (e.g., a parent) who retains a copy of the document.

A number of similar guidelines have been produced by international organizations such as the World Medical Association's *Helsinki Declaration*, the Council for International Organizations of Medical Sciences' (CIOMS) *International Ethical Guidelines for Biomedical Research Involving Human Subjects*, and the World Commission on the Ethics of Scientific Knowledge and Technology, which was established by UNESCO to advise it on the ethical dimensions of all matters relating to science and technology. CIOMS guidelines cover not only planned interventions on human subjects but also research in which environmental factors are manipulated in a way that could jeopardize the well-being of incidentally exposed individuals (CIOMS 2002, revised).

The main mechanisms for applying these guidelines are research ethics committees or institutional review boards (IRBs), which decide whether or not the proposed research violates the rights of subjects. Written experimental protocols in general contain at least the following: the aim of the research; the reasons it is to be undertaken on human subjects; the nature and severity of known dangers due to the research; the participant recruiting sources; the voluntary nature of participation; and the means for ensuring informed consent. Protocols are to be scientifically and ethically appraised in both sponsoring and host countries by a suitable body independent of the investigators.

All U.S.-funded research—wherever it is conducted—is required by law to be reviewed by IRBs, which evaluate protocols for investigations dealing with human subjects, including fetuses, tissues, body fluids, and so on. Many countries and health ministries have mandated analogous review panels to consider outside requests to conduct investigations within their jurisdictions (Indian Council for Medical Research 2000). Yet a 2004 survey found that one-fourth of clinical trials conducted in developing countries do not undergo ethical review (Hyder et al. 2004). As of 2007, 36% of countries in Africa did not have research ethics committees and the capacity and expertise of members in countries with established committees was weak (Kass et al. 2007).

Diversity in IRB membership is important to ensure that a range of perspectives is represented in the ethical evaluation of the research proposal. Most review boards are composed of physicians, nurses, lawyers, and administrators. In both Africa and Latin America there is a shift toward including "lay people" (Rivera and Ezcurra 2001; Kass et al. 2007).

Ethics committees can suffer from the following limitations: they may be composed of fellow researchers who may be more sympathetic to the cause of research than the rights of subjects; in small institutions, committee members may be collaborators with the authors of the proposal on other research projects; they may lack representatives of the subjects' background (class, race, ethnicity, culture, religion, etc.); or they may be thousands of miles away from the location of the research and therefore not fully understand the context of the research. For example, a recent review of ethics committees in South Africa showed that more than a decade after apartheid ended, most are still composed of white males—not representative of the racial, gender, and other characteristics of the general population (Moodley and Myer 2007).

The ethics of international health research and practice often transpires in a gray zone not explicitly covered by legal codes in either sponsoring or hosting nations, and ethics procedures may need to be negotiated iteratively with local populations rather than rely strictly on international guidelines (Harper 2007). Standard informed consent documents may be either inappropriate or impractical in many developing country settings, for example, among persons who for reasons of age, education, or world experience may not be in a position to evaluate the potential benefits and risks of experimental procedures. Special efforts must be made to inform non-literate subjects about the purpose of the study, the need for their consent, and their freedom to withdraw. The situation may be even more complex for persons living in certain traditional communities, where informed consent may be meaningless whether or not a signature or witnessed mark is obtained (Bhutta 2004).

As well, the practice of paying study participants may negate all pretense of informed consent in poor communities, serving as an unethical inducement to participation. Community compensation or ex post facto payment may serve as an alternative, but one that may turn developing country study subjects into a "cheap bargain" for researchers.

A further problem in the United States and elsewhere is that data collection for public health programs usually does not live up to the same ethical standards expected of research studies. While data are not always collected in the context of particular studies, many public health departments around the world gather personal information, store it, and use it to solve problems, whether or not they call these activities research. Few protections are offered to the "subjects," making surveillance and other related public health activities areas of growing concern (Mariner 1997).

In addition to the issues arising in studies involving individual consent, community-level trials also pose ethical challenges. For experimental treatment of water supplies, health services research, studies on environmental pesticides or nutritional supplementation of everyday foods, and similar broadscale research interventions, individual consent may not be feasible. Entire communities may be randomized to experimental or control status, and the decision to undertake the research is in the hands of political authorities on behalf of the community. Some societies put greater stress on the embeddedness of the individual within the community and define a person by his or her relations to others (Christakis 1988). In such contexts, the consent process may shift from the individual to the family or to the community (LaVertu and Linares 1990). Consent through a community leader "proxy," however, could be susceptible to inducement or fraud, and individuals could be reluctant to disagree with the selected community leader, even if they have grave reservations about participation in the trial.

Some of these problems pose insurmountable dilemmas to research; consultation with a wide array of community representatives, researchers, and political leaders may prove helpful but will not necessarily resolve ethical concerns or make research meaningful and relevant to developing country contexts (Bhutta 2002).

Why Are Research Ethics Important?

Flagrant violations of research ethics in the past led to the establishment of IRBs, yet similar episodes have continued to occur in the international research context. Perhaps most controversial was the AIDS/AZT trial of the mid-1990s. By then, it was well established that a small proportion of infants of HIV-infected mothers are born with the infection, and that the drug AZT can reduce maternal transmission to infants. In 1995, a series of experiments were undertaken in nine sub-Saharan African countries, as well as in Thailand and the Dominican Republic (with funding support from the U.S. government, the UNAIDS program, and health ministries of some of the countries involved) to determine whether there were less expensive ways to achieve similar benefits in developing countries. Approximately 12,000 pregnant women participated as research subjects. According to the project design, half of the women received AZT in varying dosages and half received an inert placebo. Critics of the study pointed out that under this protocol hundreds of infants would needlessly contract HIV. They demanded that the study be halted on ethical grounds, given that there was already evidence of AZT's effectiveness: in such circumstances, the new regimen ought to have been compared to the existing medication, not to a placebo.

Indeed, in a classic double-blinded, placebo-controlled randomized clinical trial, a vaccine or medication is tested against an inert substance (placebo) to assess its efficacy in preventing or treating the disease among participants. The trials of the Salk polio vaccine in the mid-1950s, and of the first measles vaccine in the early 1960s, were of this type. At the time of those trials, there was no other available method of preventing polio or measles. But once a safe and effective vaccine or medication becomes available, a simple placebo-controlled trial is no longer ethically acceptable: an effective intervention cannot be withheld just to see if a new product might be in some way better, because this would expose subjects unnecessarily to what has become a preventable disease. All subjects in the next generation trial would normally be randomized to receive either the new candidate intervention or the existing one, without any placebo. Such a trial using what is called an "active control" is rational and ethical though far more costly than the original one that tested the initial intervention against a placebo. It was this extra cost that researchers and their funders were seeking to avoid in the AZT study.

An article and an editorial in the *New England Journal of Medicine* agreed that the AZT trial was unethical and compared it to the Tuskegee study of untreated syphilis (Angell 1997; Lurie and Wolfe 1997). These pieces touched off an intense debate about the ethics of placebo-controlled randomized clinical trials in developing countries. U.S. officials, including the directors of the NIH and CDC, countered that the use of placebos was the only way to get quick, reliable results, and that the women in the study were not deprived of any therapy that they would otherwise have received since most of them did not have access to AZT outside of the trial context (Varmus and Satcher 1997). In the end, the study was forced to abandon the use of placebos and all women were given the drug.

The HIV/AIDS pandemic, with the understandable rush to find a vaccine or medication to prevent transmission of the virus, has added to the challenges of adhering to research ethics in clinical trials. Because these trials are conducted largely in sub-Saharan Africa, where the incidence and prevalence are highest but IRBs are often suboptimal, there are concerns that researchers may be taking ethical responsibilities lightly. The WHO has published guidelines for research on HIV that call for investigators to take additional care when dealing with issues such as informed consent, selecting criteria for eligibility for care, the provision of antiretrovirals (ARVs) post-trial, the need to involve local communities in research, and so on (WHO 2003a).

Of course, unethical practices are not confined to the developing world. There are numerous examples of clinical trials being manipulated to serve commercial interests—even where IRBs are mandated. In the United States there has been growing concern about the collaboration between the pharmaceutical industry and university-based researchers since the Bayh-Dole Act of 1980, which granted permission to federally funded researchers to patent and license inventions (Sharav 2002). This opened the gate to significant conflict of interests between researchers and industry (Angell 2004).

In recent decades, the independence of the U.S. Food and Drug Administration (FDA), which approves pharmaceutical products, has also been brought into question. Bowing to pressure from the pharmaceutical industry, the FDA has shortened the approval process for new drugs and delayed withdrawing drugs from the market even after they have been banned (due to side effects) by European health agencies (Sharav 2002). The influence of lobbyists on the political process has also soared: in 2001 there were an estimated 625 lobbyists for the pharmaceutical industry who were paid exorbitant salaries to influence the U.S. federal government (Claybrook 2001).

Most recently, in 2008, the FDA abandoned its adherence to the 1989 Declaration of Helsinki protecting human subjects in clinical research for foreign clinical trials. Instead, a looser standard will hold, which does not require new treatments to be tested against existing ones, only against placebos. In effect, this will push more trials to developing countries, where research subjects are likely to be denied access to effective treatments (http://www.cspinet.org/integrity/watch/index.html).

Other Ethical Dimensions of International Health

Although much of bioethics in wealthy countries is driven by the financial or individual implications of new technologies and procedures—such as in vitro fertilization, "fertility drugs," surrogate parenting, DNA fingerprinting, gene therapy—all aspects of (international health) are riddled with ethical dilemmas.

Immunization programs might seem to be morally unassailable, but even the eradication of diseases such as polio poses ethical dilemmas. On one level, eradication is endorsed by all WHO member states, and most developing countries are enthusiastic in their support since polio eradication attracts donor funding. Eradication programs help build a "culture of prevention" even if health infrastructure is not always adequately addressed. Yet on another level, arguments against the polio campaign are valid: countries are pressured to defer their own priorities (such as infant and maternal mortality, which are much greater contributors to premature death and disability) and to divert resources and efforts at the expense of other health activities; the financial benefits of eradication are greatest to wealthier countries; and poor countries bear the major costs and negative effects of the campaign, such as polio outbreaks. Indeed, oral vaccine-associated polio outbreaks still occur, generating resistance and resentment in some countries. In parts of Nigeria and Pakistan, some religious leaders have spearheaded opposition to the campaign due to real and perceived harms; elsewhere there is suspicion that early polio vaccine trials in Congo contributed to the spread of simian viruses (potentially linked to HIV). Moreover, although the oral polio vaccine is more effective at eliminating the disease, it is more dangerous than the killed vaccine now used in most developed countries, raising concerns about double standards.

Many ethical conundrums revolve around the asymmetries within and between countries, such as unequal power and resources; inequitable regulations concerning patents and drug-marketing policies; exploitative trade in infant formulas and harmful products; the migration of health professionals from low-income to high-income countries; the shipment of toxic waste in the reverse direction; and many similar matters. Cultural and religious differences in societal goals, moral teachings, the meaning of justice, and perceptions of individual autonomy also create ethical quandaries: attitudes vary among populations about the treatment of children, women, the disabled, the elderly, and members of certain ethnic minorities and societal subgroups.

The activities of international workers may conflict with locally established practices regarding abortion, family planning, the position of women, and a host of other conventions. In such cases the terms of reference of any activity must be spelled out in particular detail, and the scope of work of specific project activities of foreign workers must be carefully described and monitored to maintain respect for the ethical precepts of the host country and protection of host populations. International health workers in violation of these precepts may be asked to leave; conversely, foreign health workers witnessing systematic abuse in the host country may terminate their activities so that they are not associated with repressive governments. As discussed in the human rights section ahead, denouncing such abuses is a further responsibility of international health workers and organizations.

International health workers and activities can generate competition with local health workers over provision of services and goods, making the former's contribution to local needs questionable. Contractors and suppliers from donor countries may benefit handsomely. Food aid, for example, is often criticized because the transferred products can disrupt normal markets for local producers, create a preference for imported foods, or cause a shift in agricultural production away from local foods and toward export products. Moreover, the foods shipped may represent those in surplus in the donor country, may be produced under price support programs, and may not be those requested or desired by the recipients. As discussed elsewhere, well-funded international health programs (which frequently do not coincide with locally defined priorities) often draw local workers away from routine programs, destroying the capacity of health systems to cope with numerous needs.

Finally, foreign projects and expatriate workers often have a relatively brief time commitment in a country, leaving residents to bear the long-term consequences, for good or harm, of implemented programs. On a larger scale is the question of the lasting impact on local populations, resources, and environment.

In the end, ethics are not simply a matter for research and researchers but are relevant to every international health program, worker, and instance of cooperation.

Organizational Level: Missions and Interventions

Since many readers of this text who go on in international health will seek a paid position or volunteer work in an existing agency, a few words of advice are warranted. Potential employees/contractees should learn about the sponsoring organization's mission and funding sources, as well as the larger context of its activities. For example, during the Cold War many socially committed Peace Corps volunteers in developing countries did not realize that they were perceived by local residents to be part of the U.S. (particularly the Central International Agency's) response to the "communist threat."

Equally important is to understand how the activity or aid is provided, whose interests it serves, how it relates to the stated organizational mission and implicit intentions, what strings are attached, and the extent to which resources actually reach the most needy. By simply pursuing these issues in an ongoing fashion, a political economy of health perspective can be infused in almost any work setting. While challenging an organization to be true to its mission, better define its goals, or demonstrate how it is publicly accountable can be threatening to both the challenger and the agency, it is one of the most important means of effecting change.

One key question is: what proportion of funding actually reaches intended beneficiaries? A 2006 report by ActionAid International noted that of total US$79 billion in development aid provided in 2004, US$37 billion (47%) was "phantom aid," including funds double-counted as debt relief, funds spent on international consultants and in the home country, tied funds, and so on (ActionAid International 2006). Of the US$37 billion of phantom aid, $11.8 billion was spent on "overpriced and ineffective technical assistance" (ActionAid International 2006, p. 9). The ActionAid report cited the failure of technical assistance as caused by: donor driven (political) priorities; development models that do not work; local capacity-building being overlooked; and the high cost and ineffectiveness of consultants. In some settings, outside consultants are paid hundreds of times more than local government employees.

Before deciding to work or volunteer with an organization, you might examine its rating according to ActionAid or www.CharityNavigator.org, which gauge the proportion of resources that actually reach programs versus administrative and fund-raising activities. For example, organizations that emphasize partnerships—Partners In Health, CARE, and Save the Children—score high on efficiency, while organizations that sponsor medical missions, such as IHCF African Christian Hospitals and the Medical Benevolence Foundation, score very poorly.

Of course, organizations want to survive. Thus, NGOs, government agencies, and consulting firms write grant proposals and bid on contracts for things that they know how to do, or hope to learn to do, and for which funding is available. Even organizations that seek to serve needs according to local knowledge and priority-setting may be severely constrained by funders. In that sense, helping an organization to find alternative funding sources, especially sources that are locally accountable, can be enormously useful.

The Aid Milieu

In many developing countries, there is a profusion—an "unruly mélange" (Buse and Walt 1997)—of bilateral and multilateral aid agencies and the international and local NGOs they support. All are ostensibly working to improve the health of local citizens, yet these organizations often work at cross-purposes with population needs or in competition with one another. The precise role of each group may be unclear to outside observers, the host government, people using the services, and at times the agencies themselves. From Mozambique to Nicaragua to Nepal, the donor aid milieu—and, in particular, the rise of NGOs since the end of the Cold War—has proven damaging to health (Justice 1989; Panday 1999; Birn, Zimmerman, and Garfield 2000). As analyzed by James Pfeiffer:

> The Mozambique experience reveals that the deluge of NGOs and their expatriate workers over the last decade has fragmented the local health system, undermined local control of health programs, and contributed to growing local social inequality. Since national health system salaries plummeted over the same period as a result of structural adjustment, health workers became vulnerable to financial favors offered by NGOs seeking to promote their projects in turf struggles with other agencies...The multiplicity of competing organizations that duplicate program support, create parallel projects, pull health service workers away from routine duties, and disrupt planning processes has generated concern for both donors and recipients...
>
> In this engagement, the exercise of power by wealthy donors over their target populations, including local health workers, is laid bare and the disempowerment of public sector services by international agencies is most visible. Expatriate health workers employed by international agencies can be found at all levels of many developing world health systems; from Ministry of Health offices in capital cities to remote villages where they are involved in health program implementation. These agencies' activities may be integrated into Ministry programs, or conducted completely outside the public system. In addition to their expatriate staff, agencies usually employ small armies of 'nationals,' from trained health professionals and office workers to drivers and guards. Usually these workers are paid far more than their counterparts in the public sector (Pfeiffer 2003, pp. 725–726), leading to hierarchies of inclusion, exclusion, and favoritism.

Expatriate health workers may wittingly or unintentionally play a part in these problems. Good intentions are insufficient: international workers should ensure that they do not contribute to chaos and local vulnerability but rather assist in strengthening the host country's ability to organize and deliver services and activities on its own terms. Indeed, health professionals can have a powerful voice in insisting that local public health agendas be set in the spirit of "cooperative actions and solutions" (Institute of Medicine 1997, p. 20), for example, through an international code of conduct emphasizing accountability, respect, local agenda-setting, and building capacity based on "long-term equitable professional relationships in a sustainable adequately funded public sector" (Pfeiffer 2003, p. 725), and on codes developed for humanitarian crises (Thieren 2007; Pfeiffer et al. 2008).

A cardinal rule for international health work is the same as it is for medicine: *primum non nocere*—first do no harm. Organizations and individuals involved in international health must be prepared to shed their own prejudices and opinions, work together with organizations and people from the host country as true partners, and understand that the appropriate role of outside groups is supportive and subsidiary to what the country wishes to achieve.

Some individuals, perhaps due to frustrations with other organizations or motivated by unfilled needs, decide to found their own NGO. While starting an international NGO may seem appealing, the proliferation of small and large agencies in recent years with literally thousands of organizations operating at local, national, and international levels has had numerous negative consequences, including duplication of efforts, the draining of enormous logistical and administrative resources, and lack of sustainability. In many settings, NGOs form a "state within a state," adding new layers of bureaucracy but without any pretense of democratic representation. UN bodies, NGOs, and donor-funded programs often lure health care professionals away from the public system because they offer higher salaries, which puts long-term pressure on strapped health care systems. Moreover, NGOs often become dependent on funding and interests of larger donors, turning them into unwitting interlocutors or implementers of dominant priorities (Pfeiffer 2003) and displacing social movements (Roy 2004).

Before starting an NGO, it is thus important to consider: what its long-term role might be; what need it is fulfilling and why that need is not currently being served; why an international NGO is preferable to a local organization or a publicly funded effort; and what other avenues might be pursued.

One alternative to the founding of new organizations is the formation of coalitions and networks of existing political movements that pressure for fair trade, universal access to water and other basic human needs, worldwide occupational health protections, and so on. The Third World Network, based in Penang, Malaysia, with offices in Delhi, Montevideo, Accra, and Geneva, and affiliates in various other developing country settings, is an independent, nonprofit research and activist network that effectively focuses attention on trade, development, health, and other social and political issues that affect the lives and livelihoods of the majority of people in developing countries. National and transnational alliances against militarism (as discussed in Chapter 8), or in favor of the Tobin tax—a proposed tax on cross-border currency transactions that would be channeled to environmental and human needs—also have enormous potential for improving global health (equity). In most instances, building on existing local and international efforts is likely to be more effective and sustainable than founding countless new organizations.

Yet even the most sensitive, noble, and knowledgeable persons and organizations cannot single-handedly transcend the larger context—or world order—of economic exploitation and inequality.

The Logic of the World Order and Its Relation to International Health

Over 100 years ago, the Polish revolutionary and socialist philosopher Rosa Luxemburg posed the question of whether reform (change from within) was useful and possible or whether it impeded revolution (change from without). Her espousal of the latter position, leading to her participation in the Berlin revolution, cost her her life in 1919 when she was captured by German authorities and tortured to death. The "reform versus revolution" question continues to be evoked today. Davidson Gwatkin, consultant on health and poverty to the World Bank, recently argued that "The health of the world's poor would be best served by a series of revolutions that bring into power national leaderships that are centrally concerned about the well-being of disadvantaged groups within their borders" (Yamey 2007, p. 1558). The World Bank, however, has long supported private enterprise, not socialist revolution, as the formula for progress. How might we reconcile this paradox?

Today, many regard the reform versus revolution dichotomy to be false or at least exaggerated, instead viewing effective redistributive reforms—especially the creation of a welfare state with universal rights to safe housing, employment, neighborhoods, environments, water and sanitation, education, health care, and nondiscrimination—as the scaffolding of structural change. To return to the previous example, another such effort would call for reform of the World Bank itself (as an alternative to more revolutionary calls for its elimination), so that it democratically represents not only all countries but all social classes. In this way, the World Bank could become a people's bank, rather than a bank representing elite interests. Indeed, every multilateral or UN agency should have such democratic policy processes, allowing an integration of scientific expertise and representative decision making. How would a democratization reform change the World Bank? The widespread misery caused by loan conditionalities could be addressed, for example, not through small-scale or symbolic debt forgiveness and "mutual" reform efforts (as crafted by one-sided lenders cushioned from the effects of "adjustment" programs), but through: total and unconditional debt cancellation; abolition of loan conditionalities; payment of reparations for enslavement, plundering, and exploitation; and the creation of reverse conditionalities (i.e., no loan would be allowed unless it decreased the Gini index, increased access to water or education, etc.), as decided through democratic and accountable governance processes (Jubilee South 2008).

So, too, might you see your own work in international health as a reform effort en route to improving the determinants of health at each level of the political economy of international health framework explored in this book. Should you find yourself working—or advocating for change—within an organization that follows "business as usual" in international health, your efforts, together with those of colleagues and supporters, could help reform the organization in a variety of ways. For example, as an epidemiologist employed by an international epidemiologic surveillance agency, you might insist that surveys of AIDS prevalence include variables regarding living conditions, nutritional well-being, employment and income security, and other factors. Or if you live in a high-income country, you may decide that your efforts will be more effective at home through activism with a political movement that calls for changes in trade and commodity pricing rules, challenges foreign aid strategies that further entrench power imbalances, or defends occupational health conditions worldwide.

How can people concerned with reforming international health reconcile the larger world order with the reality of practicing international health day to day in an organization? Approaches include:

1. Working with/for an organization in whose modus operandi you believe. Many progressive-minded agencies are listed in Chapter 3 and the Appendix. For example, Doctors for Global Health (DGH) goes only where it is invited, and uses the concepts of "health as reconciliation" and "anti-colonization" as its guiding principles when setting up cooperative projects in marginalized communities (Smith 2007) (see Fig. 14–1).

A key to effective international health work, either by individuals or organizations, is commitment over long time periods to a specific population or country. Health Alliance International has been working in Mozambique for decades (just as has Partners In Health in Haiti), maintaining its support over the very long term, through war, political strife, government change, funding challenges, and so on (see Box 13–5 and Fig. 14–2). This contrasts considerably with larger international NGOs that often pursue high-profile "relief" efforts rather than making long-term investments in communities.

Other organizations that prioritize local sustainability include Healthnet/TPO, based in Amsterdam (www.healthnettpo.org), which focuses on establishing primary health care for mental health and psychosocial needs through local organizations. Its aim is to enable services to operate entirely independent of international staffing. TPO has worked with local partners to establish organizations in Cambodia, Burundi, Uganda, Sri Lanka, Indonesia, Pakistan, and Nepal; the majority of these are now run autonomously.

Sometimes the most effective organizations are not involved in community activities but in monitoring the work of organizations that are or claim to be providing aid. ActionAid International, based in South Africa, is a good example of a social auditing group that works to hold leaders accountable for guaranteeing access to services, participation, etc. ActionAid's Washington, DC office is working to

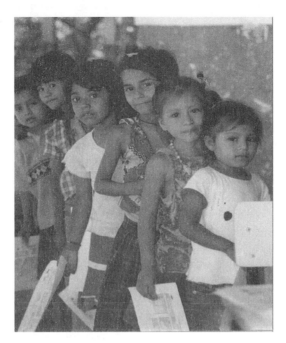

Figure 14–1 Schoolchildren in Santa Marta, El Salvador, awaiting their annual check-up performed by health promoters and doctors supported by Doctors for Global Health. DGH first started supporting Santa Marta in 1999. Photo courtesy of Shankar LeVine, 2004.

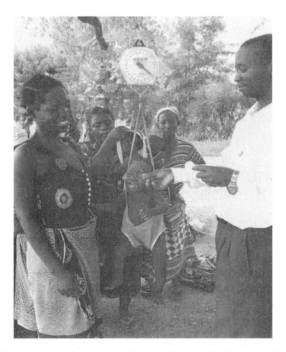

Figure 14–2 Well-baby clinic outside a public health center in Nhamatanda, Sofala Province, Mozambique. Health Alliance International has supported the Ministry of Health in Sofala since 1995. Photo courtesy of Wendy Johnson, 2005.

change IMF policies that restrict spending on health in developing countries. On a regional level, India's Centre for Health and Social Justice also carries out social auditing and presses for public health policies to be formulated and implemented on the basis of social justice principles.

2. Working from within an organization, questioning and challenging it to change its practices. Individuals working within mainline international health agencies can also play a major role in reforming international health endeavors to be true to their stated mission, rooted in local agenda-setting, and sensitive to the international political economy context. For example, the struggle against unaccountable private sector influences through PPPs at the WHO has been spearheaded by WHO employees themselves, supported by international activists and researchers. In recent years, Red Cross workers have pushed their organization to take a stance against war. On another front, health professionals from the WHO and the Christian Children's Fund have worked with many others to develop culturally appropriate mental health guidelines for emergency health activities (www.humanitarianinfo. org/iasc).

Individuals may also press their own organizations to become involved in campaigns that challenge the foreign policy of powerful donor governments to reform aid priorities and eliminate arms sales. This effort may be enhanced through the first-hand witnessing by the organization of the untoward health effects of a particular country's foreign policy. While there are many social movements engaged in reforming trade, aid, and debt systems (see ahead), organizations (especially those that are large and well-funded) often have more resources and access to power than do social movements and can serve as influential and "respectable" advocates for change.

CHANGING PATTERNS OF INTERNATIONAL HEALTH: CHALLENGING THE WORLD ORDER

Much current activity in international health still follows the traditional framework, focusing with great confidence on medical dimensions of the problems of ill health and magic tools to alleviate these problems, divorced from either the social or larger geopolitical context. This is not to deny that standard international health activities can be useful—for example, in building health centers or carrying out certain disease campaigns. Yet the failure to integrate technical and social approaches—and the widespread reluctance to address the underlying local and global political economy determinants of health—has limited the effectiveness, reception, and legitimacy of these efforts and of the field writ large.

If international health were simply an issue of diffusing effective measures to combat ill health—ranging from good nutrition to boost immunological resistance, universal water and sanitation access to diminish waterborne disease, eliminating the industrial use of carcinogens, averting war, and many others—it would have long ago been folded into national health efforts operated by democratically elected sovereign governments. But, as we have discussed throughout the book, the equal distribution of these measures and their determinants is rarely an aim of international health activities. How might those who decide to work in the international health field redress this situation?

As we have seen, in traditional international health approaches, "experts" go to look, see, learn, provide some technical assistance, and then leave (no sustainable impact behind). Here it is important to remember that *how* assistance is provided is as important as *what* assistance is provided. Crucial issues that need to be incorporated include:

1. as full an understanding as possible of the socioeconomic and political context of the country and its impact on health services and health outcomes;
2. a willingness to learn from local communities and local experts;
3. a nonjudgmental attitude to local problems; and
4. a willingness to share and learn from expertise in ways that empower local people and contribute to sustainable change.

Box 14–4 presents critical questions any individual (or organization) should ask before embarking on international health work.

Box 14–4 Key Questions to Consider in Carrying Out International Health Work

- How are problems conceptualized by local stakeholders, local policymakers, and international health workers?
- How are the population and country selected?
- Who defines the agenda for work and how are priorities selected?
- What is the approach to cooperation? Is it technical, environmental, social, or a mixture?
- Is this a one-time intervention or is it sustained over time? What are its environmental effects?
- How is the program funded and over what time frame? To what extent do national health expenditures and priorities get determined by outside programs?
- Does the program strengthen or weaken existing institutions?
- What are the benefits and drawbacks for the population, organizations, and health workers involved in the initiative?
- How much aid reaches designated beneficiaries and how are their health needs addressed?
- Is the program tackling the underlying determinants of health (in the specific or larger context)?
- How is the program evaluated, by whom, and when? (What constitutes success? Who decides?)
- What is the potential for the program to do harm? (Could the program stigmatize participants or local implementing organizations?)
- What are the safety and ethical concerns for participants and implementers?

ALTERNATIVE APPROACHES TO TRADITIONAL INTERNATIONAL HEALTH

South-to-South Partnerships

Of course, most international health efforts are carried out through organizations, many of which, as we examined in Chapter 3, reflect powerful political and economic interests or carry out work supported by these interests. Yet alternate approaches to international health have a long history. One of the most notable instances of alternative international health was the medical solidarity provided by health worker brigades from Europe and the Americas to democratic forces during the Spanish Civil War of the 1930s. With the growth of grassroots health projects over the past quarter century, other new approaches to international health have emerged, some inspired by the success of locally run health programs (such as Doctors for Global Health, the Voluntary Health Association of India, Hesperian Foundation, etc.). We will return to these efforts shortly.

But first, one of the most important international health developments of recent years has been the proliferation of developing to developing country—so-called South-to-South—efforts, which are providing increasing health aid in terms of health care services and larger infrastructural efforts. The most widely known example is that of Cuba: over 20,000 Cuban doctors have been working in recent years as primary care practitioners and specialists in Venezuela, South Africa, Haiti, Pakistan (following the disastrous 2005 earthquake), Angola, Guatemala, Bolivia, and other countries (De Vos et al. 2007). Like any aid program, Cuba's health cooperation efforts provide the donor country with certain political benefits (Feinsilver 1993). Yet most countries it has helped, including Ethiopia, The Gambia, and Haiti, provide no quid pro quo in the form of goods, services, or strategic alliances. Moreover, unlike many donor programs, Cuba's placement of "physicians where none have practiced before has been overwhelmingly well received by the local communities" (Cooper, Kennelly, and Orduñez-Garcia 2006, p. 821). A related effort is Operation Miracle, through which Cuban and Cuban-trained doctors have treated, for free, the eye conditions of over 750,000 people since 2004, either in Cuba or at several dozen eye hospitals in Latin America and Mali.

As discussed in Chapter 12, Cuba's Latin American School of Medicine (ELAM) trains thousands of students from numerous developing countries and from marginalized communities in the United States. Students are provided medical education as well as board and lodging at no cost to themselves or their country of origin. ELAM's curriculum emphasizes serving marginalized populations and encourages students to go into primary care or community medicine. (See http://www.elacm. sld.cu/historia.html and http://www.medicc.org/index.php.)

Brazil also sends physicians and other health care personnel (e.g., lab technicians) to Portuguese-speaking countries in sub-Saharan Africa (such as Angola and Mozambique) to assist in the capacity-building of their HIV/AIDS and tuberculosis programs.

At the time this book went to press, Venezuelan President Hugo Chávez had begun a massive effort to use his country's petrodollars to provide strings-free aid and financing within Latin America. Venezuela's Bolivarian Alternative for Our American Peoples (ALBA) is a cooperative regional development and economic integration effort that seeks to redress the imbalances generated by mainstream development agencies, emphasizing local interests in fighting against poverty and social exclusion (People's Health Movement, Medact, and Global Equity Gauge Alliance 2008). Aid has been used to prevent factory closures in Brazil, build health clinics in Bolivia, and provide low interest loans to farmers in Nicaragua. Venezuela pledged to provide aid totaling US$8.8 billion for 2007 (www.iht.com/ articles/ap/2007), larger than the 2006 combined total of OECD countries' aid of US$6.9 billion to Latin America in all sectors. The United States has increased its promise of aid to Latin America to counter the growing influence of the left-leaning Chávez (Wagner 2007).

At first glance, such aid may appear to be a continuation of mainstream aid patterns. However, it differs on at least three counts: first, South-to-South aid decreases dependence on aid channels from industrialized countries and multilateral agencies, which constrain sovereignty by attaching conditions to receipt of aid. Aid is a priori invited on equal terms; with power and resource differentials between donor and recipient much reduced, aid is turned into bona fide cooperation or exchange. Second, much South-to-South aid seeks to be transformative, for example in building social infrastructure, training primary health care practitioners, and working hand in hand with government agencies to create lasting and equitable means of providing essential needs. Third, even while convening international partners, many of these efforts are community-based: not only are priorities defined through local agenda-setting, but local populations are integral to shaping cooperative activities through their ideas, labor, and decision making.

Regional networks have also been formed to challenge aid paradigms. In Africa, for example, the African Union and regional economic communities, such as the Southern African Development Community, have adopted health strategies that emphasize regionally based priority-setting.

The notion that developing countries should find ways to help one another is not new. In 1978 the UN General Assembly adopted the Buenos Aires Plan of Action for Promoting and Implementing Technical Cooperation among the Developing Countries. Its objectives included self-reliance and finding local solutions (UNDP 1994). By 2003 cooperation had increased significantly, including efforts by China, India, Malaysia, Turkey, and Nigeria in areas such as training, administration, economic development, and scientific and technological research (United Nations' High-level Committee on the Review of Technical Cooperation among Developing Countries 2003). The WHO adopted similar resolutions, leading member countries to cooperate in three main areas: immunization (including the loan of vaccines in emergencies), emergency preparedness and disaster relief, and provision of essential drugs and technology (PAHO 1998). While successful, none of these programs have challenged the international financial architecture or gone beyond the scope of technical assistance.

In addition to South-to-South partnerships, South-to-North instances of aid are evolving, sometimes in unexpected ways. Following Hurricanes Katrina and Rita in 2005, Cuba's President Castro offered the United States 1,586 Cuban doctors and 26 tons of medicine—part of its highly developed disaster response network (see Chapter 8)—to assist the United States in coping with the medical and public health consequences. The United States did not respond to Cuba's offer, given the diplomatic and political tensions that have existed since Cuba's 1959 revolution (Special to the World 2005), but the U.S. government did accept a $25,000 donation from Sri Lanka.

Aid previously destined for medically underserved populations in developing countries is also being redirected to address inequalities in wealthier countries. For example, the NGO Remote Access Medical, which has sent medical expeditions to Haiti, Guyana, India, and Tanzania, now operates medical and dental clinics in rural West Virginia in the United States (Corbett 2007).

Alternatives to the traditional approach—small as they are in most regions—offer some useful ideas on how international health efforts might provide more "cooperative actions and solutions" (Institute of Medicine 1997, p. 2) but also show the limits of technical cooperation.

Emerging lessons from new international health approaches include the following:

- Understanding—from multidisciplinary perspectives—why problems exist, what forces create and maintain them, and how they might be resolved are key to making international health activities sustainable.
- Working to strengthen the efforts of organizations (both national and international) that facilitate local decision making and the use of local knowledge to solve problems is imperative.
- Solutions to health challenges can be found in both developed and developing country settings, but it is important to bear in mind that international health's underlying problems stem as much, or even more, from the unequal distribution of power and resources *within* countries as *between* them.

Health and Human Rights Approaches

In Chapter 4 we explored the potential of human rights approaches to secure and promote health. Central to this endeavor is the recognition of "health as a human right," including:

1. The impact (positive and negative) of health policies, programs, and practices on human rights.
2. The health effects of violations of rights.

3. The inextricable link between the promotion and protection of health and of human rights and dignity (Mann et al. 1999).
4. The role of health determinants, including decent living, working, and other social conditions.

Although the actions of the private sector and civil society have enormous bearing on human health, it is governments that are responsible for enabling their populations to achieve better health through respecting, protecting, and fulfilling rights (i.e., not violating rights, preventing rights violations, and creating policies, structures, and resources that promote and enforce rights) (Gruskin and Tarantola 2004). This obligation extends beyond the provision of essential medical care to tackling the social determinants of health, such as adequate education, housing, food, and favorable working conditions.

The first step in a rights-based approach to international health is to review how and to what extent policies and programs (governmental and nongovernmental) are respectful of human rights and of benefit to public health in their design, implementation, monitoring, and evaluation. In addition to the questions in Box 14–4, a health and human rights approach asks (using the relevant international human rights documents covered in Chapter 4): what and whose rights are affected positively and negatively by the policy or the program (Gruskin and Tarantola 2005)? The review can be conducted by policy makers and public health officials to help develop, implement, and evaluate policies and programs or by NGOs and activist networks to hold governments accountable for the ways in which they are and are not in compliance with international legal obligations to respect, protect, and fulfill public health and human rights. Health and human rights reviews also extend to the role and effects of foreign policy and global policymaking (e.g., by the WTO): governments, multilateral bodies, and transnational corporations can be held accountable for the global impact of their actions and decisions through human rights assessments (as part of larger health impact assessments) (Scott-Samuel and O'Keefe 2007).

Advocacy and Bearing Witness

A number of organizations monitor and report on violations of human rights. The most prominent of these are Amnesty International, Human Rights Watch, and Physicians for Human Rights, as well as the International Federation of Health and Human Rights Organisations. There are also numerous local and regional human rights organizations in developing countries. These include African Rights—Working for Justice, Algeria Watch, Al-Haq in Palestine, the Arab Association for Human Rights, Madre (fighting for women's rights) and FEDEFAM (focused on forced disappearances) in Latin America, the Asian Human Rights Commission, INSEC (a Nepali NGO that documents human rights violations related to conflict and state-sponsored atrocities), and Human Rights in China. In addition to monitoring violations such as torture, ill-treatment of prisoners, disappearances, violence against women, and the death penalty, these organizations are increasingly monitoring access to medical care, most notably to HIV/AIDS treatment.

Countless other organizations around the world focus on violations of economic, social, and cultural rights including the right to adequate housing, shelter, and social security. A small sampling includes: the Asian Coalition for Housing Rights, the People's Health Movement, the Confederation of Human Rights Organizations (India), Food First, Kensington Welfare Rights Union, and the Center for Economic and Social Rights.

In the context of conflict and where human rights are being abused, international health workers and humanitarian organizations may be the only witnesses who can document and direct wider attention to these abuses. In these circumstances, staying silent is tantamount to condoning abuses and allowing them to perpetuate. Yet health workers may also find themselves forced to remain neutral given their ethical obligation to alleviate suffering, including among those abusing human rights (Burnham and Robinson 2007).

Many humanitarian agencies are moving away from a neutral and impartial stance toward one that is explicitly political. Dr. James Orbinski (who was international president of MSF when it won the Nobel Peace Prize) and colleagues categorize three approaches to the role of monitoring abuses. The first is a "state reportage model" employed by the International Committee of the Red Cross, which uses its "influence within the corridors of power and mainly report to government officials" (Orbinski, Beyrer, and Singh 2007, p. 698). If governments fail to respond, the organization(s) can choose to publicize the report, potentially damaging their reputed neutrality. Amnesty International, Human Rights Watch, and Physicians for Human Rights, meanwhile, follow a "wide-dissemination model," reporting internationally on abuses of human rights in the belief that such reports will pressure states to stop or curb abuses. Because such dissemination tactics generate antagonism, governments may bar these organizations from entering countries. The third, hybrid, model, developed by MSF, provides aid *and* reports on human rights abuses in health. This hybrid approach faces the same challenges as both of the other two models, at sometimes great peril to its work and workers.

A human rights-based approach is not simply a checklist to ensure the protection of human subjects or maintain patient confidentiality, important as these issues are. Nor does it entail perfunctory attention to the idea of health as a human right in theoretical terms but which lacks enforcement mechanisms or political legitimacy (Skolnik 2007). Instead, human rights, when anchored by broad social and political movements, can be central to the political economy perspective portrayed in this book.

Application of Legal Standards

Applying human rights to health requires using internationally accepted and nationally agreed upon norms, standards, and accountability mechanisms. For example, the civil society AIDS advocacy group Treatment Action Campaign successfully brought suit against the South African government in the early 2000s to compel it to provide nevirapine to pregnant women by arguing for the unborn child's right to health (Singh, Govender, and Mills 2007). In Latin America, individuals and NGOs have undertaken multiple lawsuits against their governments regarding access to ARVs. In Argentina, one such successful suit resulted in assurances of provision of care for 15,000 people.

The right to health has also been used outside of the court system to stimulate health care reform. In 2002 the AIDS Law Project, a human rights advocacy organization working in South Africa, filed a complaint with the Competition Commission against the high prices of ARVs made by GlaxoSmithKline and Boehringer Ingelheim. They argued that high prices prevented needed drug access to the general public, resulting in large-scale, "premature, predictable, and preventable death" (Singh, Govender, and Mills 2007, p. 524) The chief argument was that excessive drug pricing violated both national competition legislation and constitutional and international rights to life and health. In 2003 the case was referred to the Competition Tribunal, after the Commission determined that the companies had violated the law. The companies settled the case before it proceeded to the tribunal, agreeing to issue voluntary licenses to generic manufacturers to produce the drugs. Due to this action and several others against pharmaceutical manufacturers, the price of ARVs has fallen substantially, and hundreds of thousands of persons with HIV/AIDS now have access to life-saving treatment. Of course, the South African population—like most populations—still does not enjoy universal access to clean water, shelter, adequate food and employment, and many other determinants of health.

A rights-based approach can go well beyond access to health care services, as evidenced by the work of CARE (which was founded in 1945 to deliver food packages to World War II survivors and now operates in 70 countries with 13,000 staff). For several decades CARE has focused on poverty; it moved from poverty alleviation, to poverty reduction, and now to poverty eradication strategies (i.e., institutional reforms, structural causes of poverty, empowerment of civil society relative to political elites). This evolution has been accompanied, in turn, by a shift from a symptoms-based approach, to a needs-based development model, to a rights-based transformative framework (Sinho 2006). CARE defines this as a "deliberate and explicit focus on people achieving the minimum conditions for living with dignity by exposing the roots of vulnerability and marginalization and expanding the range of responses" (CARE International 2005, p. 39).

Another key aspect of human rights approaches to health has to do with challenging the voluntaristic and charitable ideologies/mentalities that have come to characterize many international health efforts and replacing them with the language and action of rights. For example, in recent years, corporations have been urged to engage in international health and poverty alleviation efforts by making charitable donations, complying with working condition standards, and establishing "policies that improve the business climate and foster shared growth." The Washington think tank, Center for Global Development, recently sponsored a report encouraging corporations to consider a "menu of options" in joining the fight against global poverty that offer "win-win opportunities of commercial leverage." Accordingly, the report notes that improving "worker training, health care, day care, and other benefits can enhance employee productivity and aid in talent retention." At the same time, companies are reminded that they can sell their products to new low-income markets and "appeal to socially conscious consumers in their home countries" (All quotations in this paragraph are from Warden 2007, p. 13). The report even suggests that the poverty reduction business is ripe for entrepreneurship!

What this glossy, feel-good report omits is that complying with worker health and safety standards is not a matter of corporate largesse but one of worker and citizen rights, rights that were fought for and won as a result of enormous sacrifice and loss of life. A rights approach insists that every corporation comply with local and international laws protecting worker and environmental safety and health, and that violators be prosecuted. Accordingly, protecting the social well-being of workers must be understood and implemented not as a question of choice on a corporate "menu of options" but rather as an issue of human rights.

Practicing International Health "Without a Passport"

Up to this point, we have discussed approaches in international health that focus on activities in low-income settings. We have shown how careful consideration of individual motivations, organizational missions, and the logic of the world order can prevent many of the pitfalls of the traditional approach. However, it is also important to point out that activities carried out within high-income countries are crucial to addressing international health problems. In this section, we describe careers and activities in international health problems that can be practiced "without a passport."

Because improvements in international health hinge on policies, activities, and politics across the world, effective international health work likewise needs to take place across the world. In many ways, working to influence the policies of high-income countries and donor governments, which have sway over the international trade regime, may have a greater impact than working in a foreign country. Such visible activism includes:

- lobbying at home and participating in political movements that focus on reforming foreign policy;
- working against patent protections that limit access to needed drugs at affordable prices;
- working to change health system policies to meet local needs without poaching professionals from other countries;

- assisting health needs and movements in other countries through supportive campaigns, logistical help, collecting funds, supplies, and information;
- working toward cooperative approaches to health that are "of, for, and by the people," rather than prioritizing foreign policy or commercial goals;
- participating in struggles for fair systems of commodity pricing, trade, currency exchange, and worker protection *instead* of international aid;
- working on "global health" issues at home—for example, classist, sexist, and racist violence; access to medical care, housing, and quality education; cutbacks to social security; and migrant and refugee population needs;
- working to combat climate change and other environmental health problems by fighting for stronger standards—and enforcement mechanisms—for the reduction of greenhouse gas emissions and industrial pollution;
- working to reform international organizations;
- revealing the human rights violations caused by one's home country; and
- publicizing and contesting corporate policies and practices that harm the health of workers and communities (e.g., sweatshops or Bechtel's role in water privatization in Bolivia) and putting pressure on boards of directors.

Successful examples of these approaches include the activities of Nobel laureates International Physicians for the Prevention of Nuclear War, and the International Campaign to Ban Landmines. They have had dramatic international health impact, but their work is primarily conducted with political leaders in high-income countries rather than "in the field." As well, For an Independent WHO, formed in 2007, "urges WHO to recover its independence in line with its constitution, in particular in relation to ionising radiation" (For an Independent WHO 2008) and the conflict of interest inherent in its 1959 agreement with the International Atomic Energy Agency. Another highly effective international activist network involves the People's Health Movement, Medact, and the Global Equity Gauge Alliance. These groups have brought together hundreds of health practitioners, scholars, and advocates to produce *Global Health Watch: An Alternative World Health Report*, now in its second edition. The report critically assesses the state of global health and the current paradigm of development and provides an alternative array of achievable solutions "to ensure that all people have their basic and essential health needs met" (People's Health Movement, Medact, and Global Equity Gauge Alliance 2008, p. xiv).

Ronald Labonte and Ted Schrecker (2007) argue that (people in) donor countries should focus on how their own governments' policies negatively affect the performance of developing countries. Besides addressing issues of tied aid, complicated reporting systems, short-term financial assistance for long-term problems, priorities unrelated to need, and the imposition of public sector expenditure ceilings, they suggest that donor countries should focus on debt relief, the elimination of agricultural subsidies paid to farmers in developed countries, and reform of unfair trade policies. Organizations such as Jubilee 2000, 50 Years is Enough, Centre

Europe Tiers Monde, and the People's Health Movement (PHM) argue further that the international financial institutions should be completely revamped—if not entirely eliminated—to reduce the damages caused by loan conditionalities and the imposition of market-oriented policies on developing countries (see Chapters 3, 4, and 9 for further details on these efforts). PHM was founded in Bangladesh in 2000 as an international movement, with national affiliates, struggling for health as a human right (see Fig. 14–3). Its *People's Charter for Health* (www.phmovement.org/charter/pch-english.html), translated into dozens of languages, uses a political economy of health analysis as a call for multilevel action to collectively tackle the broad determinants of health in order to achieve Alma-Ata's vision of "health for all."

People at the beginning of their careers may not recognize that working on these issues is as significant as going abroad under the auspices of a humanitarian agency. Participating in international health struggles without leaving home may not seem as exciting as an overseas experience, but these struggles have the potential to be just as—perhaps even more—effective at addressing the root causes of ill health across the world.

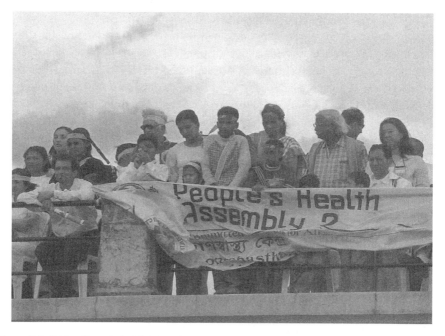

Figure 14–3 The Bangladeshi delegation at the Ceremony of the Native Peoples of the World, Savar, First People's Health Assembly, held near Dhaka, 2000. Photo courtesy of Arturo Quizhpe Peralta and María Hamlin Zúniga, copyleft 2006. *Voices of the Earth: From Savar to Cuenca.* People's Health Movement—Latin America, Facultad de Ciencias Médicas de la Universidad de Cuenca, Ecuador, People's Health Assembly 2, and Third World Network.

What Constitutes Success in International Health?

"Shared problems, sharing solutions" (Thompson 2001). This new definition of global health should not be left at the level of rhetoric. How might it be harnessed to transform the field? Individual motives of social justice and shared well-being are a good start but they are not enough. Pushing organizations to improve the accountability and equity of their actions is also important, yet still not enough. Understanding the nature of power and how the distribution of political and economic resources affects the determinants of well-being—and participating in efforts to democratize this power—are key to achieving success in global health.

There are a number of ways in which success in international health can be measured, some more narrowly focused than others. At a purely technical level, one can measure the number of cataract surgeries performed by a team of doctors and nurses from a developed country in a developing country. It may be argued that in a country with a significant backlog of cataracts that require removal, even one successful operation is beneficial (albeit to only one person and not to the millions more who are still affected by the condition). Continuing with this example, a more important indicator of success might be how many local health workers have been trained by the team to provide cataract surgeries. At another level, success might by measured by the team's efforts to lobby for developed countries to refrain from recruiting ophthalmologists from developing countries and to provide aid to increase the remuneration of health workers in developing countries. At yet another level, success may be gauged by the team's participation in efforts to create equitable trade relations so that there are more resources in public coffers to fund comprehensive and universal health services. The ultimate goal, of course, is to prevent premature death and disability, alleviate suffering, and improve living conditions to allow all people to thrive.

> "If we are serious about ending poverty, we have to be serious about ending the system that creates poverty by robbing the poor of their economic wealth, livelihoods, and incomes. Before we can make poverty history, we need to get the history of poverty right. It's not about how much wealthy nations can give so much as how much less they can take."
>
> —Vandana Shiva (Shiva 2005)

Some analysts, such as Jeffrey Sachs, argue that increasing and transforming foreign aid is the key to global health success. An estimated US$25 to $70 billion in donor spending per year between 2005 and 2015 would be required to assist developing countries to meet the health-related Millennium Development Goals, as compared to actual total MDG-related donor aid in 2004 of US$12 billion (Labonte and Schrecker 2007). Others call for good governance and better absorptive capacity by aid recipients (Roodman 2006; World Bank 2008). Although aid in the form of donor funds—especially from donors that employ aid in cooperative terms—can be helpful under particular circumstances, alternative strategies, such as the development of fair trade rules and debt relief, may offer a far more sustainable approach to human welfare (Mandel 2006; Blouin 2007; Oxfam International 2007). For example, the Norwegian government has eliminated duties and quotas on products from low-income countries, is set to abolish national export subsidies, has written off 100% of HIPC debt to Norway, has increased ODA to 1% of total GNI, has established ethical and human rights screening procedures for Norwegian mining companies wishing to invest abroad, and has reduced carbon emissions through carbon taxes (Eurodad 2006; CBC 2006; Trade Watch 2007).

Success in international health may also be measured in terms of the field's ability to integrate political economy, human rights, and collective health approaches with public health's technical tools. In the end, international health success will be gauged by *how* and *how well* we have reduced—or eliminated— social inequalities in health within and between countries.

At this point it is useful to revisit the three levels at which international health work can be conceptualized: individual actions and motivations, organizational missions and interventions, and the logic and structures of the world order. It is not uncommon to become frustrated that your own heartfelt motivations and hard work are not changing the public health reality in a marginalized community. Yet given the complexity of political, social, and economic forces that affect health at local, national, and global levels, this is to be expected. On the other hand, your own work, and that of the organizations and networks in which you participate, can also influence the logic of the world order, whether by pushing for a comprehensive welfare state, fair rules of international trade and finance, or human rights accountability. Much vital international health work should be aimed at industrialized countries, donor agencies, and multilateral organizations. This kind of activity requires long-term commitment and patience, as change usually occurs slowly. That said, being part of such an effort is the most human, humane, and human rights-infused endeavor imaginable.

Ultimately, the international health community should be:

a catalyst, a world health conscience behind national change, and, when requested, a helper giving visible expression to progressive ideas and decisions within national social policies....this means the end of well-intentioned international technical paternalism in health and its replacement by an era of international collaboration and cooperation (WHO 1976, pp. 80–81).

CONCLUSION

Learning Points:

- In contrast to traditional models, new approaches to international health make health aid "of, for, and by the people," following the dictum: cooperate, do not dictate.

- Alternative approaches to international health often focus on South-to-South partnerships, human rights-based approaches, and doing international work "without a passport."
- At the international level, priorities should include debt relief, ending loan conditionalities, creating equitable trade rules, and ensuring worker standards and protections.
- At national, transnational, and local levels, there is a need to balance priorities within the public health sector (primary care infrastructure, health personnel, sanitation, access to medicines, universal health coverage) and priorities outside the direct purview of the health sector (redistribution of resources, wealth, power; climate change).

Before or while reading this textbook, you may have asked yourself: who could possibly oppose international health aid, a heartwarming arena involving committed advocates, specialized practitioners, and glamorous celebrities? Yet aid that is uneven, that comes with conditions, that interferes with democratic processes, that increases stigma or vulnerability among communities receiving support, and that perpetuates dependency and power differentials offers more hindrance than help. Paradoxically, such aid violates the ethic of "do no harm" despite good intentions of the individuals and agencies involved. To put it differently, imagine if public services in your own community were dependent on the charity of an international group, the whims of a famous performer, or the foreign policy priorities of another country.

We have closed the book with a few examples of how international health is or could be better practiced in the 21st century, and how a political economy approach, cognizant of the structural reasons for ill health among populations, is valuable—or rather invaluable—for a keen appreciation of these issues. Personal and institutional motivations and principles to combat discrimination, exploitation, and harm at an interpersonal and organizational level are necessary to improve international health. But they are not sufficient. Understanding how to make international health transformative for the billions of people beset by poverty, inequality, ill health, and premature death requires a further set of conceptual and analytic tools and perspectives, which are not often taught in international health programs or to health professionals. It is our hope that this book will serve as a primer for this understanding and help inspire readers' lifelong commitment to equitable cooperation in health. Now it is up to you to harness your imagination, passion, persistence, knowledge, and skills to bettering international health for the benefit of future generations.

REFERENCES

ActionAid International. 2006. Real Aid2: Making Technical Assistance Work. http://www. actionaid.org/docs/real_aid.pdf. Accessed February 5, 2007.

Angell M. 1997. The ethics of clinical research in the Third World (Editorial). *New England Journal of Medicine* 337(12):847–849.

Angell M. 2004. *The Truth About the Drug Companies: How They Deceive Us and What to Do About It.* New York: Random House.

Belmont Report. 1979. The National Commission for the Protection of Human Subjects of Biomedical and Behavioral Research, Department of Health, Education, and Welfare, U.S. Government.

Bezruchka S. 2000. Medical tourism as medical harm to the Third World: Why? For whom? *Wilderness and Environmental Medicine Journal* 11(2):77–78.

Bhutta ZA. 2002. Ethics in international health research: A perspective from the developing world. *Bulletin of the World Health Organization* 80(2):114–120.

————. 2004. Beyond informed consent. *Bulletin of the World Health Organization* 82(10):771–777.

Birn A-E, Zimmerman S, and Garfield R. 2000. To decentralize or not to decentralize, is that the question?: Nicaraguan health policy under structural adjustment in the 1990s. *International Journal of Health Services* 30(1):111–128.

Bjerneld M, Lindmark G, Diskett P, and Garrett MJ. 2004. Perceptions of work in humanitarian assistance: Interviews with returning Swedish health professionals. *Disaster Management Response* 2(4):101–108.

Blouin C. 2007. Trade policy and health: From conflicting interests to policy coherence. *Bulletin of the World Health Organization* 85(3):169–173.

Burnham G and Robinson C. 2007. Protecting the rights of those in conflict. *Lancet* 370(9586):463–464.

Buse K and Walt G. 1997. An unruly mélange? Coordinating external resources to the health sector: A review. *Social Science and Medicine* 45(3):449–463.

CARE International. 2005. Principles into Practice: Learning from innovative rights-based programmes. London, UK: CARE International.

CBC. 2006. The carbon tax: The pros and cons of a tax on fossil fuels. http://www.cbc.ca/news/background/kyoto/carbon-tax.html. Accessed February 7, 2008.

Cheung YW and New PK. 1985. Missionary doctors vs Chinese patients: Credibility of missionary health care in early twentieth century China. *Social Science and Medicine* 21(3):309–317.

Christakis A. 1988. The ethical design of an AIDS vaccine trial in Africa. *Hastings Center Report* 18:31–37.

CIOMS. 2002, revised. *International Guidelines for Biomedical Research on Human Subjects.* Geneva: Council for International Organizations of Medical Sciences.

Claybrook J. 2001. Drug Companies Wage War on Consumers; win billions in excess profits with insider lobbying, campaign cash. *Public Citizen,* November 30.

COHRED. 2007. *Statement: Responsible Programming of Global Health Research.* Geneva: COHRED.

Collier P. 2007. *The Bottom Billion: Why the Poorest Countries are Failing and What Can Be Done about It.* New York: Oxford University Press.

Cooper RS, Kennelly JF, and Orduñez-Garcia P. 2006. Health in Cuba. *International Journal of Epidemiology* 35(4):817–824.

Corbett S. 2007. Patients without borders. *New York Times Magazine,* November 17, 62–65.

De Vos P, De Ceukelaire W, Bonet M, and Van der Stuyft P. 2007. Cuba's International Cooperation in Health: An Overview. *International Journal of Health Services* 37(4):761–776.

Department of Health. 2003. *International Humanitarian and Health Work: Toolkit to Support Good Practice.* London: Department of Health.

Easterly W. 2006. *The White Man's Burden*. Oxford: Oxford University Press.

Eurodad. 2006. Norway makes groundbreaking decision to cancel illegitimate debt. http://www.eurodad.org/whatsnew/articles.aspx?id=302. Accessed February 7, 2008.

Feinsilver JM. 1993. *Healing the Masses: Cuban Health Politics at Home and Abroad*. Berkeley and London: University of California Press.

Fèvre E, Picozzi K, and Fyfe J. 2005. A burgeoning of epidemic sleeping sickness in Uganda. *The Lancet* 366(9487):745–747.

For an Independent WHO. 2008. http://independentwho.info. Accessed February 12, 2008.

Ford J. 1971. *The Role of Trypanosomiasis in African Ecology*. London: Oxford University Press.

Gamble V. 1997. Under the Shadow of Tuskegee: African Americans and health care. *American Journal of Public Health* 87(11):1773–1778.

Global Health Education Consortium. 2008. www.globalhealth-ec.org. Accessed February 5, 2008.

Gruskin S and Tarantola D. 2004. Health and Human Rights. www.hsph.harvard.edu/fxbcenter/FXBC_WP10--Gruskin_and_Tarantola.pdf. Accessed April 9, 2007.

———. 2005. Health and Human Rights. In Gruskin S, Grodin M, Annas G, and Marks S, Editors. *Perspectives on Health and Human Rights*. New York: Routledge Press.

Gupta AR, Wells CK, Horwitz RI, Bia FJ, and Barry M. 1999. The International Health Program: The fifteen-year experience with Yale University's Internal Medicine Residency Program. *American Journal of Tropical Medicine and Hygiene* 61(6):1019–1023.

Gupta R and Farmer PE. 2005. International electives: Maximizing the opportunity to learn and contribute. *Medscape General Medicine* 7(2):78.

Harper I. 2007. Translating ethics: Researching public health and medical practices in Nepal. *Social Science and Medicine* 65(11):2235–2247.

Harrison M. 1994. *Public Health in British India: Anglo-Indian Preventive Medicine, 1859–1914*. Cambridge: Cambridge University Press.

Hoppe KA. 2003. *Lords of the Fly: Sleeping Sickness Control in British East Africa, 1900–1960*. Westport, CT: Praeger.

Hyder AA, Wali SA, Khan AN, Teoh NB, Kass NE, and Dawson L. 2004. Ethical review of health research: A perspective from developing country researchers (Global Research Ethics). *Journal of Medical Ethics* 30(1):68–72.

Indian Council for Medical Research. 2000. *Ethical Guidelines for Biomedical Research on Human Subjects*. New Delhi: Indian Council for Medical Research.

Institute of Medicine. 1997. *America's Vital Interest in Global Health: Protecting Our People, Enhancing Our Economy, and Advancing Our International Interests*. Washington, DC: The National Academies Press.

Intergovernmental working group on public health, innovation and intellectual property. 2007. Second session: Provisional agenda item3. A/PHI/IGWG/2/INF.DOC./2, August 28, 2007.

Jubilee South. 2008. Don't Owe, Won't Pay! http://www.jubileesouth.org/. Accessed February 12, 2008.

Justice J. 1989. *Policies, Plans, and People*. Berkeley, CA: University of California Press.

Kass NE, Hyder AA, Ajuwon A, Appiah-Poku J, Barsdorf N, Elsayed DE, et al. 2007. The structure and function of Research Ethics Committees in Africa: A case study. *PLoS Medicine* 4(1):26–31.

Kassalow JS. 2001. *Why Health Is Important to U.S. Foreign Policy*. New York: Council on Foreign Relations and Milbank Memorial Fund.

Kauchali S, Rollins N, and Solarsh G. 2002. Traditional beliefs of diarrhoeal illness in children in an area of high HIV seroprevalence—implications for design and interpretation of epidemiological surveys. XIV International AIDS Conference. July 7–12, Barcelona, Spain; 14: Abstract no. MoPeE3747. University of Natal, Durban, South Africa.

Krogh C and Pust R. 1990. International health: A manual for advisers and students. In *The Society of Teachers of Family Medicine*. Leawood, KS: Society of Teachers of Family Medicine.

Krumeich A, Weijts W, Reddy P, and Meijer-Weitz A. 2001. The benefits of anthropological approaches for health promotion research and practice. *Health Education Research* 16(2):121–130.

Labonte R and Schrecker T. 2007. Foreign policy matters: A normative view of the G8 and population health. *Bulletin of the World Health Organization* 85(3):185–191.

LaVertu DS and Linares AM. 1990. Ethical principles of biomedical research on human subjects: Their application and limitations in Latin America and the Caribbean. *Bulletin of the Pan American Health Organization* 24(4):469–479.

Lurie P and Wolfe SM. 1997. Unethical trials of intervention to reduce perinatal transmission of the human immunodeficiency virus in developing countries. *New England Journal of Medicine* 337(12):853–856.

Mandel S. 2006. Debt relief as if people mattered: A rights-based approach to debt sustainability. London: New Economics Foundation.

Mann JM, Gruskin S, Grodin MA, and Annas GJ, Editors. 1999. *Health and Human Rights—A Reader*. New York: Routledge.

Mariner WK. 1997. Public confidence in public health research ethics. *Public Health Reports* 112(1):33–36.

Matlin S. 2005. Introduction. In Burke M and de Francisco A, Editors. *Monitoring Financial Flows for Health Research 2005: Behind the Global Numbers*. Geneva: Global Forum for Health Research.

Moodley K and Myer L. 2007. Health research ethics committees in South Africa 12 years into democracy. *BMC Medical Ethics* 8:1.

Ncayiyana DJ. 2007. Combating poverty: The charade of development aid. *British Medical Journal* 335(7633):1272–1273.

Nicholson B, Lewis G, and Martineau F. 2007. International Health Foundation Programmes. *British Medical Journal Career Focus* 334:23–25.

Orbinski J, Beyrer C, and Singh S. 2007. Violations of human rights: Health practitioners as witnesses. *Lancet* 370(9588):698–704.

Oxfam International. 2007. *The World is Still Waiting: Broken G8 Promises are Costing Millions of Lives*. Oxford, UK: Oxford Publishing.

Ozgediz D, Roayaie K, Debas H, Schecter W, and Farmer D. 2005. Surgery in developing countries: Essential training in residency. *Archives of Surgery* 140(8):795–800.

PAHO. 1998. Technical cooperation amongst countries: Panamericanism in the twenty-first century. Provisional Agenda Item 4.3. 25th Pan American Sanitary Conference, 50th Session of the Regional Committee Washington DC. September 21–25, 1998. CSP25/9 (Eng.).

Panday DR. 1999. *Nepal's Failed Development: Reflections on the Mission and the Maladies*. Kathmandu: Nepal South Asian Centre.

People's Health Movement, Medact, and Global Equity Gauge Alliance. 2008. *Global Health Watch 2: An Alternative World Health Report*. London: Zed Books.

Pfeiffer J. 2003. International NGOs and primary health care in Mozambique: The need for a new model of collaboration. *Social Science and Medicine* 56(4):725–738.

Pfeiffer J, Johnson W, Fort M, Shakow A, Hagopian A, Gloyd S, et al. 2008. Strengthening health systems in poor countries: Do we need an NGO code of conduct? *American Journal of Public Health* 98(12): 2134–2140.

RedR Australia. 2008. Training Courses. http://www.redr.org.au/index.php?option=com_c ontent&view=article&id=50:training-courses&catid=13:training&Itemid=50. Accessed February 5, 2008.

Reverby SM, Editor. 2000. *Tuskegee's Truths: Rethinking the Tuskegee Syphilis Study.* Chapel Hill: University of North Carolina Press.

Rivera R and Ezcurra E. 2001. Composition and operation of selected research ethics review committees in Latin America. *IRB: Ethics and Human Research* 23(5):9–12.

Roodman D. 2006. *Aid Project Proliferation and Absorptive Capacity.* Washington, DC: Center for Global Development.

Roy A. 2004. Help that hinders. *Le Monde Diplomatique.* November. http://mondediplo. com/2004/11/16roy. Accessed February 14, 2008.

Sachs JD. 2005. *The End of Poverty.* London: Penguin Books.

———. 2008. Primary health for all: Ten resolutions could globally ensure a basic human right at almost unnoticeable cost. *Scientific American,* December 16, 34–36.

Sarfaty S and Arnold LK. 2005. Preparing for international medical service. *Emergency Medicine Clinics of North America* 23(1):149–175.

Scott-Samuel A and O'Keefe E. 2007. Health impact assessment, human rights and global public policy: A critical appraisal. *Bulletin of the World Health Organization* 85(3):212–217.

Sharav VH. 2002. Conflicts of interest. Paper presented at the 14th Tri-Service Clinical Investigation Symposium, May 5–7, 2002.

Shaw J and the CFHI Team. 2007. *Professionalism 101.* San Francisco, CA: Child Family Health International.

Shiva V. 2005. New Emperors, Old Clothes. *The Ecologist,* July 1.

Singh JA, Govender M, and Mills EJ. 2007. Do human rights matter to health? *The Lancet* 370(9586):521–527.

Sinho S. 2006. CARE's adoption of rights-based approaches. Paper read at the 134th Annual Meeting of the American Public Health Association, Boston, MA.

Skolnik R. 2007. *Essentials of Global Health.* Sudbury, MA: Jones & Bartlett.

Smith CL. 2007. Building health where peace is new in near post-war El Salvador. *Development* 50(2):127–133.

Special to the World. 2005. Cuba offers assistance. *People's Weekly World Newspaper,* September 10. http://www.pww.org/article/articleview/7684/1/285/. Accessed February 5, 2008.

Thieren M. 2007. Health and foreign policy in question: The case of humanitarian action. *Bulletin of the World Health Organization* 85(3):218–224.

Thompson T. 2001. America's Commitment to Global Health, Speech by US Secretary of Health and Human Services. *54th World Health Assembly.* Geneva. http://www.hhs. gov/news/speech/2001/010515.html. Accessed November 18, 2007.

Trade Watch. 2007. Norway Country Brief. http://www.dfat.gov.au/geo/norway/norway_ brief.html. Accessed February 7, 2008.

Turshen M. 1984. *The Political Ecology of Disease in Tanzania.* New Brunswick: Rutgers University Press.

UNDP. 1994. *Buenos Aires Plan of Action for Promoting and Implementing Technical Cooperation amongst Developing Countries*. New York: UNDP.

United Nations' High-level Committee on the Review of Technical Cooperation among Developing Countries. 2003. Review of progress in the implementation of the Buenos Aires Plan of Action, the new directions strategy for technical cooperation among developing countries, and the decisions of the High-level Committee. Thirteenth session, 27–30 May, New York. http://tcdc.undp.org/HLCdocs/TCDC%2013%20 L.2.pdf. Accessed December 12, 2007.

Varmus H and Satcher D. 1997. Ethical complexities of conducting research in developing countries. *New England Journal of Medicine* 337(14):1003–1005.

Wagner B. 2007. US acts to counter Venezuela's clout in Latin America. http://www. voanews.com/english/archive/2007-03/2007-03-07-voa1.cfm?CFID=37830370&CFTO KEN=58021103. Accessed February 5, 2008.

Warden S. 2007. *Joining the Fight Against Global Poverty: A Menu for Corporate Engagement*. Washington, DC: Center for Global Development.

WHO. 1976. *Introducing WHO*. Geneva: WHO.

———. 2003a. Principles and practices: The implementation of ethical guidelines for research on HIV. http://www.who.int/hiv/strategic/mt020603/en/. Accessed February 5, 2008.

———. 2003b. Traditional Medicine. www.who.int/mediacentre/factsheets/fs134/en. Accessed February 5, 2008.

World Bank. 2008. Governance and Anticorruption: Strategy. http://web.worldbank.org/ WBSITE/EXTERNAL/TOPICS/EXTGOVANTICORR/0,,contentMDK:21096079~page PK:210058~piPK:210062~theSitePK:3035864,00.html. Accessed February 7, 2008.

Yamey G, on Behalf of the Interviewees. 2007. Which single intervention would do the most to improve the health of those living on less than $1 per day? *PLoS Medicine* 4(10):1557–1560.

Appendix: Some World Wide Web Sites of Interest for International Health[a,b]

(Main list is followed by lists of websites of Universities and Training Programs, Government and Bilateral, and UN agencies)

Name	URL
A	
Academy for International Health Studies Inc.	http://www.AIHS.com/
Action by Churches Together (ACT)	http://act-intl.org/
Action Aid International	http://www.actionaid.org/
Adventist Development and Relief Agency	http://www.adra.org/site/PageServe
Afrique Verte	http://www.afriqueverte.org/
African Union	http://www.africa-union.org/
Aga Khan Foundation	http://www.akdn.org/
Agencies in International Aid	http://www.interaction.org/
Agency for Cooperation and Research in Development (ACORD)	http://www.acordinternational.org
ALAMES (Latin American Social Medicine Association)	http://www.geocities.com/alamesgeneral/
Alternative Information and Development Centre (AIDC)	http://aidc.org.za
American Association of Health Plans	http://www.aahp.org
American Federation of Labor	http://www.afl-cio.org
American Friends Service Committee	http://www.afsc.org/
American International Health Alliance	http://www.aiha.com/en/
American Jewish World Service	http://www.ajws.org/
American Medical Student Association	http://www.amsa.org/
American Public Health Association	http://www.apha.org

(continued)

Name	URL
American Society for Tropical Medicine and Hygiene	http://www.astmh.org/
Amnesty International	http://www.amnesty.org/
Antiwar.com	http://www.antiwar.com/
Appui Forim	http://www.forim.net/
Asian Development Bank	http://www.adb.org/
The Australian Demographic & Social Research Institute	http://adsri.anu.edu.au/
B	
Basic Needs	http://www.basicneeds.org/
Basic Social Services for All	http://www.un.org/esa/population/pubsarchive/bss/fbsstoc.htm
Behrhorst Partners for Development	http://www.behrhorst.org/
Bill and Melinda Gates Foundation	http://www.gatesfoundation.org
BIREME, Latin American and Caribbean Center on Health	http://www.bireme.br
Bolivarian Alternative for the Americas (ALBA)	http://www.alternativabolivariana.org/
BRAC	http://www.brac.net/index2.htm
Bridderlech Deelen	http://www.cathol.lu
Bridges to Community	http://www.bridgestocommunity.org
Bristol-Myers Squibb Foundation	http://www.bms.com/sr/foundation/data/index.html
Broederlijk Delen	www.broederlijkdelen.be
Burden of Disease Unit	http://www.hsph.harvard.edu/organizations/bdu/
C	
Catholic Agency for Overseas Development (CAFOD)	http://www.cafod.org.uk
Canada World Youth	http://www.cwy-jcm.org
Canadian Centre for Policy Alternatives	http://www.policyalternatives.ca
Canadian Institute for Health Information	http://www.cihi.ca
Canadian Society for International Health	http://www.csih.org/
CARE	http://www.care.org
Caritas International	http://www.caritas.org/
Carso Health Institute	http://www.salud.carso.org/index_ing.html
Catholic Relief Services	http://crs.org/
Center for Global Development	http://www.cgdev.org/
Center for Health, Environment and Justice	http://www.chej.org/
Center for Health Information and Technology	http://www.healthnet.org

(continued)

Name	URL
Center for Policy Analysis on Trade and Health: San Francisco	http://www.cpath.org
Center of Concern	http://www.coc.org
Centre de Recherche et d'Information pour le Developpement (CRID)	http://www.crid.asso.fr/
Centre for Health and Social Justice	http://www.chsj.org/
Centre for Science and Environment	http://www.cseindia.org/index.html
Center for Social and Economic Rights	http://www.cesr.org/
Centre for World Indigenous Studies (CWIS)	http://www.cwis.org/index.php
"Charity Village"	http://www.charityvillage.com
Christian Connections for International Health	http://www.ccih.org/
Church World Service	http://www.churchworldservice.org/
CIVICUS	http://www.civicus.org
Cochrane Collaboration	http://www.cochrane.org
Comité Catholique contre la Faim et pour le Développement (CCFD)	http://www.ccfd.asso.fr/
Comité de la Charte	http://www.comitecharte.org/
Committee for Asian Women (CAW)	http://www.cawinfo.org/
Comprehensive Rural Health Project Jamkhed	http://www.jamkhed.org/
Confédération européenne des ONG d'urgence et de développement (CONCORD)	http://www.concordeurope.org/
Consumers International	http://www.consumersinternational.org/homepage.asp
Coordination du Sud	http://www.coordinationsud.org/
Council of Canadians	http://www.canadians.org
Council on Health Research for Development (COHRED)	http://www.cohred.org/main/
Cordaid	http://www.cordaid.nl/
Corporate Watch	http://www.corpwatch.org/
D	
Dag Hammarskjold Foundation (DHF)	http://www.dhf.uu.se/
DATA—Debt, AIDS, Trade, Africa	http://www.data.org/
Data for Decision Making Project	http://www.cdc.gov/cogh/descd/otherProject/dataDM.htm
David and Lucille Packard Foundation	http://www.packard.org/home.aspx
Democracy Center	http://www.democracyctr.org
Demographic and Health Surveys	http://www.measuredhs.com/

(*continued*)

Name	URL
Development Alternatives with Women for a New Era (DAWN)	http://www.dawnnet.org
Development and Peace	http://www.devp.org
Development Information	http://www.eldis.org
Diakonia World Federation	http://www.diakonia-world.org/
Dignitas International	http://www.dignitasinternational.org/articles.aspx?aid=12
Doctors for Global Health	http://www.dghonline.org
Doctors Without Borders	http://www.doctorswithoutborders.org
E	
Emergency Life Support for Civilian War Victims	http://www.emergency.it/index.php?ln=En
Emerging Infectious Diseases Home Page	http://www.cdc.gov/ncidod/eid/index.htm
Emerging Infections Information Network	http://info.med.yale.edu/EIINet/—— link broken
EngenderHealth	http://www.engenderhealth.org/
Entraide et Fraternité	http://www.entraide.be/
Environmental Defense	http://www.environmentaldefense.org/home.cfm
Epi Info	http://www.cdc.gov/epiinfo/
Equidad listserv	http://listserv.paho.org/archives/equidad.html
Equinet	http://www.equinetafrica.org/
Essential Information	http://www.essential.org/index.html
European Centre for Disease Prevention and Control	http://www.ecdc.eu.int/
European Community Humanitarian Aid (ECHO)	http://ec.europa.eu/echo/
European Health Management Association	http://www.ehma.org
European Union	http://europa.eu/
Exchange	http://www.healthcomms.org/
F	
FADSP (Federación de asociaciones para la defensa de la sanidad pública)	http://www.fadsp.org/
Fair Trade Federation	http://www.fairtradefederation.com/
Family Health International	http://www.fhi.org/en/index.htm
Fastenopfer	http://www.fastenopfer.ch/
Fifty Years Is Enough	http://www.50years.org/issues/health.html
Filipino/American Coalition for Environmental Solutions (FACES)	http://www.facessolidarity.org
Focus on the Global South	http://www.focusweb.org/
Food and Water Watch	http://www.foodandwaterwatch.org/

(continued)

Name	URL
Food First: Institute for Food and Development Policy	http://www.foodfirst.org
Ford Foundation	http://www.fordfound.org/
Friedrich Ebert Stiftung Foundation	http://www.fes.de/intro_en.html
Fundacao Evangelizacao e Culturas	http://www.fecongd.net/
Fundação Oswaldo Cruz	http://www.fiocruz.br

G

Name	URL
G-77 (Group of 77)	http://www.g77.0rg/
G-8 Information Centre	http://www.g7.utoronto.ca/
GAVI Alliance	http://www.gavialliance.org/
Global AIDS Alliance	http://www.globalaidsalliance.org/
Global AIDS Interfaith Alliance (GAIA)	http://www.thegaia.org/
Global Alliance for Improved Nutrition	http://www.gainhealth.org/
Global ChildNet	http://www.gcsltdc.com/gcnb_p.html
Global Development Network (GDN)	http://www.gdnet.org/
Global Exchange	http://www.globalexchange.org
Global Forum for Health Research	http://www.globalforumhealth.org/Site/000__Home.php
Global Fund to fight AIDS, Tuberculosis and Malaria	http://www.theglobalfund.org/en/
Global Health Action Group American Medical Students Association	http://www.amsa.org/global/
Global Health Council	http://www.globalhcalth.org/
Global Health Education Consortium (GHEC)	http://www.globalhealth-ec.org/
Global Health Network Supercourse	http://www.pitt.edu/~super1/
Global Health Watch	http://www.ghwatch.org/
Global Impact	http://www.charity.org/type.html
Global Issues	http://www.globalissues.org/
Global Justice Center	http://www.globaljusticecenter.org/
Global Population Database	http://infoserver.ciesin.org/datasets/cir/gpopdb-home.html
Global Technology Network	http://www.usgtn.org
Global Trade Watch (GTW)	http://www.tradewatchoz.org/
Grameen Bank	http://www.grameen-info.org/
The Greenbelt Movement	http://www.greenbeltmovement.org/
Greenpeace International	http://www.greenpeace.org/homepage/
GuideStar Guide to Nonprofit Organizations	http://www.guidestar.org/

H

Name	URL
Hadassah	http://www.hadassah.org/

(continued)

Name	URL
Haut Conseil de la Coopération Internationale (HCCI)	http://www.hcci.gouv.fr/
Health Action International	http://www.haiweb.org
Health Alliance International	http://depts.washington.edu/haiuw/
Health, Development, Information and Policy Institute (HDIP)	http://www.hdip.org/
Health and Health Statistics Websites	http://www.who.int/whosis/database/national_sites/index.cfm
Health Canada	http://www.hc-sc.gc.ca/
Health Global Access Project (Health GAP)	http://www.healthgap.org
Health Information Forum discussion list	http://www.inasp.info/file/200/hif-net.html
Health Systems Trust	http://www.hst.org.za/
Health Volunteers Overseas	www.hvousa.org/sg.cfm
Healthlink Worldwide	http://www.healthlink.org.uk/
HealthWrights—Workgroup for People's Health and Rights	http://www.healthwrights.org/
The Hesperian Foundation	http://www.hesperian.org
Helps International	http://www.helpsintl.org
HLSP	http://www.hlsp.org/
Human Rights Library	http://www.umn.edu/humanrts/
Human Rights Watch	http://www.hrw.org/
I	
ICD-10	http://www.who.int/classifications/icd/en/
Independent Media Center	http://www.indymedia.org/en/index.shtml
India, Brazil, South Africa (IBSA) Trilateral Agreement	http://www.ibsa-trilateral.org/
Influenza Centers	http://www.who.int/csr/disease/influenza/centres/en/
Institute for Agriculture and Trade	http://www.iatp.org//
Institute for Global Communication (PeaceNet, EcoNet, LaborNet, ConflictNet and WomensNet)	http://www.igc.org/
Institute of Medicine (National Academy of Sciences) Board on Global Health	http://www.sica.net/incap http://www.iom.edu/CMS/3783.aspx
Institute of Nutrition of Central America and Panama (INCAP)	http://www.sica.net/incap
Institut Pasteur	http://www.pasteur.fr/ip/index.jsp
InterAction (the American Council for Voluntary International Action)	http://www.interaction.org/

(continued)

Name	URL
Inter-American Development Bank	http://www.iadb.org/
International Affairs Network list of international agencies	http://www.ucis.pitt.edu/iacnet/
International AIDS Vaccine Initiative	http://www.iavi.org/
International Association of Health Policy	http://www.healthp.org/
International Association for Medical Assistance to Travellers	http://www.iamat.org/
International Association of Physicians in AIDS Care (IAPAC)	http://www.iapac.org
International Baby Food Action Network	http://www.ibfan.org/site2005/Pages/index2.php?iui=1
International Center for Diarrheal Disease Research, Bangladesh (ICDDR, B)	http://www.icddrb.org/
International Clinical Epidemiology Network (INCLEN)	http://www.inclen.org
International Cooperation for Development and Solidarity	http://www.cidse.org/
International Council of Voluntary Agencies	http://www.icva.ch/
International Development Research Centre (Canada)	http://www.idrc.ca
International Federation for Alternative Trade (IFAT)	http://www.ifat.org/
International Federation of Medical Students	http://www.ifmsa.org/
International Federation of Pharmaceutical Manufacturers Associations	http://www.ifpma.org/
International Federation of Red Cross and Red Crescent Societies	http://www.ifrc.org/
International Forum on Globalization (IFG)	http://www.ifg.org
International Health Central American Institute Foundation	http://www.ihcai.org
International Healthcare Opportunities Clearinghouse	http://library.umassmed.edu/ihoc/index.cfm
International Healthcare Volunteer Opportunities	http://www.brynmawr.edu/healthpro/international.htm
International Health Economics Association	http://www.healtheconomics.org/
International Institute for Sustainable Development (IISD)	http://www.iisd.org/
International Medical Corps	http://www.imc-la.com/index.htm

(continued)

Name	URL
International Monetary Fund	http://www.imf.org/
International People's Health Council	http://www.healthwrights.org/politics/iphc.htm
International Planned Parenthood Federation	http://www.ippf.org/en/
International Public Health Watch	http://www.ldb.org/iphw/index.htm
International Red Cross	http://www.icrc.ch
International Relief Teams	http://www.irteams.org
International Rescue Committee	http://www.theirc.org/
International Society for Equity in Health (ISEqH)	http://www.iseqh.org/
International Society for Infectious Diseases	http://www.isid.org/
International Union Against Cancer	http://www.uicc.org/
International Union for Health Promotion and Education (IUHPE)	http://www.iuhpe.org/
Islamic Relief Worldwide	http://www.islamic-relief.com/
Italian Association Raoul Follereau's Friends (Aifo)	http://www.aifo.it/index.htm
J	
JHPIEGO (John Hopkins Program for International Education in Gynecology and Obstetrics)	http://www.jhpiego.org/
John D. and Catherine T. MacArthur Foundation	http://www.macfound.org/site/c.lkLXJ8MQKrH/b.3599935/
John Snow Inc.	http://www.jsi.com/JSIInternet/
K	
Kabissa-Space for Change in Africa	http://www.kabissa.org/index.php
Koordinierungsstelle	http://www.koo.at
Kresge Foundation	http://www.kresge.org/
L	
Lalmba	http://www.lalmba.org
Landless Workers Movement (MST) (Brazil)	http://www.mstbrazil.org
Latin American Social Medicine Database	http://hsc.unm.edu/lasm/
Library of Congress Country Studies	http://lcweb2.loc.gov/frd.cs
Living Routes Study Abroad Programs for a Sustainable Future	http://www.LivingRoutes.org
Lutheran World Relief	http://www.lwr.org/
M	
Management Sciences for Health	http://www.msh.org/

(continued)

Name	URL
Manos Unidas	http://www.manosunidas.org
Marie Stopes International	http://www.mariestopes.org/Home.aspx
Medact	http://www.medact.org/
Médecins du Monde	http://www.medecinsdumonde.org/fr/faire_un_don
Médecins Sans Frontières (MSF)	http://www.msf.org/
Medical Education Cooperation with Cuba (MEDICC)	http://www.medicc.org/index.php
Medical Research Council	http://www.mrc.ac.uk/index.htm
Medicus Mundi International	http://www.medicusmundi.org/
Mennonite Central Committee	http://mcc.org/
Merck Company Foundation	http://www.merck.com/corporate-responsibility/approach/philanthropy
Merlin	http://www.merlin.org.uk/
Millennium Villages Initiative	http://www.unmillenniumproject.org/press/gov_japan.htm
Ministries of Health, Various	See "Web sites of Some Ministries of Health"
Misereor	http://www.misereor.org
Multilaterals Project	http://fletcher.tufts.edu/multilaterals.html
Muslim Aid	http://www.muslimaid.org/
N	
National Societies of the Red Cross & Red Crescent	http://www.icrc.org/Web/Eng/siteeng0.nsf/htmlall/info_res_othersites_rc
Navdanya and the Research Foundation for Science, Technology and Ecology	http://www.vshiva.net
NETWORK- A National Catholic Social Justice Lobby	http://www.networklobby.org
Norwegian Church Aid	http://english.nca.no/article/archive/449/
Nuffield Foundation	http://www.nuffieldfoundation.org/
O	
Office of Population Research (OPR), Princeton University Data Archive	http://opr.princeton.edu/archive/
Organization for Economic Cooperation and Development (OECD)	http://www.oecd.org/
One World Action	http://www.oneworldaction.org/
OneWorld International	http://www.oneworld.net
Overseas Development Institute	http://www.odi.org.uk/
Oxfam International	http://www.oxfam.org
P	
Packard Foundation	http://www.packard.org
Palestinian Medical Relief Society	http://www.upmrc.org

(*continued*)

Name	URL
Panos Institute	http://www.panos.org.uk/
Partners in Health	http://www.pih.org
Pathfinder Fund	http://www.pathfind.org/site/PageServer
Peoples' Global Action	http://www.nadir.org/nadir/initiativ/agp/index.htm
People's Health Movement	http://phmovement.org/
Pesticide Action Network International	http://www.pan-international.org/panint/?q=node/33
Pesticide Action Network North America (PANNA)	http://www.panna.org/
Physicians and Scientists for Responsible Application of Science and Technology (PSRAST)	http://www.psrast.org/
Physicians for Human Rights	http://www.phrusa.org
Physicians for a National Healthcare Program	http://www.pnhp.org
Physicians for Social Responsibility	http://www.psr.org
Physicians for Peace	http://www.physiciansforpeace.org
POPIN Worldwide Directory of Population Institutions	http://www.un.org/popin/other4.htm
Popnet (Global population information)	http://www.un.org/popin/
Population Council	http://www.popcouncil.org/
Population Index	http://popindex.princeton.edu
Population Reference Bureau (PRB)	http://www.prb.org/
PRB Glossary of Population Terms	http://www.prb.org/Educators/Resources/Glossary.aspx
Positive Deviance Approach	http://www.positivedeviance.org/
Positive Futures Network	http://www.futurenet.org/index.htm
Prayas	http://www.prayaspune.org/
Program for Appropriate Technology in Health (PATH)	http://www.path.org
Project Hope	http://www.projecthope.org
ProMed: Program for Monitoring Emerging Diseases	http://www.fas.org/promed/index.html
Public Citizen	http://www.citizen.org/index.cfm
Public Citizen Global Trade Watch	http://www.publiccitizen.org/trade
Public Health Policy Unit	http://www.ucl.ac.uk/spp/about/
Public Services International	http://www.world-psi.org
R	
Rachel's Democracy & Health Weekly Newsletter	http://www.rachel.org/home_eng.htm
ReliefWeb, UN Department of Humanitarian Affairs	http://www.reliefweb.int/

(continued)

Name	URL
ReproLine (Reproductive Health Online)	http://www.reproline.jhu.edu
Resource Centres on Urban Agriculture & Food Security (RUAF)	http://www.ruaf.org/
Results Washington	http://www.results.org
Robert Wood Johnson Foundation	http://www.rwjf.org/main.html
Rockefeller Foundation	http://www.rockfound.org
Roll Back Malaria	http://www.rbm.who.int/
Royal Netherlands TB Association	http://www.tuberculose.nl/Site/Public.aspx

S

Safe Motherhood	http://www.safemotherhood.org
Save the Children	http://www.savethechildren.org/
Science and Development Network	http://www.scidev.net/en/
Scottish Catholic International Aid Fund (SCIAF)	http://www.sciaf.org.uk
SOCHARA (Society for Community Health Awareness, Research and Action)	http://www.sochara.org
Social Medicine Portal	http://www.socialmedicine.org/
Social Security Programs Throughout the World	http://www.ssa.gov/policy/docs/progdesc/ssptw/
Social Watch	http://www.socwatch.org.uy/en/portada.htm
Society for International Development	http://www.sidint.org
Southeast Asia Ministers of Education Organization (SEAMEO), Regional Tropical Medicine and Public Health Network (TROPMED)	http://www.tm.mahidol.ac.th/seameo/home.htm
Southern African Development Co-operation (SADC)	http://www.sadc.int/
Spirit of 1848	http://www.spiritof1848.org/
STISSS Salvadoran Health Worker's Union	http://stissselsalvador.blogspot.com/
Stop TB Partnership	http://www.stoptb.org/
Sustainable Development Sources	http://www.ulb.ac.be/ceese/meta/sustvl.html

T

Teaching Aids at Low Cost	http://www.talcuk.org/
Third World Network	http://www.twnside.org.sg/
Toxics Action Center	http://www.toxicsaction.org/
Transcultural Psychosocial Organization	http://www.healthnettpo.org/
Transcultural Psychosocial Organization-Cambodia	http://www.camnet.com.kh/tpo/
Transparency International	http://www.transparency.org

(continued)

Name	URL
Treatment Action Campaign	http://www.tac.org.za/
Trócaire	http://www.trocaire.org
U	
Unite for sight	http://www.uniteforsight.org/
United for a Fair Economy	http://www.faireconomy.org
United Nations Agencies	see separate section below
Urmul Trust	http://www.judypat.com/india/urmul.htm
V	
Via Campesina	http://viacampesina.org/main_en/index.php
Virtual Library—Public Health	http://www.sphcm.med.unsw.edu.au/SPHCMWeb.nsf/page/WWWVLPH
Volontari nel Mondo—FOCSIV	http://www.focsiv.it
W	
Weizmann Institute	http://www.weizmann.ac.il/
Wellcome Trust	http://www.wellcome.ac.uk/
Wemos Foundation	http://www.wemos.nl/
William J. Clinton Foundation	http://www.clintonfoundation.org/index.htm
William and Flora Hewlett Foundation	http://www.hewlett.org/Default.htm
W.K. Kellogg Foundation	http://www.wkkf.org/Default.aspx?LanguageID=0
Women's Global Network for Reproductive Rights (WGNRR)	http://www.wgnrr.org/
World Bank	http://www.worldbank.org/
World Bank/Health, Nutrition and Population	http://www.worldbank.org/hnp/
World Bank PovertyNet	http://www.worldbank.org/poverty/
World Factbook (CIA)	https://www.cia.gov/library/publications/the-world-factbook/index.html
World Federation of Public Health Associations	http://www.wfpha.org/
World Fertility Surveys	http://opr.princeton.edu/archive/
World Social Forum: São Paulo, Brazil	http://www.forumsocialmundial.org.br
World Trade Organization (WTO)	http://www.wto.org/
World Vision	http://www.worldvision.org/
Worldwatch Institute	http://www.worldwatch.org/
Universities and Training Programs	
Aga Khan University—Community Health	http://www.aku.edu/CHS/
Boston University School of Public Health	http://sph.bu.edu/

(*continued*)

Name	URL
Center for Global Health and Economics	http://www.cghed.columbia.edu/
Center for International Public Health Policy	http://www.health.ed.ac.uk/CIPHP/
Center on Globalization and Sustainable Development	http://www.earthinstitute.columbia.edu/cgsd/
Columbia University Mailman School of Public Health—Global Health Track	http://www.cumc.columbia.edu/dept/sph/globalhealth/globalhealth-ms.html
Escola Nacional de Saúde Pública Sergio Arouca FIOCRUZ, Brazil	http://www.ensp.fiocruz.br/
Escuela de Salud Pública, Universidad de Chile	http://www.med.uchile.cl/salud_publica/esapu.html
Escuela de Salud Pública, Universidad Nacional de Córdoba, Argentina	http://www.saludpublica.fcm.unc.edu.ar/
Escuela Nacional de Salud Pública, Cuba	http://www.ensap.sld.cu/
Escuela Nacional de Salud Pública de México	http://www.insp.mx/Portal/Espm/index-espm.html
Emory Task Force for Child Survival and Development	http://www.taskforce.org/
Emory University Global Health Institute	http://whsc.emory.edu/globalhealth.cfm
George Washington University, School of Public Health, Department of Global Health	http://www.gwumc.edu/sphhs/academicprograms/graduate.cfm
Hanoi School of Public Health	http://www.hsph.edu.vn/english/
Harvard Initiative for Global Health	http://www.globalhealth.harvard.edu/icb/icb.do
Harvard University School of Public Health	
Department of Population and International Health	http://www.hsph.harvard.edu/departments/population-and-international-health/
Francois-Xavier Bagnoud Centre for Health and Human Rights	http://www.hsph.harvard.edu/fxbcenter/
Hebrew University, Hadassah School of Public Health and Community Medicine	http://www.md.huji.ac.il/depts/occenvmed/about.html
Johns Hopkins Center for Clinical Global Health Education	http://www.ccghe.jhmi.edu/ccg/index.asp
Johns Hopkins Center for Global Health	http://www.hopkinsglobalhealth.org/
Johns Hopkins University, Bloomberg School	http://www.jhsph.edu/dept/IH/index.html
Karolinska Institute	http://www.ki.se/
Liverpool School of Tropical Medicine	http://www.liv.ac.uk/lstm/

(continued)

Name	URL
Loma Linda University, School of Public Health, Department of Global Health	http://www.llu.edu/llu/sph/glbh/index.html
London School of Hygiene and Tropical Medicine	http://www.lshtm.ac.uk/prospectus/masters/msphdc.html
WHO Collaborating Center on Global Change and Health	http://www.lshtm.ac.uk/cgch/
Mahidol University (Thailand), Faculty of Public Health	http://www.ph.mahidol.ac.th/
Mansoura University (Egypt), Community Medicine	http://www.mans.edu.eg/facmed/english/Dept/Com_ Medi/Community.htm
New York University, Program in Global Public Health	http://www.nyu.edu/mph/
Peking University, School of Public Health	http://sph.bjmu.edu.cn/eng/index.htm
Queen Margaret University	http://www.qmced.ac.uk/cihs/
Tulane University, International Health and Development	http://www.sph.tulane.edu/IHD
Universidad Peruana Cayetano Heredia, Faculty of Public Health	http://www.upch.edu.pe/faspa/
Université Libré de Bruxelles, Ecole de Santé Publique	http://www.ulb.ac.be/facs/esp/index.html
University of Alabama at Birmingham, International Health and Global Studies Program	http://www.soph.uab.edu/
University of California at Berkeley, International Health Program	http://sph.berkeley.edu/degrees/areas/spec_ih.html
University of California at Los Angeles, International Health Program	http://www.ph.ucla.edu/emph/faculty.html
University College London, Centre for International Health and Development	http://www.ihmec.ucl.ac.uk/
University of Edinburgh	http://www.health.ed.ac.uk/CIPHP/postgraduate/ globalhealth.htm
University of Iowa, Global Health Studies Program	http://international.uiowa.edu/centers/global-health/ default.asp
University of Michigan International Health	http://www.sph.umich.edu/epid/programs/international_ health.html
University of New South Wales	http://www.handbook.unsw.edu.au/postgraduate/ plans/2008/PHCMIS9045.html
University of New South Wales, School of Public Health	http://www.sphcm.med.unsw.edu.au/
University of North Carolina, Chapel Hill Office of Global Health	http://www.sph.unc.edu/globalhealth/

(*continued*)

Name	URL
University of Pennsylvania, Global Health Programs	http://www.med.upenn.edu/globalhealth/links.shtml
University of Pittsburgh, Graduate School of Public Health, Global Health Certificate Program	http://www.publichealth.pitt.edu/interior.php?pageID=82
University of South Florida, Department of Global Health	http://www.usf.edu/Academics/USF-Health/Public-Health/Global-Health.asp
University of Sussex, Institute of Development Studies Knowledge Services	http://www.ids.ac.uk/go/ids-knowledge-services
University of Sydney	http://www.health.usyd.edu.au/future/coursework/internatpublichealth/master.php
University of Texas, School of Public Health, Global Health Concentration	http://www.sph.uth.tmc.edu/ghc/
University of Tokyo, Department of Public Health	http://publichealth.m.u-tokyo.ac.jp/intro.html
University of Toronto, Centre for International Health (CIH)	http://intlhealth.med.utoronto.ca/
University of Toronto, Global Health Focus	http://www.phs.utoronto.ca/Global.asp
University of Uppsala, Sweden International Health Programmes	http://www.healthtraining.org/schools/uppsala.php
University of Washington, Department of Global Health	http://depts.washington.edu/deptgh/
University of the Witwatersrand, South Africa	http://web.wits.ac.za/Academic/Health/PublicHealth/
University of York, Center for Health Economics	http://www.york.ac.uk/inst/che/
Yale University, School of Public Health, Global Health Division	http://www.med.yale.edu/eph/ghd/index.html

Websites of Some Ministries of Health and Bilateral Aid Agencies[c]

Argentina: Ministry of Health	http://www.msal.gov.ar/
Australia: Department of Health and Ageing	http://www.health.gov.au/
Austria: Ministry of Labor, Health and Social Affairs	http://www.bmsk.gv.at/
Bahrain: Ministry of Health	http://www.moh.gov.bh/
Bolivia: Ministry of Health and Sport	http://www.sns.gov.bo/
Brazil: Ministry of Health	http://portal.saude.gov.br/saude/
Canada: Health Canada/Santé Canada	http://www.hc-sc.gc.ca/index_e.html
Canadian Institutes of Health Research	http://www.cihr-irsc.gc.ca/

(*continued*)

Name	URL
Canadian International Development Agency (CIDA)	http://www.acdi-cida.gc.ca/index-e.htm
Chile	
Health Ministry	http://www.minsal.cl/
Institute of Public Health	http://www.ispch.cl/
China: Ministry of Health	http://www.moh.gov.cn/
Colombia: Ministry of Social Welfare	http://www.minproteccionsocial.gov.co/
Costa Rica: Ministry of Health	http://www.ministeriodesalud.go.cr/
Croatia: Ministry of Health and Social Welfare	http://www.mzss.hr/
Cuba	
Ministry of Foreign Relations (Cooperation)	http://www.cubaminrex.cu/Cooperacion/inicio_cooperacion.asp
Ministry of Public Health	http://www.dne.sld.cu/minsap/
Czech Republic: Ministry of Health	http://www.mzcr.cz/
Denmark: Ministry of Social Welfare	http://www.social.dk/
Ecuador: Ministry of Public Health	http://www.msp.gov.ec/
Estonia: Ministry of Social Affairs	http://www.sm.ee/eng/pages/index.html
Finland: Ministry of Social Affairs and Health	http://www.stm.fi
France	
Agence Française de Développement (AFD)	http://www.afd.fr/jahia/Jahia/lang/en/home
Ministry of Health	http://www.sante.fr
Germany	
GTZ	http://www.gtz.de/en/
Ministry of Health	http://www.bmgesundheit.de/
Guatemala: Ministry of Public Health and Welfare	http://www.mspas.gob.gt/
Guyana: Ministry of Health	http://www.health.gov.gy/
Hong Kong: Department of Health	http://www.info.gov.hk/dh/
Hungary: Ministry of Health	http://www.eum.hu/
India	
Ministry of Health and Family Welfare	http://mohfw.nic.in/
State of Kerala Department of Health and Family Welfare	http://www.kerala.gov.in/dept_health/health.htm
Indonesia: Ministry of Health	http://www.depkes.go.id/index.php
Ireland: Department of Health and Children	http://www.doh.ie/
Israel: Ministry of Health	http://www.health.gov.il/

(continued)

Name	URL
Italy: Ministry of Health	http://www.ministerosalute.it/
Japan	
Japanese International Cooperation Agency (JICA)	http://www.jica.go.jp/
Ministry of Health, Labor and Welfare	http://www.mhlw.go.jp/index.html
Jordan: Ministry of Health	http://www.moh.gov.jo:7778/MOH/arabic/home.php
Kenya: Ministry of Health	http://www.health.go.ke/
Kingdom of Saudi Arabia	http://www.moh.gov.sa/ar/index.php
Lithuania: Ministry of Health	http://www.sam.lt/en/
Luxembourg: Ministry of Health	http://www.ms.etat.lu/
Malaysia: Ministry of Health	http://www.moh.gov.my/
Malta: Ministry of Health	http://www.sahha.gov.mt/
Mexico	
Instituto Nacional de Salud Pública (INSP)	http://www.insp.mx/
Ministry of Health	http://www.ssa.gob.mx/
Morocco: Ministry of Health	http://www.sante.gov.ma/
Namibia: Ministry of Health and Social Service	http://www.healthnet.org.na/mhssindex1.htm
New Zealand: Ministry of Health	http://www.moh.govt.nz/moh.nsf
Netherlands: Ministry of Health, Welfare and Sport	http://www.minvws.nl/
Norway: Ministry of Health and Care Services	http://www.regjeringen.no/nn/dep/hod.html?id=421
Palestine: Ministry of Health:	http://www.moh.gov.ps
Philippines: Council for Health Research and Development	http://www.pchrd.dost.gov.ph/
Peru: Ministry of Health	http://www.digesa.sld.pe/
Portugal: Ministry of Health	http://www.dgs.pt/
Russia	
Ministry of Public Health and Social Development	http://www.mzsrrf.ru/health/
Priority program on primary health care	http://www.mzsrrf.ru/razv_pev_med/
Public Health Research Institute	http://whodc.mednet.ru/eng/index.php
Senegal: Ministry of Health and Prevention	http://213.154.85.37/
Singapore: Ministry of Health	http://www.moh.gov.sg
Slovak Republic: Ministry of Health	http://www.health.gov.sk/

(continued)

Name	URL
South Africa: Department of Health	http://www.sacs.org.za/level4/heal.htm
Spain: Ministry of Health	http://www.msc.es/
Sri Lanka: Ministry of Healthcare & Nutrition	http://www.health.gov.lk/
St. Lucia: Ministry of Health Wellness, Family Affairs, National Mobilisation, Human Services and Gender Relations	http://www.stlucia.gov.lc/agencies/ministry_of_health.htm
Sweden	
Ministry of Health and Social Affairs	http://www.regeringen.se/sb/d/2061
Swedish International Development Cooperation Agency (SIDA)	http://www.sida.se/sida/jsp/sida.jsp?language=Sv_se
Taiwan: Department of Health	http://www.doh.gov.tw/cht2006/index_populace.aspx/
Thailand: Ministry of Public Health	http://www.moph.go.th
Turkey: Ministry of Health	http://www.saglik.gov.tr
United Arab Emirates: Ministry of Health	http://www.moh.gov.ae/
United Kingdom	
British Department for International Development (DFID)	http://www.dfid.gov.uk/
Ministry of Health	http://www.dh.gov.uk/en
Uruguay: Ministry of Public Health	http://www.msp.gub.uy/index_1.html
Venezuela	
Ministry of Popular Power for Health	http://www.barrioadentro.gov.ve/
Mission Barrio Adentro (social welfare program)	http://www.mpps.gob.ve/ms/index.php
Vietnam: Ministry of Health	http//www.moh.gov.vn/
United States Government Agencies	
Agency for Health Care Research and Quality (AHRQ)	http://www.ahcpr.gov/
Centers for Disease Control and Prevention (CDC)	http://www.cdc.gov/
CDC Coordinating Office for Global Health	http://www.cdc.gov/cogh/index.htm
CDC Diseases and Conditions Page	http://www.cdc.gov/DiseasesConditions/
CDC Epidemic Information Exchange	http://www.cdc.gov/epix/
CDC Morbidity & Mortality Weekly Report	http://www.cdc.gov/mmwr/
CDC Travel Information	http://wwwn.cdc.gov/travel/
Census Bureau International Data Base	http://www.census.gov/ipc/www/idbnew.html

(continued)

Name	URL
American Factfinder	http://factfinder.census.gov/home/saff/main.html?_lang=en
Food and Drug Administration (FDA), FDA International Agencies Page	http://www.fda.gov/oia/agencies.htm
Healthy People 2010 Home Page	http://www.healthypeople.gov/
Library of Congress Country Studies	http://lcweb2.10c.gov/frd/cs/cshome.html#toc.
National Center for HIV, STD, and TB Prevention (NCHSTP)	http://www.cdc.gov/nchhstp/
National Institute for Occupational Safety and Health (NIOSH)	http://www.cdc.gov/niosh/
National Institutes of Health	http://www.nih.gov/
National Library of Medicine	http://www.nlm.nih.gov/
NLM Online Databases and Electronic Resources	http://www.nlm.nih.gov/databases/index.html
Pubmed (formerly MEDLINE)	http://www.ncbi.nlm.nih.gov/sites/entrez/
PEPFAR (President's Emergency Plan for AIDS Relief)	http://www.pepfar.gov/
THOMAS—U.S. Congress on the Internet	http://thomas.loc.gov/
U.S. Agency for International Development (USAID)	http://www.usaid.gov/
U.S. Department of Health and Human Services	http:/dhhs.gov/
U.S. Public Health Service	http://www.usphs.gov/
U.S. State Department Travel Warnings and Consular Information Sheets	http://www.travel.state.gov/travel/warnings.html
United Nations Agency Websites	
Food and Agriculture Organization (FAO)	http://www.fao.org/
International Labour Organization (ILO)	http://www.ilo.org/global/lang—en/index.htm
UN NGO Link (DPI-NGO)	http://www.un.org/dpi/ngosection/index.asp
UNAIDS	http://www.unaids.org/en/
UN Conference on Trade and Development (UNCTAD)	http://www.unctad.org/Templates/StartPage.asp?intItemID=2068
UN Development Fund for Women (UNIFEM)	http://www.unifem.org
UN Development Programme (UNDP)	http://www.undp.org
UNDP HIV/AIDS Publications	http://www.undp.org/hiv/pubs.htm
UN Economic and Social Council (ECOSOC)	http://www.un.org/ecosoc/

(*continued*)

Name	URL
UN Educational, Scientific and Cultural Organization (UNESCO)	http://www.unesco.org
UN Environmental Programme (UNEP)	http://www.unep.org
UN High Commission for Refugees (UNHCR)	http://www.unhcr.org
UN Human Settlements Programme (UN-HABITAT)	http://www.unhabitat.org/
UNICEF (UN Children's Fund)	http://www.unicef.org/
UN Inter-Agency Network on Women and Gender Equality (IANWGE)	http://www.un.org/womenwatch/ianwge/
United Nations	http://www.un.org/
UN Millennium Development Goals	http://www.un.org/millenniumgoals/
UN Office of the High Commissioner for Human Rights (OHCHR)	http://www.ohchr.org/EN/Pages/WelcomePage.aspx
UN Population Fund (UNFPA)	http://www.unfpa.org/
Population & Family Planning Bookshelf	http://www.un.org/popin/books.htm
UN Volunteers	http://www.unv.org
UN World Food Programme (WFP)	http://www.wfp.org/english/
World Health Organization (WHO)	http://www.who.int/
Library and Information Networks For Knowledge	http://www.who.int/library/en/
Pan American Health Organization (PAHO)	http://www.PAHO.org
Regional Offices Around the World	http://www.who.int/regions/
WHO Statistical Information System	http://www.who.int/whosis/en/

[a]This is a sampling of some useful Web sites as of early 2008. Many of these include links to other sites. New sites are added constantly. Web addresses (universal resource locators) and organization names may change.

[b]Numerous initiatives around the world—some of which have very long histories in primary health care (e.g. Gonoshasthaya Kendra [GK] in Bangladesh)—do not have Web sites. In general, the most grassroots groups do not appear on the list as they are less likely to have access to the Internet.

[c]Most Web pages are in the respective national language.

Index

Note: Page numbers with "f" denote figures and those with "t" denote tables.

3 by 5 Initiative, 107
10/90 gap, 118, 639, 707
50 Years is Enough Network, 89, 459, 731

Abortion, 674
  definition, 222
  international legality of, 261
  and maternal mortality, 261
Abt Associates, 97
Accessibility:
  as a principle of health care systems, 618
Action by Churches Together (ACT), 109
Acute respiratory tract infections. *See*
  Respiratory tract infections
Adolescent health, 254, 667
Adult health, 254, 255–265, 381t
  ARV therapy and, 294f
  HIV prevalence and, 288f
  and productivity, 255
Adventist Development and Relief
  Agency, 108t
Advocacy, 63, 115–116, 118, 353, 640,
  727–728
Aedes aegypti. See Mosquitoes
Affordability:
  as a principle of health care
  systems, 619

Afghanistan, 93, 97, 388, 404, 452
  child soldiers, 385
  humanitarian workers, 376, 403
  maternal mortality rate, 219, 252
  refugees, 378t
Africa, 21, 23
  aid, 98
  and China, 96
  debt, 94, 96
  HIV/AIDS relief efforts, 144, 178
  malaria in, 77
  medical schools in, 634
  regional offices, 74t
  river blindness in, 665
  Southern African Development
    Community, 98, 725
  Stanley expedition in, 29
  sub-Saharan. *See* Sub-Saharan Africa
  trypanosomiasis in, 29
African Development Bank, 83
African Medical Research Foundation
  (AMREF), 97
African sleeping sickness/trypanosomiasis,
  270t, 698. *See also* Neglected
  tropical diseases
  and imperialism, 29
African Union, 98, 625, 725

Africa Rights, 727
Aga Khan Foundation (AKF), 102, 704
  endowment and priorities, 100t
Age adjustment, 220
  age standardized mortality rate between
    countries, 249f
Agencies. *See also* individual agencies as
    listed on, 68t, 70t, 91t, 100t, 108t,
    121t
  aid, 94, 113, 374, 717
  definition, 62
  spending and activities, 108t
Agenda 21, 509t, 511–512
Agent Orange, 392
Age-productivity profile, 227, 228
Age pyramids, 205, 206f. *See also*
    Population pyramids
Aging:
  health needs, 256
  illnesses associated with, 256
  and long-term care, 622
  quality of life, 256–257
Agriculture, 158. *See also* Food security;
    Food sovereignty
  and climate change, 478
  and environmental degradation, 428, 495,
    500, 502, 504
  Green Revolution, 158
  historical development, 472
  and pesticide use, 424, 445, 494, 500, 671
  social movements, 71, 180–181, 526
  subsidies, 148t, 316, 317
  sustainable agriculture, 520t, 526
  and trade, 311, 317
  urban agriculture, 510t, 526–527
  workers, 325, 334, 336, 338
Aid, 119–125, 155–161. *See also*
    Development; Global health;
    International health
  0.7% GNI to ODA, 94, 160
  agencies, 94, 113, 374, 717
  bilateral, 86, 89–97, 374, 559, 615
  and debt, 86, 94, 96, 166
  food aid, 96, 374, 402, 406–407, 715
  humanitarian assistance, 181

  multilateral, 90, 632, 717
  Official Development Assistance.
    See Official Development Assistance
  phantom aid, 90, 716
  South–North, 726
  South–South, 96, 724–726
  tied aid, 90, 159, 731
AIDS. *See* HIV/AIDS
AIDS Law Project, 729
Air pollution:
  burning of biomass fuels, 482t, 493–494,
    518
  health effects, 484t
  indoor, 493–494
  London Smog (1952), 490
  outdoor, 490–493
  particulate matter, 490–491
ALAMES (Asociación Latinoamericana de
    Medicina social), 676, 702.
ALBA. *See* Bolivarian Alternative for Latin
    America and the Caribbean
Alejandro Prospero Reverend School
    of Medicine, 117
Al-Haq, 727
Allende, Salvador, 142, 675
Alliance for Progress, 158
Alma-Ata Conference and Declaration, 76t,
    79–80, 171, 351, 353, 354, 603,
    625, 643, 644–646, 659, 681, 732.
    See also Primary health care
Aloha Medical Mission, 110
American Friends Service Committee, 108t
American Jewish World Service, 108t, 110
Amnesty International, 114, 705, 727, 728
Angola:
  health worker migration from, 634
Annan, Kofi, 176, 459
Anopheles. See Mosquitoes
Anthrax, 390, 391
Antibiotics, 140, 285
  antibiotic resistance, 277
Anti-colonization, 720
Antiretroviral drugs (ARVs), 93, 101, 107,
    113, 150, 289, 291, 656, 729.
    See also 3 by 5 Initiative; HAART

access to, 292, 428, 429, 445, 457, 628
people using ARVs, by region, 292, 293f
and pharmaceutical companies, 101
rights to, 729
sex and, 149
unmet need, sub-Saharan Africa, 292, 294f
and XDR TB, 285
Appropriate technology, 626
Arab Association for Human Rights, 727
Aral Sea, 495, 496f
Arbenz, Jacobo, 406
Argentina, 45
debt, 457
financial crisis, 439
human rights to health, 729
IMF conditionalities, 85
water privatization in, 169
Arsenic:
exposure and health effects, 486t
ARVs. See Antiretroviral drugs
Asbestos, 279, 431, 447–448, 487, 509t,
    515. See also Hazardous waste
Asia, 23. See also Central Asia; East Asia;
    South Asia; Southeast Asia
air quality and motor vehicles, 491
avian influenza, 299
birth registration, 213
CO$_2$ emission, 477t
energy consumption, 476
infant mortality rate, 216, 660
land tenure, 336
maternal death, 261
medical schools in, 634
neoliberal economic model, 439
outdoor air pollution, 491
smallpox eradication campaign
    (South Asia), 78, 659
tsunami in, 370–371
Asian Development Bank, 83
Asian Human Rights Commission, 727
Asthma, 252
and air pollution, 490–491, 493, 494
Australia:
aboriginal residential schools,
    265, 335

foreign-trained doctors in, 635
harmful products, bans on, 515
indigenous health, 263t, 335
light bulbs, ban on, 515
Austria:
health care system, 597
Avian influenza. See Influenza
Azerbaijan:
complex humanitarian emergency, 376f
refugees, 378t

Bacille Calmette-Guérin (BCG) vaccine.
    See Tuberculosis
Badiano, Juan, 23
Bamako Initiative (BI):
cost recovery, 549
Bandung Conference, 67
Bancrji, Debabar, 143
Bangladesh, 117, 409. See also BRAC
"A Kind of Childhood" documentary
    film, 417
Bengali famine (1943), 316
comparison of health measures, health
    expenditures, and inequities,
    573–574, 574t
disparity in measles immunization, 275
Grameen Bank, 114
Grameen Foundation, 114
health system typology (Roemer), 588t
health workers, 634
measles vaccination, 275
People's Health Movement in, 63,
    116, 731
prostituted children, 452t
Barrio Adentro. See Misión Barrio Adentro
Basel Convention, 488
Bearing witness, 727–728
Behavioral approach to health and disease,
    134, 146, 150, 178, 250, 312–313,
    346–348
Behring, Emil von, 39
Bendana, Alejandro, 174
Benzene:
exposure and health effects, 485t
Bertillon, Jacques, 213

Beveridge Report, 598
Bhopal:
    Union Carbide leak (1984), 441, 487
Bhutan:
    gross national happiness, 321
Bifurcated needles, 658
Big Pharma. *See also* Pharmaceutical
        industry
    international health, role in, 103–104
    political economy of, 628–629
Bilateral:
    definition, 62
Bill and Melinda Gates Foundation, 62, 82,
        99–101, 121t, 124, 562
    critique of, 101, 665–666
    endowment and priorities, 100t
    Grand Challenges in Global Health
        Initiative, 101, 665–666
Biodiversity, 478, 501, 502, 507, 511, 526
Biofuels, 502, 520t
    Agenda 21, 512
    and food insecurity, 512
Biological weapons. *See* Weapons
Biomedical model of health and disease,
        133, 135, 136, 139, 146, 147t,
        148t, 150, 152, 178, 181, 315,
        345–346, 701
Birth registration. *See* Registration
Black, Sir Douglas, 343
Black Death. *See* Plague
Black Report:
    class differences in health, 236,
        342–343, 343f
Bolivarian Alternative for Latin America
        and the Caribbean (ALBA),
        68t, 96, 725
Bolivia, 725
    GDP, debt, and health expenditures, 563t
    indigenous health, 263t
    nationalization of energy, 457
    privatization of water in Cochabamba,
        169, 431
Bosnia:
    gender-based violence, 382
    refugees, mental health, 381t

Botswana:
    age pyramid, 206f
    health system typology (Roemer), 588t
    HIV prevalence, 287, 290
    private expenditures in health, 592t
Bovine spongiform encephalopathy.
        See Emerging infectious diseases
BRAC, 111, 114, 115
Brain drain, 453, 634–636, 639. *See also*
        Health care workers
Brandt Commission, 174
Brazil:
    Amazon deforestation, 502
    ARVs. *See* Antiretroviral drugs
    biomass fuels, 512
    child mortality under SAPs, 438
    Curitiba, 521
    FIOCRUZ, 117
    health reform in, 610
    health system, 5
    health system typology (Roemer), 588t
    HIV/AIDS, access to ARVs, 92
    IBSA, 97
    income inequality, 328
    indigenous health, 263t
    infant mortality rate by region, 219t
    international assistance, 96
    Landless Workers' Movement (MST),
        336
    National AIDS Program, 291–292
    participatory budgeting, Porto Alegre,
        524, 678
    private health insurance plan penetration,
        104t
    prostituted children, 452t
    TRIPS, 429, 457
Brazilian purpuric fever. *See* Emerging
        infectious diseases
Breast feeding, 79, 253, 254, 289, 329f,
        433, 659. *See also* Infant formula
Breilh, Jaime, 143
Brennan, Richard, 373
Bretton Woods, 65
    agreement, 164
    institutions, 437–438, 459

Bristol-Myers Squibb Foundation, 102
Britain. *See* England; United Kingdom
Brown, Michael, 368
Buenos Aires Plan of Action, 725
Buffet, Warren, 101
Built environment, 471, 479, 482,
    507, 519
Burma:
    refugees, mental health, 401
Buruli ulcer. *See* Neglected tropical
    diseases
Burundi:
    indigenous health, 264t
    private expenditures in health, 592t
    refugees, 378t
Business interests in health, 102–105

Cadmium:
    exposure and health effects, 486t
Cambodia:
    comparison of health measures, health
        expenditures, and inequities,
        573–574t
    GDP, debt, and health expenditures, 563t
    indigenous health, 264t
    private expenditures in health, 592t
    refugees, mental health, 381t
    toxic waste dumping, 448
Cameron, Lovett, 25
Cameroun:
    indigenous health, 264t
Campylobacter:
    exposure and health effects, 486t
Canada:
    aboriginal residential schools, 335, 682
    asbestos, exporting of, 447–448
    Bill C-9, 104
    biomass fuels, 512
    birth registration problems, 223
    Canadian Institute for Advanced
        Research, 5
    CIDA. *See* Canadian International
        Development Agency
    Canadian Society for International
        Health, 118, 704

disparities in smoking-related
    deaths, 682
financing and delivery of health
    care, 587t
foreign aid priorities, 181
foreign-trained doctors and
    nurses in, 635
health economics/health insurance model,
    546, 547, 548t
health system typology (Roemer), 588t
homeless health indicators, 318
IDRC. *See* International Development
    Research Centre
indigenous health, 263t
Lalonde Report, 346
MAI resistance, Council of Canadians,
    116, 458
Ministry of Health (Health Canada/Santé
    Canada) mission statement, 584
private expenditures in health, 592t
safe injection sites, 258
voting power at the IMF and World
    Bank, 82t
Canadian International Development
    Agency (CIDA), 68t, 704
Cancer, 278 280
    and aging, 256
    bowel, 279
    breast, 246f, 278, 279
    cervical. *See* Cervical cancer
    colon, 278
    deaths due to, 278
    determinants, 279
    esophageal, 279
    and infectious disease, 279
    interventions, 279
    as a leading cause of death, 229t, 245f,
        246f
    liver, 278, 279
    lung, 198, 278, 279, 313, 490, 491
    pancreatic, 279
    screening, 279
    stomach, 278
Capital flows, 164, 166, 167f, 168,
    427, 439

Capitalism, 141, 147. *See also* Economics;
    Globalization; Neoliberalism
  capital, 137, 157, 162, 163, 164,
    165, 424t
  and the Cold War rivalry, 66, 120
  definition, 137, 183
  and environmental degradation, 507, 528
  exploitation, 35
  and health and disease, 137, 142, 143
  and international health, 11
  and Keynesian model, 156
  and *laissez-faire* economics, 167
  and modernization theory, 161
  and organization of health systems, 586
  and power, 330, 349, 356
  and social inequalities, 327, 342, 443
  transition from feudalism, 30–31,
    472–473
  transition to, in former Soviet Union,
    145, 151–152
  and underdevelopment, 164
  world order, 9, 10, 50, 54, 698
  and world system theory, 163
Carbon dioxide, 522. *See also* Climate
    change; Greenhouse gases
  emissions by region, 476–477
Carbon monoxide:
  exposure and health effects, 368, 484t
Cardiovascular disease (CVD), 277–278.
    See also Coronary heart disease
  and aging, 256
  as cause of death, 277
Caribbean:
  disasters, preparation for, 406
  health care system, 609–611
  health workforce migration, 635
  slave trade in, 25, 26
Caribbean Development Bank, 83
Caritas International, 109
Carso Health Institute, 102
Carson, Rachel:
  Silent Spring, 510
Castro, Fidel, 85, 142, 726
Catholic Relief Services (CRS), 108t, 112
Census, 202–209, 243t

  essential features, 204–205
  global, 205, 208
  history, 202
  limitations, 208–209
  procedures and cost, 202–205
  requirements, 202t, 203–204t
Center for Global Development (CGD),
    115, 630, 660, 730
Center for Global Health and Economic
    Development, 117
Center for Policy Analysis on Trade and
    Health (CPATH), 115, 460
Center for Social and Economic
    Rights, 114
Centers for Disease Control and Prevention
    (CDC), 97, 198, 295, 704, 713
  and Hurricane Katrina, 368–369
Central African Republic:
  indigenous health, 264t
Central American Bank for Economic
    Integration, 83
Central American Free Trade Agreement
    (CAFTA), 429, 447
Central Asia. *See also* Asia; East Asia;
    South Asia; Southeast Asia
  avian influenza in, 299
  behavioral approach to health and
    disease, 150
  International Rescue Committee in, 113
  plague in, 19
  tuberculosis in, 285
Centre Europe Tiers Monde, 731–732
Centre for Health and Social Justice,
    701, 722
Cerebrovascular disease, 277–278
  and aging, 256
  consequences, 277
  deaths due to, 229t, 247f, 248f, 249f
  determinants, 278
  interventions, 278
Certificates:
  birth, 210t, 212, 213, 223
  death, 211t, 214, 215, 215f, 221, 224
  marriage, 210t, 211t, 212
Cervical cancer, 280

in developing countries, 279
vaccine for human papilloma virus, 279
Chadwick, Edwin, 35
    Poor Law, England, 34
    *Report on an Inquiry into the Sanitary
        Condition of the Labouring
        Population of Great Britain*, 34,
        341–342
Chagas disease, 318, 708. *See also*
    Neglected tropical diseases
Chan, Margaret, 74, 352, 353
Chávez, Hugo, 85, 725
Chemical contamination:
    exposure and health effects, 484t
    toxic building materials, 482, 487, 494
Chemical weapons. *See* Weapons
Chernobyl. *See* Ukraine
Chikungunya fever. *See* Emerging infec-
    tious diseases
Child Family Health International, 700
Child and infant health, 193, 250–254,
        329f, 646. *See also* Infant mortality;
        Under-5 mortality
    bureaucratic and resource barriers, 618
    causes of death and illness, 251–254
    child survival, 254. *See also* Child
        Survival campaigns
    and environment, 483
    inequalities in health care facilities, 623
    infrastructural and economic
        barriers, 621
    interventions, 253–254
    and quality care, 620
Child labor, 419, 422, 435t, 449–450, 462
Child soldiers, 385–386
Child Survival campaigns, 79–80, 438,
        659–660
Chile, 142, 438. *See also* Allende, Salvador
    comparison of health measures, health
        expenditures, and inequities,
        573–574t
    military dictatorship, 172
    private health insurance plan
        penetration, 104t
China:

age pyramid, 206f
aid, 96
    artemisinin, antimalarial treatment, 28,
        275, 708
    barefoot doctors, 79, 603
    biomass fuels, 494, 512
    census, 202
    CO_2 emissions, 477
    development assistance from, 96
    health care system, 602–605
    health system typology (Roemer), 588t
    HIV/AIDS, 288
    indigenous health, 263t
    life expectancy, differences, 340–341
    marginalization, diseases of, 281
    pollution, 282, 488t, 494
    poverty reduction in, 337
    private expenditures in health, 592t
    private health insurance plan
        penetration, 104t
    prostituted children, 452t
    SARS, 298
    Shanghai, urban agriculture, 526
    socialist market, 602–605
    Three Gorges Dam, 505–506
    tuberculosis program, 661
    voting power at the IMF and World
        Bank, 82t
Chlorofluorocarbons (CFCs), 513–514
    Montreal Protocol, 511, 514
    ozone hole, 514
Cholera, 42, 267, 267f, 268t, 269, 297t, 498
    exposure and health effect, 296t, 484t
    history of, 33, 39, 46–47, 48–49, 473
    international conferences, 48, 49
    John Snow, 35–36
    mortality, 267, 267f
    trade and quarantine, 47
Christian Connections for International
    Health, 110
Chronic disease. *See* Noncommunicable
    disease
Chronic obstructive pulmonary disease
    (COPD), 282–283, 491, 493
    and aging, 256

Chronic obstructive pulmonary disease
     (COPD) (*Cont.*)
   consequences, 282
   determinants, 282–283
   and indoor air pollution, 282, 493
   interventions, 283
   mortality, 227t, 229t, 245f, 246f, 247f
   prevalence, 282
Civil society movements. *See* Social
     movements
Clapp, Jennifer, 479–480
Class. *See also* Marx, Karl; Social class
   Classism, 369
   class struggle, 163
Cleanliness, 21
Climate change/global warming,
     475–479, 478t
   causal factors, 475–477
   CO_2 emissions, by region, 477t
   greenhouse effect, 476
   health consequences, 477–478
   heat and heat waves, 476, 477,
     485t, 501
   and human development, 478
   Intergovernmental Panel on Climate
     Change (IPCC), 476
   Kyoto Protocol, 509t, 511, 512–513
   process, 476
   responses, 478–480
Codex Badianus, 23
Cold War:
   context of health and development
     policies, 66–67, 120–121, 153, 156,
     160, 161
   and disease control efforts, 64, 75, 77
   and population control, 91–92
Collective health, 5, 143, 351, 671,
     680, 686
Colombia:
   healthy cities, Bogotá, 683
   malaria in, 275
   war on drugs programs, 392
Colombo Plan, 65, 158
Colonialism, 18–25, 28, 30, 66–67, 161,
     162, 169, 339, 695, 697. *See also*
     Imperialism; Tropical medicine

   and Christian missions, 109, 697–698
   colonial medicine, 22, 23, 39, 41, 65,
     698, 708
   colonists' mortality, 24, 43
   exchange of diseases, 24
   health, and trade, 42
   and indigenous mortality, 22, 24, 335
   motives for health measures, 30, 41, 50
Comité International de la Croix Rouge, 52.
     See also International Committee of
     the Red Cross
Commission on Intellectual Property Rights
     (WHO), 78
Commission on Macroeconomics and Health
     (CMH) (WHO), 352, 559–562
   "basket" of interventions, 561
   critique of, 560–562
   and Disease Control Priorities Project,
     279, 562
   health as productivity, 559–562
   investments in health, 560
   Jeffrey Sachs, 171, 560
Commission on Social Determinants of
     Health (CSDH) (WHO), 236,
     352–354
   action areas, 203, 352
   critique of, 353–354
Communicable disease, 225, 228, 246,
     266. *See also* Child and infant
     health; Chronic obstructive pulmo-
     nary disease; Emerging infectious
     diseases; HIV/AIDS; Influenza;
     Malaria; Neglected tropical diseases;
     Respiratory tract infections; Severe
     Acute Respiratory Syndrome;
     Sexually Transmitted Infections;
     Tuberculosis
   definition, 243t
Complex humanitarian emergency (CHE),
     374–386, 408, 409
   in the Balkans, 382
   constraints and approaches, 386
   definition, 366, 377
   in East Timor, 377
   effects on health and health care services,
     380–382, 383f

gender-based violence, 382–384
history of, 376–377
in Kosovo, 377
malnutrition and, 379–380
map of, 376f
mental health, 380–382
response, 377–379
in Sudan, 379–380
violence and war effects, on children,
    384–386
in Zaire, 377, 379
Comprehensiveness:
as a principle of health care systems, 619
Conflict and health, 393–399
Congo-Brazzaville:
indigenous health, 264t
Consumer movements, 524–525
Contract providers and consulting firms,
    68t, 97, 715–717
Convention on the Rights of the Child
    (CRC), 178t, 179, 212, 452
Convention on Tobacco Control. See
    Framework Convention on Tobacco
    Control
Coopération Internationale pour le
    Développement et la Solidarité, 109
Coronary heart disease (CHD). See also
    Cardiovascular disease
and aging. See Aging
consequences, 277
deaths due to, 245f, 246f, 247f, 248f
determinants, 278
interventions, 278
Corporate accountability/social
    responsibility, 517–518
Corporate foundations, 68t, 102
Corruption in health sector, 565–566
Cortés, Hernán, 22
Costa Rica, 669
comparison of health measures, health
    expenditures, and inequities,
    573–574t
features of welfare state, 668, 669
health care reform, 320
health indicators, 669
health system typology (Roemer), 588t

selected determinants of health and mor-
    tality rates, 668t
Cost-benefit analysis (CBA), 550–553
benefits of, 555t
critique of, 552–553
definition, 551
Dorothy Rice, 553
ethical considerations, 553–554
opportunity cost, 554
smallpox, 552
and WHO, 552
willingness to pay, 554
Cost-effectiveness and cost-effectiveness
    analysis (CEA), 554–557,
    566–567, 570
benefits of, 555t
and Commission on Macroeconomics
    and Health, 560–561
critique of, 555–557
definition, 554
disability-adjusted life years, 232,
    555, 556t
and Disease Control Priorities Project,
    559, 562
and donors, 564
and health financing in Georgia, 539
limitations of, 556–557
WHO, use by, 555
and World Bank, 558, 567
and World Development Report 1993:
    Investing in Health, 558
Côte d'Ivoire:
complex humanitarian emergency, 376f
toxic waste dumping in, 449
Council on Health Research for
    Development (COHRED), 118, 707
Critical medical anthropology, 321
Croatia:
complex humanitarian emergency, 376f
war and civilian casualties, 389
Cuba. See also Latin American School of
    Medicine
aid, 96
Civil Defense System, 369
comparison with United States and
    Sweden, 591t

Cuba (*Cont.*)
    features of welfare state, 668, 669
    financing and delivery of health care, 587t
    health indicators, 152
    hurricane preparedness, 369
    medical missions, 96
    post-USSR dissolution, 152
    private expenditures in health, 592t
    reductions in childhood diarrhea, 269
    selected determinants of health and mor-
        tality rates, 668t
    social services, 670
    South–South aid, 725
    special period in peacetime, 670
    trade embargo, 671
    urban agriculture, 671
Culture, 320–321, 706, 711
    influences on health, 701
    religion and health, 320–321
Currency devaluation and stabilization, 64,
        84, 85, 164, 166, 425t

Dams:
    in China, 505–506
    environmental effects, 505
    in Ghana, 505
    in India, 506
    resistance movement against, 506
DATA (Debt, AIDS, Trade, Africa):
    Bono, 115
Dauvergne, Peter, 479–480
David and Lucille Packard Foundation:
    endowment and priorities, 100t
DDT, 485t
    birds, effect on, 510
    environmental effects, 77, 527
    malaria control, 53, 77, 272, 273,
        657, 663
Death. *See also* Mortality
    causes of, 245–249, 245f, 246f, 247f,
        248f, 249f
    certified, 220
    in children, 251t, 253f
    globally, 227t, 245f
    by income level, 229t

medical certification of, 214–215
    definition, 222
    limitations of certification, 221
    rate definitions, 201t, 243t
    records, 212
    registration, 221f
    road traffic, 280
    verbal autopsy, 222–223
    war-related, 389–390
Debt, 83–85, 159, 339. *See also*
        International Monetary Fund; World
        Bank
    and aid, 86, 94, 96, 166
    due to health spending, 439, 607
    and health systems, 558, 559, 607
    resource transfers, from developing coun-
        tries, in billions, 166f
    resource transfers, from developing coun-
        tries, by region, 167f
Debt cancellation/relief, 87t, 88, 94, 96,
        169, 174, 182, 438–439, 462, 514,
        716, 731, 735. *See also* Heavily
        Indebted Poor Countries Initiative;
        Multilateral Debt Relief Initiative;
        Policy Support Instrument
    campaigns for, 458–459, 719, 734
Debt crises, 164–166, 166f,
        167f, 437–439
    capital flight, 165
    effect on infrastructure/services,
        426–427, 437–439
    Mexico, 83
Decentralization, 558, 596, 600, 602,
        613, 675
    and district health systems, 643
Decolonization, 66, 157
Deforestation:
    of Amazon, 502
    and health, 501–502
Deindustrialization, 266, 436
de la Cruz, Martin, 23
de las Casas, Bartolomé, 22
Democratic Republic of the Congo (DRC),
        367, 397–399, 419
    Civil war and mortality, 339

diarrheal disease and conflict,
    Goma, 379
gold mining and war, 501
indigenous health, 264t
mortality surveys, 398
Demographic and health survey (DHS),
    210, 212, 287
Demographic transition, 31–32, 256
Dengue fever, 270t, 295t, 297t. *See also*
    Neglected tropical diseases
Denmark:
    0.7% GNI in aid, 94
    health/disease profile, 246–247
    indigenous health, 264t
    mortality rates, 667t
    top ten causes of death, 246f
    wind energy, 519
Dependency theory of development,
    161–162
Deregulation, 167, 168, 424t, 427f, 431.
    See also Neoliberalism
Desert flowers, 504
d'Espine, Marc, 213
Detection of disease, 198, 279, 554–555
Developing countries. *See* Low-income
    countries
Development, 152–164
    aid (critique of), 697, 715–718, 722
    definition, 152, 153
    "development blocks disease"/"disease
        blocks development," 170–171
    dilemmas of, 504–505
    as freedom, 172
    and health, 67, 152, 170
    institutional, 47
    modernization theory of, 158, 161,
        163–164
    sustainable, 511–512
Development Assistance Committee
    (DAC), 89, 94f, 95f. *See also* Aid;
    Official Development Assistance;
    Organization for Economic
    Cooperation and Development
Development Bank of Southern
    Africa, 83

Diabetes mellitus, 145, 146, 148t, 152,
    281–282
    aboriginal and indigenous populations,
        281
    and aging, 256
    consequences, 282
    determinants, 281
    interventions, 282
    mortality, 227t, 229t, 246f, 281
    Type I, 281
    Type II, 281, 282
Diarrhea, 267–269, 314, 315
    and breast feeding, 253, 269
    causes, 268, 482t
    and CHEs, 378–379, 398
    child health, 700
    consequences, 268
    contrasting health models for
        understanding, 147t
    control and interventions, 254, 269,
        378–379
    enteric agents, 268t
    mortality, 267, 269, 379, 495
    oral rehydration therapy, 269
Dickens, Charles, 340, 341
Dignitas International, 114
Disability-adjusted life years (DALYs),
    230–232, 555
    and cost-effectiveness analysis, 555, 556t
    critique of, 231–232
    definition, 230, 243t
    distribution of disease burden, 230f
    global burden of disease, 228
    leading causes, globally, 231t
    and *World Development Report 1993:
        Investing in Health*, 230–231
Disability/impairment, 255. *See also*
    Disability-adjusted life years
Disasters, 252, 379
    aid, 96, 112–113
    definition, 366
    ecological, 366
    industrial, 441
    natural, 365, 367–374
    political economy of, 405–407

Disasters (*Cont.*)
    preparedness and preparation, 365, 376,
        402–403
Disease. *See also* Communicable dis-
    ease; Emerging infectious disease;
    Infectious diseases; Neglected
    tropical diseases; Noncommunicable
    disease
    defining illness/disease, 133–134
    primary, secondary, tertiary
        prevention, 250
Disease Control Priorities Project, 279, 559,
    562. *See also* Cost-effectiveness
Disease-development dialectic, 170
District Health Systems, 549, 643
Doctors for Global Health (DGH), 113,
    720, 721f
Doctors of the World. *See* Médecins
    du Monde
Doctors Without Borders. *See* Médecins
    Sans Frontières
Doha Declaration, 104, 429, 462
DOTS strategy, 235, 286, 662. *See also*
    Tuberculosis
Doyal, Lesley, 143
Dracunculiasis. *See* Guinea worm;
    Neglected tropical diseases
Drinking water. *See* Water
Drug resistance, 272, 275, 661
Drug use, 258, 311, 318
    harm reduction, 258
    health effects, 258
    injecting drug use, 258
    stigma, 258
Dunant, Jean-Henri, 48, 112

Earthquakes, 365, 371–373. *See also*
    Disasters
East African Development Bank, 83
East Asia. *See also* Asia; Central Asia;
    South Asia; Southeast Asia
    cholera in, 42
    dependency theory of development, 162
Eastern Europe. *See also* Europe; Western
    Europe

avian influenza in, 299
behavioral approach to health and
    disease, 150
epidemiologic transition, 40
tuberculosis in, 285
Ebola. *See* Emerging infectious diseases
E. coli, 268t, 296t, 297t, 486t, 498, 499
Ecological design, 519, 521
Ecological footprint, 480–481, 508, 519
Ecology, 471
    political, 471–474
Economic development, 157, 162, 171,
    432, 519
Economics, 537
    equity-efficiency trade-off, 557
    genuine progress indicator (GPI), 572f
    of maldistribution, 316, 373
    marginal benefit, 551
    market, 583
    neoliberal, 121, 143, 144, 166–170,
        172, 479
    working of markets, 540–543, 544t
Ecosystem, 470, 474, 475f, 478, 501, 504,
    516, 525, 528
    damage from Exxon Valdez oil spill, 507
    definition, 471
    thinking, 523
Ecuador, 438
    oil drilling and health, 440
    water privatization and contamination,
        431–432
Education and health, 462
Egypt:
    comparison of health measures, health
        expenditures, and inequities,
        573–574t
    female genital cutting, 685
    health/disease profile, 75
    health system typology (Roemer), 588t
    health worker migration from, 635
    life expectancy, 247
    top ten causes of death, 245, 247t
    under-5 mortality rate, disparities, 193
E-health, 627
Einstein, Albert, 113

Eli Lilly and Company Foundation, 102
El Salvador:
  social inequalities, indigenous, 335
  civil war, 396
Embargoes/economic sanctions, 395–396
Embodiment, 350
Emerging infectious diseases (EIDs), 267,
    295–297, 296t, 297t
  contributing factors, 295–296t
  listing of EIDs, 295t
Engels, Friedrich, 34–36, 142, 342
  *The Condition of the Working Class in
    England*, 35, 141
  food quality and societal determinants
    of health, 316
  and Karl Marx, *The Communist
    Manifesto*, 35
EngenderHealth, 110
England. *See also* United Kingdom
  as colonial power, 25–26, 66
  industrial revolution in, 32–33, 47, 473
  mortality rates, 37
  Poor Law, 212
  Public Health Act (1848), 35
  sanitary reform, 34–36
Enumeration, 200–201, 204, 208. *See also*
    Census
Environment. *See also* Air pollution;
    Climate change; Ecological
    footprint; Garbage; Recycling;
    Sanitation; Water
  built. *See* Built environment
  dams. *See* Dams
  debt swaps, 509t, 514
  definitions, 470
  deforestation, 472, 474, 476, 478, 482t,
    501–502, 506
  and human interactions, 471
  land, 499–500
  and market-driven pressures, 506
  mining. *See* Mining
  natural, 470, 480, 507, 519
  political ecology. *See* Political ecology
  political economy of environmental
    health. *See* Political economy

  social, 471
  social movements, 525–528
  technologies and practices for
    improvement, 520t
Environmental contamination, 484
Environmental conferences and agreements,
    71, 72t, 511
Environmental Defense Fund (EDF), 527
Environmental dilemmas:
  and development, 504
Environmental disease burden:
  by WHO sub-region, 483f
Environmental health. *See* Environment;
    Environment and health
Environmental improvements:
  agriculture, 520t
Environment and governmental responsibil-
    ity, 479, 506–507, 509t, 514
  local government actions, 509t,
    519–524
  national government actions, 509t, 511,
    512–513, 514–516
Environment and health, 4, 470–471,
    528–529. *See also* Climate change;
    Environment; Precautionary
    principle; Toxins, exposure to
  child health, 483
  framework, 470
  health problems, 481
  and industry, 472, 476, 483–489, 520t
  pollution, 470
  problems, 481–506. *See also* Mining
  solutions, 506–528
  toxic waste, 437, 440, 448–449, 488, 489
Environmental impact assessment (EIA),
    509t, 516
Environmental movements:
  bioenvironmentalists, 480
  social movements, 525
Environmental racism, 489
Environmental regulations, 426, 482, 488,
    509t, 515, 518, 520t, 525, 528
Environmentally sustainable approaches:
  eco-building and eco-housing, 509t, 518,
    520t, 521, 529

Environmentally sustainable approaches:
(*Cont.*)
green taxes, 509t, 516–517
renewable energy, 518–519, 520t
sustainable cities, 523
sustainable development, 479, 511, 523
Environmental world views, 479
Environment and Socially Sustainable
Network, 81
Epidemiologic transition, 266
critique of, 40–41
Epidemiology:
role in crises, 393, 394–395, 399
terms and definitions, 243t
and toxicology, 489
Equinet, 115
Equity-efficiency trade-off, 557
Equity in health. *See* Health equity
Ergotism, 21
Escherichia coli. See E. coli
Essential drugs program and essential
medicines, 78–80, 292, 628, 645
Ethics:
dilemmas, 714
importance, 712–714
informed consent, 709–712
international ethical guidelines for
biomedical research, 710
of international health, 707–709, 714–715
in international settings, 706
principles, 709
Ethiopia, 421
famine, 380, 403
Ethnicity, 199, 202t, 203, 208, 209, 237,
320, 326, 332–333, 341, 350, 355.
See also Race
Europe, 19, 21, 49, 139. *See also*
European Union
plague, 18–21
reconstruction post-WWII, Marshall
Plan, 156
European Bank for Reconstruction and
Development, 83
European Centre for Disease Prevention
and Control (ECDC), 100
European Environment Agency, 97

European Food Safety Authority, 97
European Medicines Agency (EMEA), 97
European Union (EU), 98
banning asbestos, 448
development assistance mandate and
priorities, 182
ECHO (European Community
Humanitarian Aid Office), 118
GMO ban, 430–431
hormone-treated beef dispute, 429
jet fuel tax, 491
E-waste, 489
Expanded Program on Immunization (EPI),
78, 107
Export of hazardous materials. *See*
Hazardous waste
Export processing zones (EPZs), 424t,
428, 437
ExxonMobil Foundation, 102
Exxon Valdez:
oil spill, 507–508

FAME (Fellowship of Associates of
Medical Evangelism), 110
Family Health International (FHI), 97, 110
Famine, 141, 316, 373, 402, 403
Farmer, Paul, 704
Farming, 33, 158, 500. *See also*
Agriculture
farm workers and health, 526
Farr, William, 213
Female circumcision. *See* Female genital
cutting
Female genital cutting, 259, 685
anti-colonial resistance, 685
Female genital mutilation. *See* Female
genital cutting
Financial liberalization, 439–440. *See*
also Neoliberal globalization;
Neoliberalism
and inequality, 439
speculation, 439
Finland:
healthy cities, Helsinki, 684
Finlay, Carlos, 39, 43
First International Congress on Statistics, 48

Fleas:
  exposure, health effects of, 484t
Flies:
  exposure, health effects of, 484t
Focus on the Global South, 115, 702
Food aid, 96, 374, 406–407, 715
Food and Agricultural Organization (FAO),
    70, 374
Food and Drug Administration, U.S.
    (FDA):
  approvals process, 93, 714
Foodborne illness, 268, 271t, 279, 316, 317,
    499. See also Cholera; Diarrhea;
    E. coli; Food safety
Food safety, 498–499
  Codex Alimentarius, 499
  genetically modified organisms, 499. See
    also Genetically modified organisms
Food security, 315–317, 373, 526, 670
  and biofuels, 512
  and HIV/AIDS, 315
Food sovereignty, 71, 108t, 315, 373, 526
Ford Foundation:
  endowment and priorities, 100t
Foreign direct investment, 425t
Foreign exchange market, 425t
Foreign reserves, 425t
Forests, 499
Former Soviet Union. See Russion
    Federation; Soviet Union
Foundations, 98–99. See also individ-
    ual foundations as listed on 100t;
    Philanthropy
  definition, 62
  endowments and priorities, 100t
Fracastoro, Girolamo, 20
Framework Convention on Tobacco Control
    (FCTC) (WHO), 79
  promises and limitations, 683
France, 36, 48, 52, 431
  Agence Française de Développement
    (AFD), 91t
  colonialism, 24, 47
  Institut Pasteur, 47, 117
  revolution and social protection, 36
  sanitary reform in, 36

voting power at the IMF and World
    Bank, 82t
Franco, Generalissimo Francisco, 142
Franco, Saúl, 143
Frank, Johann Peter, 31, 38
Free trade, 88, 425t
  pesticide use and, 445
  zones. See Export processing zones
Friedrich Ebert Stiftung Foundation:
  endowment and priorities, 100t
Funds, 98–102
  definition, 62
  for global health, 563, 707

Gabon:
  health system typology (Roemer), 588t
Gambia, The, 51
  environmental trade, 517
  international aid and health
    expenditures, 563
  private expenditures in health, 592t
Garbage, 319, 503–504
  disposal, 503
  environmental impacts, 503
  health effects, 504
  liquid sewage and waste water,
    504, 520t
  waste minimization, 517, 520t
  waste regulation, 509t
Gastrointestinal diseases. See Cholera;
    Diarrhea
Gates Foundation. See Bill and Melinda
    Gates Foundation
GAVI Alliance, 107, 656
Gender, 204, 259–262, 290. See also
    Prostituted children; Women's health
  as a determinant of health, 330–332
  as a determinant of health in Sri Lanka, 671
  and development, 173
  Fourth World Conference on Women,
    Beijing, 71
  gender-based violence, 331, 382–384
  Green Belt Movement, 525
  and humanitarian emergencies, 372
  Millennium Development Goals, 173
  and water, 169, 315

General Agreement on Tariffs and Trade
(GATT), 88
General Agreement on Trade in Services
(GATS), 431
Genetically modified organisms
(GMOs)/food, 499
  bans on trade, 515
  exposure and health effects, 486t
  and the precautionary principle,
  430–431
Genuine progress indicator, 571, 572f
Georgia:
  health financing post-USSR, 539
Gerber:
  unethical marketing of formula, 433–434
Germany:
  biogas plants, 512
  comparison of health measures, health
    expenditures, and inequities,
    573–574t
  German Organization for Technical
    Cooperation (GTZ), 91t
  health system, 595–597
  health system typology (Roemer), 588t
  national health insurance, 595–597
  packaging law, 517
  sickness funds, 596–597
  voting power at the IMF and World
    Bank, 82t
  waste reduction, 392
Ghana, 228, 496, 538
  Akosombo Dam, 505
  financing and delivery of health
    care, 587t
  GDP, debt, and health expenditures, 563t
Giardia:
  exposure, and health effects of, 484t
GINI coefficient, 155
GlaxoSmithKline, 101
Global AIDS Alliance, 79, 116
Global AIDS Interfaith Alliance, 109
Global burden of disease, 228–231, 559.
  See also Disability-adjusted life
  years; Disease Control Priorities
  Project

disease burden estimates by risk
  factors, 229
disease groupings, 228
and HIV, 287
Global Forum for Health Research, 118
Global Fund to Fight AIDS, Tuberculosis
  and Malaria (Global Fund),
  4, 62, 106
GlobalGiving, 119
Global health, 6–8, 11, 170, 177, 181–183.
  See also Agencies; Bill and Melinda
  Gates Foundation; International
  health
  definition, 6
  and globalization, 7
  governance, 63, 125
  and international health, 6
  successes in, 657, 659, 660–661,
    733–734
  total international funding, 563
Global Health and Foreign Policy Initiative,
  182–183, 697
Global health tourism, 699
Global Health Watch, 731
Globalization, 7, 417. See also Neoliberal
  globalization
Global Malaria Eradication Campaign. See
  Malaria
Global Outbreak Alert and Response
  Network (GOARN), 295
  and SARS, 298–299
Global public goods for health, 567–568
Global sex survey, 149
Global Trade Watch (GTW), 460
Global warming. See Climate change
GOBI/GOBI-FFF, 79, 659
Good Health At Low Cost, 590
Gore, Albert, 508
Gorgas, William C., 44
Grameen Bank, 114. See also Bangladesh
Granda, Edmundo, 143
Grand Challenges in Global Health
  Initiative. See Bill and Melinda
  Gates Foundation
Grassi, Giovanni, 29

Graunt, John, 213
Great Britain. *See* England; United
    Kingdom
Greece:
    comparison of health measures, health
        expenditures, and inequities,
        573–574t
    private expenditures in health, 592t
Green cities, 509t, 519–522, 684
    Curitiba, Brazil, 521, 522f
Greenhouse gases, 476, 479, 490–491,
    503–506, 508, 512
Greenland:
    indigenous health, 264t
Greenpeace, 527–528
Green Revolution, 158
Griscom, John, 39
Gross national happiness (GNH), 321
Gross national income (GNI), 153–154
Gross national product (GNP), 424t
Group of 8 (G-8), 78, 98, 109, 116
Group of 77, 67
Guatemala, 406, 434
    breast milk substitutes, 433
    indigenous health, 263t
Guinea:
    private expenditures in health, 592t
Guinea worm. *See also* Neglected tropical
        diseases
    exposure and health effects, 484t
    Guinea-Worm Eradication Program, 272
Gunder Frank, Andre, 162
Gwatkin, Davidson, 719

H-8, 109
HAART (highly active antiretroviral
        therapy), 113, 292
Hadassah, 108t
Haiti, 322, 396
    deforestation, 502
    embargo, 396
    GPS survey, 399
    Hurricane Jeanne, 369
    Khian Sea toxic waste dumping, 448–449
    private expenditures in health, 592t

refugees and HIV/AIDS, 287
Hanta virus. *See* Emerging infectious
        diseases
Haq, Mahbub ul, 173
Harvard Initiative for Global Health, 117
Hazardous waste:
    asbestos, 447, 515
    dumping, 448–449, 488, 504
    export of, 447–449, 462, 488, 494,
        500, 513
    exposure and health effects, 484t
    and *Khian Sea*, 448
    pesticides, 445. *See also* Pesticides
    workplace, 442–447
Health:
    definition, 3
Health Alliance International (HAI), 674
    in Mozambique, 113, 674
Health and human rights, 114, 177–178,
        327, 726–730
    and Alma-Ata, 644–646
    critique of approach, 179–180
    governmental obligations, 178–180, 179t,
        727, 728
    instruments, 177, 178t
    rights-based approach, 179, 726–727
    and transnational corporations, 432–436,
        435t. *See also* Trade-Related
        Intellectual Property Rights
        Agreement; Water
Health and social justice. *See* Social justice
Health as reconciliation, 720
Health care:
    policy, 454, 552, 583–584, 585,
        587–589, 640
        as distinct from health policy, 583
    as a right, 179–180, 584, 585, 594, 599,
        600–601, 602, 610, 612, 728. *See
        also* Health and human rights
    systems. *See* Health care systems
Health care administration. *See also* Health
        care financing; Health care reform;
        Health care systems
    cost comparison, United States and
        Canada, 547, 614

Health care administration (*Cont.*)
　　costs of, in the United States, 543,
　　　　607–608
Health care delivery mechanisms, 560, 624
Health care equipment, 624
Health care expenditures, 545, 546, 571f,
　　　　563, 563t. *See also* Health care
　　　　financing
　　comparison of single-payer and
　　　　multiple-payer systems, 548, 548t
　　controlling, 547
　　global, 538t, 563
　　and health outcomes, 571, 572, 573t,
　　　　575, 591
　　personal, 542, 543, 545
　　private, % of total health spending, 592
　　third-party/insurance, 542
　　total, per capita, 590–591
Health care facilities, 372, 622, 641
Health care financing, 544–547, 632
　　as aid, 563–564
　　in developing countries, 562
　　health insurance model, 546–547
　　and international agencies, 562–565
　　mechanisms, 545
　　progressive, 545
　　regressive, 545
　　role of international agencies in,
　　　　562–565, 563t
　　single-payer and multiple-payer systems,
　　　　comparison between, 547, 548t
　　trends, 563
　　user fees, 548–550
Health care markets, 540–544
　　and limits, 542–543, 544t
　　in underdeveloped countries,
　　　　558–559
Health care reform, 608–616
　　in Brazil, 610
　　characteristics of, 609t
　　cost management, 613–615
　　in emerging economies, 612–613
　　in India, 613
　　in Latin America and the Caribbean,
　　　　609–611

　　in Mexico, 610–611
　　in OECD countries, 613–615
　　in post-socialist states, 611–612
　　in South Africa, 612–613
　　in South Korea, 612
　　in stratified systems, 609–611
　　in sub-Saharan Africa, 615–616
　　in under-resourced settings, 615–616
Health care systems, 583–585.
　　　　See also Health care reform
　　building blocks, 585, 621–631
　　characteristics of, 585
　　in China, "market socialism",
　　　　602–605
　　corruption in, 565–566
　　definition, 583
　　delivery, 586
　　evolution of, 594t
　　financing, 544, 548, 586, 587t, 609t, 632.
　　　　See also Health care financing
　　in former Soviet Union, centrally
　　　　planned, 600–602
　　and % of GDP spent on health care,
　　　　589–590
　　in Germany, national health insurance,
　　　　595–597
　　in Great Britain, National Health Service,
　　　　597–600
　　health spending comparisons, 589–593
　　management of, 641–643
　　organizational coherence and
　　　　intersectoral cooperation, 621
　　organization of, 585
　　origins, 595
　　policy and planning of, 640–641
　　political economy of, 586
　　principles, 585, 616–621
　　regulation of, 633–634
　　Roemer's typology, 587–589, 588t
　　typologies, 586–589, 593–594
　　in the United States, private, pluralistic,
　　　　unsystemic, 605–608
　　and values, 585
　　World Health Report 2000, 593–594
Health care workers, 623–625, 634–636

brain drain and shortage of, 634–635
density, globally, 633f
migration of, 634–636
nurses, 624
pharmacists, 599, 624
physicians/doctors, 623–624
and SARS, 298
shortage of, 634–636
technicians and other health
    professionals, 624
traditional healers, 624–625.
    See also Traditional healers
Health data, 192–195, 195t, 200t. *See also*
    Census; Health services statistics;
    Mortality; Registration; Social
    inequalities in health; Vital statistics
assumptions, 194
challenges in collection, 193
limitations, 198–199
types, 199–202
uses, 194–198
Health disparities, 196, 209, 231, 236–237,
    311, 350, 355. *See also* Health
    equity; Social inequalities in health
Health economics, 537–540. *See also* Cost-
    benefit analysis; Cost-effectiveness
    and cost-effectiveness analysis
comparison of single-payer and
    multiple-payer systems, 548t
definition, 537
global public goods, 567–568
global spending on health, 538
health care markets, 540–543, 544t
international comparisons, 573t
versus political economy, 570–575
politics of, 149–151, 566–567
Preston Curve applied to health
    spending, 571f
social and redistributive approaches,
    569–570, 569t
and underdeveloped countries, 566–567
Health equity, 341, 550, 618–619, 675
Health for All by 2000, 354, 681.
        See also Alma-Ata Conference
        and Declaration

Health impact assessment (HIA), 196, 516
Health indicators, 86, 200t, 201t, 320, 328,
    566, 591t
Health insurance, 546–547, 631
community-based, 547, 549
cost sharing, 548
insurance companies, 542, 544t, 546
premiums, 544t, 545, 546, 547, 548t,
    592, 607, 610, 632
risk pooling, 546
risk selection, 546
social insurance, 539, 540, 546, 547
Health maintenance organizations
    (HMOs), 606
HealthNet/TPO, 720
Health promotion, 680–682, 733
Health services statistics, 234–235
resources for collection, 234
type of data collected, 199
Health Systems Trust, 97
Health transition, 40
Healthy Cities Program (HCP), 351, 519,
    523, 682–685
in Bogotá, 683
in Helsinki, 684
in Iran, 683, 684
in The Netherlands, 684
in Portland, 684
in Toronto, 682, 684
Healthy societies, 656, 666
Healthy years equivalent (HYE), 227
Heart attack. *See* Coronary heart disease
Heavily Indebted Poor Countries (HIPC)
    Initiative, 86–88, 439, 462
Hegemony, 163, 174, 418
Helminths. *See* Neglected tropical
    diseases
Helsinki Declaration, 710
Hemolytic uremic syndrome, 296t
Hemorrhagic fever. *See* Emerging infectious
    diseases
Henderson, DA, 552, 659
Hepatitis B virus (HBV), 252, 258, 296t
Hepatitis C virus (HCV), 258, 296t
Hesperian Foundation, 114

High-income countries, 153, 322, 330, 339,
    348, 365, 524–525, 545, 591, 632,
    636, 666, 695, 699, 720, 730
  leading causes of death in, 229t, 231
Hippocrates, 474
HIV/AIDS, 286–293. *See also* Bill and
    Melinda Gates Foundation; DATA;
    Global Fund to Fight AIDS,
    Tuberculosis and Malaria; HAART;
    President's Emergency Plan for
    AIDS Relief; UNAIDS
  and advocacy groups, 115–116
  ARVs, 93, 150, 289, 292, 428, 429, 457,
    628, 729. *See also* Antiretroviral
    drugs
  AZT trials with pregnant women,
    712–713
  consequences, 290
  and corporate foundations, 102
  and demographic health surveys,
    210, 287
  determinants, 289
  and human rights, 114, 115, 178
  interventions, 290–291
  and labor, 635
  mortality, 149, 205, 253f, 286–287
  mother-to-child transmission
    (MTCT), 289
  orphans, 290
  prevalence, global and in sub-Saharan
    Africa, 93, 144, 149, 176, 287,
    290, 321, 665
  prevention of mother-to-child
    transmission (PMTCT), 291
  and public–private partnerships,
    106, 107
  and societal determinants of health, 321
  stigma/discrimination, 287
  WHO Global Program on AIDS,
    76, 79, 287
Homelessness, 318–319, 326
Honduras, 421
  health system typology (Roemer), 588t
Hookworm, 24, 28, 233, 657
Host–agent–environment interaction, 149

Housing conditions, 284, 311, 312, 313,
    317–320, 327, 328, 334, 335,
    339, 340, 342, 347, 348. *See also*
    Homelessness
Human Development Index (HDI), 155,
    172–173
Human Development Report, 111, 154,
    172–173
Humanitarian aid/assistance, 384
  ICRC guidelines, 112
  politics of, 48, 404–405
  workers, 403–404
Human rights, 114. *See also* Health and
    human rights
  civil and political rights, 178
  economic, social, cultural rights,
    178, 434
  governmental obligations, 178–181
  health and human rights-based approach,
    181, 728
  and political freedoms, 327–328
  in refugee populations, 402
Human Rights Watch, 114, 727, 728
Human trafficking/sex trafficking:
  prostituted children, 452, 453
  of women and children, 451–453
Human and household waste, 487,
    503–504, 509t, 512. *See also*
    Environment and health; Garbage;
    Recycling
  exposure, health effects of, 484t
Hungary:
  post-USSR health system reform, 611
Hurricane Jeanne, 369
Hurricane Katrina, 367–370
Hurricane Mitch, 405–406

Iceland:
  infant mortality rate, 252
Immigration, 39
Immunization, 235, 552, 568, 657
  ethical debates, 714
Impairment. *See* Disability
Imperialism, 28, 29, 30, 64, 66, 157, 158,
    162, 163, 339, 695, 704, 708

definition, 163
European, 21–25
and health, 26–28, 29, 30, 41–47, 54,
    143. *See also* Tropical medicine
motives for health measures, 30
Import Substitution Industrialization
    (ISI), 161
Income distribution, 328, 348, 538,
    571, 573t
Income inequality, 237, 328
and population health, 330
India:
age pyramid, 206f
ARVs, 429
Bhopal disaster, Union Carbide, 441
biomass fuels, 512
Chipko movement, 525
generic medication, 429
health care system, 613
homeless populations, 318
IBSA, 97
indigenous health, 263t
infant mortality rate, by state, 218t
informal labor, 450–451
Kerala. *See* Kerala, India
maternal death, 259
Million Death Study, 223
Narmada river dams, 506
physician migration from, 635
private expenditures in health, 592t
private health insurance plan
    penetration, 104t
prostituted children, 452t
selected health outcomes, Kerala, 673t
suicide among farmers, 336
tuberculosis in Assam, 664
voting power at the IMF and World
    Bank, 82t
waste dumping, 449
India-Brazil-South Africa Trilateral
    Agreement (IBSA), 97
Indigenous and aboriginal health, 262–265,
    333–334, 335–336
access to services, 237
colonialism, 335

health disparities, 263t
health indicators, selected, 263t
populations, selected, 262–265
Indonesia:
female genital cutting, 685
financial crisis, 440
integrated swamps development, 527
tsunami in, 371
Yayasan Duta Awam, 527
Industrialization, 294, 487, 503
and health, 137
and public health, 30–41, 474, 487,
    503, 511
rise of capitalism, 143
Industrial Revolution:
in England, 32–33, 47
environmental effects, 473
factories and worker health, 33
Inequalities in health. *See* Social inequali-
    ties in health
Infant formula, 433–434
International Code of Marketing of
    Breast Milk Substitutes, 433
unethical marketing of, 433
Infant health. *See* Child and infant health
Infant mortality, 342
causes, 53
under colonialism, 24
and demographic transition, 31–32
determinants of, 216, 233
distribution, 251t
in Georgia, 539
and infant formula in Guatemala, 433
in Kerala, 575
and the LNHO, 53
and population assistance, 91
prevention packages, 274
reduction, 85
under slavery, 26
social class and, 343f
underreporting, 216
by wealth quintile, 329f
and welfare states, 155, 338, 667, 667t
Infant mortality rate (IMR), 212, 215–219,
    247, 252, 573t, 591t, 668t

Infant mortality rate (IMR) (*Cont.*)
  among African Americans, 332, 591t
  in Brazil, by region, 219t
  in Chile, 438
  in China, 341
  in Costa Rica, 320, 669
  definition, 201t, 215–216, 244t
  and economic growth, 560
  in former Soviet bloc countries, 611
  global rates, 216
  and health of indigenous
      populations, 263t
  and health status, 212
  highest and lowest national rates, 217t
  increases, 438
  in India, by state, 218t
  as indicator of development, 252
  in Jamaica, 438
  in Kerala, compared to India, 673t
  lower limit, 216
  measurement, 216
  miscarriages, abortion, and stillbirth, 216
  and the Misión Barrio Adentro program
      (Venezuela), 678
  in Nicaragua, 85–86
  in Nigeria, 247
  and piped water access, 314–315
  and social democratic principles, 667
  in South Africa, 333
  in the United Kingdom, 342, 343f
  in Uruguay, 672
  by wealth quintile, 329f
Infectious diseases, 41, 47, 137, 252, 279,
    294, 428. *See also* Communicable
    disease
Influenza, 299–300
  avian influenza, 299
  vaccine, 299
Informal sector, 424t
Informal work, 610
Injuries. *See* Occupational health;
    Road traffic injuries and death
Institute of Nutrition of Central America
    and Panama (INCAP), 73–74
Instituto Nacional de Salud Pública, 117

Instituto Oswaldo Cruz, 117
Institut Pasteur, 117
InterAction (American Council for
    Voluntary International Action), 110
Inter-American Development Bank, 83
Internally displaced persons (IDPs), 366,
    377, 381, 384, 386, 399–401, 400f,
    400t, 408, 409
  definition, 366
International:
  definition, 62
International AIDS Vaccine Initiative, 106
International Baby Food Action Network
    (IBFAN), 116, 433
International Bank for Reconstruction and
    Development (IBRD). *See* World
    Bank
International Campaign to Ban Landmines,
    731. *See also* Land mines
International Center for the Settlement
    of Investment Disputes, 81
International Classification of Diseases
    (ICD), 194, 213, 215, 320
International Classification of Health
    Interventions (ICHI), 235
International Code of Marketing of Breast
    Milk Substitutes, 116, 433
International Commission on
    Epidemics, 48
International Committee of the Red Cross
    (ICRC), 61, 112
  history, 48
  and human rights, 727
  stance on war, 125, 722
International Federation of Red Cross and
    Red Crescent Societies (IFRC),
    52, 112–113, 404, 405
International Council of Voluntary
    Agencies, 110
International Decade for Clean Drinking
    Water, 71
International Development Association
    (IDA), 81. *See also* World Bank
International Development Research Centre
    (IDRC), 118, 705

International Federation of Pharmaceutical Manufacturers (IFPMA), 103
International Finance Corporation, 81. *See also* World Bank
International financial institutions (IFIs), 437. *See also* International Monetary Fund; World Bank; World Trade Organization
  critique of, 7, 82, 82t, 84–85, 87–89, 169, 337–338, 438–439
  and health financing and organization, 171, 539, 558, 562, 570, 610, 611, 613, 615, 619. *See also World Development Report 1993: Investing in Health*
  movements to counter, 457–459
International health. *See also* Aid; Global health; International health research; International health work
  activity, eras of, 64
  and Cold War, 6
  and colonialism, 6, 66–67
  conceptualizations, 8–11
  definition, 61–63
  distinguishing features, 5
  early priorities, 5
  ethics, 699–715
  evolution, after WWII, 63–67
  funders, 121t
  and global health, 6
  historical background, 5, 17
  imperatives, 41
  and INGOs in developing countries, 716, 718
  measuring success in, 733–734
  organizational missions, 699, 701, 715–716, 722, 733. *See also* individual agency missions discussed throughout 68–119
  organizations and actors, 61–125
  technical approaches to, 665–666
  traditional approach to, 696, 698, 730
  "without a passport", 730–734
  and the world order, 719–722
International health aid, 85–86, 119–125, 182
  critique of, 92, 123–126, 686–687, 730, 733–734
  priorities, 109, 181
  total funds, 563
International Health Board, 50. *See also* Rockefeller Foundation
International Health Division. *See* International Health Board
International Health Regulations/ International Sanitary Regulations, 196–198
International health research, 707–709
  10/90 gap, 118, 639, 707
  agenda setting, 707
  costs, 708
  ethics, 706, 710–712
  research imperialism, 708
International health work, 62, 99, 694, 696, 707, 714–715, 718
  ethnocentrism, 700
  funding, 707
  at home, 706, 720
  and human rights, 698, 726–727
  key questions in, 723
  key skills, 703
  motivations for, 699, 701
  organizational values, 715–719
  traditional work, 696–698
  training, 702–707
  work experience/internships, 702–707
International Labour Organization (ILO), 7, 70, 418, 449–450, 454–455
International Monetary Fund (IMF), 65, 83–85, 122, 155, 439, 457, 462. *See also* Debt; Heavily Indebted Poor Countries Initiative; International financial institutions; Policy Support Instrument; Poverty Reduction Strategy Papers; World Bank
  critique of, 7, 10, 82t, 84–85, 89, 168–169, 437–438, 722
  history, 85
  loans and conditionalities, 10, 65, 169
  recent anti-poverty strategies, 86–88

International Monetary Fund (IMF) (*Cont.*)
   repayment of debts to, 85, 457
   role, 168
   structural adjustment programs, 83. *See also* Structural adjustment programs
   voting power, 82t
   work with World Bank, 86, 88
International nongovernmental organization (INGO), 62, 701, 705, 718, 719
International Physicians for the Prevention of Nuclear War (IPPNW), 731
International Planned Parenthood Federation, 110
International public health, 8, 12, 250. *See also* International health; Global health
International Rescue Committee (IRC), 113
International Sanitary Bureau, 45. *See also* Pan American Sanitary Bureau
International Sanitary Conferences, 48–49
International Sanitary Conventions, 45, 49
International sanitary cooperation, 42
"Investing in Health", 558. *See also* Commission on Macroeconomics and Health; Disease Control Priorities Project; *World Development Report 1993: Investing in Health*
   critique of, 559, 561–562
   through social and redistributive approaches, 569–570
Iran:
   earthquake, 371
   healthy cities, Tehran, 683–684
   private expenditures in health, 592t
Iraq, 97, 315
   civilian mortality survey, 394
   humanitarian workers, 403
   infant mortality rate, 314f
   internally displaced persons, 401
   refugees, 378t
   war, 394–395
Ireland:
   potato famine, 501
Islamic Development Bank, 83

Islamic Relief Worldwide, 108t, 110
Israel:
   as aid recipient, 125
   community health movement, 695
   national health program, 597
   and Palestinian Occupied Territories, 397
Italy, 22
   plague, quarantine, 19

Jamaica, 407
   under-registration of infant deaths, 216
Japan:
   CO_2 emission, 477t
   epidemiologic transition, 40
   health system typology (Roemer), 588t
   hospital stays, 622
   Japanese International Cooperation Agency (JICA), 91t
   life expectancy, 193
   nuclear weapons, 392, 487
   post-WWII reconstruction, 153
   voting power at the IMF and World Bank, 82t
Jebb, Eglantyne, 112. *See also* Save the Children
Jenner, Edward, 23, 47
John D. and Catherine T. MacArthur Foundation:
   endowment and priorities, 100t
John Snow Inc., 97
Jordan:
   private expenditures in health, 592t
Jubilee 2000 movement, 89, 458–459, 731

Kabila, Joseph, 398
Katz, Alison, 561
Kazakhstan. *See also* Alma-Ata Conference and Declaration
   Aral Sea, 495
Kellogg Foundation:
   endowment and priorities, 100t
Kenya:
   compulsory licensing for ARVs, 429
   female genital cutting, 685
   GDP, debt, and health expenditures, 563t

Greenbelt Movement, 510t, 525
tobacco licensing, 429, 683
Kerala, India, 309, 331–332, 339, 572, 575.
    See also India
  features of welfare state, 339
  female empowerment, 674
  health indicators, 673t
  as welfare state, 673–675
Kiva, 119
Koch, Robert, 39, 46
Kresge Foundation:
  endowment and priorities, 100t
Krieger, Nancy, 237–238, 350. *See also*
    Embodiment
  eco-social model, 350–351
Kuwait:
  health system typology (Roemer), 588t
Kyoto Protocol, 509t, 511, 512–513

Labonte, Ronald, 731. *See also*
    Globalization
Labor, 424t
  child, 419, 422, 435t, 449–450, 462
  wage, 437
Labor conditions. *See also* Occupational
    health
  export processing zones, 437
  and inequalities, 436
  maquiladoras, Mexico, 437
Labor markets, 436–437
Lalonde Report, 346
Land:
  and agriculture, 502
  degradation, 499–500
  and food security, 512
  landless movement, Brazil, 116, 180
  pesticide use, 500
  tenure, 311, 328, 336
Land mines, 384, 385f, 388–389
  1997 Mine Ban Treaty, 389
Lassa fever. *See* Emerging infectious
    diseases
Latin America. *See also* individual
    countries
  and Cold War, 159

decolonization, 64
health care system, 609–611
Healthy Cities Program, 683
lost decade, 166
malaria control, 75, 77
medical schools in, 634
PAHO, 45
polio eradication, 665
SAPs, 86
slums/informal settlements, 482
street children, 318
Latin American School of Medicine
    (ELAM), 117, 636, 724
Latin American Social Medicine (LASM).
    See Social Medicine
Laurell, Cristina, 143, 677
Laveran, Charles, 29
Lead:
  contamination and poisoning, 491–492
  exposure and health effects, 486t
League of Nations Health Office (LNHO),
    52, 53, 99
League of Red Cross Societies, 52. *See
    also* International Federation of Red
    Cross and Red Crescent Societies
Leishmaniasis. *See* Neglected tropical
    diseases
Leprosy. *See* Neglected tropical diseases
Lesbian, gay, bisexual, and transgender
    (LGBT):
  health issues, 262
  stigma and discrimination, 262
Levi Strauss Foundation, 102
Liberalization, 425t. *See also* Neoliberalism
Liberia:
  refugees, 378t
Libya:
  health system typology (Roemer), 588t
Lifecourse perspective, 213, 256, 312, 333,
    345, 346, 350
Life expectancy, 246, 247, 255, 259, 263t,
    265, 287, 340
  and annual per capita expenditure on
    health, 146, 570–571
  causation, 26, 135

Life expectancy (*Cont.*)
  decreases, Russian Federation,
    sub-Saharan Africa, 146, 151–152
  definition, 244t
  global increases, 340
  inequalities in, 149
  intracountry variation, 193
  problems in data collection, 193
  regional trends, 145f
  by social class, 344f
Lifestyle and health, 133, 134, 313,
    346–347, 351
Lind, James, 47
Living conditions, 313–322, 342
Loans. *See also* Debt; International
    Monetary Fund; World Bank
  conditionalities, 10, 337–338, 719
  health effects, 558, 559
  structural adjustment programs, 337. *See
    also* Structural adjustment programs
London School of Hygiene and Tropical
    Medicine (LSHTM), 117, 703
Louis-Philippe, King of France, 36
Low-income countries/developing countries/
    low-resource settings, 136, 153, 156,
    228, 246, 247, 249, 251, 255, 266,
    322, 339, 422, 423, 538, 558, 560,
    567, 669, 671, 695, 696, 730, 734
  with high levels of health, 439, 590
  leading causes of death in, 229t
  post-WWII development assistance, 32
Lutheran World Relief, 108t
Luxembourg:
  0.7% GNI in aid, 94
Luxemburg, Rosa, 719
Lyme borreliosis. *See* Emerging infectious
    diseases
Lymphatic filiariasis. *See* Neglected tropical
    diseases

Maathai, Wangari:
  Greenbelt Movement, 525
Macro International, 97
Madagascar:
  health expenditure, 590
Malaria, 272–275, 657

bednets, 556
  campaigns, 75, 77
  cases in proportion to population
    size, 274f
  consequences, 273
  DDT, 77, 272, 273, 657, 663
  determinants, 301, 482t
  drug resistance, 77, 275, 657
  Global Malaria Eradication Campaign,
    75–77, 273, 657–658
  and imperialism, 28
  interventions, 77, 273–274, 657–658
  quinine, 28, 44
Malawi:
  bed nets for malaria, 275
  ecological footprint, 481
  health worker mortality due to AIDS,
    635
  maternal mortality, 625
Malaysia:
  financial controls, 457
  financial crisis, 440
  health system typology (Roemer), 588t
Malnutrition, 379–380
  child health, 252
  in crisis, 379
  determinants, 482t
  and health, 315–316, 378
  rates, 316, 374
Managed care organizations (MCOs), 606
Management Sciences for Health (MSH), 97
Mann, Jonathan, 287
  health and human rights approach to
    HIV/AIDS, 178
Manson, Patrick, 28–29, 39
Marburg virus. *See* Emerging infectious
    diseases
Markets:
  failure, 567
  health markets, 540–544
  neoclassical economic theory, 540
Marmot, Sir Michael, 319, 344, 352.
    See also Commission on Social
    Determinants of Health
Marshall Plan/European Recovery
    Program, 156

Martinez cobo, J, 262
Marx, Karl, 140, 330, 349
    and Friedrich Engels, *The Communist
        Manifesto*, 35
Maternal health, 32, 46, 78, 254, 259, 260f,
        312, 313, 329f, 618, 620, 621, 623,
        625, 632, 638, 641, 645, 646.
        See also Child and infant health
    abortions, 261
    access to health services, 260
    barriers to care, 259, 260
    and BRAC, 114
    and MDGs, 174
    and social policy, 135, 138f, 570, 589,
        661–662, 671
Maternal mortality, 219–220, 253, 257, 259,
        260f, 261, 300–301, 331, 667t
    definition of maternal death, 219, 244
    in Denmark, 246
    in Egypt, 247
    in Georgia, 539
    leading causes, 261
    maternal mortality rate, 201t, 219
    maternal mortality ratio (MMR),
        201t, 219
    in Mexico City, 677
    in Nigeria, 248
    in Sri Lanka, 661–662, 671
Mauritania:
    HIV/AIDS prevalence, 287
McKeown, Thomas:
    mortality declines, 37–38
McNamara, Robert, 174
MDR TB, 285–286, 661. *See also*
        Tuberculosis
Measles, 248, 248f, 251, 251t, 253f, 275–
        276, 277, 301. *See also* Respiratory
        tract infections
Médecins du Monde (MDM)/Doctors of the
        World, 113
Médecins Sans Frontières (MSF)/Doctors
        Without Borders, 113, 292, 374,
        698, 728
Medical Research Council (UK), 117
Medical tourism, 636
Mennonite Central Committee, 108t

Men's health:
    gender roles, 262, 331
Mental health:
    of adults, 261
    and aging, 256
    during CHEs, 380–382
    and conflict, 395
    determinants, 261
    health services, 261
    prevalence, 381t
    and refugees, 381
    suicide, 261
Mercantilism, 473
Merck Company Foundation, 102, 104
Mercury:
    exposure and health effects, 486t
Merhy, Emerson, 143
Mexico:
    air pollution, Mexico City, 491
    Aztec sanitary system, 472–473
    CONACyT, 709
    health reform, federal, 610
    health system typology (Roemer), 588t
    indigenous health, 263t
    informal work, 610
    maquiladora, health conditions, 462
    Mexican Society for Public Health, 119
    National Public Health Institute
        (INSP), 117
    neoliberal economics, 170
    private expenditures in health, 592t
    Rockefeller Foundation, 35f, 51,
        158, 233
    rural health posts unfilled, 634
    social inequalities, indigenous, 335
    social medicine, Mexico City (Integrated
        Territorial Social Program), 677
Miasma/miasmatic causes of disease,
        34, 47
Micronutrient deficiency. *See also*
        Malnutrition
    consequences, 253t
Middle-income countries, 153, 228, 246,
        247, 251, 322, 524–525, 558, 560,
        567, 627, 632, 671
    leading causes of death in, 229t

Migration, 321, 334. *See also* Immigration;
    Refugees
  health effects, 139
  of health workers, 634–636
Milbank Memorial Fund, 99
Militarism, 386–388, 408, 409
  arms trade, 387–388
Military:
  expenditures, 387, 387f
  responses to natural disasters, 371
  targeted aid, 159
Millennium Challenge Corporation, 92
Millennium Development Goals (MDGs),
    71, 173–177. *See also* Brandt
    Commission
  critique of, 73, 174–176
  and health, 173–174
  Millennium Declaration, 173, 174,
    176, 177
  $1/day international poverty line,
    175–176, 175f
Millions Saved report, 660–661, 665
Mining, 472
  deaths and health effects, 369, 398, 435t,
    436, 441, 445, 446, 501
  environmental health effects, 470, 484t,
    488t, 491–492, 500–501, 502
  movements to curb, 436t, 526, 527
Mining Watch, 527
Misión Barrio Adentro, 678–680. *See also*
    Venezuela
Missionary groups, 697–698
  and colonialism, 23, 109
Mission Doctors Association, 110
Mission Exchange, 110
Modernization theory of development, 158,
    161. *See also* Dependency theory of
    development; World systems theory
  challenge to, 162, 163
Montreal Protocol, 511
Morbidity statistics, 224–234
  collection of data, 224–225
  definition of disease/illness, 224
  and international health regulations, 225
  notifiable diseases, 225–226

  sources, 224
  uses, 224, 225
Mortality, 213–223. *See also* Death;
    specific diseases
  civil war and, 339
  death registration, 220–221
  among homeless, 318
  indigenous, 22, 265, 334, 335
  infant. *See* Infant mortality
  international comparisons of, 213
  limitations of mortality data, 220–223
  maternal. *See* Maternal mortality
  statistics on, 215
  surveys, 394, 398
Mosquitoes. *See also* Dengue fever;
    Malaria; Yellow fever
  Aedes aegypti, 44, 495
  Anopheles, 44, 51, 77, 272, 273
  breeding sites, 473, 495, 504
  and climate change, 473, 478
  and deforestation, 502
  exposure, health effects, 484t
  scientific discoveries, 29
  as vectors of disease, 44, 44, 272
Mother-to-child transmission. *See* HIV/AIDS
Mozambique:
  aid and health fragmentation, 717
  aid proliferation, 96
  ARVs, compulsory licenses, 429
  dependency theory of development, 162
  Health Alliance International (HAI),
    113, 674
  HIV treatment program, 674
Multilateral:
  definition, 62
Multilateral Agreement on Investment
    (MAI), 116
  and Council of Canadians, 458
Multilateral Debt Relief Initiative
    (MDRI), 87t
Multilateral Investment Guarantee Agency, 81
Multinational corporations, 424t. *See also*
    Transnational corporations
Muslim Aid, 108t
Mustard gas, 390, 391t

Namibia:
 private health insurance plan penetration,
  104t
National health accounts (NHAs), 234
National Institutes of Health (NIH), 561, 704
Natural environment, 470
Navarro, Vicente, 142–143, 144t, 163–164,
  586, 587, 593, 667
Neglected tropical diseases (NTDs),
  269–272
 consequences, 271
 determinants, 269
 individual diseases, 270t
 interventions, 272
 and pharmaceutical companies, 272
 Special Program for Research and
  Training in Tropical Diseases
  (TDR), 698
Neighborhood conditions and health, 311,
  313, 317, 319, 324, 342, 349
Neoliberal globalization, 418, 419–421, 561
 definition, 417–418
 effect on poor economies, 422
 and the environment, 426
 eras, 419
 and health, 7, 421, 422, 425
 and health pathways, 425, 426–441, 427f
 and occupational health and safety, 424
 opponents, 423
 and regional responses, 510
 and trade, 418, 421–425, 428–432, 430t
Neoliberalism, 7, 166–169, 337. See also
  International financial institutions;
  Structural adjustment programs;
  World Bank
 compared to social justice approaches to
  health, 569t
 critique of, 121–122, 144, 353, 684
 economic model, 166–170, 172. See also
  Economics
 features of, 167–168
 ideology, 144, 167, 647
 political economy approaches to health,
  143, 144
 resisting, 669, 676, 678, 686, 687

Nepal:
 biomass fuels, 512
 health system typology (Roemer), 588t
 prostituted children, 452t
Nestlé:
 Foundation, 102
 and unethical marketing of infant formula, 433
Netherlands, The:
 0.7% GNI in aid, 94
 health system typology (Roemer), 588t
 needle exchange programs, 258
 quinine plantations, 28
 safe injection sites, 258
 transit programs, 684
New International Economic Order
  (NIEO):
 Charter of Economic Rights and Duties
  of States, 67
New Zealand:
 death registration, 220
 financing and delivery of health
  care, 587t
 foreign trained doctors in, 635
 Framework Convention on Tobacco
  Control, 683
 ill-defined deaths, 221
 indigenous health, inequalities, 263t
 private expenditures in health, 592t
 Treaty of Waitangi, 335
Nicaragua:
 banana workers and health, 526
 conflict, 85, 390
 debt, 86
 economic conditions exacerbating storm
  effects, 406
 fragmentation of health aid, 85–86, 717
 GDP, debt, and health expenditures, 563t
 Sandinista advances in health and
  welfare, 85
Niger:
 famine and food insecurity, 373–374
 oil drilling and environmental degradation, 440–441
 stunting, 477

Nigeria:
　Biafra War, 376
　census, 205
　health/disease profile, 246
　health system typology (Roemer), 588t
　measles vaccination, 276
　oil exploitation and health, 440–441
　opposition to polio vaccine, 714
　top ten causes of death, 249f
　user fees, 549
Nitrogen dioxide:
　exposure and health effects, 484t
Nixon, Richard, 164
Non-aligned movement, 67, 160
Noncommunicable disease/chronic disease,
　　228, 229, 249–250, 266. *See also*
　　Cancer; Cardiovascular disease;
　　Cerebrovascular disease; Coronary
　　heart disease; Diabetes mellitus
Nongovernmental organizations (NGOs),
　　62, 110–116, 717–718
　advocacy groups/campaigns, 115–116
　critique of, 111–112, 124–125, 717–719
　definition, 62
　developing country, 114–115
　human rights and health groups, 114
　international health and development
　　think tanks, 115
　large humanitarian, 112
　relief groups, 112–113
　social rights/service provision, 113
North America. *See also* Canada, Mexico,
　　United States
　abortion in, 261
　cholera in, 33
　energy consumption, 476
　environmental movements in, 527–528
　epidemiologic transition in, 40
　e-waste, 489
　malaria control in, 273
　neoliberal globalization, 419
　revolutionary movements in, 30
　sanitary reform in, 38–39
　sanitation and garbage in, 503
　taxes on air travel, 491

　tuberculosis in, 284
　waste minimization in, 517
North American Free Trade Agreement
　　(NAFTA), 98, 432
Norway:
　0.7% GNI in aid, 94
　fair trade/aid regulations, 734
　health system typology (Roemer), 588t
　transit, Oslo, 523
Notestein, FW, 31–32, 31f. *See also*
　　Demographic transition
Nuclear waste, 393, 484t
　dumping, 448–449
　exposure and health effects, 484t
Nuclear weapons. *See also* Weapons
　arms race, 393
　Nuclear Non-Proliferation Treaty, 393
Nuffield Foundation:
　endowment and priorities, 100t
Nuremberg war crimes trials, 709
Nurses, 372, 591t, 601, 608, 624, 625, 635.
　　See also Health care workers
　migration of, 635, 646
Nussbaum, Martha:
　capabilities approach, 172
Nutrition. *See also* Food security;
　　Malnutrition
　and agricultural subsidies, 316
　child health, 315
　during crisis, 316
　and food system, 315–317
　and industrialization, 317
Nyerere, Julius, 656–657

Obesity:
　contrasting health models for
　　understanding, 148t
Occupational health, 325, 338, 434
　consequences, 443
　in developing countries, 442–447
　health workers, 453
　international labor standards, 454–455
　international policy, 337, 454
　mortality and morbidity due to, 259, 278,
　　283, 424, 453

services, 453–454
L'Office Internationale d'Hygiène Publique
(OIHP)/Paris Office, 49–50, 52, 53, 63
limitations, 49–50
Official development assistance (ODA),
89–90, 92–94, 158, 166, 734. *See
also* Organization for Economic
Cooperation and Development
0.7% GNP/GNI plan, 160
for health by source, 122f
long term trends, 159f, 160f
net amounts, 95f
net as percentage of GNI, 95f
Oil:
alternatives to (biofuels), 512
burning of, 484t, 485t
consumption, 479
debt crisis, 165
drilling/exploitation/mining and health,
440–441, 500, 502
OPEC, 164
shocks, 165
spills, 440, 507–508. *See also* Exxon
Valdez
Omran, Abdel, 40
Onchocerciasis. *See* Neglected tropical
diseases
Oral rehydration therapy (ORT), 147, 254,
269. *See also* Diarrhea
Orbinski, James, 728
Organization:
definition, 62
Organization for Economic Cooperation
and Development (OECD), 458, 614
benefits to donors, 90
Development Assistance Committee,
89–90
membership, 93, 590
Official Development Assistance. *See*
Official Development Assistance
priorities for spending, 91t
Outbreaks, 50, 53
cholera, 42
early detection of, 198
hepatitis A, 432

malaria, 51
plague, 19
polio, 714
SARS, 298–299
typhus, 141
yellow fever, 43
Out-of-pocket spending, 548–550. *See also*
Health insurance; User fees
Overseas Development Institute, 115
Oxfam, 113, 376
Ozone, 491. *See also* Chlorofluorocarbons
and air pollution, 490–491, 574
exposure and health effects, 484t

Pacini, Filippo, 46
Packard Foundation. *See* David and Lucille
Packard Foundation
Pakistan, 452
earthquake, 371–373
health workers, 376
opposition to polio vaccine, 714
Palestinian Occupied Territories:
health and social status, 397
refugees, 378t
Panama Canal:
and yellow fever and malaria,
43–45, 45f
Pan American Health Organization (PAHO),
45, 376
Pan American Sanitary Bureau (PASB),
45, 46, 52, 63, 74t. *See also* Pan
American Health Organization
Papua New Guinea:
GDP, debt, and health
expenditures, 563t
Paradox of plenty, 164
Paris Declaration on Aid Effectiveness, 564
Participation:
as a principle of health care systems, 620
Particulate matter (PM), 490. *See also* Air
pollution
exposure and health effects, 484t
Partners In Health, 113, 292, 716
Pasteur, Louis, 39
Pathfinder Fund, 110

Pearson, Lester B:
  0.7% GNP to ODA plan, 160
  and Commission on International
    Development, 421
People's Health Movement (PHM), 63, 116,
  525–526, 702, 728, 732, 732f
  and Commission on Social Determinants
    of Health, 353
  environmental advocacy, 510t, 525–526
  Global Health Watch: An Alternative
    World Health Report, 82, 731
  People's Charter for Health, 732
PepsiCo, 104–105
Persistent organic pollutants (POPs):
  exposure and health effects, 485t
Peru:
  child mortality, inequalities in, 329
  cholera, 267
  debt-for-nature swap, 514
  pollution, 488t
Pesticide Action Network, 527
Pesticides, 44t, 45t. *See also* Agriculture;
  DDT; Farming
  actions to confront, 509t, 510, 520t,
    526, 527
  environmental degradation, 487, 500
  export of banned pesticides, 500, 526
  exposure and health effects, 424, 445,
    446f, 485t, 494, 499
  and Rhine river, 487
  Union Carbide explosion in Bhopal,
    441, 487
Pettenkofer, Max von, 38, 550, 551
Pharmaceuticals, 583, 627–631. *See also*
  Antiretroviral drugs; Essential drugs
  program and essential medicines
  counterfeit medicines, 629–630
Pharmaceutical industry, 78, 101, 103–105,
  105t, 428, 429, 456, 457, 490. *See*
  also Big Pharma; Trade-Related
  Intellectual Property Rights
  Agreement
  involvement in international health,
    103–104
  pharmaceutical development, 629t,
    630–631

  political economy of, 628–629
Philanthropy, 98–99. *See also* Foundations
  corporate, 102, 104, 105
  critique of, 51–52, 99, 101, 107, 120,
    122–124, 666
  current funding, 98–102
  history, 50
Philippines, The:
  environmental contamination, 435
  health system typology (Roemer), 588t
  migration of nurses from, 635
  prostituted children, 452t
Physical Quality of Life
    Index (PQLI), 227
Physicians/doctors, 623–624. *See also* Brain
    drain; Health care workers
  remuneration mechanisms, 637–638
Physicians for Human Rights, 114, 389,
  705, 728
Physicians for Social Responsibility, 114
Pinochet, Augusto, 160
Placebo-controlled trials, 712–714
Plague, 18–21
  Black Death, 19–21
  early public health measures, 20–21
  Justinian Plague, 19
  quarantine, 19–20
Pneumonia. *See* Respiratory tract infections
Poland, 249f, 601, 611, 661
  civilian casualties, WWII, 390
Policy Support Instrument (PSI), 87t
Polio, 13. *See also* Expanded Program on
    Immunization
  controversies around, 664, 701, 714
  eradication program, 76t, 78, 665
  Salk vaccine trial, 713
Political ecology, 471–474
  definition, 471
Political economy:
  approach to health and disease, 12–14,
    134, 145, 149–151, 311, 327, 345,
    349–350, 356, 474, 584, 682, 684,
    694, 695, 716, 719, 722, 728,
    732, 734
  of Big Pharma, 628–629
  classification of countries, 153f

of environmental health, 474, 475f, 480, 506, 528–529
framework, 12–13, 309
versus health economics, 570–572, 575
of health systems, 586–589, 591
and international health training, 703
major tenets, 140
and neoliberalism, 160–170
theorists, 141–143
Political economy disease typology:
  diseases of modernization and marginalization, 280–293
  diseases of modernization and work/ production patterns, 277–280
  diseases of modernization/deprivation, 266–277
Polycyclic aromatic hydrocarbons (PAHs), 484t
Popular epidemiology, 527
Population Council, 110
Population health, 5
Population pyramids, 207f, 256f
Portability:
  as a principle of health care systems, 618
Portugal:
  imperialism, 21–22, 24
Poverty, 34, 725. *See also* Low-income countries; Millennium Development Goals; Poverty Reduction Strategy Papers
  absolute versus relative, 323, 328, 330, 342
  anti-poverty efforts, 169–170
  and capabilities approach, 172
  as cause of diarrhea, 147t
  as determinant of health, 237, 285, 289, 313, 322–323, 340, 342, 346
  and disability, 255
  and disease, 266–267, 285, 289, 301
  feminization of, 331, 451
  global rates, 175f
  Human Poverty Index, 173
  and human rights, 178, 179
  international poverty line, 175–176
  level wages, 436t, 437

and MDGs, 173
and neoliberal economic model, 420, 423, 439
pro-poor programs, 680
and racism, 333, 334, 335
reduction, 86–89, 337, 351, 352, 437–439
and social medicine, 143
and tuberculosis in South Africa, 139–140
Poverty Reduction Strategy Papers (PRSPs), 88, 438–439
Prebisch, Raúl, 161
Precautionary principle, 509t, 516
  and genetically modified organisms, 499
  and WTO, 430–431
President's Emergency Plan for AIDS Relief (PEPFAR), 92–93, 121t, 292
  budget, 92, 121t
  critique of, 93
  priorities, 92–93
Preston Curve. *See* Health economics
Prevention:
  primary, secondary, tertiary, 250
Primary health care (PHC), 64, 76t, 79–80, 106, 594, 643–646. *See also* Alma-Ata Conference and Declaration; Selective primary health care
  affordability, 547, 550, 590
  in Brazil, 610
  and child survival, 79–80
  China and barefoot doctors, 603
  in Costa Rica, 669
  Declaration of Alma-Ata, 644–645
  and health effects, 320, 646
  and health systems, 608, 609t, 643
  integrated with economic and social redistribution, 538
  Mexico City, 677
  Misión Barrio Adentro, 679
  in Mozambique, 674
  principles, 645
  in South Africa, 612–613
Private sector involvement in health, 102–103, 588, 612

Privatization of services, 425t
    health care, 169, 559, 611
    structural adjustment programs, 169. *See
        also* Structural adjustment programs
    water, Bolivia, 169, 431
Program:
    definition, 62
Progressive taxation, 183, 425t, 545
Project:
    definition, 62
Prostituted children, 452, 453. *See also*
        Human trafficking/sex trafficking
Protectionism, 425
Prussia:
    sanitary reform in, 38
    typhus, 141
Public health:
    definition, 4
    emergency, definition, 197
    historical antecedents, 18–26
    industrialization and emergence of,
        30–41
Public–private partnerships (PPPs),
    105–109
    definition, 62

Quality:
    as a principle of health care systems, 620
Quality-adjusted life years (QALYs), 227
Quarantine:
    and plague, 19–20
    and SARS, 298

Race, 199, 332–334. *See also* Ethnicity
    and class, 333, 334, 355
    and gender, 331, 355
    and health data, 199, 203, 204, 209,
        233, 237
    racial determinants and inequalities in
        health, 332–334, 350
Racism, 25, 209, 233, 328, 332, 350, 369
    environmental, 489
    and health, 332–334
Radiation, 501, 513
    ionizing, 485t, 487

    nonionizing, 485t
Rajchman, Ludwik, 52
Rapid jet vaccinators, 658. *See also*
        Smallpox eradication campaign
Rats. *See* Plague
Rape:
    during conflict and displacement, 382,
        383–384
Rawls, John, 172
Recycling, 489, 503–504, 506, 517, 520t,
        521, 524. *See also* Environment and
        health
    in Curitiba, 521
Red Cross. *See* International Committee
        of the Red Cross; International
        Federation of Red Cross and Red
        Crescent Societies
RedR-IHE, 703
Reed, Walter, 43
Refugees, 377, 386, 396, 399–405, 409
    complex humanitarian emergencies, 381t
    definition, 366
    disaster prevention/preparedness and,
        402–403
    environmental refugees, 401–402
    humanitarian aid workers and, 403–405
    human rights and, 402
    main countries of origin and
        asylum, 378t
    population trends, 401
    and public health, 315
    status, 334
    total numbers, 399–400, 400t, 400f
Registration, 202, 210
    birth, 212–213
    death, 220, 221f
    marriage, 202, 210, 211t, 212
    non-registration of birth, 216
Remote Access Medical, 726
Remuneration mechanisms. *See* Physicians/
        doctors
Research. *See* International
        Health Research
Resource Centers on Urban Agriculture and
        Food Security (RUAF), 526

Respiratory tract infections/acute respiratory
    tract infections, 275–277
  and CHEs, 378–379, 398
  and child/infant health, 275–277
  consequences, 276–277
  deaths, 245f, 246f, 247f, 248f, 253f,
    276f, 398
  determinants, 198, 482t
  and indoor air pollution, 493
  interventions, 276, 277
  measles, 275–276
  pneumonia, 277
Rickets, 33
Rift Valley Fever. *See* Emerging infectious
    diseases
Rio Earth Summit, 71, 72t, 511. *See also*
    Environmental conferences and
    agreements
Road traffic injuries and death, 145–146,
    280, 322, 331
  consequences, 280
  determinants, 280
  interventions, 280
Rockefeller, John D., 50
Rockefeller Foundation, 5–6, 35f, 53, 65,
    79, 99, 233, 603
  endowment and priorities, 100t
  history, 50–51
  international cooperation, 49, 123,
    170, 657
  in Mexico, 35f, 51, 158
  new international health, 51
  strategies, 51–52
  yellow fever vaccine, 51
Rodents:
  exposure and health effects, 484t
Roemer, Milton I:
  typology of health systems,
    587–589, 588t
Roll Back Malaria Global Partnership, 106
Rome Declaration on Harmonization, 564
Ross, Ronald, 29, 43, 170
Rostow, Walter W., 163
  modernization theory, 161
Rotary International, 78

Roux, Emile, 39
Royal Netherlands TB Association, 97
Russian Federation. *See also*
    Soviet Union
  coal mining explosion, 446, 501
  and Cold War, 66–67, 122, 160
  diphtheria, 151
  growing health inequalities, 323f,
    324f, 340
  health system typology (Roemer),
    588t
  indigenous health, 264t
  industrial pollution, 488t
  life expectancy, decreasing, 144,
    151–152
  mortality, gendered, 151–152
  pollution, 488t
  private expenditures in health, 592t
  prostituted children, 452t
  shock therapy capitalism, 145
  voting power at the IMF and World
    Bank, 82t
Rwanda, 517
  and community/environmental
    clean-up, 517
  gender-based violence, 383
  genocide, 367, 383
  indigenous health, 264t
  refugees, 402

Sachs, Jeffrey, 560, 697, 733
  Millennium Development Goals, 733
  WHO Commission on Macroeconomics
    and Health, 171, 560
Salmonella:
  exposure and health effects, 486t
Sand, René, 675
Sanitary and Phytosanitary Measures (SPS),
    agreement on, 429, 430t
Sanitation, 21, 314–315, 319, 496.
    See also Environment and health
  access/coverage, 497f, 498
  cost, 496
  environmental impact, 503–504
  and health, 482t, 600

Sanitation (*Cont.*)
  improved, 497f
  infant mortality rates, 314–315
  lack of facilities, 496, 498
  Mexico, 472–473
  reform, globally, 36–40
Saudi Arabia:
  private expenditures in health, 592t
Save the Children, 52, 78, 112, 314f,
  376, 716
Scaling up, 662–663
Schistosomiasis. *See* Neglected tropical
  diseases
Sector expenditure programs (SEPs), 86
Sector-wide approaches (SWAps), 86, 87t,
  88, 615
Seko, Mobutu Sese, 398
Selective interventions:
  and health, 660–662
  Millions Saved report, 660,
    661, 665
Selective primary health care (SPHC), 79.
  See also Child survival campaigns;
  Primary health care
  critique of, 79, 645, 660
September 11, 2001 (9/11):
  emergency response, 395
  World Trade Center attacks, 395
Sen, Amartya, 316, 373
  capabilities approach, 172
  development as freedom, 172
  Human Development Index, 172–173
  WHO Commission on Social
    Determinants of Health,
    203–204, 353
Severe Acute Respiratory Syndrome
  (SARS), 197, 298–299, 639
Sexually transmitted diseases (STDs).
  See Sexually transmitted infections
Sexually transmitted infections (STIs), 254,
  257–259, 297t
  herpes simplex virus, 257
  HIV/AIDS. *See* HIV/AIDS
  infection rates, 257
  prevention, 257

Shared responsibility, 523
Shattuck, Lemuel, 39
Shell Foundation, 102
Shigella:
  exposure and health effects, 268t, 486t
Shiva, Vandana, 336, 733. *See also*
  Biodiversity
Sickness funds (Germany), 596–597,
  631, 638
Sierra Leone, 378t, 382
  infant mortality rate, 217t
  life expectancy, 193
  maternal mortality rate, 219
Singer, Hans, 161
Single disease campaigns. *See also* Malaria;
  Polio; Smallpox eradication
  campaign
  limitations of, 663–666
Slavery:
  mortality, 25
  and racism, 25
  slave trade, 24, 25–26
  wage labor, 437
Slim, Carlos, 102. *See also* Carso Health
  Institute
Slums, 319, 496
Smallpox, 22, 196, 552
  1804 vaccination, 23
  eradication campaign, 77–78, 657,
    658–659, 663
  prevention, 23
  WHO eradication program, 23, 77–78,
    552, 658–659
Snow, John, 36
  John Snow Inc., 97
  On the Mode of Communication of
    Cholera, 35
Social capital, 327
Social class, 134, 183, 209, 236, 237, 330,
  476. *See also* Class
  Black Report, 343–344
  and health, 312, 330, 341, 349, 355
  and infant mortality (UK), 343f
  life expectancy by, 344f
  stratification, 330

Whitehall studies on social gradient in
    health, 344, 345, 347
Social cohesion, 327, 382
Social determinants of health, 4, 236. *See
    also* Societal determinants of health
    definition, 310
    distinguished from societal determinants,
        310
    measurement, 203–204
    WHO Commission on Social
        Determinants of Health, 77, 116,
        203, 236, 352–354. *See also*
        Commission on Social Determinants
        of Health
Social environment, 471
Social exclusion, 327, 725
Social gradient in health, 344
Social inclusion, 326–327
Social inequalities in health, 265, 309,
    340–344
    addressing, 351–355
    Black Report, 236, 342–344
    data, 199–200, 236–237
    definition, 311
    documentation, history of, 341–342
    evidence of, 342
    explanatory models, 344–350
    measurement, 203–204
    policy implications of, 351
Social justice, 352, 733. *See also* Social
    movements
    approaches to development, 180, 561
    approaches to health, 10, 63, 99, 124,
        538, 569t, 698, 722
    and neoliberalism, 10, 569t
    organizations and actors, 63, 108t, 109,
        113, 118
Social medicine, 5, 38
    key tenets, 676
    Latin American Social Medicine,
        8, 675–680
    main theorists, 142
Social movements. *See also* Social
    medicine
    community health, 695–696

environmental health, 487, 488, 506,
    509t, 510t, 525–528. *See also*
    individual movements listed on
    525–528; Healthy Cities Program
    labor, 443, 444t
    non-aligned, 66–67, 69t
    social justice, 63, 89, 116, 119, 124,
        458–459, 460, 687, 702, 718, 719,
        722, 728, 730, 731
Social security, 135, 136, 310, 311, 312,
    327, 328, 338, 349, 350, 632, 687,
    707, 731. *See also* Welfare state
    concept of, 596
    dismantling of Soviet, 145
    in Germany, 596–597
    in Latin America, 609–610, 642
    in Sweden, 667
Social selection and health, 345–346
Social supports, 327
Societal determinants of health, 309–312. *See
    also* Social determinants of health
    and behavioral understanding of health,
        312–313
    class stratification, 330
    colonialism, 339–340
    definition, 310
    factors, influencing, 310–312
    gender, 330–332
    imperialism, 339–340
    income/wealth distribution, 328–330
    indigenous status, 335–336
    international financial instruments and
        policies, 337–338
    international trade regimes, 337
    land tenure, 336
    lifecourse trajectories, 312
    living conditions, influence of, 313–322
    measurement, 203–204
    militarism, 339–340
    political system, 338–339
    race and racism, 332–334
    social policies and government
        regulations, 322–328
Socioeconomic status (SES), 279, 330
Solidarity, 319, 320, 325, 356, 675

Somalia:
  complex humanitarian emergency, 376f
  refugees, 378t
Somoza, Anastasio, 406
South Africa, 96
  ARVs, 292
  census and apartheid, 209
  cholera outbreak, 498
  Department of Health mission statement,
    625
  health care services, 546
  health care system, 612–613, 627, 642
  health system typology (Roemer), 588t
  HIV/AIDS, population effects of, 205,
    207f
  homeless population, 318
  IBSA, 97
  international assistance, 720
  private expenditures in health, 592t
  private health insurance plan
    penetration, 104t
  Public Health Association of South
    Africa, 119
  publicly-covered health services, 546
  racist apartheid system, 333
  Treatment Action Campaign, 115, 729
  tuberculosis and mines, 139
  water privatization in, 498
  XDR TB, in HIV-infected persons, 285
South Asia. See also Asia; Central Asia;
    East Asia; Southeast Asia
  birth registration, 213
  cholera in, 42
  complex humanitarian emergency, health
    impact of, 377
  energy consumption, 476
  infant mortality rate, 216, 660
  International Rescue Committee in, 113
  land tenure, 336
  maternal and child health, 641
  modernization theory of development, 161
  neoliberal economic model in, 439
  outdoor air pollution, 491
  smallpox eradication campaign, 78, 659
  tsunami in, 370–371
  waste minimization, 517

Southeast Asia. See also Asia; Central Asia;
    East Asia; South Asia
  acute respiratory tract infections in, 276f
  avian influenza in, 299
  cholera in, 46, 267
  complex humanitarian emergency, health
    impact of, 377
  dental health in, 258
  pharmaceutical industry in, 629, 630
  tuberculosis in, 283
  war-related injury/death in, 389
Southern African Development
    Community, 98, 725
South Korea:
  CO$_2$ emissions, 477t
  financial crisis and health care system,
    440, 457
  health care system, 612
  private expenditures in health, 592t
South–North aid, 726
South–South partnerships and aid, 695–696,
    724–726. See also Latin American
    School of Medicine; Misión Barrio
    Adentro
  ALBA, 96, 725
  from Brazil, 96
  from China, 96
  from Cuba, 96, 724
  IBSA, 97
  principles, 724
  from South Africa, 96, 696
  from Venezuela, 96, 724
Soviet Union (former). See also Russian
    Federation
  CO$_2$ emission, 477t
  and Cold War, 6
  Communist Party, 600
  dissolution of, 126, 151–152, 602
  health model, features of, 602
  government-to-government health
    cooperation, 96
  health care system, 600–602, 611–612
  life expectancy, 340
  outdoor air pollution, 490
  political and economic crises,
    121–122, 166

religious missions and health-related
activities, 110
tuberculosis in, 97, 284
Spain:
Civil War, 389, 724
colonialism, 21–23
financing and delivery of health care,
587t
Inquisition, 22
Panama canal, 43
Spanish-American War, 43
wind energy, 519
Sri Lanka, 671–672
Colombo Plan, 65, 158
comparison of health measures, health
expenditures, and inequities,
573–574t
features of welfare state, 668
health system typology (Roemer), 588t
ill-defined deaths, 221
infant mortality rate, 314f, 315
maternal health, 641, 661–662, 671
selected determinants of health and
mortality rates, 668t
Stanley, Henry Morton, 29
Starfield, Barbara, 646
Stiglitz, Joseph, 438
Stockholm Conference, 511
Stop TB Partnership, 106, 286
Streptococcus group A ("flesh-eating"
disease), 296t
Stroke. See Cerebrovascular disease
Structural adjustment programs (SAPs),
81, 83–84, 337, 406, 438,
558, 615
critique of, 84, 86, 169–170, 338,
438–439, 450, 459
health effects, 86, 169, 409, 462
Sub-Saharan Africa:
ARVs, 294f
birth registration, 213
complex humanitarian emergency, 376f,
377, 401
debt crisis, 166
disease burden in, 231
economic growth with globalization, 560

energy consumption, 476
and global trade, 423
health sector reform in, 615–616
HIV/AIDS in, 41, 287, 288f, 321
prevalence rates of, 149
social cost of, 290
hospitals in, 109
infant mortality rate, 216, 251, 660
injecting drug use, 258
life expectancy, 144
maternal death, 216, 261
neoliberalism, poverty and inequality,
175, 176, 439
water access, 496
Subsidiary/foreign affiliate, 425t
Subsidies, 148t, 425t, 460. See also
Agriculture
green, 517, 518, 520t, 523, 525
Sudan:
complex humanitarian emergency, 379
gender-based violence, 401
refugees, 378t
Suez Canal, 42, 49
Summers, Lawrence, 448
Surinam:
expenditure on health, external
financing, 563
Sustainable technologies, 518, 619.
See also Environmentally
sustainable approaches
Swaziland:
HIV prevalence, 287
life expectancy and HIV/AIDS, 290
Sweden:
0.7% GNI in aid, 94
age pyramid, 206f
comparison of health indicators with
United States and Cuba, 591t
features of welfare state, 667
institution-based medical care
system, 622
private expenditures in health, 592t
public health strategy, 667
societal determinants of health, 667
Swedish International Development
Cooperation Agency (SIDA), 91t

Switzerland:
  chemical contamination of Rhine
    River, 487
  HIV/AIDS policy, 106
  takeback waste program, 489

Tajikistan:
  health system typology
    (Roemer), 588t
Tanzania. *See also* Nyerere, Julius
  child mortality, inequalities in, 330
  comparison of health measures, health
    expenditures, and inequities,
    573–574t
  pesticide use and free trade, 445
  SAPs and undermining of training
    capacity, 635
Tariffs and duties, 423, 424t, 425t. *See also*
    General Agreement on Trade in
    Services
Task Force for Child Survival, 79.
    See also Child and infant health;
    Child survival campaigns
Technical Barriers to Trade Agreement
    (TBT), 430t, 431, 462
Technology, 520t
  appropriate, 626
  communication, 439
  equipment and, 625–627
  transfer, 437, 626
Telemedicine, 627. *See also* E-health
Texaco:
  and oil and toxic waste discharge in
    Ecuador, 440
Thailand:
  ARVs, 429
  avian influenza, 299
  financial crisis, 440
  financing and delivery of health care,
    587t
  health system typology (Roemer), 588t
  ill-defined deaths, 221
  malaria in, 275
  prostituted children, 452t
Theiler, Max, 51

Third World Network, 115, 163, 718
Tobacco:
  and cancer, 279
  and cardiovascular disease, 278
  and cerebrovascular disease, 278
  Framework Convention on Tobacco
    Control, 79, 683
Tobin tax, 718
Toxic agents, hostile use, 391t. *See also*
    Weapons
Toxins, exposure to, 266–267. *See also*
    Environment and health
Trachoma. *See* Neglected tropical diseases
Trade, 417, 418, 420, 421–425, 424t. *See*
    also Export processing zones;
    Transnational corporations; World
    Trade Organization
  fair, 88
  food aid and subsidies, 406–407
  free, 88, 425t, 445
  and health, 31, 42, 47, 48, 428–432,
    430t, 460
  liberalization, 84, 426
  slave, 24, 25–26, 27
  social movements working on trade and
    health, 460–461, 718, 719, 722, 730,
    731, 733, 735
Trade-Related Intellectual Property Rights
    (TRIPS) Agreement, 104, 428–429,
    430t, 462, 628
  and access to medication, 104, 429
  and Brazil, 456–457
  generic medication, 428–429
  and India, 456
Traditional healers, 18, 23, 110, 321,
    624–625
Traditional medicine, 78, 97, 603, 624, 625,
    701, 706
  African traditional medicine, 625
  and Alma-Ata Declaration, 625
  Ayurveda, 706
  Chinese traditional medicine, 23, 603, 706
  homeopathy, 625
  Islamic medicine, 18, 706
  and malaria treatment, 28

Siddha medicine, 625
and smallpox prevention, 23, 658
Tibetan medicine, 706
traditional healers, *See* Traditional
    healers
Unani medicine, 625
Trafficking. *See* Human trafficking
Transition. *See* Demographic transition;
    Epidemiologic transition; Health
    transition
Transnational corporations (TNCs), 71,
    432–434, 461, 727, 729
and human rights, 434
labor standards, 436
Transportation, 522–523
cycling, 524
environmentally friendly, 517
Treatment Action Campaign, 115, 729
Trinidad:
green sales taxes, 517
TRIPS Agreement. *See* Trade-Related
    Intellectual Property Rights
    Agreement
Tropical medicine, 5, 28–30
and malaria, 27, 28–29
Tropics, 26, 41
Truman, Harry:
and development, 157
doctrine, 156
Point IV aid program, 157
Trypanosomiasis. *See* African sleeping
    sickness; Neglected tropical diseases
Tsunami, 112, 365, 366, 367
relief efforts, 371
in South Asia, 370–371
Tuberculosis (TB), 283–286. *See also*
    Global Fund to Fight AIDS,
    Tuberculosis and Malaria; Stop TB
    Partnership
BCG (Bacille Calmette-Guérin) vaccine,
    75, 76t, 284
consequences, 283
determinants, 285
DOTS strategy, 286
drug resistance, 285

in Eastern Europe/former Soviet Union,
    285
funding for, 102, 105, 106
history, 283
and HIV/AIDS, 286
incidence rates, by country, 284f
interventions, 285
multidrug-resistant tuberculosis (MDR
    TB), 285
in South African miners, 139–140
XDR TB, 285
Turkey, 590, 636
Turkish Public Health Association, 119
Tuskegee syphilis study, 709

Uganda, 29
child soldiers, 385
indigenous health, 264t
user fees, 549
Ukraine:
Chernobyl, 487
pollution, 488t
UNAIDS (Joint United Nations Programme
    on HIV/AIDS), 70, 107, 287, 292.
    See also HIV/AIDS
UNCTAD (United Nations Conference on
    Trade and Development), 67, 70, 460
Underdevelopment, 142, 143, 153,
    157, 162, 163–164. *See also*
    Development
Under-5 mortality, 193. *See also* Child
    and infant health
and MDGs, 173
in Nigeria, 246
in Pakistan, 438
rates of change, 252f
UNDP (United Nations Development
    Programme), 70, 79, 90, 671
and climate change, 478
Human Development Index (HDI).
    See Human Development Index
and income inequalities, 421
Unemployment, 5, 141, 165, 167, 176,
    316, 319, 325, 334, 338, 339,
    426, 438, 451

UNFPA (United Nations Population Fund), 70, 205, 208, 254
UNHCR (United Nations High Commissioner for Refugees), 70, 70t, 113, 378t, 399–401, 400t, 400f
UNICEF (United Nations Children's Fund), 70, 76, 78, 107, 210, 212, 213, 673
and child survival programs, 79, 659–660
United Jewish Agency, 110
United Kingdom, 27–28, 36, 48, 139, 182, 336. See also England
Beveridge Report, 598
Black Report, 236, 342
class-based mortality, 343
Department for International Development (DFID), 91t
financing and delivery of health care, 587t
health system typology (Roemer), 586, 588t
health workers, 635
inequalities in health, 236, 341–342, 343
National Health Service, 236, 343, 597–600
private expenditures in health, 592t
safe injection sites, 258
voting power at the IMF and World Bank, 82t
Whitehall studies, 342
United Nations (UN), 61, 65–66, 69–73, 369. See also individual UN Specialized Agencies and UN Organizations
agencies, 70t, 71, 80, 106
conferences and summits, 71, 72t
development decades, 71
founding of, 65
membership, 71
role of, 65
United Nations Monetary and Financial Conference, 65
United Nations Office of the High Commissioner for Human Rights (OHCHR), 70, 685

United Nations Relief and Rehabilitation Administration (UNRRA), 65
United States Agency for International Development (USAID), 85, 90–92, 91t, 182, 210, 403, 701. See also President's Emergency Plan for AIDS Relief
budget, 91t
priorities, 91t
United States Environmental Protection Agency (EPA), 488
United States/United States of America (U.S./U.S.A.):
American Yellow Fever Commission, 43
bilateral assistance, 90–94
biomass fuels, 512
carbon footprint, 481
census taking, 205
Centers for Disease Control and Prevention, 97. See also Centers for Disease Control and Prevention
CO_2 emissions, 522
and Cold War, 91–92, 398
comparison of health indicators with Cuba and Sweden, 591t
corruption in health care, 565
Department of State, 92
early immigration and health reports, 39
environmental racism, 489
Exxon Valdez spill, 507
financing and delivery of health care, 587t
foodborne illness, 317
foreign aid priorities, 92, 181
foreign-trained doctors and nurses in, 635
and global/international health, 143, 670, 674, 695
health care expenditures, 543, 590, 591, 591t
health care system, 605–608
health insurance, 104t, 546, 605–607
health maintenance organizations (HMOs), 606
health system typology (Roemer), 588t
healthy cities, Portland, 684
hegemony, 46

homeless, health indicators of, 318
Hurricane Katrina, 367–370
indigenous health, 264t
infant mortality, 332
Institute of Medicine, 6
life expectancy, disparities in, 237, 309
marine hospital service, 42
National Institutes of Health (NIH), 704
PEPFAR, 92–93, 121t, 292
private expenditures in health, 592t, 614
prostituted children, 452t
Public Health Service, 45
role in organization of international
    health in the Americas, 41–46
selected determinants of health and
    mortality rates, 668t
Superfund program, 488
uninsured populations, 610
USAID. *See* United States Agency for
    International Development
voting power at the IMF and World
    Bank, 82t
war on drugs program, 392
Washington, DC, health indicators, 591t
Union of Soviet Socialist Republics
    (USSR). *See* Soviet Union; Russian
    Federation
Universal Declaration of Human Rights
    (UDHR), 4, 177, 434
Universality:
    as a principle of health care systems,
        616–618
Urbanization, 294
Urmul Trust, 115
Uruguay, 672–673
    age pyramid, 206f
    features of welfare state, 672
    Framework Convention on Tobacco
        Control, 667t, 683
    PANES (Plan to Address the Social
        Emergency), 672–673
    private health insurance plan
        penetration, 104t
User fees, 548–550
    critique of, 549

and World Bank, 548
Uzbekistan, 512
    Aral Sea, 495

Vehicles
    emissions, 476, 479, 490, 491, 508,
        518, 520t
    passenger vehicles, 492f, 493f
Venezuela:
    aid activities, 96
    ALBA, 96, 725
    Alejandro Prospero Reverend School of
        Medicine, 117
    Bank of the South, 85
    health system typology (Roemer), 588t
    Misión Barrio Adentro, 679
    private expenditures in health, 592t
    prostituted children, 452t
    South–South cooperation, 96
    vertical disease programs, 75–78,
        664–665
Via Campesina (La), 180, 526
Vietnam, 564
    Agent Orange, 392
    civilian casualties, 389
    health system typology (Roemer), 588t
    refugees, 378t
    War, 392
Villermé, Louis-René, 36, 236, 341
Violence, 326, 335, 339
    effects on children, 382–386, 437, 451
    gender-based violence, 331
    and health, 326
    mortality, 331
Virchow, Rudolf:
    social medicine, 38, 142
    typhus, Prussia, 141–142
Vital statistics, 199, 210–212
    problems with, 223–224

Wage labor slavery, 437. *See also* Capitalism;
    Transnational corporations
Waitzkin, Howard, 143, 676
Wallerstein, Immanuel:
    world systems theory, 163

War, 386–399. *See also* Complex
    humanitarian emergency
  civilian casualties, 389
  civil wars, 26, 160, 339, 386,
    389, 409
  Cold, 66, 67, 77, 88, 120, 153, 159, 161,
    177, 392, 507
  and environment, 392
  low-intensity conflicts, 390
  military casualties, 389
  public health effects, 392
  World War II, international health focus,
    63–64
Waste disposal. *See* Garbage
Water, 314–315, 494–498, 505
  access and infant mortality rates, 315
  agricultural use, 494, 498, 500, 504
  breeding sites, 478, 484t
  contaminants and contamination, 473,
    484t, 485t, 486t, 487, 488t, 489,
    491, 492, 495, 499, 500, 501,
    503, 504
  cost to access, 498
  damage of freshwater supply, 478, 484t
  dams. *See* Dams
  drinking water, 314f, 315, 473, 497f, 527
  and gender, 315
  global shortage, 495
  and health, 498
  improved water sources, 315
  lack of water access/water insecurity,
    315, 478, 482, 482t, 496, 498
  liquid sewage and waste water, 504,
    520t, 526
  privatization of, 168–169, 431–432, 498
  regulation, standards, and recycling of,
    515, 516, 517, 518, 521, 524
  right to water movements, 169, 526, 527
  use, 473, 494. *See also* Ecological
    footprint
Watt, James, 33
Weapons, 387
  biological, 390, 393
  chemical, 390, 393
  control, 392–393

  of mass destruction (WMD), 392
  nuclear, 392, 393
  public health effects, 392
  toxic and infective, selected, 391t
Weber, Max, 237, 330
Welfare state, 121, 135, 154–155, 154f,
    156, 167, 176, 338–339, 686,
    698–699, 734
  challenges to, 170, 280, 294, 612.
    See also Neoliberalism
  definition, 338
  developed country, 666–668
  developing country, 668–675
  features of, 668, 719–720
  and health, 143, 155, 250, 338–339, 354
  infant mortality rates, selected, 667t
  typology, 589
Wellcome Trust:
  endowment and priorities, 100t
West African Development Bank, 83
Western Europe. *See also* Eastern Europe;
    Europe
  cholera in, 33
  cost management reforms in, 613
  energy consumption, 476
  epidemiologic transition in, 40
  local transportation, 522
Wetlands, 474, 505, 516
Wilkinson, Richard, 328, 330
William and Flora Hewlett Foundation:
  endowment and priorities, 100t
William J. Clinton Foundation, 101–102
  endowment and priorities, 100t
Willowbrook hepatitis study, 709
Whitehall studies, 342–344, 347
  employment class and health, 342–343
  social gradient in health, 344
Women's health, 259–261. *See also*
    Maternal health
  abortions, 261
  barriers to care, 259–260
  female genital cutting, 259
  health services, 259
  maternal health, 259
  societal determinants, 259

violence during conflict and
    displacement, 326
Work, 310, 324–325, 349. *See also*
    Occupational health
hazards, 442–447
occupational safety and health, 442, 443
workplace, 434, 435
World Bank (International Bank for
    Reconstruction and Development),
    7, 65, 84, 121t, 156, 169, 170, 374,
    460, 558, 562. *See also* International
    financial institutions; Neoliberalism;
    World Development Report 1993:
    Investing in Health
approach to health economics, 149–151,
    538, 555
behavioral advice, 152
critique of, 7, 86, 88, 437–439, 462
on Cuba's success, 670
and Disease Control Priorities Project,
    559
earthquake relief in Pakistan, 372
and environmental critique of role in
    development projects, 506, 527
and environmental impact
    assessment, 516
in health efforts, 82
and health financing and organization,
    558–559, 562, 567, 610, 611, 613, 615
Health, Nutrition, and Population Branch,
    81–82, 562
history, 81–83
and income inequalities and health, 330,
    329f, 348
Lawrence Summers' "dirty industries"
    memo, 448
$1/day international poverty line,
    175–176, 322, 423
proposals to reform, 459, 719–720
role, 81
structure, 81
targeting the poor, 354
user fees and cost recovery, 498,
    548–550
voting power, 82t

World Development Report 1993: Investing
    in Health, 82, 558–559. *See also*
    Commission on Macroeconomics
    and Health; Disability-adjusted life
    years; Disease Control Priorities
    Project
"basket" of interventions, 558, 619
and DALYs, 230–231
health services privatization, 559,
    610–611, 613, 615
World Economic Forum, 105, 459
World Food Programme (WFP), 70, 374, 407
World health, 6. *See also* Global health;
    International health
World Health Assembly (WHA), 74, 197,
    291, 645
World Health Day, 65
World Health Organization (WHO), 3, 53,
    99, 121t, 255, 299–300, 455. *See*
    also World Health Assembly
budget, 75
commissions, 74, 76t. *See also*
    Commission on Intellectual
    Property Rights; Commission
    on Macroeconomics and Health;
    Commission on Social Determinants
    of Health
functions, 73–74
and global campaigns, 75–78, 76t,
    657–659
governance, 74–75
International Classification of
    Diseases (ICD). *See* International
    Classification of Diseases
major activities/campaigns, 75–80
measles, 76t, 78, 275
member states, 197, 213, 714
and national health policy, 640
occupational health, 455
PRSPs, 438–439
quality of life measure, 227
regional offices, 74t
role, 122
statistical information system
    (WHOSIS), 234

World Health Report 2000, 593–594. *See also* World Health Organization
World Social Forum, 116, 459
World Summit on Sustainable Development, 511
World systems theory, 163
World Trade Organization (WTO), 7, 88–89, 421–425. *See also* individual agreements as listed on 430t; International financial institutions
    agreements/trade treaties, 103–104, 421, 430t
    critique of, 88–89, 116, 422–423, 428, 431, 460, 462
    Doha Development Round, 422
    health implications of WTO agreements, 428–432, 430t
    history, 88
    and infant formula, 434
    and precautionary principle, 430–431
    priorities, 422
    role, 88
World Vision, 108t

XDR TB, 285, 297. *See also* Tuberculosis

Years of Potential Life Lost (YPLL), 227
Yellow fever, 24, 39, 42, 43, 296t
    and building of the Panama Canal, 43–45, 45f
    and international sanitary agreements, 45, 48, 49
    and occupation of Cuba, 43–44
    and Rockefeller Foundation, 50–51
Yunus, Mohammed, 114

Zaire. *See* Democratic Republic of the Congo
Zambia:
    GDP, debt, and health expenditures, 563t
    genetically modified organisms, 515
    life expectancy and HIV/AIDS, 287
    prostituted children, 452t
Zimbabwe, 438
    ARVs, 429
    life expectancy and HIV/AIDS, 287
    private health insurance plan penetration, 104t
    SAPs and pesticides, 445
Zoonotic diseases, 500